# Critical Care Nursing of Older Adults
## Best Practices

3
ION

**Marquis D. Foreman, PhD, RN, FAAN,** is Professor and Chair, Department of Adult Health and Gerontological Nursing, Rush University College of Nursing. Dr. Foreman was formerly Professor and Associate Dean for Nursing Science Studies at the University of Illinois at Chicago College of Nursing. He has been actively engaged in efforts to improve the care of hospitalized older people for more than 30 years. He earned a diploma in nursing from the St. Vincent Hospital School of Nursing, Toledo, OH, a BSN from the University of Toledo, an MSN from the Medical College of Ohio at Toledo, and a PhD in nursing science from the University of Illinois at Chicago (UIC). Dr. Foreman also completed a postdoctoral fellowship at UIC before joining the faculty. Foreman is known best for his research about delirium in hospitalized older people. He is a fellow of the American Academy of Nursing, and the Institute of Medicine–Chicago, and has received numerous awards for his work, including the Mary Opal Wolanin Award for Excellence in Gerontological Clinical Nursing Research, the Harriet H. Werley New Investigator Award, and the Mosby-Cameo Nursing Research Award—all for his work on delirium in hospitalized older people.

**Koen Milisen, PhD, RN,** is an Associate Professor of Geriatric Nursing at the Centre for Health Services and Nursing Research, Katholieke Universiteit Leuven (Belgium), a Clinical Nurse Specialist at the Division of Geriatric Medicine at the University Hospitals of Leuven (Belgium), President of the Flemish Center of Expertise for Falls Prevention, and President of the European Nursing Academy for Care of Older Persons. Dr. Milisen has extensive research and clinical expertise in the management of frail older persons having conducted numerous studies focusing on delirium in hospitalized older patients over the past 15 years. More recently, he has also been actively engaged in the area of falls prevention in hospitalized and community-dwelling older persons. Dr. Milisen obtained his diploma of bachelor hospital nurse at the Department of Healthcare, Katholieke Hogeschool Limburg, Belgium (1988–1991). After this training, he obtained a master's degree in medical and social science with an option in nursing science (1991–1994) from the Katholieke Universiteit Leuven. Dr. Milisen was visiting scholar at the College of Nursing, University of Illinois at Chicago (1997 and 1998), and obtained his doctoral degree in social health science at the Katholieke Universiteit Leuven (June 1999). Dr. Milisen received the Borgerhoff Award for Geriatrics for his work on falls prevention and the Award of the Belgian Psychogeriatric Association for his endeavors on delirium prevention.

**Terry T. Fulmer, PhD, RN, FAAN,** is The Erline Perkins McGriff Professor and Dean of the College of Nursing at New York University. She received her bachelor's degree from Skidmore College, her master's and doctoral degrees from Boston College, and her Geriatric Nurse Practitioner Post-Master's Certificate from New York University. Dr. Fulmer joined the faculty of New York University in 1995 and is currently a member of the Executive Committee for the new medical school curriculum and also serves as an attending in nursing at the NYU Langone Medical center. Her annual honors colloquium entitled "Comfort and Suffering," an interdisciplinary course in the College of Arts and Sciences as well as the College of Nursing, is highly subscribed. Dr. Fulmer's program of research focuses on acute care of the elderly and specifically, elder abuse and neglect. She served on the National Research Council's panel to review risk and prevalence of elder abuse and neglect and has published widely on this topic. She has received the status of Fellow in the American Academy of Nursing, the Gerontological Society of America, and the New York Academy of Medicine. She has served as a member of the National Committee for Quality Assurance geriatric measurement assessment panel and is currently on the Veterans Administration Geriatrics and Gerontology Advisory Committee. She completed a Brookdale National Fellowship and is a Distinguished Practitioner of the National Academies of Practice. Dr. Fulmer was the first nurse elected to the board of the American Geriatrics Society and the first nurse to serve as the president of the Gerontological Society of America. She is a trustee of Skidmore College, Bassett Hospital, and the New York Academy of Medicine.

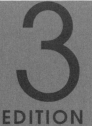

# Critical Care Nursing of Older Adults
## Best Practices

Editors

Marquis D. Foreman, PhD, RN, FAAN
Koen Milisen, PhD, RN
Terry T. Fulmer, PhD, RN, FAAN

**SPRINGER PUBLISHING COMPANY**
New York

Springer Publishing Company, LLC
11 West 42nd Street
New York, NY 10036
www.springerpub.com

*Acquisitions Editor: Allan Graubard*
*Production Editor: Pamela Lankas*
*Cover design: TG Design*
*Composition: International Graphic Services*
Ebook ISBN: 978-0-8261-1097-8

9 10 11 12 13 / 5 4 3 2 1

The author and the publisher of this Work have made every effort to use sources believed to be reliable to provide information that is accurate and compatible with the standards generally accepted at the time of publication. Because medical science is continually advancing, our knowledge base continues to expand. Therefore, as new information becomes available, changes in procedures become necessary. We recommend that the reader always consult current research and specific institutional policies before performing any clinical procedure. The author and publisher shall not be liable for any special, consequential, or exemplary damages resulting, in whole or in part, from the readers' use of, or reliance on, the information contained in this book. The publisher has no responsibility for the persistence or accuracy of URLs for external or third-party Internet Web sites referred to in this publication and does not guarantee that any content on such Web sites is, or will remain, accurate or appropriate.

**Library of Congress Cataloging-in-Publication Data**

Critical care nursing of older adults : best practices / Marquis D. Foreman, Koen Milisen, Terry T. Fulmer, editors.—3rd ed.
    p. ; cm.
  Rev. ed. of: Critical care nursing of the elderly / Terry T. Fulmer, Marquis D. Foreman, Mary Walker, editors. 2nd ed. c2001.
  Includes bibliographical references and index.
  ISBN 978-0-8261-1096-1 (alk. paper)
  1. Geriatric nursing. 2. Intensive care nursing. I. Foreman, Marquis D. II. Milisen, Koen. III. Fulmer, Terry T. IV. Critical care nursing of the elderly.
[DNLM: 1. Critical Care. 2. Aged. 3. Geriatric Nursing. WY 152 C9339 2009]
  RC954.C75 2009
  618.97′0231—dc22
                2009037676

Printed in the United States of America by Hamilton Printing

# Contents

# Contributors

**Cheryl M. Bradas, BSN, RN**
Vanderbilt University, School of Nursing
Nashville, TN

**Alexandra J. Brock, RN, BSN, CCRN**
The Pennsylvania State University, School of Nursing
State College, PA, and
Geisinger Medical Center
Danbury, PA

**Carol Dealey, PhD, MA, BSc (Hons), RGN, RCNT**
Senior Research Fellow
Research Development Team
University Hospital Birmingham NHS Foundation Trust
Birmingham, UK

**Tom Defloor, RN, PhD**
Professor Nursing Science, Department of Public Health
Ghent University
Ghent, Belgium

**Carol L. Delville, PhD, RN, ACNS-BC**
Assistant Professor
University of Texas at Austin, School of Nursing
Austin, TX

**Judy Dillworth, MA, RN, CCRN, NEA-BC**
Director of Nursing, Critical Care/ED/Medicine/Neurology
NYU School of Nursing, New York University
New York, NY

**Elizabeth H. Enfield, RN, BSN**
Staff Nurse, Coronary Care Unit
University of Virginia Health System
Charlottesville, VA

**Donna M. Fick, PhD, GCNS-BC, FGSA**
Associate Professor of Nursing, College of Health and Human Development
Associate Professor of Medicine, Department of Psychiatry
Penn State University
State College, PA

**Céline Gélinas, RN, PhD**
Postdoctoral Trainee, School of Nursing
McGill University
Montreal, Quebec
Canada

**Nalaka S. Gooneratne, MD, MSc**
Assistant Professor of Medicine
University of Pennsylvania Medical Center
Philadelphia, PA

**Polly Beckwith Hawkes, RN, MSN, FNP**
Geriatrics and Palliative Care
University of Virginia Health System
Charlottesville, VA

**Keela Herr, RN, PhD, FAAN, AGSF**
Professor and Area Chair, Adult and Gerontology
University of Iowa College of Nursing
Iowa City, IA

**Ronald Hickman, Jr., PhD, RN, ACNP-BC**
Lecturer, Frances Payne Bolton School of Nursing
Clinical Research Scholar, Clinical and Translational Science (NIH/CSTA-KL2)
Eleanor Lambertsen RN Scholar, American Nurses Foundation
Case Western Reserve University
Cleveland, OH

**Rita A. Jablonski, PhD, CRNP**
Assistant Professor, School of Nursing
Pennsylvania State University
State College, PA

**Jill Kamen, MA, RN**
Clinical Nursing Instructor, NYU College of Nursing
New York University
New York, NY

**Karen Kehl, PhD, RN, ACHPN**
Postdoctoral Research Scholar and the Institute of Clinical and Translational Research
School of Nursing
Postdoctoral Research Scholar and the Institute of Clinical and Translational Research
University of Wisconsin–Madison
Madison, WI

**Karin T. Kirchhoff, PhD, RN, FAAN**
Professor Emerita, School of Nursing
University of Wisconsin–Madison
Madison, WI

**Ruth M. Kleinpell, PhD, RN, FAAN, FAANP**
Director, Center for Clinical Research and Scholarship
Rush University Medical Center
Chicago, IL

**Jane S. Leske, PhD, CNS-BC**
Professor, University of Wisconsin Milwaukee
Milwaukee, WI

**Courtney H. Lyder, ND, GNP, FAAN**
Professor and Dean
University of California at Los Angeles, School of Nursing
Los Angeles, CA

**Elisabeth Marie, MA**
Research Coordinator
Center for Sleep and Respiratory Neurobiology
University of Pennsylvania
Philadelphia, PA

**Kathleen M. McCauley, PhD, APRN-BC, FAAN, FAHA**
Associate Professor, Cardiovascular Nursing
University of Pennsylvania, School of Nursing
University of Pennsylvania
Philadelphia, PA

**Graham J. McDougall, Jr., PhD, APRN, FAAN**
Professor of Nursing, Gerontological Nurse Practitioner
The University of Texas at Austin
Austin, TX

**Lorraine C. Mion, PhD, RN, FAAN**
Independence Foundation Professor of Nursing, School of Nursing
Vanderbilt University
Nashville, TN

**Ethel L. Mitty, EdD, RN**
Adjunct Clinical Professor, Nursing
NYU School of Nursing
New York University
New York, NY

**Debra K. Moser, DNSc, RN, FAAN**
Professor, Gill Chair of Cardiovascular Nursing
University of Kentucky, College of Nursing
Lexington, KY

**Mary H. Palmer, PhD, RNC, FAAN**
Helen W. & Thomas L. Umphlet Distinguished Professor in Aging
School of Nursing at UNC-Chapel Hill
Chapel Hill, NC

**Nirav Patel, MD**
Assistant Professor, Clinical Medicine
University of Pennsylvania Medical Center
Philadelphia, PA

**Barbara Resnick, PhD, CRNP, FAAN, FAANP**
Professor of Nursing
University of Maryland School of Nursing
Baltimore, MD

**Michael W. Rich, MD**
Professor of Medicine, Washington University School of Medicine
Washington University in St. Louis
St. Louis, MO

**J. Mark Ruscin, Pharm D, BCPS**
Professor, Department of Pharmacy Practice
SIU-E School of Pharmacy
Southern Illinois University at Edwardsville
Springfield, IL

**Marc Sabbe, MD, PhD**
Professor, Department of Acute Medicine, University Hospitals
Katholeike Universiteit Leuven
Leuven, Belgium

**Marieke Schuurmans, PhD, RN**
Professor, Nursing Sciences
University Medical Center Utrecht
Utrecht, Netherlands

**Jeffrey H. Silverstein, MD, CIP**
Professor of Anesthesiology, Surgery, and Geriatrics & Adult Development
Vice Chairman for Research
Department of Anesthesiology
Associate Dean for Research
Mount Sinai School of Medicine
New York, NY

**Matthew R. Sorenson, PhD, RN**
Instructor, Feinberg School of Medicine
Northwestern University
Evanston, IL

**Dorothy F. Tullmann, PhD, CNL, RN**
Assistant Professor, School of Nursing
University of Virginia
Charlottesville, VA

**Joris Vandenberghe, MD**
Psychiatrist, Department of Psychiatry, Division of Liaison Psychiatry
University Hospital Gasthuisberg / UPC K.U. Leuven
Katholieke Universiteit Leuven
Leuven, Belgium

**Katrien Vanderwee, RN, PhD**
Assistant Professor, Department of Public Health
Faculty of Medicine and Health Sciences
Ghent University
Ghent, Belgium

**Clareen Wiencek, PhD, ACNP**
Assistant Professor, Frances Payne Bolton School of Nursing
Nurse Practitioner, Palliative Care Consult Service
University Hospitals
Case Western Reserve University
Cleveland, OH

**Kathryn A. Wilt, RN, BSN, MAS, NP (c)**
The Pennsylvania State University
University Park, PA

# Foreword

How important is this book? It's simple to answer this question if my words are not considered to be hyperbole. When one writes a foreword to a book it is expected that he or she will be enthusiastic and very complimentary. For why else would the authors ask for a foreword if not for an endorsement?

But in this case my enthusiasm is closer to excitement than to any other emotion; well, perhaps excitement and gratitude. The contents of this book, read serially or in pieces, are vitally needed right now. Our hospitals are filled with older people who, more often than not, are in critical care units for part of their hospital stay. The myriad problems they experience are described in detail with theoretical and evidence-based interventions. The experts—who are academics/clinicians—have been close to geriatrics for much of their professional lives. They are sharing with the reader the wisdom they have gained and this knowledge, applied by others, will improve the care of our older patients immeasurably.

The book's contents run the gamut of elder problems and care: physiology, pharmacology, nutrition, restraints, substance abuse, family involvement, sepsis, and so on; it is a compendium that can be used as a text or a resource. My preference would be for readers to become familiar with the contents and approach sections when you need them most so that their value will be immediately accessible. Written by nurses and physicians, the material covered is aided by the use of numerous case studies that illustrate and exemplify emblematic problems and solutions.

I would like to point out something that we often overlook when considering hospitalized patients of all ages. This is the importance of family visiting; attendance is vital wherever the patient is on the health–illness continuum. Years ago, in looking for a subject for my doctoral dissertation, my 1 $^1$/$_2$-year-old son had an emergency herniorrhaphy. Having studied and worked in psychiatric nursing I was very familiar with the works of Anna Freud and John Bowlby concerning separation of young children from parents during hospitalization (or war time). I chose this area of study and later, after publication of the monograph (Fagin, 1966), which led to national changes in hospital visiting privileges for parents, I thought and wrote about the importance of families during other times of life as well. This book touches on the subject of family visitation and acknowledges the deficits for patients in critical care because of restricted visiting. This resonated strongly with me because of my past work, but also because of dealing with my older sister's illness and repeated admissions to the ICU. Knowing I was there for her made a huge difference in her recovery.

The reader will find other areas of particular interest because of their own professional and personal backgrounds. But all health care providers need part or all of the content of this book. We must get acute and critical care nursing "right" for the sake of the patient and the health care system. Currently, hospitals are places that are more often feared than seen as places of refuge and healing. I believe nursing can and must change this perception. Older people are the prime "business" of our health care system today. The book will be my reference of choice, and I strongly recommend it for all aware nurses, physicians, and other colleagues.

Claire M. Fagin, PhD, RN, FAAN
New York

## Reference

Fagin, C. M. (1966). *The effects of maternal attendance during hospitalization on the behavior of young children.* Philadelphia: F. A. Davis.

# Acknowledgment

The editors wish to acknowledge Mary Walker, PhD, RN, FAAN, for her contributions to a previous edition of this book.

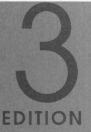
3
EDITION

# Critical Care Nursing of Older Adults
## Best Practices

# Part I

# The Context for Critical Care Nursing of Older Adults

# Introduction and Overview

1

Marquis D. Foreman
Koen Milisen
Terry T. Fulmer

Older adults overwhelmingly represent the majority of patients receiving critical care worldwide. In response to the health care needs of this population, in 1992 Fulmer and Walker published their groundbreaking book on critical care nursing of the elderly; one of the first of its kind. Seventeen years later, the need for a clinical reference for improving the care of older adults with critical illness is even more important. At the beginning of the 21st century, in most developed countries we find ourselves amid an explosion of older people, especially the old-old. With greater longevity, more people are growing older and dealing with chronic health conditions, many with multiple comorbid conditions, which creates a unique set of challenges as much for the care provided as for the complexity of that care. Nurses and associated health professionals must consider the usual physiologic changes that accompany aging, the frequent comorbid conditions that exist in this population, the interaction among these factors, and the treatment provided. Here, expertise in geriatric care is a must. Although efforts to prepare for the graying of the world's population began in the 1960s, now, early in the 21st century, clearly these efforts have fallen short—the number of health care providers trained to care for older adults is gravely insufficient. Nowhere is this insufficiency more evident than in critical care. As a result, in a 2008 report from the Institute of Medicine (IOM), John Rowe suggested that all health care providers must become competent in the care of older adults. To that end, this book was written.

This volume presents the collective thinking of international experts who are striving to address current questions regarding how to better provide critical care to older adults. We have organized the content into 26 chapters arranged in four parts. In all but a few of these chapters, you find the state of the science organized around a real-life case study, which is intended to provide application of the ideas presented to the real world and to bring these ideas to life. This structure enables the book to serve as a reference on major clinical issues for nurses working at the forefront in providing care to critically ill older adults and their families: from nurses working in critical care and step-down units to nurses in trauma and emergency departments. Nurse educators for all degree levels, interdisciplinary team members, and researchers will find this book of great use because it highlights gaps in knowledge with regard to the care of critically ill older adults.

Here is a brief look at the material covered in this book. Part I: The Context for Critical Care Nursing of Older Adults, is comprised of four chapters. This chapter Introduction and Overview, written by Foreman, Milisen, and Fulmer, describes the volume's intent.

Chapter 2: Standards of Practice for Gerontological and Critical Care Nursing, written by Kleinpell, presents an overview of standards of practice for geriatric nursing care. One of the challenges here is that there are a number of standards in use that are presented by several august groups: the American Nurses Association, the American Association of Critical Care Nurses, and the Emergency Nurses Association, among others. Kleinpell describes how these standards interface to complement care of critically ill older adults, and highlights resources available to guide care of this patient population.

Chapter 3: The Critical Care Environment, by Tullmann, Hawkes, and Enfield, accentuates the need to appropriately modify the intensive care unit (ICU) environment to promote or preserve functional ability for the older adult population. They recommend successful strategies for an optimal physical, interpersonal, and social milieu, leading to a more healing environment for older adults in critical care.

Chapter 4: Patient Safety: Safety and quality are the mantra now and will be for the foreseeable future until we can prove to the public that "never" events are no longer detectable. In 2009, The National Quality Forum published its safe practices and set a "blueprint" for the way in which organizations should improve safety and quality of care for the patients they serve. This chapter, which is written by Dillworth and Fulmer, reflects the standards and practices of that document (Hughes, 2008; Institute of Medicine, 2000). The chapter addresses key areas for safety and provides a lexicon of resources for practicing nurses as they strive to eliminate error for the benefit of the critically ill older patient.

Part II: Social Aspects of Critical Care Nursing of Older Adults has seven chapters beginning with chapter 5: Ethical Decision Making. In this chapter, Mitty discusses central aspects of the approach of care for critically ill older individuals within a framework of caring and shared decision making. Who should receive care? Who should pay? When should care be withdrawn or, in fact, at what point should new care regimens be discontinued? All these are serious issues that are likely to overwhelm the health care system unless careful, proactive thinking evolves.

In chapter 6, Continuity of Care, McCauley profiles critically ill older adults likely to be at risk for readmission. She describes the common types of adverse events and the outcomes that occur with these patients. To prevent complications or detect early causes of deterioration, McCauley urges nurses and other health care providers to manage not only the care in each setting but also to proactively integrate the transition between settings. She gives an overview of effective care models that have been proven to promote continuity and benefit for older patients and describes concrete examples on how to implement these models.

Chapter 7: Family Responses to Critical Care of the Older Adult—here Leske emphasizes family-centered care as a strategy for improving outcomes of care for critically ill older adults. Consequently, in this chapter, she focuses on family assessments, interventions, and theories to better comprehend the influence of critical illness on the family.

Chapter 8: End-of-Life Care: Caring for critically ill older adults who are facing end-of-life issues is challenging at best. Kehl and Kirchhoff provide strategies for making the shift from a curative to a comfort focus by attending to the elements that make for good end-of-life care. These strategies include methods for improving communication, symptom management, and preparation for death.

Chapter 9: Becoming Frail: McDougall and Delville update the work of Wolanin on frailty in critically ill older adults. They provide an overview of the cascade of events terminating in a critically ill older adult becoming frail and how this adds to the complex issues that arise in providing care to such patients. Strategies for assessing the status of these patients and perspectives for improving outcomes of care for this vulnerable patient population are presented.

In chapter 10: The Chronically Critically Ill, Wiencek and Hickman depict a new way of describing the patient, *the chronically critically ill patient*, which has evolved from the extraordinary interventions and strategies now available in health care. The Office of Technology Assessment's classic 1987 report on life-sustaining technologies in the elderly was a harbinger for how we would be able to provide care in 2010. That report warned us that, within the foreseeable future, hospitals would become intensive care units, and in fact, this is so today. All of us need to think about our approach to care for individuals who will need our critical care skills over an extended period of time.

In chapter 11, Function of Older Adults in Acute Care: Optimizing an Opportunity, Resnick contributes to one of the most important responsibilities that nurses may have in caring for older adults, especially those enduring a critical illness—optimizing function. In this chapter, she addresses the importance of function among older hospitalized individuals to optimize their clinical outcomes as well as to decrease the cost of care. She does so by reviewing extensively the contributing factors for functional decline, by illuminating the differences between function and physical activity and functional decline and disability, and by describing care approaches such as integrated restorative care, which nurses can use as an effective strategy in the rehabilitation process of the older patient.

Part III of the volume—Foundations for Clinical Care of Critically Ill Older Adults—begins with chapter 12, Physiology of Aging: Impact on Critical Illness and Treatment. Physiologic changes associated with aging may be usual but are anything but normal. Brock and Jablonski examine these usual physiologic changes by organ system and discuss how these changes affect the presentation of disease as well as the response to treatment.

Chapter 13: Pharmacotherapy—the principles outlined in this chapter by Ruscin remind us that with technology, pharmaceutical advancements, and biotechnologies more intervention is now possible than heretofore could be imagined. The author then describes underlying concepts of appropriate pharmacologic intervention for critically ill individuals.

Chapter 14: Nutrition and Hydration: Wilt and Fick explore nutrition and hydration in the context of critically ill older individuals, some of whom have severely altered patterns of ingestion and elimination over brief or sustained periods of time. Again, reflecting on the notions of ethical care, humane care, and care that provides comfort and safety, one needs to realize that these domains intersect in an ongoing, complex, and profound way.

Chapter 15: Physical Restraints in Critical Care: Practice Issues and Future Directions: The use of physical restraints remains a controversial and challenging practice, especially within the critical care environment. Although the use of physical restraints in critical care has received scant attention in the literature (in contrast to other settings), Mion and Bradas have identified and described essential values, norms, best practice principles, and recommendations for changing practice within an interdisciplinary patient-centered fashion.

Chapter 16: Infection, Sepsis, and Immune Function—In this chapter, Sorenson identifies age-related changes in immune function, discusses the interaction between comorbid conditions and immunity, describes immunological biomarkers that may facilitate the detection of those frail elders at greater risk for chronic disease and functional decline, and finally concludes with interventions to prevent, alleviate, or manage problems associated with immunosenescence.

Chapter 17: Understanding and Managing Sleep Disorders in Older Adult Patients in the Intensive Care Unit—It is generally agreed that sleep in the ICU is poor, but this problem is compounded among older patients. Marie, Patel, and Gooneratne present the many-factored origins of poor sleep in the ICU with strategies for promoting sleep.

Chapter 18: Pain in the Critically Ill Older Adult: Pain is a major concern because of its complexity, high prevalence, and impact on older persons in all settings, but especially in the critical care setting. Gélinas and Herr comprehensively describe important issues such as problems associated with attitudes and misperceptions regarding untreated pain and pain assessment, and how to manage these in both a pharmacological and nonpharmacological manner. Special attention goes to those critically ill older patients who are unable to communicate pain because of a diminished level of consciousness (e.g., intubation, sedative agents, and/or cognitive decline).

The final section of this book, Part IV: Approaches to Complex Clinical Issues in Critically Ill Older Adults, describes specific treatment approaches for this population.

In chapter 19: Pressure Ulcer Prevention and Management, Defloor, Vanderwee, and Dealey remind us about the high costs associated with decubitus, both in terms of patient suffering and financial burden. Fortunately, nurses might use the many evidence-based strategies available nowadays for effective prevention and management, leading to improved safety and quality of care for the patients.

Chapter 20: Wound Healing in the Elderly: The consequences of chronic wounds are devastating for critically ill older patients, as they are more likely to experience greater morbidity, such as loss of an extremity, as well as greater mortality, than do other patients. For institutions, critically ill older patients with chronic wounds or hospital-acquired wounds create financial havoc, as these are considered indicators of poor quality care for which the Centers for Medicare and Medicaid Services no longer pay. Lyder provides information essential for preventing the occurrence of such wounds as well as the information necessary for promoting the normal wound-healing cascade.

Chapter 21: Substance Abuse and Withdrawal: Psychoactive substance use, abuse, and withdrawal are an interdisciplinary challenge. In their extensive overview, Sabbe and Vandenberghe highlight the importance of knowledge and insights about physical and mental dependency, tolerance, abstinence reactions, and withdrawal effects of various chemical substances affecting the central nervous system. Special emphasis is given to the observation and management of symptoms and behaviors as contributors to the patient's complex diagnostic and treatment plan.

In chapter 22, Urinary Incontinence in Critically Ill Older Adults, Palmer reminds us that although seemingly benign, urinary incontinence is a potentially life-threatening condition, a condition frequently overlooked during a critical illness. Palmer provides background information about urinary incontinence and discusses evidence-based approaches for meeting the continence needs of critically ill older adults.

Chapter 23: Heart Failure in the Critically Ill Older Patient: In this chapter, Moser and Rich provide an overview of the unique care needs of critically ill older adults with heart failure. They bring clarity to the important contribution critical care nurses make with respect to the chain of education and advocacy leading to appropriate health care and improved outcomes for this patient population.

Chapter 24: Perioperative Care—this chapter examines perioperative care of older adults, which is a new focus for research. Yet, despite the fact that the knowledge on which to found perioperative best practices is limited, older patients are successfully undergoing extensive operative procedures that were previously restricted to younger patient populations. Silverstein discusses these issues and the state of the science of perioperative care for critically ill older adults.

Chapter 25: Acute Respiratory Failure and Mechanical Ventilation in the Elderly: Respiratory failure is the primary reason for the majority of admissions to critical care units. In this chapter, Kamen discusses the major factors contributing to respiratory failure in critically ill older adults. Mechanical ventilation is the mainstay treatment for this problem; however, she also addresses alternatives to such treatment and strategies for improving outcomes for this vulnerable patient population.

Chapter 26: Delirium in Critical Illness: Delirium is one of the most complex issues facing critically ill older adults, their families, and those providing care to these patients. It is a clinical condition that frustrates and strains care providers, frightens families, dehumanizes older patients, and costs billions of dollars annually. In this chapter, Foreman, Schuurmans, and Milisen discuss the nature of delirium and how this adds to the challenges of recognition and diagnosis, factors that place patients at risk for developing delirium with critical illness, methods of assessment for its identification, and currently accepted strategies for preventing and managing delirium in older critically ill patients.

We are indebted to these authors for their efforts in helping us to bring this book to life. We thank them for these contributions, to their lifelong dedication to improving the quality of care for this vulnerable patient population, and their friendship.

**Marquis D. Foreman**
**Koen Milisen**
**Terry T. Fulmer**

# References

Fulmer, T. T., & Walker, M. K. (1992). *Critical care nursing of the elderly*. New York: Springer Publishing Company.

Hughes, R. G. (Ed.). (2008). *Patient safety and quality: An evidence-based handbook for nurses* (AHRQ Publication No. 08-0043). Rockville, MD: Agency for Healthcare Research and Quality. Retrieved July 29, 2009, from www.ahrq.gov/QUAL/nursehdbk

Institute of Medicine. (2000). *To err is human: Building a safer health system*. Washington, DC: National Academy Press.

Institute of Medicine. (2008). *Retooling for an aging America. Building the health care workforce*. Washington, DC: National Academy Press.

National Quality Forum. (2009). *Safe practices for better healthcare 2009 update: A consensus report*. Washington, DC: Author.

Office of Technology Assessment. (1987). *Life-sustaining technologies and the elderly*. Washington, DC: U.S. Government Printing Office.

# Standards of Practice for Gerontological and Critical Care Nursing

# 2

Ruth M. Kleinpell

## Introduction

Focusing on best care practices for geriatric nursing care requires an awareness of available resources within current standards of practice. A number of standards exist to guide critical care nursing of the elderly, including standards from the American Nurses Association (2001, 2004), the American Association of Critical Care Nurses (2005), and the Emergency Nurses Association (http://www.ena.org/education/ GENE/default.asp). This chapter presents an overview on standards of practice for geriatric nursing care, highlighting resources that are available to guide nursing practice that is focused on evidence-based care. Discussion of how the standards interface and can be used to complement care for critical care nursing of the elderly is also provided.

## Standards Defined

Standards are defined as authoritative statements by which the nursing profession outlines nursing care responsibilities (American Nurses Association, 2004). Standards provide a framework for evaluating nursing practice, provide direction for nursing

# Exhibit 2.1

## Nursing Standards of Practice

**Standard 1:** Assessment: The registered nurse collects comprehensive data pertinent to the patient's health or the situation.
**Standard 2:** Diagnosis: The registered nurse analyzes the assessment data to determine the diagnosis or issues.
**Standard 3:** Outcomes Identification: The registered nurse identifies expected outcomes for a plan individualized to the patient or the situation.
**Standard 4:** Planning: The registered nurse develops a plan that prescribes strategies and alternatives to attain expected outcomes.
**Standard 5:** Implementation: The registered nurse implements the identified plan.
**Standard 6:** Evaluation: The registered nurse evaluates progress toward attainment of outcomes.

*Note.* Adapted from American Nurses Association (2004).

practice, and outline responsibilities that nurses are accountable for as well as recommended outcomes (American Nurses Association). Standards also serve as guidelines and provide a framework by which care is measured (Hanson, 2009). The document *Nursing: Scope and Standards of Practice* (American Nurses Association) outlines six generic standards of practice (Exhibit 2.1).

These six standards of practice indicate that nursing care is framed around the critical thinking model known as the nursing process, which forms the foundation for nursing decision making (American Nurses Association, 2004). As outlined in *Nursing: Scope and Standards of Practice*, several fundamental aspects of standard nursing practice include:

■ Providing age-appropriate and culturally and ethnically sensitive care
■ Maintaining a safe environment
■ Educating patients about healthy practices and treatment modalities
■ Assuring continuity of care
■ Coordinating the care across settings and among caregivers
■ Managing information
■ Communicating effectively
■ Using technology

## Standards of Practice for Gerontological Nursing

Persons aged 65 and older are a growing proportion of the population who have specific health care and nursing related needs. In 2006, there were an estimated 37 million people aged 65 and older in the United States, representing just over 12% of the population, with growth projections predicted to reach nearly 20% by 2030 (Federal Interagency Forum on Aging Related Statistics, 2008). As a result, planning for the health care needs of the aging population has become a priority area for nursing as well as for the spectrum of health care clinician disciplines. Professional nurses play a significant role in developing, implementing, and evaluating standards of nursing practice (Stanley & Blair, 2005). In 1987, the American Nurses Association Standards of Gerontological Nursing Practice were revised from the original generic standards to serve as a model for gerontological nursing practice. The standards recommend similar areas of focus as the generic standards of practice, but are focused on gerontological nursing care. Several areas of focus include comprehensive assessment of the older adult's functional, psychological, and psychosocial status; response to the aging process; history of health conditions; and the importance of individualization of care; among other areas of focus. Exhibit 2.2 provides a listing of the standards of practice for gerontological nursing.

## Using Standards of Practice to Promote Evidence-Based Practice

As practice guidelines for care, standards of practice are derived from evidence-based practice and are continuously evolving (Hanson, 2009). For the specialty area of gerontological nursing practice, a number of resources exist for developing and revising standards of practice, including federally based resources such as the Agency for Healthcare Research and Quality (www.ahrq.gov) and the Nursing Quality Forum (www.qualityforum.org); geriatric specialty organizations such as the Hartford Institute for Geriatric Nursing (www.hartfordign.org), American Geriatrics Society (www.americangeriatrics.org), National Institute on Aging (www.nia.nih.gov), among others; and quality-based organizations such as the Institute for Healthcare Improvement (www.ihi.org). Exhibit 2.3 outlines a number of resources for geriatric best care practices that can be used to develop and revise standards of practice for gerontological nursing. Exhibit 2.4 provides a listing from another geriatric care resource entitled ConsultGeriRN, the geriatric clinical nursing Website of The Hartford Institute for Geriatric Nursing (www.consultgerirn.org), which has a variety of evidence-based protocols for managing common geriatric syndromes and conditions.

A number of health care disciplines are promoting evidence-based standards of practice for gerontology practice. The National Association of Professional Geriatric Care Managers' standards of practice outline that geriatric-focused care practice guidelines should address several areas, including fostering self-determination, right to privacy, and personal integrity of the older person (2003). Medical standards of care for geriatric practice also highlight recommendations for standards of care that focus on comprehensive geriatric assessments, effective disease prevention and early detection, individualized prevention, encouraging compliance, respect for decisional capacity and justice, integration of care using local resources, team-based care, effective end-of-life care, effective palliative care, coordination with hospice care, and effective care in nursing homes (Luchi, Gammack, Marcisse, & Porter Storey, 2003).

Specialty geriatric organizations can also serve as sources of information to inform standards of practice. The National Gerontological Nursing Association (www.ngna.org) has published position statements that outline best care practices for geriatric patients that can be used to formulate and revise standards of practice. Additionally, institutional resources focusing on geriatric care best practices such as the University of Pennsylvania School of Nursing's GeroTIPS online (http://www.nursing.upenn.edu/

# Exhibit 2.2

## Standards of Practice for Gerontological Nursing Practice

**Standard 1:** Assessment: The gerontological nurse collects patient health data. The data may include information on:

■ Functional abilities (activities of daily living)
■ Physical, psychological, psychosocial, economic, cognitive, cultural, and spiritual status
■ Environmental assessment, including safety issues and identification of available and accessible support systems and material resources
■ Response to the aging process
■ History of health patterns and illness
■ Prescribed medication, self-medication, and complementary/integrative therapies and practices
■ Current self-care and health-promotion activities
■ Past and current lifestyles
■ Individual coping patterns
■ Perception of and satisfaction with health status
■ Health beliefs, values, and practices
■ Advanced directives for health care

**Standard 2:** Diagnosis: The gerontological nurse analyzes the assessment data in determining diagnoses
**Standard 3:** Outcomes Identification: The gerontological nurse identifies expected outcomes individualized to the older adult. Expected outcomes:

■ Reflect the diagnoses
■ Belong to the older adult and are mutually formulated with the older adult, family, or significant others and the interdisciplinary team
■ Are culturally appropriate and realistic in relation to present and potential capabilities
■ Are attainable in relation to resources available to the older adult and care setting
■ Include a time frame for attainment
■ Are identified with consideration of the associated benefits and costs
■ Provide direction for continuity of care
■ Are documented as measurable goals

**Standard 4:** Planning: The gerontological nurse develops a plan of care that prescribes interventions to attain expected outcomes
**Standard 5:** Implementation: The gerontological nurse implements the interventions identified in the plan of care. Interventions may include:

■ Facilitation of self-care and optimal functioning
■ Health promotion and maintenance
■ Disease prevention
■ Health teaching
■ Counseling
■ Psychobiological interventions
■ Consultation
■ Data collection and assessment
■ Exploration of treatment choices including integrated interventions/modalities such as nutrition, therapeutic touch, relaxation techniques, and exercise
■ Palliative care for the chronically ill or dying older adult
■ Referral to community resources
■ Case management
■ Evaluation and education of caregivers

**Standard 6:** Evaluation: The gerontological nurse evaluates the older adult's progress toward attainment of expected outcomes.

*Note.* Adapted from the American Nurses Association (2001).

# Exhibit 2.3

## Geriatric Best Practice Resources

University Geriatric Websites
University of Iowa www.medicine.uiowa.edu/igec

University of Pennsylvania
www.nursing.upenn.edu/centers/hcgne/default.htm

Hartford Institute for Geriatric Nursing/NYU site
www.hartfordign.org

Try This Series:
http://www.hartfordign.org/resources/education/tryThis.html

**Additional Geriatric Websites**

Alzheimer's Association
www.alz.org

Alzheimer's Association Resource Center
www.alz.org/ResourceCenter/ResourceCenter.htm

American Geriatrics Society Nursing Review Syllabus
www.americangeriatrics.org/products/gnr_syllabus.shtml

*Merck Manual of Geriatrics*
www.merck.com/pubs/mm_geriatrics/contents.htm

National Institute on Aging
www.nia.nih.gov/health

> Age Pages
> www.niapublications.org/shopdisplayproducts.asp?id=15&cat=Age+
> Pages+and+Fact+Sheets

> Communicating with Older Patients
> www.nia.nih.gov/health/pubs/clinicians-handbook/index.htm#content

**Coalition of Geriatric Nursing Organizations**
www.hartfordign.org/resources/policy/coalition.html

American Academy of Nursing (AAN)—Expert Panel on Aging

- The American Association of Nurse Assessment Coordinators
- National Association of Directors of Nursing Administration in Long Term Care (NADONA/LTC)
- National Conference of Gerontological Nurse Practitioners (NCGNP)
- National Gerontological Nursing Association (NGNA)
- The John A. Hartford Foundation Institute for Geriatric Nursing

John A. Hartford Foundation Gerontological Nursing Initiative
www.gerontologicalnursing.info

**Geriatric Nursing Journals**

*Geriatric Nursing*
www2.us.elsevierhealth.com/scripts/om.dll/serve?action=searchDB&s earchDBfor=home&id=gn

*Journal of Gerontological Nursing*
www.slackinc.com/allied/jgn/jgnhome.htm

*Geriatric Emergency Nursing Education*
http://www.ena.org/education/GENE/default.asp
   A series of educational modules addressing geriatric care including discharge planning, abuse and neglect, attitudes and ageism, polypharmacy, physical and psychological changes, palliative care, pain management, and triage and assessment

*Note*: From Emergency Nurses Association: See http://www.ena.org/nursing/geriatric/top10-resources. asp/ and http://www.ena.org/education/GENE/default.asp

# Exhibit 2.4

## Evidence-Based Geriatric Protocols and Topics

Atypical Presentation

Delirium

Dementia

Depression

Elder Mistreatment and Abuse

Falls

Family Caregiving

Function

Hydration Management

Iatrogenesis

Mealtime Difficulties

Medication

Normal Aging Changes

Nutrition in the Elderly

Oral Health in Aging

Pain

Palliative Care

Physical Restraints

Pressure Ulcers

Sensory Changes

Sexuality Issues in Aging

Sleep

Substance Abuse

Treatment Decision Making

Urinary Incontinence

*Note.* Retrieved from http://consultgerirn.org/resources/geriatric_topics

centers/hcgne/gero_tips/RES_Best_Practice.htm) and the Emergency Nurses Association's Geriatric Best Practice Resources (http://www.ena.org/nursing/geriatric/top10-resources.asp) provide educational and clinical practice references that can be used to update standards of practice to ensure alignment with current best practice recommendations.

## Standards of Practice Relating to Critical Care

The American Association of Critical Care Nurses (AACN) is a resource for standards of practice relating to critical care. A number of standards have been created for critical care nursing practice, including AACN's Standards of Care for Acute and Critical Care Nursing (Exhibit 2.5), Standards of Professional Practice for Acute and Critical Care Nursing (Exhibit 2.6), as well as clinical practice standards focusing on specific clinical conditions such as deep vein thrombosis prevention, verification of feeding-tube placement, preventing catheter-related bloodstream infections, ventilator-acquired pneumonia prevention, and severe sepsis. The AACN standards of care and professional practice for acute and critical care nursing provide examples of the roles and responsibilities expected of the critical care nurse and include both standards of care, which prescribe a competent level of nursing practice, and standards of professional performance, which articulate the roles and behaviors expected of nursing professionals. These standards are directly applicable to the critical care nursing of the elderly as they outline considerations for general care of acute and critically ill patients with respect to assessment, diagnosis, outcome identification, planning, implementation, and evaluation as well as quality-of-care considerations.

The AACN standards for establishing and sustaining healthy work environments outline several standards, including communication, collaboration, effective decision making, appropriate staffing, recognition, and leadership (Exhibit 2.7). As broad-based standards, they can be applied to care of the critically ill elder to promote evidence-based and relationship-centered principles of professional practice.

The Emergency Nurses Association is an additional resource for standards of practice relating to emergency care. Standards of practice for emergency care outline clinical standards for direct patient care and include considerations related to assessment, diagnosis, treatment plan, implementation, and evaluation/outcome, as well as quality-of-care aspects (http://www.ena.org/pdf/Standards.pdf). These standards can also be applied to critical care nursing of the elderly patient with urgent or emergent care conditions.

## Interface of Standards

The standards of practice for gerontological nursing interface in several ways with the critical care and emergency nursing standards. The standards provide direction for nursing practice and outline responsibilities for aspects of critical care nursing, including general considerations for assessment, diagnosis, outcome identification, planning, implementation, and evaluation, which can readily be applied to care of the elderly patient.

The standards can be used in conjunction to promote best practices for critical care nursing of the elderly. For example, the standards of practice for gerontological

# Exhibit 2.5

## Standards of Care for Acute and Critical Care Nursing

**Standard of Care I: Assessment**

THE NURSE CARING FOR ACUTE AND CRITICALLY ILL PATIENTS COLLECTS RELEVANT PATIENT HEALTH DATA.
Measurement Criteria

1. Data collection involves the patient, family, and other health care providers as appropriate to develop a holistic picture of the patient's needs.
2. The priority of data collection activities is driven by the patient's immediate condition and/or anticipated needs.
3. Pertinent data are collected using appropriate assessment techniques and instruments.
4. Data are documented in a retrievable form.
5. Data collection process is systematic and ongoing.

**Standard of Care II: Diagnosis**

THE NURSE CARING FOR ACUTE AND CRITICALLY ILL PATIENTS ANALYZES THE ASSESSMENT DATA IN DETERMINING DIAGNOSES.
Measurement Criteria

1. Diagnoses are derived from the assessment data.
2. Diagnoses are validated throughout the nursing interactions with the team consisting of the patient, family, and other health care providers, when possible and appropriate.
3. Diagnoses are prioritized and documented in a manner that facilitates determining expected outcomes and developing a plan of care.
4. Diagnoses are documented in a retrievable form. ·

**Standard of Care III: Outcome Identification**

THE NURSE CARING FOR ACUTE AND CRITICALLY ILL PATIENTS IDENTIFIES INDIVIDUALIZED, EXPECTED OUTCOMES FOR THE PATIENT.
Measurement Criteria

1. Outcomes are derived from actual or potential diagnoses.
2. Outcomes are mutually formulated with the patient, family, and other health care providers, when possible and appropriate.
3. Outcomes are individualized in that they are culturally appropriate and realistic in relation to the patient's age and present and potential capabilities.
4. Outcomes are attainable in relation to resources available to the patient.
5. Outcomes are measurable and should include a time estimate for attainment, if possible.
6. Outcomes provide direction for continuity of care so that the nurse's competencies are matched with the patient's needs.
7. Outcomes are documented in a retrievable form.

**Standard of Care IV: Planning**

THE NURSE CARING FOR ACUTE AND CRITICALLY ILL PATIENTS DEVELOPS A PLAN OF CARE THAT PRESCRIBES INTERVENTIONS TO ATTAIN EXPECTED OUTCOMES.
Measurement Criteria

1. The plan is individualized to reflect the patient's characteristics and needs.
2. The plan is developed collaboratively with the team, consisting of the patient, family, and health care providers, in a way that promotes each member's contribution toward achieving expected outcomes.
3. The plan reflects current acute and critical care nursing practice.

*(continued)*

**Exhibit 2.5** *(continued)*

4. The plan provides for continuity of care.
5. Priorities for care are established.
6. The plan is documented to promote continuity of care.

**Standard of Care V: Implementation**

THE NURSE CARING FOR ACUTE AND CRITICALLY ILL PATIENTS IMPLEMENTS INTERVENTIONS IDENTIFIED IN THE PLAN OF CARE.
Measurement Criteria

1. Interventions are delivered in a manner that minimizes complications and life-threatening situations.
2. The patient and family participate in implementing the plan of care based upon their ability to participate in and make decisions regarding care.
3. Interventions are documented in a retrievable manner.

**Standard of Care VI: Evaluation**

THE NURSE CARING FOR ACUTE AND CRITICALLY ILL PATIENTS EVALUATES THE PATIENT'S PROGRESS TOWARD ATTAINING EXPECTED OUTCOMES.
Measurement Criteria

1. Evaluation is systematic, ongoing, and criterion-based.
2. The team consisting of patient, family, and health care providers is involved in the evaluation process as appropriate.
3. Evaluation occurs within an appropriate time frame after interventions are initiated.
4. Ongoing assessment data are used to revise the diagnoses, outcomes, and plan of care as needed.
5. Revisions in diagnoses, outcomes, and plan of care are documented.
6. The effectiveness of interventions is evaluated in relation to outcomes.
7. The patient's responses to interventions are documented.

*Note.* Retrieved from http://www.aacn.org/WD/Practice/Content/standards.for.acute.and.ccnursing. practice.pcms?menu=Practice

nursing can be used to establish a general framework for critical care nursing, whereas the standards of practice for critical care and emergency care can be used to focus care specific to stabilization of critical care or emergency care conditions. Put together, these standards can be used to structure care processes to improve nursing care for elderly patients with acute, critical, and emergent care conditions.

# Summary

Nursing standards of practice are beneficial in guiding nursing care. As the scope of practice in gerontological nursing is ever evolving, it becomes important that nursing standards of practice for gerontological nursing incorporate evidence-based practice concepts and promote best practices. A number of standards of practice exist that pertain to critical care nursing of the elderly, including the American Nurses Association's standards of practice for gerontological nursing, the American Association of

# Exhibit 2.6

## Standards of Professional Practice for Acute and Critical Care Nursing

**Standard of Professional Practice I: Quality of Care**

THE NURSE CARING FOR ACUTE AND CRITICALLY ILL PATIENTS SYSTEMATICALLY EVALUATES THE QUALITY AND EFFECTIVENESS OF NURSING PRACTICE.
Measurement Criteria

1. The nurse participates in quality-of-care activities.
2. The nurse uses the results of quality-of-care activities to initiate changes in nursing practices and the health care delivery system as appropriate.
3. The nurse assures that quality-of-care activities incorporate the patient and family's perspective as appropriate.

**Standard of Professional Practice II: Individual Practice Evaluation**

THE PRACTICE OF THE NURSE CARING FOR ACUTELY AND CRITICALLY ILL PATIENTS REFLECTS KNOWLEDGE OF CURRENT PROFESSIONAL PRACTICE STANDARDS, LAWS, AND REGULATIONS.
Measurement Criteria

1. The nurse evaluates his or her own nursing practice in relation to the professional practice standards and relevant statutes and regulations.
2. The nurse engages in a self-assessment and/or a formal performance appraisal on a regular basis, identifying areas of strength as well as areas where professional development would be beneficial.
3. The nurse seeks and reflects on constructive feedback from the team consisting of patient, family, and other health care providers regarding his or her own practice.
4. The nurse takes action to achieve performance goals.

**Standard of Professional Practice III: Education**

THE NURSE ACQUIRES AND MAINTAINS CURRENT KNOWLEDGE AND COMPETENCY IN THE CARE OF ACUTE OR CRITICALLY ILL PATIENTS.
Measurement Criteria

1. The nurse participates in ongoing educational activities to acquire knowledge and skills needed to care for acute and critically ill patients.
2. The nurse seeks experiences that reflect current clinical practice in order to maintain current clinical skills and competencies needed to care for acutely and critically ill patients.
3. The nurse participates in ongoing educational activities related to professional issues.

**Standard of Professional Practice IV: Collegiality**

THE NURSE CARING FOR ACUTE AND CRITICALLY ILL PATIENTS INTERACTS WITH AND CONTRIBUTES TO THE PROFESSIONAL DEVELOPMENT OF PEERS AND OTHER HEALTH CARE PROVIDERS AS COLLEAGUES.
Measurement Criteria

1. The nurse shares knowledge, skills, and experiences with colleagues.
2. The nurse provides peers and other health care providers with constructive feedback regarding their practice, as appropriate to their level of expertise.
3. The nurse interacts with colleagues to enhance his or her own professional nursing practice.
4. The nurse contributes to a learning environment that is conducive to health care education.
5. The nurse contributes to an effective team environment by working with others in a way that promotes and encourages each person's contribution.

*(continued)*

## Exhibit 2.6 *(continued)*

**Standard of Professional Practice V: Ethics**

THE NURSE'S DECISION AND ACTIONS ON BEHALF OF ACUTELY AND CRITICALLY ILL PATIENTS ARE DETERMINED IN AN ETHICAL MANNER.
Measurement Criteria

1. The nurse's practice is guided by the ANA's Code for Nurses, AACN's Ethic of Care, and ethical principles.
2. The nurse maintains patient confidentiality within legal and regulatory parameters.
3. The nurse acts as a patient advocate and assists others in developing skills so they can advocate for themselves.
4. The nurse delivers care in a nonjudgmental and nondiscriminatory manner that is sensitive to patient diversity.
5. The nurse delivers care in a manner that meets the diverse needs and strengths of the patient and preserves patient autonomy, dignity, and rights.
6. The nurse uses available resources in formulating ethical decisions.

**Standard of Professional Practice VI: Collaboration**

THE NURSE CARING FOR ACUTE AND CRITICALLY ILL PATIENTS COLLABORATES WITH THE TEAM, CONSISTING OF PATIENT, FAMILY, AND HEALTH CARE PROVIDERS, IN PROVIDING PATIENT CARE IN A HEALING, HUMANE, AND CARING ENVIRONMENT.

Measurement Criteria

1. The nurse communicates with the team regarding patient care and the nurse's role in providing care.
2. The nurse works with the team to formulate the plan of care and to make decisions related to the care and delivery of services.
3. The nurse consults with other health care providers and initiates referrals as appropriate to promote continuity of care.

**Standard of Professional Practice VII: Research**

THE NURSE CARING FOR ACUTE AND CRITICALLY ILL PATIENTS USES CLINICAL INQUIRY IN PRACTICE.
Measurement Criteria
The nurse continually questions and evaluates practice and uses best available evidence or research findings to develop appropriate plans of care. The nurse participates in activities to support clinical inquiry appropriate to the nurse's level of expertise.

**Standard VIII: Resource Utilization**

THE NURSE CARING FOR ACUTE AND CRITICALLY ILL PATIENTS CONSIDERS FACTORS RELATED TO SAFETY, EFFECTIVENESS, AND COST IN PLANNING AND DELIVERING PATIENT CARE.
Measurement Criteria

1. The nurse evaluates factors related to safety, effectiveness, availability, and cost when choosing among two or more practice options that would result in the same expected outcome.
2. The nurse assists the patient and family in identifying and securing appropriate and available services to address health-related needs.
3. The nurse assigns or delegates aspects of care as defined by the state nurse practice acts.
4. If the nurse assigns or delegates aspects of care, the decision is based upon an assessment of the needs and condition of the patient, the potential for harm, the stability of the patient's condition, the predictability of the outcome, and the competencies of the health care provider.
5. The nurse assists the patient and family in becoming informed consumers about costs, risks, and benefits of treatment and care.

*Note.* Retrieved from http://www.aacn.org/WD/Practice/Content/standards.for.acute.and.ccnursing.practice. pcms?menu=Practice

# Exhibit 2.7

## AACN Standards for Establishing and Sustaining Healthy Work Environments

**Skilled Communication**

Nurses must be as proficient in communication skills as they are in clinical skills.

**True Collaboration**

Nurses must be relentless in pursuing and fostering true collaboration.

**Effective Decision Making**

Nurses must be valued and committed partners in making policy, directing and evaluating clinical care, and leading organizational operations

**Appropriate Staffing**

Staffing must ensure the effective match between patient needs and nurse competencies.

**Meaningful Recognition**

Nurses must be recognized and must recognize others for the value each brings to the work of the organization.

**Authentic Leadership**

Nurse leaders must fully embrace the imperative of a healthy work environment, authentically live in that environment, and engage others in its achievement.

*Note.* Retrieved from http://www.aacn.org/WD/Practice/Content/PublicPolicy/workenv.pcms?menu=Practice

Critical Care Nurses standards, and the Emergency Nurses Association standards of practice. These standards can assist nurses in evaluating and improving nursing practice to promote optimal care for critically ill elders. Standards of practice have been identified as objective criteria for assessing nurses' performance, for determining staffing needs of a clinical unit, for identifying educational and staff development programs, and for identifying areas of clinical practice for research (Stanley & Blair, 2005). As the aging population continues to increase, it is expected that the critical care needs of the elderly will also increase. Critical care nursing will need to continue to focus on promoting high standards of gerontological nursing practice to ensure that nursing care continues to meet standards of practice for high-quality care that promote best outcomes for critically ill elders.

# References

American Association of Critical Care Nurses (n.d.). *Standards for acute and critical care nursing practice.* Retrieved August 12, 2009, from http://www.aacn.org/WD/Practice/Content/standards.for. acute.and.ccnursing.practice.pcms?menu=Practice

American Association of Critical Care Nurses. (2005). *AACN standards for establishing and sustaining healthy work environments.* Retrieved August 12, 2009, from www.aacn.org

American Nurses Association. (2001). *Scope and standards of gerontological nursing practice.* Washington, DC: Author.

American Nurses Association. (2004). *Nursing: Scope and standards of practice.* Washington, DC: Author.

Emergency Nurses Association. (n.d.). Retrieved August 12, 2009, from http://www.ena.org/education/GENE/default.asp

Federal Interagency Forum on Aging Related Statistics. (2008). *Older Americans 2008: Key indicators of well-being.* Hyattsville, MD: Federal Interagency Forum on Aging Related Statistics.

Hanson, C. M. (2009). Understanding regulatory, legal and credentialing requirements. In A. B. Hamric, J. A. Spross, & C. M. Hanson (Eds.), *Advanced practice nursing: An integrative approach.* Philadelphia: Saunders Elsevier.

Luchi, R. J., Gammack, J. K., Marcisse, J., & Porter Storey, C. (2003). Standards of care in geriatric practice. *Annual Review of Medicine, 54,* 185–196.

National Association of Professional Geriatric Care Managers. (2003). *Standards of practice for professional geriatric care managers.* Tucson, AZ: Author.

Stanley, M., & Blair, K. (2005). *Gerontological nursing: Promoting successful aging with older adults.* Philadelphia: F.A. Davis.

# The Critical Care Environment

# 3

Dorothy F. Tullmann
Polly Beckwith Hawkes
Elizabeth H. Enfield

## Introduction

The fundamental focus of care for a geriatric patient lies not only with medical diagnosis and intervention, but also with promoting or preserving functional ability. Older adults (> 65 years) comprise more than 40% of intensive care unit (ICU) admissions and almost 60% of all ICU days (Marik, 2006). The older adult is likely to present to the ICU with multiple comorbidities intermingled with the admitting diagnosis, which can significantly reduce functional status. Even without a critical illness, intrinsic changes associated with normal physiologic aging alter or diminish the function of many organ systems, thus increasing the complexity of diagnosis and treatment and prolonging the recovery time from a critical illness. Unstable social and economic situations such as worrying about mounting hospital bills, how a pet is faring at home, the condition of an unwell spouse visiting every day can increase the stress associated with illness, compounding the patient's already fragile response. As a result of these phenomena, older patients incur a much higher risk of malnutrition, functional decline, and iatrogenesis than their younger counterparts (Palmer, Counsell, & Landefeld, 1998). The potentially preventable problems acquired during the hospitalization greatly increase mortality and morbidity rates associated with ICU admissions. Older patients who survive an acute illness can concurrently suffer a remarkable deterioration of functional status. It is estimated that one third to one half of older adult patients experience complications that prolong their hospital stay and increase the need for institutionalization after discharge (Behroozi, Brennan, & Bellantonio, 2007). It is widely accepted that accurate diagnosis and treatment are not always sufficient for the geriatric patient unless close attention is paid to the hospital environment. Patients who function independently in one setting can become dependent in another setting, even in the absence of disease (Duthie, 2007). Factoring in the physiologic responses to stress and critical illness accentuates the need to appropriately modify the ICU environment to improve care to the older adult population.

In this chapter, we will first explore the general role of the environment in the functional status of older adults. We will then address the various aspects of the critical care environment and how those influences can negatively affect the older person's recovery and long-term functional status. Next we will explore evidence-based interventions critical care nurses can implement to create a more healing environment for older adults in critical care. Finally, we will envision how ICU environments of the future might be changed to maximize long-term functional status for older adults.

## Functional Status in Older Hospitalized Adults

The term *functional status* refers to the ability of a person to live and act independently, both physically and psychologically. Tools designed to address activities of daily living (ADLs) measure physical abilities such as bathing, dressing, and feeding. Skills assessed by instrumental activities of daily living (IADLs) scales address the ability to plan for and orchestrate an individual's independence (Lawton & Brody, 1969). The ability to manage finances, organize and plan for meal preparation, medication adherence, and so on is crucial in safe, independent functioning. Functional status can be a barometer of well-being for an older patient, reflecting the impact of an illness on a patient's life (Kresivic, 2008). An acute illness will often initially express itself as a change in functional status. For example, an older adult woman in the early stages of pneumonia might develop dizziness or a decline in coordination long before she has other symptoms. A patient with dehydration may present only with a change in mental status that impedes her ability to balance her checkbook. If these illnesses are severe enough to warrant hospitalization, the potential for further functional decline increases dramatically (Kresevic). Early interventions by the medical team, especially nurses, are pivotal both in restoring functional status and preventing further decline.

Negative consequences of hospitalization revolve around the physiologic, psychological, and social circumstances that are often associated with advanced age. Very common occurrences associated with hospital care and its environment can lead to a cascade of problems in the older adult patient. Reduced accessibility to fluids in addition to frequent orders of "nothing by mouth" (NPO) for medical tests can result in marked dehydration, which in turn, can lead to delirium. Immobilization and deconditioning can lead to psychological dependence and depression. Vasomotor instability related to normal cardiac changes, medication side effects, or dehydration can lead to dizziness and then to falls and fractures. Fragile skin combined with immobilization will often lead to skin tears or serious pressure ulcers. Approximately

25% of patients with Foley catheters develop bacteriuria after even short-term use (Leduc et al., 2007). Older adults admitted to ICUs face additional challenges and often experience a severe decline in functional status as a result.

# The Critical Care Environment: Impact on the Functional Status of Older Adults

In this chapter the "critical care environment" refers to the external conditions surrounding patients in an ICU. This environment may include physical factors such as noise and sleep disruption; interpersonal factors such as busy, preoccupied nurses, physicians, and other health care workers; social factors such as limited contact with family members; and medical treatment factors, including invasive procedures and cognition-altering medications. The ICU environment, with its endless activity and adrenaline-producing drama, is attractive to many nurses; viewing the environment from an older patient's perspective, however, produces a different and potentially troubling picture.

The nature of the ICU environment makes it a hostile place for older patients, with loud noises from equipment and monitors, bright lights, and 24-hour activity (Jastremski, 2000). Distractions from high acuity of the patients often prevent the ICU staff from recognizing the adversity of the environment from the patient's perspective (I. Dyer, 1995). The ICU lacks the familiarity of even the acute care hospital units, with fewer interactions with families and other patients. In addition, the ICU lacks familiar routines such as regular mealtimes and a clearly defined day and night (C. B. Dyer, Ashton, & Teasdale, 1995; I. Dyer, 1995). In the typical ICU, patients have restricted mobility related to invasive tubes and lines, disturbed sleep–wake cycles, continuous lighting and unfamiliar noises that cause sensory overload. At the same time, the isolation from all that is familiar, including their families, their routines, and even the ability to distinguish night from day can cause a sense of isolation and deprivation (Jastremski, 2000). These characteristics of the critical care environment can prove to be detrimental to any patient, but most especially to the older adult whose physiologic and psychologic ability to adapt to stress is markedly impaired.

## Sensory Overload

Excessive stimuli in the form of bright lights and noise can be detrimental to the older adult in the ICU. The continuous light exposure found in the ICU environment can affect a patient's rhythm and the natural day–night cycle (Drouot, Cabello, d'Ortho, & Brochard, 2008). In the typical ICU patient room, there are lights both above the patient's bed, which are tailored for convenience and visibility to caregivers, and lights behind the bed for visibility of the patients. Ceiling lights should be used only when essential for patient care and should be dimmed for patient comfort, especially at night, and whenever possible throughout the day. Sleep masks can be offered to provide a sense of darkness for the older adult.

For over 30 years noise level in critical care units has been the focus of investigation. In 1974 the Environmental Protection Agency (EPA) recommended that the noise level in hospitals be limited to fewer than 45 decibels (dB) during the day and under 35 dB at night (Environmental Protection Agency, 1974). More recently, the World Health

Organization's (WHO) guidelines for sound levels in hospitals lowered the recommended level to not greater than 35 dB at night and 40 dB during daytime hours (WHO, 1999). Despite the earlier EPA recommendations, Dracup (1988) reported the ICU noise level to be consistently greater than 70 dB over a 24-hour period, which is comparable to the hospital cafeteria at noon. Jastremski (2000) more recently found the average noise level in the ICU to still be 45 dB with spikes greater than 70 dB every 9 minutes. It has been reported that the sound of three people talking in normal tones at the foot of a patient's bed can be measured to be between 60 to 80 dB, well above the EPA and WHO recommendations. Indeed, the biggest complaint from patients related to the noise in intensive care units is from the loud voices of hospital employees, and not from alarms or other equipment (Jastremski, 2000).

The environment of the ICU not only contains intermittent spikes of noise from monitors, alarms, and other loud noises that are disquieting and even startling to patients, but it also contains an abundance of "white noise." The continuous background hum and reverberation such as that from suction devices and intravenous (IV) pumps can cause sensory overload for the older adult, which then block reception of meaningful stimuli such as voices of family or health care providers. Sensory overload and decreased ability to interpret meaningful stimuli in the form of altered sensory inputs may be a factor in the development of ICU delirium in the older adult (C. B. Dyer et al., 1995).

In the ICU sudden noises are often caused by alarms, resulting in frequent sharp spikes of noise that are particulary noxious to patients (Jastremski, 2000). Most patients do not recognize that many of the alarms are caused by mundane activities, such as scratching near an electrocardiogram (ECG) monitoring wire. Without frequent reassurance and explanation, the older adult will often become anxious, exhibiting displaced fear from knowing neither the source nor the significance of the intrusion (I. Dyer, 1995). It is crucial for the nurse to envision the perspective of the patient in this unfamiliar and hostile environment so that the inevitable fears can be allayed and misperceptions can be clarified.

## Sleep Disruption

The ICU atmosphere changes little over a 24-hour period; there are few variations in light, noise, or activity level to allow patients to distinguish day from night, much less encourage a normal sleep pattern. Many patients in the ICU experience sleep disorders related to anxiety, noise, light, and frequent nursing interventions, and disrupted sleep is one of the most frequent complaints from ICU patients (Drouot et al., 2008). Although some older adults are hearing impaired and may not react to increased noise levels, it should not be assumed that this is a uniform disability. Even with moderate hearing loss, the extreme variations in sound levels can be very disturbing to older adults patients, thereby preventing adequate sleep (Tullmann & Dracup, 2000).

The sleep disorders that occur in the ICU include lack of sleep and severe fragmentation of that sleep (Drouot et al., 2008). The older adult is especially at risk for sleep disorders while in the ICU as he or she is more prone to sleep disturbances at baseline. The critically ill older adult will often exhibit these sleep disturbances with even greater intensity, magnifying the need for careful monitoring and intervention.

## Decreased Mobility

Early mobility in older adults is recommended to prevent muscle breakdown and deconditioning, yet many patients in the ICU are placed on bed rest because of the severity of their illness (Krishnagopalan, Johnson, Low, & Kaufman, 2002). Mobility for the general ICU patient is then usually associated with passive movement on the part of the patient. The mobility of a critically ill person in the ICU is often limited to activities such as being pulled up in bed or turned for linen changes (Morris, 2007). Additional reasons for decreased mobilization of patients in the ICU can be staff fears of adverse effects such as accidental removal of an endotracheal tube or vascular access device, or concerns over the strain that mobility could have on the patient's oxygenation and hemodynamic status (Morris). For the truly immobile patient, it has been shown that despite the standard of care of turning every 2 hours, this does not happen for many patients in the ICU (Krishnagopalan et al.).

The critical care patient who is not completely immobilized because of medical condition or subsequent sedation still suffers very limited mobility as a result of the use of monitoring equipment and intravenous therapies. Immobility caused by restricted movement from tubes and lines is cited by patients as being a cause of stress while in the intensive care unit (Cornock, 1998). In addition, the older adult is already at an increased risk for pressure ulcers because of decreased muscle mass and a decrease in subcutaneous fat and the imposed immobility increases the risk for pressure ulcers, which affect almost 10% of ICU patients (Eachempati, Hydo, & Barie, 2001).

## Restricted Visitation

In many acute care hospital units visitation restrictions have been relaxed but heavy restriction on visitors and visitation hours continues to be the norm for most ICUs (Berwick & Kotagal, 2004; Kleinpell, 2008). A survey conducted by the American Association of Critical Care Nurses indicated that only 14% of ICUs had open visiting all hours of the day and 44% were open on a scheduled basis (Kirchhoff, Pugh, Calame, & Reynolds, 1993). More recently, researchers (M. D. Lee et al., 2007) found that of 171 hospital ICUs polled in their survey, only 32% did not limit the time of day or length of time for visitation. However, of those 32%, the majority (91%) set a minimum age of 12 for visitors and 78% restricted visitors to a maximum of two at a time.

ICU staff members generally cite three major concerns associated with liberalizing visiting hours: visitors interfering with care for the patient, exhaustion of family and friends, and undue physiological stress for the patient (Berwick & Kotagal, 2004). Although there may be some validity to visitors interfering with patient care, undue concern over interfering with care fosters an environment in the ICU that becomes convenient for the staff as opposed to the patients receiving care (Levy, 2007). Many ICU nurses who support liberal visitation in ICUs have found ways to alter the timing of care routines to accommodate family and friends at the bedside.

Current evidence does not validate the concerns that liberal visitation has a negative impact on family members. Rather, visitor presence provides an avenue of improved communication between patients and staff as well as increased opportunities for patient and family education (Berwick & Kotagal, 2004). In addition, increased visiting in the ICU can decrease anxiety of family and friends and improve visitor satisfaction (Simpson et al., 1996).

Finally, the belief that visitor restriction is set in place so as to reduce physical stress for the patient, implies that visitor presence evokes stress (Berwick & Kotagal, 2004). The presence of friends and families actually reassures and calms the patient, provides some familiarity in an unfamiliar environment, and helps the patient to make some sense of the overstimulation that can be found in the ICU environment (Berwick & Kotagal, 2004). The literature also suggests that there are no adverse physiological changes associated when family and friends are visiting (Berwick & Kotagal, 2004). Kleman et al. (1993) showed no cardiovascular changes to heart rate, blood pressure, ST-segment elevation or depression, oxygen saturations, and premature ventricular contractions (PVCs) before, during, or after family visits. Fumagalli et al. (2006) showed a statistically significant decrease in the rates of pulmonary edema and shock with an unrestricted visiting policy versus a restricted visitor policy. It was hypothesized that this was to the result of closer surveillance of the critical care patient by family and friends who were at the patient's bedside more frequently than the critical care staff. Based on the most compelling evidence available, the American College of Critical Care Medicine (ACCM) and the Society of Critical Care Medicine (SCCM) recommend open, flexible visitation for families of ICU patients (Davidson et al., 2007).

For nearly 150 years, nurses have laid claim to the fact that the nurse was accountable for making changes to the patient's environment. The older adult is especially vulnerable to the hostilities of the intensive care unit environment. Most nurses want to create a healing environment for patients but the ability to accomplish this often seems compromised (Kritek, 2001). By being more cognizant of the environment of the ICU as seen from the patient's perspective, the ICU nurse can make changes that can improve outcomes not only for the older adult, but for all patients in the ICU.

# Best Practice: Modifications of the Critical Care Environment

There is agreement among researchers and geriatric clinicians that implementation of evidence-based clinical guidelines and protocols to prevent, identify, and treat many common problems (geriatric syndromes) faced by older patients in an acute care setting improves outcomes (Counsell et al., 2000; Rosenthal & Kavic, 2004). In addition, providing a multidisciplinary approach to planning and executing care on an individualized basis greatly enhances the effectiveness of such protocols (Benedict, Robinson, & Holder, 2006). A detailed, multisystem assessment and ongoing surveillance by an advanced practice nurse or physician who specializes in geriatrics is crucial to identifying existing problems in older adult patients and preventing other problems.

## Environmental Responses to Physiologic Changes in the Older Adult

As the human body ages, changes occur within each body system. The extent of the changes varies from individual to individual, but the trend of the deterioration remains fairly consistent. Health care providers must be cognizant of normal physiologic changes caused by aging so that they may provide and implement adaptations to the hospital environment and the plan of care. A systems approach to these responses is presented in Table 3.1.

In addition to the suggestions posed related to the physiology of the aging adult in Table 3.1, careful attention must be also be paid to the social needs of older adults. Many times, the effect of the hospital environment, no matter what the modifications, can be detrimental to the physical and psychological well-being of a patient. The inclusion of families in patient care, as discussed previously, can be an invaluable asset to the treatment plan and can enhance positive psychosocial as well as physical outcomes (see chapter 2: Standards of Practice for Gerontological and Critical Care Nursing).

## Geriatric Resource and Consultation Services

### Comprehensive Geriatric Assessment

One of the hallmarks of geriatrics, a subspecialty of internal medicine, is its recognition that functional ability and quality of life are essential and fundamental components of medical care, not simply accessories to it. Most health care professionals would agree that functional ability and quality of life are worthy goals for older adults; yet few professionals, especially those in the ICU, consider functional ability and quality of life as important enough to incorporate into their daily practice. A comprehensive geriatric assessment is the critical first step to providing optimal care for older adults. ICU nurses may not be able to provide such a specialized assessment but need to be aware of its importance and initiate interdisciplinary collaboration so that each older adult receives such a comprehensive evaluation.

Along with diagnostic measures such as laboratory tests, radiographic scans, and other advanced physical assessment tools, the full geriatric examination should include some measure of the patient's preexisting mental, social, and functional status. In addition to alleviating a certain disease or condition, careful consideration must also be paid to preserving or improving the patient's physical and psychologic independence. Anticipation, recognition, and early treatment of "geriatric syndromes" (dementia, delirium, urinary incontinence, osteoporosis, falls/gait disorders, pressure ulcers, sleep disorders, and failure to thrive) in the ICU setting will further enhance a patient's outcome. Use of an interdisciplinary team of nurses, nurse practitioners (NPs), geriatricians, physical and occupational therapists, nutritionists, and social workers has been demonstrated to provide the optimal care environment for an older patient (Caprio & Williams as cited in Duthie, 2007).

### Acute Care of the Elderly Unit Model

An acute care of the elderly (ACE) unit is a geographically consistent hospital unit that has a specially designed physical environment as well as a multidisciplinary team of experts in geriatric care (Kresevic et al., 1998; Palmer et al., 1998). Included in the team are advanced practice nurses specializing in geriatric care, geriatricians, social workers, physical and occupational therapists, pharmacists, nurses, and nursing assistants. These experts come armed with clinical guidelines and protocols aimed at preventing, identifying, and treating negative consequences that often plague hospitalized elders. The ACE unit provides a model of care that emphasizes patient independence and rehabilitation while treating an acute illness. It is designed to help an

# 3.1 Functional Changes of Aging by Body System and Recommended Environmental Changes

| Organ System | Functional Expression of Aging | Potential Patient Response | Implication for Environmental Modification |
|---|---|---|---|
| **Neurologic** | ■ Slower processing speed<br>■ Decreased short-term memory | ■ Difficulty adapting to new environment and to understanding illness | ■ Speak slowly and clearly<br>■ Reinforce information given and provide alternate media when possible (written material, audio/visual, etc.) |
| | ■ Decreased sense of smell and taste | ■ Decreased appetite | ■ Engage nutritionist to evaluate needs and preferences<br>■ Encourage/assist with meals when appropriate |
| | ■ Diminished reflexes | ■ Increased fall risk | ■ Institute fall precautions<br>■ PT/OT Evaluation |
| | ■ Changes in sleep/wake cycle | ■ Increase in sleep disturbances in hospital | ■ Allow for long periods of uninterrupted sleep; organize care<br>■ Keep noise levels at a minimum; offer ear plugs<br>■ Provide white noise/soft music as distraction<br>■ Offer back rubs when possible<br>■ Be mindful of medication effects and interactions<br>■ Assess for s/s of delirium r/t sleep deprivation |
| **Cardiovascular** | Structural changes in heart<br>■ Decrease in muscle mass<br>■ Calcification, sclerosis, and fibrosis of valves<br>■ Fibrous deposits around SA node | ■ Increased sensitivity to fluid volume changes; dehydration AND fluid overload from HF<br>■ Orthostatic hypotension<br>■ Increased incidence of dysrhythmias | ■ Careful monitoring of I&0<br>■ Caution patients to move slowly from sitting to standing<br>■ Assess for changes in heart rhythm and address promptly<br>■ Address persistent tachycardia promptly to avoid rate-related HF<br>■ Assess for s/s delirium r/t cardiovascular changes |
| **Respiratory** | ■ Increased costal calcification<br>■ Decline in tissue elasticity<br>■ Anatomic emphysema r/t increased end expiratory pressure from insufficient exhalation | ■ Decreased vital capacity<br>■ Decreased $FEV_1$<br>■ Lower $PaO_2$<br>■ Increased risk of pulmonary complications | ■ Scrupulous attention to pulmonary hygiene<br>■ Frequent ambulation<br>■ Upright position in chair as much as possible<br>■ Maintain head of bed to at least 40 degrees as tolerated |

*(continued)*

**Table 3.1** *(continued)*

| Organ System | Functional Expression of Aging | Potential Patient Response | Implication for Environmental Modification |
|---|---|---|---|
| **Gastrointestinal** | ■ Decreased peristalsis | ■ Delayed gastric emptying<br>■ Increased constipation/ bowel obstruction | ■ Allow more time for eating<br>■ Monitor bowel function and institute appropriate therapy<br>■ Assess nutritional status |
| | ■ Decreased esophageal motility | ■ Can lead to swallowing difficulties, increased choking | ■ Assess nutritional status; problems<br>■ Use speech therapy when appropriate<br>■ Adjust food consistency if necessary |
| | ■ Decreased production of saliva | ■ Problems r/t chewing, swallowing, dentition and digestion | ■ Encourage fluid intake during meals<br>■ Adjust food consistency when necessary<br>■ Inspect oral mucosa for lesions/ dentition |
| | ■ Decreased liver function | ■ Alteration in metabolism of medication | ■ Adjust medication doses when necessary<br>■ Be aware of s/s overdose and act promptly |
| **Renal/GU** | ■ Decrease in functional nephrons<br>■ Decreased blood supply to kidneys | ■ Decrease in GFR<br>■ May lead to alteration in medication excretion | ■ Use "renal dosing" for medications when applicable<br>■ Closely monitor fluid balance and electrolyte levels |
| | ■ Decreased bladder capacity in women | ■ May lead to urgency/frequency and incontinence | ■ Suggest toileting routines<br>■ Avoid anticholinergic medications<br>■ Monitor for UTI<br>■ Avoid Foley catheter whenever possible<br>■ Promote adequate hydration<br>■ Assess for environmental barriers to self-toileting |
| | ■ Increased incidence of prostate problems in men | ■ Increased hesitancy and frequency<br>■ Increased urinary retention | ■ Monitor for urinary retention<br>■ Avoid anticholinergic medications<br>■ Monitor for UTI<br>■ Promote adequate hydration<br>■ Assess for environmental barriers to self-toileting |

*(continued)*

**Table 3.1** *(continued)*

| Organ System | Functional Expression of Aging | Potential Patient Response | Implication for Environmental Modification |
|---|---|---|---|
| **Musculoskeletal** | ■ Decreased muscle mass and strength<br>■ Deterioration of cartilage with narrowing of joint spaces<br>■ Decreased bone mass (osteoporosis) | ■ Increased incidence of falls<br>■ Decreased activity<br>■ Decrease in functional status<br>■ Rapid deterioration with any acute illness | ■ Perform functional assessment at admission and at intervals during hospitalization<br>■ Institute fall precautions<br>■ PT/OT evaluation<br>■ Encourage ambulation/activity at least three times a day<br>■ Encourage independence with ADLs<br>■ Monitor for s/s delirium |
| **Eye** | ■ Decrease in mucus production in conjunctiva<br>■ Decrease in tear secretion | ■ Potential for "dry eye syndrome"<br>■ Increase in eye infections | ■ Apply lubricating drops when necessary<br>■ Assess for eye infection |
| | ■ Flattening of cornea<br>■ Yellowing of lens<br>■ Cataract formation | ■ Decrease in visual acuity<br>■ Alteration in color perception<br>■ Decrease in functional independence | ■ Ensure pt. has accessibility to glasses<br>■ Environment should include bright colors with marked contrasts between floor and walls<br>■ Institute fall precautions for patients with significant visual difficulties<br>■ Encourage independence<br>■ OT evaluation for accommodations when necessary |
| **Ear** | ■ Degeneration of auditory nerve<br>■ Sclerosis of ossicles<br>■ Thickening of cerumen r/t dryness in external canal | ■ Decrease in hearing<br>■ Increase in delirium<br>■ Increase in social withdrawal<br>■ Potential for cerumen impaction associated with decrease in hearing and external otitis | ■ Use low-pitched tones<br>■ Ensure pt. has hearing aids with him when available<br>■ Use volume enhancer "pocket talker" when appropriate<br>■ Assess for accumulation of cerumen and initiate removal when appropriate |
| **Integumentary** | ■ Decrease in subcutaneous fat<br>■ Loss of seborrheic glands<br>■ Decrease in vascularity | ■ Alteration in temperature regulation<br>■ Increased dryness and inability to sweat<br>■ Prolonged healing<br>■ Increased susceptibility to trauma (e.g., pressure ulcers) | ■ Institute scrupulous skin care principles<br>■ Institute decubitus prevention principles<br>■ Assess entire skin surface (including skin folds and wrinkles) frequently to monitor for breakdown<br>■ Increase fluid intake to avoid dehydration |

PT/OT = Physical therapy & occupational therapy; s/s = signs & symptoms; r/t = related to; HF = heart failure; I&O = fluid intake & output; FEV$_1$ = forced expiratory volume; PaO$_2$ = partial pressure of arterial oxygen; GFR = glomerular filtration rate; UTI = urinary tract infection; ADLs = activities of daily living.

*Note:* Adapted from Rosenthal (2004) and Tullmann and Dracup (2000).

older adult patient maintain or even improve his/her baseline level of independent functioning. Discharge planning begins the day of admission, and patients in ACE units are less likely to require institutionalization at discharge. In addition, these patients may be less likely to experience geriatric syndromes such as delirium, falls, and adverse drug events.

## Geriatric Resource Nurse

Successful care for critically ill older adults cannot easily be provided outside of an ICU, thus eliminating the value of an ACE unit for these patients. However, alternative models, incorporating ACE unit principles have been developed, and show promise for utility in the critical care setting. The geriatric resource nurse (GRN) is a unit-based registered nurse who, under the leadership and guidance of an NP (nurse practitioner) who specializes in geriatrics, serves as a resource on care of the elderly for the health care team on a given acute or critical care unit (Turner, Lee, Fletcher, Hudson, & Barton, 2001). The GRN develops a set of geriatric competencies that enables the nurse to provide excellent care for older adults and role model such care for other nurses on the unit. With NP availability and ongoing continuing education for GRNs and ancillary personnel, ACE unit principles could be implemented in critical care units as well.

## Geriatric Consult Service

Another successful program that could be adopted by critical care units is a geriatric consult service (GCS), which merges the expertise of a geriatrician and nurse practitioner (geriatric NP or family NP with a focus on geriatrics) (Fletcher, Hawkes, Williams-Rosenthal, Mariscal, & Cox, 2007). Comprehensive geriatric assessments provided by such experts have resulted in beneficial outcomes for older adults seen in an emergency department and then sent home (Caplan, Williams, Daly, & Abraham, 2004) as well as those emergently admitted to acute care (Naughton, Moran, Feinglass, Falconer, & Williams, 1994). Such a consultation service made available for older adults in ICU could have a beneficial effect on their outcomes as well. Critical care nurses who are cognizant of the improvement in outcomes for patients who have access to geriatric consultants could be proactive in requesting such assistance in the provision of care.

## Changes in Sedation Practices

One recent practice development already changing the ICU environment is increased interest in, and evidence of, the detrimental effects of long-term sedation, especially for mechanically ventilated patients. ICU nurses have often thought that heavy sedation for mechanically ventilated patients would have a merciful, amnesic effect and was part of compassionate nursing care. Mounting evidence, however, indicates that heavy sedation, particularly with benzodiazepines, is associated with serious sequelae such as delirium, prolonged time on mechanical ventilation, and longer lengths of ICU stay (Pandharipande & Ely, 2006; Pandharipande et al., 2006). The resultant practice recommendations of sedation protocol use (Payen et al., 2007), daily interruption of continuous sedation (Schweickert, Gehlbach, Pohlman, Hall, & Kress, 2004), increased use of bolus dosing rather than continuous drips (Feeley & Gardner, 2006), and earlier extubation postcardiac surgery (J. H. Lee, Swain, Andrey, Murrell, & Geha, 1999) are causing nurses to take a new look at the ICU environment because they can no longer chemically shield their patients from that environment. If older patients are going to be more cognizant of the ICU environment, nurses must focus renewed energy to maximize the quality of that environment for the long-term benefit of older adults' functional status (see chapter 13: Pharmacotherapy and chapter 25: Acute Respiratory Failure and Mechanical Ventilation in the Elderly).

## Increased Focus on ICU Delirium

Another changing practice in ICU environments that may benefit older adults is an increased awareness of, and screening for, delirium. In 2002 the Society of Critical Care Medicine (SCCM; Jacobi et al., 2002) recommended that all patients in critical care units be regularly screened for delirium using the Confusion Assessment Method for the ICU (CAM-ICU; Ely et al., 2001). The vast increase in the number of studies on ICU delirium has brought the spotlight to bear on the prevalence of delirium and the serious sequelae of it, particularly for older adults. Sadly, there are no uniquely ICU-based nonpharmacologic intervention studies to prevent or decrease delirium in critically ill older adults, but an increasing number of health care providers are recognizing the importance of proactively addressing the problem of delirium. Until such investigations are completed, nurses should follow the delirium-reduction guidelines (Inouye et al., 1999) validated for acute care as they generally focus on basic principles of excellent nursing care (see chapter 26 "Delirium in Critical Illness").

## Enhancing Sleep

To help overcome the significant problem of sleep disturbance in the ICU, sleep promotion needs to be a primary focus for night nurses. One way in which this can be supported is by organizing and grouping patient treatments and interventions. Sleep cycles occur in 90-minute intervals and therefore during the hours of 2200 and 0600, gaps of 90 minutes or more should occur between nursing care (I. Dyer, 1995). This may mean decreasing frequency of vital-sign checks to every hour and a half or 2 hours in more stable patients and limiting checks on medical equipment during this 8-hour period, if at all possible.

Of course, many interventions are medically necessary and the disturbances they bring can be unavoidable, but attempts to provide a healing environment must still be a primary focus. When a patient becomes conscious in the ICU, or if he or she is admitted when conscious, a "welcoming kit" containing earplugs and eye masks to enhance sleep should be provided (Jastremski, 2000). One group of researchers (Wallace, Robins, Alvord, & Walker, 1999) found that when earplugs were provided to healthy volunteers and the volunteers were exposed to ICU noises, time spent in rapid eye movement (REM) sleep increased. The average adult needs 6 to 8 hours of sleep per night and adult ICU patients receive as little as 8 minutes of continuous sleep during an 8-hour period (Lower, Bonsack, & Guion, 2002). The use of ear plugs and eye masks can help reduce the environmental stimuli of the unit and may help promote sleep for some older adults.

Music therapy is another method used to promote sleep and create a more healing environment. All conscious patients in the intensive care unit should be offered access to a personal Motion Picture Experts Group Audio 3 (MP3) player. The MP3 players should come equipped with calming music and nature sounds; the nurse should have the ability to download the patient's musical genre of preference. Relaxing music promotes physiologic relaxation, reduces anxiety, and reverses the effects of stress responses (Jastremski, 2000; Lower et al., 2002). With the increased use of computers and technology at the bedside, providing patients with personal music players should be an easy transition into the unit, and will be easily incorporated into the patient's care plan.

# Vision for the Future: Elder-Friendly Critical Care Environments

Decades of research and clinical practice have resulted in broad knowledge regarding environmental challenges for older adults in acute and long-term care. Poor outcomes of hospitalization such as delirium, nosocomial infections, pressure ulcers, decreased functional status, and long-term cognitive decline are well known and have persisted in spite of health care providers' increased knowledge. There have been some striking examples of exemplary care of older adults in many areas throughout the United States. ACE units, described earlier, are beginning to make significant differences for some older adults in acute care (Counsell et al., 2000; Wong & Miller, 2008) and initiatives such as the Nurses Improving the Care for Healthsystem Elders (NICHE) (Fulmer et al., 2002) are stimulating more interest and action by nurses to promote better outcomes for vulnerable older adults who are under their care. However, research focused on critical care units and their impact on older adults lags far behind research in acute and long-term care. For decades critical care nurses have known intuitively that the noise, light, sleep deprivation, sensory overload, busyness, rigid visitation policies, and other common elements of ICU life are not conducive to healing for older adults, yet evidence of best practices to improve the ICU environment for this population is scarce.

A common attitude even among many ICU nurses sensitive to the need for environmental change is that nothing can be done. Critical care units necessarily focus on complex, technologically advanced life-saving activities for the immediate health crisis, often to the exclusion of more basic concerns for the long-term functional status of older adults. The systems driving hospitals in general, and critical care units in particular, are large and complex. The financial and political powers behind many decisions in critical care are often mysterious to ICU nurses, resulting in a sense of powerlessness, even in the most dedicated, compassionate nurses. They have a vision for a healing environment for older adults but lack the tools by which meaningful, lasting environmental change can be implemented.

## Healthy Work Environment Guidelines

In recent years the American Association of Critical Care Nurses (AACN) has developed guidelines for a healthy work environment to foster "care environments that are safe, healing, humane and respectful of the rights, responsibilities, needs and contributions of all people including patients, their families and nurses" (American Association of Critical Care Nurses, 2005, p. 12). Although not focused specifically on older adults, we believe that working toward the achievement of the six essential healthy work environment standards will also provide the best environment for older adults in critical care. These standards were developed primarily for the ICU work environment but also provide a framework into which our current knowledge of best practices in the care of older adults in acute care settings can be incorporated and expanded. A healthy work environment has the best potential for becoming a healing environment for older adults.

## Standard 1: Skilled Communication

**Nurses must be as proficient in communication skills as they are in clinical skills.**

In dealing with older adults, particularly those in critical care whose lives are at risk and who find themselves in environments totally foreign and frightening to them, communication is key. Ensuring that sensory aids such as glasses and hearing aids are available and functional is an intervention often overlooked by busy nurses in hectic ICU settings. Speaking slowly and clearly to accommodate older adults' slower neurologic processing speed and their decreased short-term memory will serve to easy their anxiety. Frequent reorientation has also been identified with successful delirium-prevention protocols in acute care settings and likely has the same advantage in critical care. Older adults have worries about their care and progress yet are often either not addressed directly, especially when a family member is present, or are on the receiving end of a monologue given by a health care professional, with little if any time devoted to ensuring that the message was heard, understood, and answered the older patient's questions and concerns. The communication gap is especially prevalent with mechanically ventilated patients who are unable to respond verbally. In the critical care unit committed to older patients, excellent communication will be the norm, not the exception.

## Standard 2: True Collaboration

**Nurses must be relentless in pursuing and fostering true collaboration.**

True collaboration in Standard 2 refers primarily to health care providers and other team members within health care organizations. However, in the health care environment of critical care another collaborative relationship is also essential; collaboration with the patient and family members. Often viewed as outsiders who need permission to enter the "inner sanctum" of critical care units, families have often been lost, confused, and frightened at what is happening to their loved one. Older adults, meanwhile, who have diminished coping abilities, are left alone in a frighteningly strange, high-tech environment. Involving patients and families in the plan of care is a basic and essential tenet of nursing education programs throughout the country. Yet in critical care, patients and family members are often passive receivers and observers of others' planning. Providing care and collaborating with patients and their families in decision making is often relegated to end-of-life issues. In ICUs where nurses collaborate with patients and families, allowing them to participate in both the loved one's care and decision making about that care makes the ICU experience far less alienating. Patients and family members are not just recipients of health care but should be active participants in that care. By collaborating with patients and families, educating them, and involving them in care as essential members of the health care team, the critical care environment can be transformed into a more healing place for older adults. By insisting on partnership with patients/families in every aspect of health care decision making, nurses expand effective decision making and promote better outcomes for older adults in the ICU of the future.

## Standard 3: Effective Decision Making

**Nurses must be valued and committed partners in making policy, directing and evaluating clinical care, and leading organizational operations.**

Involving nurses in the decision-making processes of health care results in better outcomes for patients (Baggs et al., 1999). With the ongoing nursing shortage, nurses have more power and influence than ever before. Now is the time for critical care nurses to expand that influence by determining what changes need to be made in the ICU environment and providing convincing evidence to hospital administrators that will compel them to support the necessary changes. If ICU nurses truly believe that having consistent geriatric consultation for their older patients would assist their patients' recovery, for example, the nurses could bring about that change. Many ICUs now have regular "quiet times" to allow patients to receive much-needed sleep in the environments where sleep is so often disrupted. This change and many other beneficial environmental changes can occur if nurses will take their knowledge, clinical expertise, and passion as far as it needs to go to change institutional, local, and national policies.

## Standard 4: Appropriate Staffing

**Staffing must ensure the effective match between patient needs and nurse competencies.**

Patient needs in critical care are typically described in terms of physiologic functioning with the most unstable patients being assigned to the most clinically competent nurses. However, rarely does nurse competence in the ICU refer to geriatric nursing. Nurses certified in geriatric nursing comprise less than 1% of the 2.2 million professional nurses nationwide (Hartford Institute for Geriatric Nursing [HIGN], 2008). The number of critical care nurses certified in geriatrics is not known (L. McNamara, personal communication, May 2008) but is presumed to be far less. Older adults comprise 60% of all ICU days (Marik, 2006) and with the aging crisis in health care rapidly approaching, encouraging geriatric nurse certification among ICU nurses is essential. AACN was 1 of 60 professional organizations that partnered in the Nurse Competence in Aging Initiative, created in 2002 to work with specialty nursing organizations to encourage nurses to gain expertise in their own specialty (e.g., critical care) as well as geriatric nursing (Stierle et al., 2006). Increasing the number of certified critical care nurses (CCRNs) who are dually certified with the Gerontological Nurse Certification (GN-C) will greatly enhance the future critical care environment for older adults as well as clearly communicate critical care nurses' competence in caring for them.

## Standard 5: Meaningful Recognition

**Nurses must be recognized and must recognize others for the value each brings to the work of the organization.**

Meaningful recognition of nurses is essential for a healthy work environment and for creating a healing environment for older adults in ICU. The ICU environment is a confusing, frightening place for the uninitiated; for older adults with compromised coping mechanisms, the environment can be even more troubling. Health care providers and technicians come in and out of patient rooms with rapid-fire regularity. With nothing familiar in the environment, older adults have no anchor to help them interpret what is happening to them. A simple gesture such as determining the older adult's preferred way of being addressed is one way to provide meaningful recognition. Also, making certain that the older adult is continually informed of the identity of the health care worker at the bedside is another way of providing meaningful recognition. When many unknown individuals enter the space of the older adult, a sense of unreality can ensue. Without properly identifying themselves to the older adult, health care workers may inadvertently communicate that the older adult is not important enough for it to matter who is providing the care. Continually acknowledging and affirming every effort the older adult makes toward his/her recovery is another means of providing meaningful recognition. In addition, many older adults carry with them an amazing history of achievements and/or service to their family, community, and even the world. By questioning the patient (when possible) and/or family members and friends of older patients, critical care nurses can uncover a wealth of information about older adults and can affirm the magnificent lifelong contributions they have made. Such recognition can be an important aspect of holistic care and a positive addition to the ICU environment for older adults.

### Standard 6: Authentic Leadership

**Nurse leaders must fully embrace the imperative of a healthy work environment, authentically live it and engage others in its achievement.**

For a critical care unit to become more of a healing environment for older adults, professional nurse leaders must be committed to and passionate about such an endeavor. By role-modeling all of the other standards of a healthy work environment and encouraging others to do the same, a nurse leads by example and becomes the catalyst for sustainable change in the ICU environment. Although contemplating a massive change of any social structure seems daunting at best, history is rife with examples of "the power of one"; how a single individual committed to necessary change brought about that change. Nurses certainly know the power Florence Nightingale exerted to benefit soldiers during the Crimean War and subsequently the entire nursing profession. Nightingale was no different than any other critical care nurse committed to the welfare of older adults under his or her care. Creating a healthy and healing environment for older adults in critical care will only happen as nurses decide it needs to happen and transform that environment unit by unit.

## Summary

The critical care environment as it currently exists does not provide the optimal physical, interpersonal, and social milieu for the best possible functioning of older adults who receive care in that environment. Some positive changes have occurred in recent years but more are needed. In this chapter we have reviewed the importance of the physical and psychosocial environment in maximizing optimal functional status for older adults in critical care. We have also examined the critical care environment and its potentially negative impact on older adults and their ability to adapt to its challenges. Although the evidence supporting specific strategies for improving the critical care environment is limited, we have recommended successful strategies supported in acute care environments. AACN's initiative on Creating a Healthy Work Environment is well known to practicing critical care nurses and also provides a helpful framework in thinking about creating a more healing environment for older adults in critical care. Increased numbers of dually certified CCRNs and GN-Cs will also help provide the expertise needed to care for the rapidly aging population of ICU patients and more quickly facilitate a more positive environment for them.

## The Patient's Perspective: Case Study and Discussion

My name is Maggie Stark. I am 85 years old and 2 months ago I spent 5 days in an intensive care unit; something with my heart was not working right. I don't really remember being admitted to the ICU but I have vague impressions of people yelling at me, being poked and prodded, not being able to breathe, lots of pain, and being cold; so very cold. I remember wishing that someone would just wrap my feet in a warm blanket; I can't sleep if my feet are cold. I also recall trying to get off my back because it was so sore but I couldn't move. When I tried to turn over something or someone held my arms down. After that, I don't remember anything until I started waking up.

My name is Lourdes Gonzales. I am an RN in the ICU, certified both in critical care (CCRN) and gerontological nursing (RN-BC). Mrs. Stark was admitted with heart failure (see chapter 23) exacerbation with respiratory failure, requiring diuresis, cardiovascular and ventilatory support (see chapter 25). It appears that prior to intubation, Mrs. Stark was extremely agitated and was given lorazepam 2 mg IV after which she was unarousable for several hours. I did not care for Mrs. Stark but in reading her story can see ways in which the ICU environment could have been more hospitable for her (see Table 3.1).

*Communication.* Speaking slowly and clearly to Mrs. Stark during her confusion would have been much more effective than raising the volume and pitch of voices. High-stress situations such as emergent intubations make this difficult but very beneficial for older adults who are already frightened and unclear as to what is happening to them.

*Ambient temperature.* ICUs are often quite cool and older adults have an altered ability to regulate temperature. Keeping Mrs. Stark covered, providing a warm blanket and bed socks would have aided in her comfort and ability to relax. Palpating foot temperature can be a clue as to whether an older adult needs increased peripheral warming, even if her or his core temperature is normal.

*Physical restraints.* Wrist restraints were applied prior to sedation, presumably because Mrs. Stark was resisting the procedure. Although restraints are sometimes necessary, they should be used only as a last resort and there should be documented evidence as to what other interventions were attempted (see chapter 15). Sometimes one person speaking quietly into the patient's ear and gently holding her hand can provide enough of a calming influence to avoid the need for restraints even in the midst of a flurry of activity.

*Sedation.* The benzodiazepine (lorazepam) given to Mrs. Stark was a poor choice as it has been associated with increased risk for delirium. Although sedation for intubation is appropriate, the nurse could have suggested a shorter half-life option such as fentanyl (see chapter 13).

*Mobility.* Turning patients every 2 hours is a well-known routine in ICUs that is sometimes neglected. Mrs. Stark was not hemodynamically unstable after her intubation, yet there is no documentation of her being turned for 6 hours. This is a serious oversight as increased mobility is necessary for optimal functioning of essentially every body system and, as important, for the prevention of pressure ulcers in the elderly (see chapter 19).

*Mrs. Stark:*      Waking up was so frightening. I was in a fog for a very long time and didn't know where I was or why I was there. I vaguely remember hearing my daughter's voice but had a hard time connecting with her. She seemed far away and I couldn't reach her. There were always loud noises and people kept shouting my name and telling me to squeeze their hands. I was afraid I was going to die.

*Lourdes:*      ICU nurses sometimes forget or underestimate how frightening the ICU environment can be for older adults. Frequent, quiet reorientation and reassurance can have a calming effect on older adults, even when they are "in a fog."

*ICU delirium.* The actual mechanisms causing delirium are unknown but there are multiple risk factors and Mrs. Stark had many of them. There was no indication of any assessment for delirium other than documenting that she "follows commands." The hypoxemia prior to admission, lorazepam administered, fluid and electrolyte fluctuations with her diuresis are all known contributors to delirium. Mrs. Stark didn't mention delusions or hallucinations, but they could have been a part of her experience as well. Consistent, regular use of a delirium instrument such as the Confusion Assessment Method for ICU (Ely et al., 2001) should be included with the usual assessment criteria for older adults in an ICU environment (see chapter 26).

*Family visitation.* Many ICU nurses still prefer to limit family visitation, in spite of the evidence supporting the benefit of visitation. Mrs. Stark's perception of "having a hard time connecting with" her daughter may have been caused by the nurses in the unit adhering to strict time limits on visitation. Although there may be exceptions, generally speaking, patients (especially older adults) are less anxious and confused when a familiar face and/or voice are readily available to them (see chapter 7).

*Mrs. Stark:*      Once the tube was out of my throat things were much better. The first time a nurse gave me a little ice chip I thought I had died and gone to heaven! After that, things got better every day. I wasn't so confused since I could actually see people's faces and communicate with them. But there were still things I didn't like. Sometimes doctors and nurses would come and talk to me but they would talk so fast that I could hardly follow what they were saying. They asked me if I had any questions but never really gave me enough time to even think about questions. I never got any decent sleep. There was always noise and sometimes I would just be dozing off and an alarm would sound. I jumped every time and never got used to it. And there was the blood pressure thing that squeezed my arm so tight and so often; I sometimes wanted to take it off just so I could sleep.

*Lourdes:*   As described earlier, clear communication is critically important whether an older adult is responding or not. Patients of the older generations are often very polite and respectful of physicians and nurses, believing that the experts should have precedence over patients; they often hesitate to ask questions or to have information repeated. When explaining anything to older adults, speaking more slowly and checking frequently with the older adult to ascertain whether or not the information is being understood is critical to a healing environment for older adults.

*Sensory overload and sleep deprivation.* ICUs are noisy places and can contribute to sleep deprivation (also a contributor to delirium) and ineffective coping. Attending to such a basic human need (sleep) should also be part of a healing environment for older adults in ICU. Alarms are a necessary part of caring for critically ill patients but the volume of those alarms can be lowered. Monitoring hemodynamic status with a noninvasive blood pressure cuff is convenient, but once the patient has stabilized, the frequency of cycling can be decreased as much as possible. Staff colleagues may need to be reminded to lower their voices at all times, especially at night, and dimming the lights as much as possible will also help to enhance sleep.

*Mrs. Stark:*   I was so happy when they let me start eating. But although I was hungry eating was a chore. Someone I had never seen before put the tray down without saying a word. There were cartons and packages to open and I was just too shaky to open them and too embarrassed to ask for help. After a successful career in advertising, raising four children, and caring for my husband before he died, one of the worst parts of being in the ICU was feeling like such a helpless invalid.

*Lourdes:*   Mrs. Stark had to deal with both physical and cognitive dysfunction, preventing her from performing her usual independent activities. Her description of being "too shaky" to open packages on her tray is just one example of how her illness caused a decreased functional status. Coming so soon after her cognitive impairment (possible delirium), recognizing her additional physical impairment might have added insult to injury. Interacting primarily with critically ill older adults, ICU nurses sometimes forget that many of these patients just a few days prior to their ICU admission were healthy, vibrant, active individuals. When the "healthy aging" perspective is lost, the nurse can begin to believe that a weak, helpless person is the norm rather than the exception. Proactively preventing circumstances that might worsen older persons' existing feelings of powerlessness is an important part of creating a healing psychosocial environment for them. In Mrs. Stark's case, the nurse or assistant could have recognized her weakened condition, asked if he/she could open the packages for Mrs. Stark, and affirm that she was getting stronger and would soon be able to resume her independent life.

Mrs. Stark:    I do remember one special person. Rick was some sort of an attendant. Whenever he took care of me, everything was great. He never yelled at me or expressed impatience, and spoke slowly so I could understand him. He was gentle and kind, always asking me about my comfort level with whatever he was doing. He encouraged me to do for myself whenever I could and he pushed me a little, but he never made me feel bad for asking for help. Rick was also a perfect gentleman. Sometimes he had to do things that were a little embarrassing but he never made a big deal about it and always reassured me that what he had to do was no problem and didn't bother him a bit.

Lourdes:    Rick provided an excellent example of nursing care of older adults, even though he was not a professional nurse. The empathy and caring he showed exemplifies that of many excellent critical care nurses and, if asked, Mrs. Stark would most certainly agree that having Rick care for her provided a very healing environment at that point in time.

Mrs. Stark:    I am more thankful for being able to be at home than ever before. I know I am alive because of all the wonderful new drugs and technology in ICU. But I'm not sure I would have wanted to live through it all if it hadn't been for Rick. I wish everyone in ICU cared for me the way he did. Who knows? I might have been able to come home even sooner!

Lourdes:    An interdisciplinary geriatrics team would have been an excellent adjunct to Mrs. Stark's care. The team would have assessed Mrs. Stark's preillness functional status, most likely contacting her children to obtain this information. The team would have instituted a plan of care that would address discharge needs as soon as Mrs. Stark was admitted. The staff of the ICU would have been notified of any special needs Mrs. Stark had and helped to institute a plan of care to prevent geriatric syndromes and to maximize the likelihood of a rapid recovery. A geriatric pharmacist would evaluate the medication interactions and recommended those that are least likely to have adverse effects (such as cognitive dysfunction). The team would encourage early mobility, frequent family visitation (perhaps staying overnight), and that familiar items be brought from home. Suggestions for maximizing sleep would also have been provided.

Mrs. Stark survived and no doubt received very good care. However, it could have been even better with the assistance of an interdisciplinary geriatric team and nurses who were knowledgeable about and committed to creating a healing critical care environment for older adults.

# References

American Association of Critical-Care Nurses. (2005). *AACN standards for establishing and sustaining health work environments: A journey to excellence.* Aliso Viejo, CA: Author. Retrieved September 11, 2008, from http://www.aacn.org/WD/HWE/Docs/HWEStandards.pdf

Baggs, J. G., Schmitt, M. H., Mushlin, A. I., Mitchell, P. H., Eldredge, D. H., Oakes, D., et al. (1999). Association between nurse-physician collaboration and patient outcomes in three intensive care units. *Critical Care Medicine, 27*(9), 1991–1998.

Behroozi, S., Brennan, M., & Bellantonio, S. (2007). Hospital care of the older adult: Part 2. recognizing common problems in hospitalized older adults. *Family Practice Recertification, 29*(8), 39.

Benedict, L., Robinson, K., & Holder, C. (2006). Clinical nurse specialist practice within the acute care for elders interdisciplinary team model. *Clinical Nurse Specialist, 20*(5), 248–251.

Berwick, D. M., & Kotagal, M. (2004). Restricted visiting hours in ICUs: Time to change. *Journal of the American Medical Association, 292*(6), 736–737.

Caplan, G. A., Williams, A. J., Daly, B., & Abraham, K. (2004). A randomized, controlled trial of comprehensive geriatric assessment and multidisciplinary intervention after discharge of elderly from the emergency department—The DEED II study. *Journal of the American Geriatrics Society, 52*(9), 1417–1423.

Cornock, M. A. (1998). Stress and the intensive care patient: Perceptions of patients and nurses. *Journal of Advanced Nursing, 27*(3), 518–527.

Counsell, S. R., Holder, C. M., Liebenauer, L. L., Palmer, R. M., Fortinsky, R. H., Kresevic, D. M., et al. (2000). Effects of a multicomponent intervention on functional outcomes and process of care in hospitalized older patients: A randomized controlled trial of acute care for elders (ACE) in a community hospital. *Journal of the American Geriatrics Society, 48*(12), 1572–1581.

Davidson, J. E., Powers, K., Hedayat, K. M., Tieszen, M., Kon, A. A., Shepard, E., et al. (2007). Clinical practice guidelines for support of the family in the patient-centered intensive care unit: American college of critical care medicine task force 2004-2005. *Critical Care Medicine, 35*(2), 605–622.

Dracup, K. (1988). Are critical care units hazardous to health? *Applied Nursing Research, 1*(1), 14–21.

Drouot, X., Cabello, B., d'Ortho, M. P., & Brochard, L. (2008, May 22). Sleep in the intensive care unit. *Sleep Medicine Reviews, 12*(5), 391–403.

Duthie, E. (2007). Comprehensive geriatric assessment. In E. Duthie, P. R. Katz, & M. L. Malone (Eds.), *Duthie: Practice of geriatrics* (4th ed.) Philadelphia: Saunders.

Dyer, C. B., Ashton, C. M., & Teasdale, T. A. (1995). Postoperative delirium. A review of 80 primary data-collection studies. *Archives of Internal Medicine, 155*(5), 461–465.

Dyer, I. (1995). Preventing the ITU syndrome or how not to torture an ITU patient! Part 1. *Intensive & Critical Care Nursing, 11*(3), 130–139.

Eachempati, S. R., Hydo, L. J., & Barie, P. S. (2001). Factors influencing the development of decubitus ulcers in critically ill surgical patients. *Critical Care Medicine, 29*(9), 1678–1682.

Ely, E. W., Margolin, R., Francis, J., May, L., Truman, B., Dittus, R., et al. (2001). Evaluation of delirium in critically ill patients: Validation of the confusion assessment method for the intensive care unit (CAM-ICU). *Critical Care Medicine, 29*(7), 1370–1379.

Environmental Protection Agency. (1974). *Information on levels of environmental noise requisite to protect public health and welfare with an adequate margin of safety* (No. 550-9-74-004). Washington, DC: U.S. Government Printing Office.

Feeley, K., & Gardner, A. (2006). Sedation and analgesia management for mechanically ventilated adults: Literature review, case study and recommendations for practice. *Australian Critical Care: Official Journal of the Confederation of Australian Critical Care Nurses, 19*(2), 73–77.

Fletcher, K., Hawkes, P., Williams-Rosenthal, S., Mariscal, C. S., & Cox, B. A. (2007). Using nurse practitioners to implement best practice care for the elderly during hospitalization: The NICHE journey at the University of Virginia Medical Center. *Critical Care Nursing Clinics of North America, 19*(3), vii, 321–337.

Fulmer, T., Mezey, M., Bottrell, M., Abraham, I., Sazant, J., Grossman, S., et al. (2002). Nurses improving care for healthsystem elders (NICHE): Using outcomes and benchmarks for evidenced-based practice. *Geriatric Nursing, 23*(3), 121–127.

Fumagalli, S., Boncinelli, L., Lo Nostro, A., Valoti, P., Baldereschi, G., Di Bari, M., et al. (2006). Reduced cardiocirculatory complications with unrestrictive visiting policy in an intensive care unit: Results from a pilot, randomized trial. *Circulation, 113*(7), 946–952.

Hartford Institute for Geriatric Nursing. (2008). *Certification*. Retrieved from http://www.consult gerirn.org/certification

Inouye, S. K., Bogardus, S. T., Charpentier, P. A., Leo-Summers, L., Acampora, D., Holford, T. R., et al. (1999). A multicomponent intervention to prevent delirium in hospitalized older patients. *New England Journal of Medicine, 340*(9), 669–676.

Jacobi, J., Fraser, G. L., Coursin, D. B., Riker, R. R., Fontaine, D., Wittbrodt, E. T., et al. (2002). Clinical practice guidelines for the sustained use of sedatives and analgesics in the critically ill adult. *Critical Care Medicine, 30*(1), 119–141.

Jastremski, C. (2000). ICU bedside environment a nursing perspective. *Critical Care Clinics, 14*(4), 723–734.

Kane, R. L., Ouslander, J. G., & Abrass, I. B. (2004). *Essentials of clinical geriatrics* (5th ed.). New York: McGraw-Hill.

Kirchhoff, K. T., Pugh, E., Calame, R. M., & Reynolds, N. (1993). Nurses' beliefs and attitudes toward visiting in adult critical care settings. *American Journal of Critical Care, 2*, 238–245.

Kleinpell, R. M. (2008). Visiting hours in the intensive care unit: More evidence that open visitation is beneficial. *Critical Care Medicine, 36*(1), 334–335.

Kleman, M., Bickert, A., Karpinski, A., Wantz, D., Jacobsen, B., Lowery, B., et al. (1993). Physiologic responses of coronary care patients to visiting. *Journal of Cardiovascular Nursing, 7*(3), 52-62.

Kresevic, D. M. (2008). *Nursing standard of practice protocol: Assessment of function in acute care*. Retrieved from http://www.consultgerirn.org/topics/function/want_to_know_more

Kresevic, D. M., Counsell, S. R., Covinsky, K., Palmer, R., Landefeld, C. S., Holder, C., et al. (1998). A patient-centered model of acute care for elders. *Nursing Clinics of North America, 33*(3), 515–527.

Krishnagopalan, S., Johnson, E. W., Low, L. L., & Kaufman, L. J. (2002). Body positioning of intensive care patients: Clinical practice versus standards. *Critical Care Medicine, 30*(11), 2588–2592.

Kritek, P. B. (2001). Rethinking the critical care environment: Luxury or necessity? *AACN Clinical Issues: Advanced Practice in Acute & Critical Care, 12*(3), 336–344.

Lawton, M. P., & Brody, E. M. (1969). Assessment of older people: Self-maintaining and instrumental activities of daily living. *Gerontologist, 9*(3), 179–186.

Leduc, J. M., Sen, S., Bertenthal, D., Sands, L. P., Palmer, R. M., Kresevic, D. M., et al. (2007). The relationship of indwelling urinary catheters to death, length of hospital stay, functional decline, and nursing home admission in hospitalized older medical patients. *Journal of the American Geriatrics Society, 55*(2), 227–233.

Lee, J. H., Swain, B., Andrey, J., Murrell, H. K., & Geha, A. S. (1999). Fast track recovery of elderly coronary bypass surgery patients. *Annals of Thoracic Surgery, 68*(2), 437-441.

Lee, M. D., Friedenberg, A. S., Mukpo, D. H., Conray, K., Palmisciano, A., & Levy, M. M. (2007). Visiting hours policies in New England intensive care units: Strategies for improvement. *Critical Care Medicine, 35*(2), 497–501.

Levy, M. M. (2007). A view from the other side. *Critical Care Medicine, 35*(2), 603–604.

Lower, J., Bonsack, C., & Guion, J. (2002). Combining high tech and high touch: Find out how two hospital units restored Florence Nightingale's vision of an oasis of rest for patients and how doing so improved outcomes. *Nursing, 32*(8), 32cc1.

Marik, P. E. (2006). Management of the critically ill geriatric patient. *Critical Care Medicine, 34*(9, Suppl.), S176–S182.

Morris, P. E. (2007). Moving our critically ill patients: Mobility barriers and benefits. *Critical Care Clinics, 23*(1), 1–20.

Naughton, B. J., Moran, M. B., Feinglass, J., Falconer, J., & Williams, M. E. (1994). Reducing hospital costs for the geriatric patient admitted from the emergency department: A randomized trial. *Journal of the American Geriatrics Society, 42*(10), 1045–1049.

Palmer, R. M., Counsell, S., & Landefeld, C. S. (1998). Clinical intervention trials: The ACE unit. *Clinics in Geriatric Medicine, 14*(4), 831–849.

Pandharipande, P., & Ely, E. W. (2006). Sedative and analgesic medications: Risk factors for delirium and sleep disturbances in the critically ill. *Critical Care Clinics, 22*(2), 313–327.

Pandharipande, P., Shintani, A., Peterson, J., Pun, B. T., Wilkinson, G. R., Dittus, R. S., et al. (2006). Lorazepam is an independent risk factor for transitioning to delirium in intensive care unit patients. *Anesthesiology, 104*(1), 21–26.

Payen, J., Chanques, G., Mantz, J., Hercule, C., Auriant, I., Leguillou, J., et al. (2007). Current practices in sedation and analgesia for mechanically ventilated critically ill patients: A prospective multicenter patient-based study article. *Anesthesiology, 106*(4), 687–695.

Rosenthal, R. A., & Kavic, S. M. (2004). Assessment and management of the geriatric patient. *Critical Care Medicine, 32*(4), S92–S105.

Schweickert, W. D., Gehlbach, B. K., Pohlman, A. S., Hall, J. B., & Kress, J. P. (2004). Daily interruption of sedative infusions and complications of critical illness in mechanically ventilated patients. *Critical Care Medicine, 32*(6), 1272–1276.

Simpson, T., Wilson, D., Mucken, N., Martin, S., West, E., & Guinn, N. (1996). Implementation and evaluation of a liberalized visiting policy. *American Journal of Critical Care, 5*(6), 420–426.

Stierle, L. J., Mezey, M., Schumann, M. J., Esterson, J., Smolenski, M. C., Horsley, K. D., et al. (2006). Professional development: The Nurse Competence in Aging Initiative: Encouraging expertise in the care of older adults. *American Journal of Nursing, 106*(9), 93–96.

Tullmann, D. F., & Dracup, K. (2000). Creating a healing environment for elders. *AACN Clinical Issues, 11*(1), 34–50.

Turner, J. T., Lee, V., Fletcher, K., Hudson, K., & Barton, D. (2001). Measuring quality of care with an inpatient elderly population. The geriatric resource nurse model. *Journal of Gerontological Nursing, 27*(3), 8–18.

Wallace, C. J., Robins, J., Alvord, L. S., & Walker, J. M. (1999). The effect of earplugs on sleep measures during exposure to simulated intensive care unit noise 1. *American Journal of Critical Care, 8*(4), 210–219.

Wong, R. Y., & Miller, W. C. (2008). Adverse outcomes following hospitalization in acutely ill older patients. *BMC Geriatrics, 8*, 10.

World Health Organization. (1999). Guidelines values. *Guidelines for community noise.* Retrieved August 7, 2009, from http://www.who.int/docstore/peh/noise/guidelines2.html

# Patient Safety for Older Patients in the Intensive Care Setting

# 4

Judy Dillworth
Terry T. Fulmer

## Case Study

Elsa Brown, 87, was admitted to the emergency department of a nursing home when she fell off the bedside commode after dinner. X-rays revealed a right hip fracture. It was 10 PM by the time Ms. Brown was prepared for surgery and 1:30 AM when she was brought to the very active recovery room. All the lights were on, there were three other postoperative cases, plus a number of monitors and machines whooshing and beeping.

Ms. Brown would awaken intermittently from her anesthesia and cry out for "Annie," her nurse from the nursing home where she had resided 6 years. The recovery-room nurses reminded her that she was at the hospital because she had broken her hip and assured her that they would take good care of her. Though this seemed to comfort the woman, she continued to thrash throughout the night.

Meperidine (Demerol) 50 mg q 2 to 3 hours PRN was prescribed to relieve pain, but the recovery-room nurses hesitated to give her much medication. They were afraid that a high dose might intensify her confusion. At 5 AM Ms. Brown was moved to the general unit, and at 5:30 AM the surgical team made rounds to check her postoperative course.

By 6:30 AM, the day shift began to arrive. At 7 AM, the primary nurse came in to introduce herself, check Ms. Brown's vital signs, and start care. Soon after, lunch activities began. Then, Ms. Brown's family came in and was very concerned about their mother. They visited for the remainder of the afternoon. That evening, Ms. Brown began to hallucinate, yelling, "Operator, operator." She was given haloperidol (Haldol) 2 mg (Fulmer, 1991).

## Overview

This case, presented and published in 1991, reflects several safety issues that can evolve when an older person comes into the hospital for care. Ms. Brown is in pain, sleep deprived, medicated with a strong narcotic, and has gone without nutrition for several hours to the point that she begins to show evidence of delirium. For this woman and for others like her, her general safety is in jeopardy. Safety is defined as "freedom from accidental injury" (Institute of Medicine, 2000, p. 4). Every time a person boards an airplane, it is expected that the pilot will arrive at the destination safely without error. When a family member becomes ill, consumers should be able to expect to get appropriate treatment in the shortest possible time, without complication. Despite the best intentions of skilled and caring health care professionals "to do no harm," mistakes or near misses occur every day in contemporary hospital settings.

In 2000, the Institute of Medicine (IOM) published the report, *To Err is Human: Building a Safer Health System*, which detailed the serious impact of medical errors on patients and triggered national attention and public awareness. It addressed issues related to patient safety and set a national agenda for reducing errors in health care (IOM). Since that time, many organizations have sought to achieve improvement through collaborative efforts. Yet, most hospitals in the United States still struggle to achieve uniform safety. According to the 2008 report of the Commonwealth Fund National Scorecard on U.S. Health System Performance, "the quality of care is highly variable with opportunities routinely missed to prevent disease, disability, hospitalization and mortality" (The Commonwealth Fund Commission on a High Performance Health System, 2008, p. 9).

An error is an act, assertion, or belief that unintentionally deviates from what is correct, right or true. "Errors are caused by faulty systems, processes, and conditions that lead people to make mistakes or fail to prevent them" (IOM, p. 2). Although these may not all cause harm, they are costly—particularly when they result in prolonged patient length of stay or disability as a result of physical and psychological discomfort, diminished patient and staff satisfaction, and loss of trust in the caregiver, the profession, and the system (IOM).

An *iatrogenic event* is "an unintended injury or harm to a patient resulting from health care management rather than the disease process" (Lehmann, Puopolo, Shaykevich, & Brennan, 2005, p. 410). Iatrogenic events are caused by technical or procedural errors, delayed or incorrect diagnoses or therapies, or adverse drug events (Lehmann et al.). "Theories about errors in high risk environments, developed by the aviation and other industries, provide insight into why ICUs are prone to errors" (Provonost, Wu, & Sexton, 2004, p. 1025).

In 2001, surveys from the Navel Postgraduate School assessing pilots' view of safety problems were adapted for hospital environments and given to 6,300 doctors, nurses, medical technicians, and hospital executives, as well as 6,900 Navy pilots. Areas of measurement included adequacy of safety backups to catch human errors and management's awareness of safety risks. "The average rate of 'problematic' responses was 5.6% for Navy pilots, 17.5% for all hospital personnel and 20.9% for hospital personnel working in hazardous settings such as the ED and ICU" (Haugh, 2003, p. 52). The best takeaway from the airline pilot model is the structure of freedom and responsibility needed within the framework of a highly developed system. The pilot has ultimate responsibility for the lives of the passengers and while operating within a very strict system, is able to make crucial decisions that stay within the established boundaries (Collins, 2001). Airline industry standards, which have a well-defined hierarchy that use redundant processes for complex tasks and technology and focus on safety, can be applied to design systems in health care to prevent error and promote patient safety (Provonost et al., 2004).

When an adverse event or medical error leads to a serious or life-threatening condition or complication, patients are often transferred to an intensive care unit (ICU)—an environment that is equipped with specialized monitoring and life-sus-taining therapies provided by a highly skilled and specialized team of professionals. Its intent is to provide the patient with a greater chance of survival when they might otherwise die. Although many patients recover and return to their prehospital state, the ICU still has the highest rate of mortality and complications.

As we review Ms. Brown's case, the risk for complications and increased recovery requirements multiply when one or more of the conditions specified in the SPICES model (sleep disorders, problems with eating and feeding, incontinence, confusion, evidence of falls and skin breakdown) are present. "The SPICES assessment, done regularly, can signal the need for more specific assessment and lead to the prevention and treatment of these common conditions. The presence of these conditions, alone or in combination, can lead to increased death rates, higher costs and longer hospital-izations in elderly patients" (Fulmer, 2007, p. 40).

## Sleep Deprivation

Sleep deprivation is associated with impaired tissue repair, decreased cellular immune function, and induction of stress in ICU patients. In the ICU setting, sleep is compro-mised by intermittent awakening for routine care, medication administration, pain, as well as the noise and lights. Invasive procedures and interventions may be required at any time and unexpected schedule changes and delays further preclude restful sleep. Further, the environment itself creates a frightening experience for those patients listening to the alarms and wondering what the noises mean in relation to their illness. They are unable to differentiate a simple alert (i.e., lead is off) from a serious warning (i.e., arrhythmia).

The ICU environment is dense with technology (computers, monitors, portable X-ray machines, video electroencephalogram, etc.) and life-supporting equipment (ventilators, intravenous pumps, dialysis machines, etc.), which have an accompanying beep or alarm to alert nurses to untoward events. These unexpected alarms all have different noise levels and pitches, to which the elderly patient with a hearing aid may be especially sensitive. Other sensory overload or deprivations related to the senses include vision problems, or the inability to wear eyeglasses. It is common to have televisions, clocks, and radios available to the patient to help with orientation; however, these adaptive strategies can also contribute to the noise-filled environment resulting in the opposite intent (see chapters 3 and 17 in this text).

The critical care setting tends to offer little privacy to facilitate monitoring, audibility of alarms, and to ensure a quick response to a sudden change in patient condition, or provide periods of rest and privacy.

## Problems With Eating and Feeding

Sick older adults may already be in a condition of undernutrition or malnutrition (see chapter 14). They may have low albumin levels and can be dehydrated. Hypoalumi-nemia is a risk factor for pneumonia (Maruyama et al., 2008) and significantly increases the risk for poor outcomes because of delayed healing and generalized weakness. Data suggest that the incidence of malnutrition is four to six times higher in patients admitted to hospitals from nursing homes compared to elderly people from the general community (Maruyama et al.). This study also showed that performance and nutritional status, oxygenation index, and the degree of dehydration are important independent prognostic factors in hospital-acquired pneumonia patients (Maruyama et al.). Enteral nutrition should be considered early (within 24 to 48 hrs of arrival to the ICU), as studies have indicated a decreased period of ventilation required, as well as decreased mortality with an increased delivery of nutrients (see chapter 14).

## Incontinence

Incontinence further contributes to an older person's feeling of loss of control as the patient has limited mobility in the ICU (also see chapter 22). Skin irritation from a wet, moist environment provides a medium for skin breakdown. Foley catheters are often inserted in the critically ill patient to accurately measure the patient's intake and output. Although there are benefits to having the catheter, which then eliminates the need for a bedpan, the patient is at risk for infection and possibly sepsis. Urinary tract infections may be caused by inattention to sterile technique on Foley catheter insertion, inadequate perineal/Foley catheter care, and prolonged length of Foley catheter days. A bladder scan can be used to detect urine in the bladder before using a straight catheter to try to reduce another potential source of infection. Fecal incontinence can be even more stressful and embarrassing to the older patient. The options of using the bedpan (and often missing) or diapers can lead to a moist environment, excoriation, and pressure ulcers if not attended to immediately and consistently (see chapters 19 and 20).

## Confusion

Confusion, the lay term for delirium, is "a common disorder among older ICU patients because of their advanced age, critical illness and multiple medical procedures and interventions. Mechanically ventilated patients are at risk for the development of delirium due to multi-system illnesses, co-morbidities, and medications" (Pisani et al., 2006, p.1). It is exacerbated by many events in the hospital, including environmental factors, excessive lights, noise, sleep interruption, medication side effects, pain, fluid and electrolyte imbalances, or infection. ICU nurses need to establish the patient's baseline and frequently assess and document fluctuations in mental status as well as to ensure detailed handoff communication from shift to shift to identify subtle changes. Providing frequent orientation to the environment, keeping the shades up day and night, applying glasses and hearing aids, promoting daytime voiding, and minimizing patient disruption during sleep are some ways to minimize the onset of confusion. Careful attention to prevention and early detection of delirium symptoms can prevent excess hospital days, demoralization of the patient, and serious injury (see chapters 3 and 26).

## Falls

Fall risk increases as the indicators of poor nutrition, incontinence, and confusion become more prevalent. For example, an older patient may have an urge to urinate and forgetting where he or she is, attempt to get out of bed. The patient may be unaware of his or her weakness and yet try to get over a side rail, which then contributes to a fall. Rhabdomyolysis is more prevalent in the elderly, and the subsequent muscle weakness further puts the patient at risk for falls. Fall risk has also been linked to insomnia and other sleep characteristics, as well as use of benzodiazepines. Poor sleep quality and fragmented sleep are an important determinant of risk of recurrent falls. Stone and colleagues (2008) studied 2,978 community-dwelling women ages 70 and up, and found that the odds of having two or more falls in a given year increased significantly for women who slept fewer than 5 hours a night (52%) compared to women who slept 7 to 8 hours.

## Skin Breakdown

Preserving a bedridden, critically ill patient's skin is a challenge in any environment. With aging, skin changes occur that include thinning, capillary fragility, and decreased sensation. With poor nutrition and hydration (which leads to drying of the skin), and the body's struggle to maintain the major organ systems' functioning, coupled with decreased resilience, skin may break down and cause pressure ulcers. Existing pressure ulcers are at risk for even further deterioration in hospitals and healing is an arduous and often slow process (see chapters 19 and 20).

Iatrogenesis and debilitation in older adults in the intensive care setting vary by institution and staffing patterns. In some institutions, the patient on the medical–surgical unit may have as many complex problems as the one in the intensive care unit. Certainly the risk for untoward events such as medication errors, falls, and pressure ulcers may even be greater when the staffing ratios (nursing, physician, respiratory therapist, pharmacy) are less favorable than in the intensive care unit. Sensitivity to the overall health status of the older patient in light of the current acute episode requiring the ICU is extremely important. Careful attention to the older patient's history can potentially avert error and risk. For example, if a patient has cancer with a low platelet count, or has had valve surgery and is on Coumadin, the outcome of hip surgery can be dramatically altered. Further, it is very important to know what alternative medicine strategies are in use. Is the patient taking St. John's wort for depression? How will it interact with other drugs/treatments? Older patients, like younger individuals, do self-medicate with over-the-counter therapies, and careful attention is required to ensure a safe and therapeutic plan of care with positive outcomes. Prolonged bed rest and immobility places a patient at risk for a deep vein thrombosis and anticoagulation is the evidence-based treatment of choice. But, if this patient has cancer, the plan will likely need to be adjusted with perhaps the use of external massage boots or adjusting the dosage of anticoagulation. All doses may need to be altered with weight loss, which can be common in older patients (see chapter 13).

Patients who require intensive care are at great risk because of the seriousness and complexity of their illness and the decreased resilience that accompanies it. The older patient has an increased propensity for adverse events as his or her overall health declines and more organ systems fail (which contributes to the complexity of the illness). Nearly 50% of patients in the ICU are age 65 or older, but age by itself has not been proven to be a reliable predictor of outcomes for the critically ill. Rather, the severity of the illness is more of a determinant (Ryan, Conlon, Phelan, & Marsh, 2008). In fact, "elderly ICU survivors appear to have a surprisingly favorable outcome and a good quality of life" (Montuclard et al., 2000 p. 3389). And this is more likely to be the case when patient safety initiatives are carried out meticulously and geriatric syndromes are anticipated and thus avoided.

The high mortality and complications may be related to the severity of the disease itself, the number of organs involved, and systemic complications. But, some complications can be attributed to "how" caregivers monitor and deliver those life-sustaining therapies. We will address some of the initiatives taken thus far, to reduce those iatrogenic events.

## Institute for Healthcare Improvement Goals to Improve Patient Care

The Institute for Healthcare Improvement (IHI) is an independent, not-for-profit organization that was founded in 1991 in Cambridge, Massachusetts. The IHI works with health professionals throughout the world to accelerate improvement by building the will for change, cultivating promising concepts for improving patient care, and helping health care systems put those ideas into action. Its goals were adapted from the IOM's six improvement aims for the health care system: safety, effectiveness, patient-centeredness, timeliness, efficiency, and equity.

In December 2004, the Institute for Healthcare Improvement (IHI) launched a nationwide initiative entitled "the 100,000 Lives Campaign," in which the following interventions were targeted: prevention of central line associated bloodstream infections (CLABS); ventilator-associated pneumonias (VAPS); surgical site infections (SSIs) and adverse drug events (ADEs); deployment of rapid response teams (RRTs) and delivery of reliable, evidence-based care for acute myocardial infarction.

Adoption of these interventions was supported by numerous national and local health care organizations whose goal was to reduce morbidity and mortality in the

United States. The IHI believed that by introducing best practices from across the country and enlisting the collective help of thousands of hospitals, 100,000 lives could be saved (http://www.ihi.org/ihi/about).

It seemed logical to select the intensive care unit to begin the patient safety initiatives specified by the IHI. Although the ICU is highly complex in terms of technology, monitoring, invasive lines, and expense, and each patient presents with his or her own unique set of problems, it is an area where some standards of care can universally be applied to improve practice. An efficacious program includes careful planning and implementation with a skilled, coordinated, and collaborative care team. The critical care nurse is particularly knowledgeable in physically assessing the patient, gathering pertinent information (vital signs, electrocardiograms, hemodynamic parameters, laboratory values and other data) and communicating with the intensivist, who provides medical management and oversees and coordinates the communication from additional medical consults (i.e., cardiology, infectious disease, nephrology, etc.) to best address the patient's overall problem. The critical care nurse must always be mindful of striking the balance among intelligence, competence, and compassion. He or she educates the family on numerous topics, including the disease process, how each piece of equipment provides information that helps validate a clinical assessment or supports an organ's function until it can resume on its own, and how the family can participate in the plan of care. The critical care nurse leads the interdisciplinary team (social work, chaplain, wound care specialist, pharmacist, physical/occupational therapy [P/OT], palliative care) and collaborates with the intensivist to ensure that all the patient's needs are addressed. As a result of better communication and synergy and standard protocols, it was hoped that fewer adverse events, greater levels of patient and family satisfaction, improved clinical outcomes, and lower cost would result.

Critical care patients are more vulnerable to iatrogenesis when they depend on invasive catheters and monitoring used to better assess and evaluate their condition (e.g., central lines, arterial lines, etc.), equipment required to support normal functions (e.g., ventilator, hyperalimentation, and dialysis) and multiple intravenous medications (e.g., antibiotics to prevent or treat sepsis, continuous infusions to sustain blood pressure or prevent arrhythmias). The intention is to provide better care, but all the treatments described introduce "foreign" media to the body and unfortunately place the patient in jeopardy of obtaining a hospital-acquired complication. This is where the IHI initiatives can be used as an opportunity for improvement. In several instances, they include a "bundle of care," which is a set of evidence-based interventions that are only effective when meticulously followed and implemented in their entirety (with no component excluded).

## Central-Line-Associated Bloodstream Infection

It has been demonstrated that implementation of a "central line bundle" can reduce the patient's risk for developing a central-line-associated bloodstream (CLAB) infection during insertion of a central venous catheter. The bundle consists of appropriate hand hygiene, using maximal barrier precautions, chlorahexidine skin antisepsis, selecting the optimal catheter site, and reviewing line necessity daily (Beaver, 2008).

The nurse is most often the observer who completes a standardized "checklist" of interventions to ensure all steps of the bundle are followed and is empowered to stop the procedure if they aren't. Although it appears to be a simple list, ensuring that all components of the bundle are performed carefully, can be a challenge:

1. Appropriate hand hygiene—Washing hands has been proven to be the single most important safeguard to preventing infections and an important first step when performing a procedure on a patient.
2. Using maximal barrier precautions—The patient is covered with a sterile drape and those present at the bedside (physician inserting the line, as well as caregivers assisting, observing, or near the sterile field), wear a sterile gown, sterile gloves, and a face mask. Similar to an operating-room setting, a "patient zone" is created to foster an environment of sterility. Technically, anybody who is not directly involved with the procedure and not wearing sterile attire (housekeepers, dieticians, X-ray technicians, visitors, etc.) should not be in the area while the central line is being inserted until the dressing has been applied. The RN is often the gatekeeper here, to ensure the environment is protected.
3. Chlorhexidine skin antisepsis—It has been proven that chlorhexidine is more efficacious than betadine (O'Grady et al., 2002). In most hospitals, preparing the skin with betadine using the traditional "circular motion" technique has changed to use of chlorhexidine applied via a vigorous back-and-forth rubbing technique (Beaver, 2008). Nurses have participated in the education of physicians in the proper technique.
4. Selecting the optimal catheter site—The subclavian vein is the most preferred site for a central line (O'Grady et al., 2002). However, less experienced physicians often choose the femoral site because it allows a large catheter and is more accessible, particularly during an emergency such as cardiac arrest. A catheter in the subclavian vein is least affected by patient movement and thus more conducive to application of a sterile dressing, which can more easily be kept dry and intact. The guidelines further suggest that if a femoral site is chosen (as is the case in emergent situations), the femoral catheter is to be removed quickly and replaced by a subclavian one.
5. Reviewing line necessity daily—The longer the line is present, the greater the chance of susceptibility to infection. Central lines are necessary for monitoring the patient's hemodynamic status and to deliver medications that might be irritating to the skin or painful or corrosive if administered peripherally (i.e., potassium, Levophed). However, as the patient improves, the necessity for the line diminishes. For example, as the patient stabilizes, medicated infusions may not be required to support his/her blood pressure, multiple blood draws are not required as frequently, and the patient may be monitored noninvasively. Patient-care rounds provide a forum for reviewing the plan of care and "daily goals" prompt reevaluation of the necessity of the line and discussion of alternatives to reduce risk (Brody, 2008; Gawande, 2007).

Although we just described the central-line bundle to be used with insertion of the line, we have found that maintenance of the central line then becomes just as integral in preventing infection. Although there is no formal bundle in line maintenance, there are several factors that the nurse must consider to protect the integrity of the insertion site and components of the intravenous system.

First, although the subclavian vein is the preferred site, it is imperative to protect the integrity of the site at all times and to maintain a clean, dry, and intact dressing, regardless of the location. Other locations such as the internal jugular (IJ) site are discouraged because the dressing/line can become dislodged with frequent movement of the neck, or the femoral site where the area is moist and susceptible to contamination when the patient is incontinent. It is generally not recommended to change the dressing until it is visibly soiled or oozing, to minimize the exposure to the air and microorganisms of the skin. Whenever the dressing is changed, sterile technique is crucial (O'Grady et al., 2002).

Second, closed-system IV administration sets should be used to minimize the tendency to disconnect the tubing. IV tubing can be disconnected to administer another medication, to change a patient gown, or can occur unintentionally as a result of not tightening the connections well enough. Whatever the circumstance, each disconnection and port of entry provides a quick vehicle for infection and vigilance must occur to keep ports closed at all times. Stopcocks on the tubing must always be capped to prevent entry of microorganisms.

Finally, access to the central line must be limited as much as possible. Every time the line is accessed to draw blood or instill meds, it is at risk for contamination. It is thus important to encourage the use of peripheral sites and lines, when possible. Sterile technique must be used whenever the central line is accessed and this technique must be enforced with others (medical students, phlebotomists, etc.). Because the older patient may have thin skin and less accessible veins as a result of multiple blood draws, there is a tendency for clinicians to use the central line for drawing blood and a resistance to suggest removing the line "just in case it is needed." It is very important to evaluate the risks against the benefits and encourage removal of the line as soon as possible while other methods of access are sought.

## Ventilator-Associated Pneumonia

By definition, hospital-acquired pneumonia (HAP) includes any case of pneumonia that starts more than 48 hours after hospital admission. Among intubated and mechanically ventilated patients, the development of HAP 48 hours or later is known as ventilator-associated pneumonia (VAP) (Kollef, 2004) (also see chapter 25). Common symptoms of VAP include fever, altered mental status, dyspnea, cough, and sputum. The diagnosis of pneumonia is often delayed in the elderly because respiratory symptoms such as dyspnea, cough, and fever are frequently absent (Maruyama et al., 2008). Confusion and delirium can mask symptoms, and the incidence of malnutrition (hypoalbuminemia) worsens the patient's clinical outcome. The degree of dehydration can also be a predictor of VAP (Maruyama et al.).

It is recommended that the VAPS bundle be implemented on all ventilated patients to prevent ventilator-associated pneumonia. The bundle consists of all of the following: 30-degree head of bed elevation, daily interruption from sedation and assessment of readiness to extubate, stress ulcer prophylaxis, and venous thromboembolism prophylaxis (www.ihi.org).

1. Elevating the head of the bed 30 degrees—Bed elevation provides for better ventilation and mobilization of secretions and prevents aspiration for a patient receiving enteral feedings. Frequent suctioning and pulmonary toilet are important nursing interventions to remove secretions. An important nursing consideration is that this position puts the patient at risk for pressure ulcers on his/her sacrum and bony prominences (particularly, the frail, elderly) if the patient is not frequently turned and positioned and/or placed on a pressure-relieving mattress. This is particularly important if the patient is sedated and

unable to say if he or she feels pressure or pain. The endotracheal tube can be a barrier to communication and the nurse must seek a yes or no response if the patient is unable to write.

2. Daily sedation vacations—Continuous sedation is held for a period of time every day until the patient "wakes up" from the sedation. The purpose is to enable the caregiver to accurately assess the patient, particularly his/her neurological status, level of pain, and ability to breathe on his/her own (or readiness to extubate). Patients are often sedated in the ICU to prevent more deleterious outcomes that may occur secondary to inadvertently pulling out a device such as an arterial line, chest tube, endotracheal tube, or falling out of bed (due to reaching for something or becoming disoriented) (Glick, Girard, & Bergese, 2008). Striking the right balance between pain control and awareness/ alertness is a challenge for the critical care nurse. A patient who is "sleeping" may still be very much in pain. Thus, a keen awareness of facial grimacing and guarding are helpful. Critical care physicians are often reluctant to treat pain because of hemodynamic instability (potential to decrease blood pressure or slow heart rate), organ dysfunction, or impaired mental status. Poorly controlled pain can lead to oversedation, which in turn contributes to decreased respiratory drive and prolonged ventilation, long-term cognitive dysfunction, and increased length of stay. Over time, sedation has a cumulative effect, especially with the elderly (related to weight loss of malnutrition, kidney/liver impairment) who then are at greater risk for disorientation and subsequently confusion, delirium, and agitation. The priority is to remove the source of VAP, the endotracheal tube, as soon as possible. Management of the agitated patient becomes the challenge afterward.

Oral care was not originally part of the VAP bundle recommended by the IHI, but nurses routinely maintain the integrity of the endotracheal tube and tracheostomy (check position, change tape/dressing) and provide mouth care whether the patient is vented or nonvented. Recent research has suggested that comprehensive oral care reduces the oral bacterial load and can minimize the probability of infection, particularly if chlorhexidine is used (Case et al., 2008). Chlorhexidine can be irritating to the mucosa, so frequent nursing assessment and other interventions may be needed.

3. Stress-ulcer prophylaxis—The critical illness, the environment, disorientation, inability to communicate well, and immobility all contribute to the patient's stress. Gastrointestinal ulcerations and bleeding are stress-related complications. As the number of systems involved increase, the disease process can be further exacerbated. Stress-ulcer prophylaxis (H2 antagonists, antacids) is thus incorporated into the plan of care. The RN's role is to provide psychological support to the patient by orienting him or her to the environment, anticipating needs, providing information prior to procedures being implemented, providing music, television, and encouraging visits from family and friends as appropriate. These are difficult to measure, but certainly can reduce the patient and family's stress levels.

4. Venous thromboembolism (VTE) prophylaxis—VTE prophylaxis (i.e., heparin, sequential compression devices) is the last component of the VAP bundle. The spectrum of VTE ranges from deep-vein thrombosis (DVT) to pulmonary embolism (PE)—all of which are commonly missed diagnoses because the common symptoms of hypotension and hypoxemia are often attributed to

congestive heart failure, acute respiratory distress syndrome, sepsis, pneumonia, and so on, instead of VTE. The patient is at risk because he or she is often bedridden, and may be sedated to prevent dislodgment of the ventilator tubing, EKG (electrocardiogram) leads, wires, access/lines, and other forms of monitoring equipment—all of which limit the patient's ability to move. Sedation and paralysis prevent the patient from describing the symptoms, which hinders the diagnosis. Furthermore, DVT and PE tend to occur during the first 7 to 10 days in the ICU.

The nurse plays an important role in administering anticoagulant therapy safely. Heparin is weight-based, so ensuring accurate weight, judicious use of intravenous fluid administration, and vasoactive medications (as the treatment of VTE can result in hemodynamic instability and hypotension), while paying attention to laboratory values are crucial to maintaining the right metabolic balance. When the sequential compression devices (SCDs) are the treatment of choice, performing regular skin assessments of the legs (checking pulses, color, and temperature), providing comfort (protect skin from SCD "sleeves"), and ensuring compliance of use are important, as is providing patient/family education.

Antimicrobial resistance is also associated with an increase in morbidity, mortality, and health care costs. Investigators have reported that longer (15 days vs. 8 days) antimicrobial therapy for VAP had no impact on survival. Other researchers found that 50% of patients who had no evidence of infection were still receiving antimicrobial therapy 1 week later, indicating unnecessary, prolonged antibiotic use. The clinician should use the shortest course of therapy that is clinically adequate for the infection and thus narrow the therapy to the microbiological results. When evaluating the "daily goals of care" and collaborating with the physician, discontinuation of antibiotic therapy after an 8-day regimen is suggested (Glick et al., 2008).

Any infection, but in particular, the two most frequently acquired hospital infections (pneumonia and urinary tract infection) can result in sepsis, a life-threatening systemic infection. Diagnosis is difficult because the early symptoms of fever, tachycardia, and dyspnea are very general and can represent other disease processes. Specific parameters of sepsis identified by the Society of Critical Care Medicine (SCCM, 2008) include (a) identification of patients who are susceptible (the elderly, the malnourished, the chronically ill, the immunosuppressed, recipients of surgery or invasive procedures, those with invasive lines or tubes, the mechanically ventilated or aspirated); (b) monitoring hemodynamic parameters for fever, tachycardia, tachypnea, elevated white blood cell count; (c) and identifying signs of organ hypoperfusion (altered mental status, abnormal peripheral circulation, oliguria, and increased lactate levels) or organ dysfunction (delirium, acute renal failure, acute respiratory distress syndrome, thrombocytopenia). It is important for the nurse to recognize and treat the signs of sepsis early because it can trigger abnormal clotting and bleeding, multiple organ failure, and death. The critical care nurse plays a vital role in the resuscitation and management of patients with severe sepsis and shock (www.sccm.org/surviving-sepsis campaign).

## Monitoring Glycemic Levels

Tight glycemic control, using continuous infusions of insulin and glucose (target ranges vary but generally are between a glucose level of 80 to 120 mg/dL and always less than 150 mg/dL), has been found to reduce mortality and morbidity in the critically ill (Amin, 2008). By correcting hyperglycemia, often a metabolic response to stress, the risk for infections, acute renal failure, prolonged mechanical ventilation, congestive heart failure, and increased length of stay can be reduced. There are many studies that have shown tight glycemic control to be effective in surgical patients. However, achieving normoglycemia in critically ill patients is a challenge, particularly in the elderly, when they are already undernourished, may have a meal delayed or enteral feeding held, and could be diabetic. This poses an increased risk of hypoglycemia, which is equally concerning (Holzinger et al., 2008). Tight glucose control can be extremely dangerous if not accompanied by other safety processes that include proper staff education on explicit protocols and procedures for accurately obtaining blood samples (central line vs. peripheral stick, obtaining results from the lab vs. bedside point-of-care testing); glucose monitoring; titrating insulin; and identifying, preventing, and correcting hypoglycemia. It is important to provide nutritional support and maintain the patient's metabolic status to minimize the elderly's susceptibility for further complications such as pneumonia and sepsis (Martindale, Wischmeyer, & Heyland, 2008).

Over the past decade, multiple organizations have dedicated time and resources to eliminate iatrogenic events. We have selected just a few examples of how these strategies can be applied to the elderly critically ill patient. A brief overview and evolution of the organizations' work in promoting patient quality and safety are described. Each group approached the objective slightly differently (either building on another initiative, working jointly with another group, or by grouping all the elements into "promoting a healthy work environment") but the overall objective is the same: to create a safe environment for our patients.

# Key Organizational Leaders in Patient Safety Initiatives

## The Institute of Medicine

The Institute of Medicine, a nonprofit organization within the National Academy of Sciences, was chartered in 1970 to secure the services of eminent members of appropriate professions in the examination of policy matters pertaining to public health. The Institute serves as an advisor to the federal government and, on its own initiative, identifies issues of medical care, research, and education. (http://www.iom.edu/CMS/AboutIOM.aspx).

In 1997, as a result of a large study conducted in Colorado and Utah and another in New York, it was reported that adverse events occurred in 2.9% and 3.7% of hospitalizations, respectively (Brennan, Leape, & Laird, 1991). It was suggested that at least 44,000 and as many as 98,000 Americans die each year as a result of medical errors that could have been prevented. Those errors were identified as occurring more frequently during the course of providing health care and included adverse drug events, restraint-related injuries, falls, pressure ulcers, and mistaken patient identities. The corresponding increased cost could be as high as $2 billion based on a $4,700 cost per hospital admission or $2.8 million annually for a 700-bed teaching hospital (Brennan et al.). Because hospital patients only represent a fraction of the general population at risk, the figures appeared to be a modest estimate of the magnitude of the problem nationally. And the cost of hospitalization has escalated over the past 10 years.

In June 1998, The IOM Quality of Health Care in America Committee was formed to strategize how to better the quality-improvement threshold, address the issues related to patient safety as a subset of overall quality-related concerns, and create a national agenda for reducing errors in health care to improve patient safety within a 10-year timeframe (IOM, 2000).

"In developing its recommendations, the committee sought to strike a balance between regulatory and market-based initiatives, and between the roles of professionals and organizations" (IOM, 2000, p. 6). Essentially the committee based its recommendations on three key motivators: internal, external, and organizational.

*The committee believes that a major force for improving patient safety is the intrinsic motivation of health care providers, shaped by professional ethics, norms and expectations. External factors include availability of knowledge and tools to improve safety, strong and visible professional leadership, legislative and regulatory initiatives, and actions of purchasers and consumers to demand safety improvements. Factors inside health care organizations include strong leadership for safety, an organizational culture that encourages recognition and learning from errors, and an effective patient safety program. (IOM, 2000, pp. 5–6)*

The recommendations were published in 2000 using a four-tiered approach:

1. Establish a national focus to create leadership, research, tools and protocols to enhance the knowledge base about safety
2. Identify and learn from errors through immediate and strong mandatory reporting efforts as well as the encouragement of voluntary efforts, both with the aim of making sure the system continued to be made safe for patients
3. Raise standards and expectations for improvements in safety through the actions of oversight organizations, group purchaser, and professional groups and
4. Create safety systems inside health care organizations through the implementation of safe practices at the delivery level. This level is the ultimate target of all the recommendations (IOM, 2000, p. 6).

The response to the IOM Report was swift and positive, within both government and private sectors. Almost immediately, the Clinton administration issued an executive order instructing government agencies that conduct or oversee health-care programs to implement proven techniques for reducing medical errors, and creating a task force to find new strategies for reducing errors. Congress soon launched a series of hearings on patient safety and in December 2000, it appropriated $50 million to the Agency for Healthcare Research and Quality (AHRQ) to support a variety of efforts targeted at reducing medical errors. (IOM, 2000, p. 5)

## Agency for Healthcare Research and Quality

The Agency for Healthcare Research and Quality (AHRQ) is a federal agency with the mission to improve the quality, safety, efficiency, and effectiveness of health care for all Americans (http://www.ahrq.gov/about). It concurrently developed and implemented an action plan which focused on the following:

1. Develop and test new technologies to reduce medical errors.
2. Conduct large-scale demonstration projects to test safety interventions and error-reporting strategies.
3. Support new and established multidisciplinary teams of researchers and health care facilities and organizations, located in geographically diverse locations, that will further determine the causes of medical errors and develop new knowledge that will aid the work of the demonstration projects.
4. Fund researchers and organizations to develop, demonstrate, and evaluate new approaches to improving provider education in order to reduce errors.

AHRQ has contributed to the funding of many of the studies related to patient safety and to promote improvement. In one AHRQ study, published July 28, 2008, researchers identified 14 patient safety indicators (PSIs) to define errors. They were grouped into seven categories: technical problems, infections, pulmonary and vascular problems, acute respiratory failure, metabolic problems, wound problems, and nurse-sensitive events. "The 14 PSIs were involved in 11% of all deaths within 90 days of a major surgery. Costs of post-discharge care were higher than initial hospitalization expenses according to the report. This large difference in the return on patient safety could make many interventions more cost-effective than previously thought" (retrieved July 29, 2009, from www.modernhealthcare.com/, p. 1). Although this study focused on a sample of 161,000 patients between 18 and 64 years old, it was suggested that when Medicare stops paying for certain medical errors and hospital-acquired infections in October 2008, the hospital industry stands to lose at least $91 million a year (retrieved July 29, 2009, from www.modernhealthcare.com, p. 1).

In addition to supporting research, the AHRQ provides education for individual consumers on their Website (www.ahrrq.gov/consumers&patients), which addresses how to stay healthy, how to choose quality care, and questions to ask when selecting and evaluating care.

The AHRQ also contracted with the National Quality Forum (NQF) to produce a list of "never events" that individual states might use as the basis of a mandatory reporting system.

According to the National Quality Forum, "never events" are errors in medical care that are clearly identifiable, preventable, and result in serious consequences, which may indicate a real problem in the safety and credibility of a health care facility. Examples of "never events" include surgery on the wrong body part, foreign body left in a patient after surgery, mismatched blood transfusion, major medication error, severe "pressure ulcer" acquired in the hospital, and preventable postoperative deaths. NQF developed this list with support from Centers of Medicare and Medicaid Services (CMS) (http://www.cms.hhs.gov/apps/media/press/release.asp?Counter=1863).

## National Quality Forum

"The National Quality Forum (NQF) is a not-for-profit membership organization created to develop and implement a national strategy for health care quality measurement and reporting. A shared sense of urgency about the impact of health care quality on patient outcomes, workforce productivity, and health care costs prompted leaders in the public and private sectors to create the NQF as a mechanism to bring about national change" (http://www.qualityforum.org/about/, p. 1). They identified and categorized safe practices that could be universally implemented in clinical settings. By focusing on faulty processes, systems, or environments of care, rather than the individual, they could reduce the risk of error and subsequent patient harm. The intent was not to capture all activities that might reduce health care events but to focus on practices that:

1. have strong evidence that they are effective in reducing the likelihood of harming a patient,
2. are generalizable and can be applied in multiple clinical care settings and/or multiple types of patients,
3. are likely to have a significant benefit to patient safety if fully implemented, and
4. have knowledge about them that is usable by consumers, purchasers, providers and researchers (National Quality Forum, 2007, p. v).

Thirty safe practices were initially endorsed by the NQF in 2003 and were updated three years later to expand the practices' scope. Some examples of the safe practice elements are: Creating and sustaining a culture of safety, informed consent and disclosure, matching needs with service, communication (e.g., handoff, readback, computerized physician-order entry), medication management (medication reconciliation, high-alert medications), prevention of health care-associated infections (HAIs) (aspiration and ventilator-associated pneumonia, central venous catheter-associated bloodstream infection prevention, hand hygiene, surgical site prevention) and condition and site-specific practices (pressure ulcer prevention, deep vein thrombosis prevention, anticoagulation therapy) (http://www.qualityforum.org/about/). These practices were developed with support from the Centers of Medicare and Medicaid Services (CMS) and reappear under the Joint Commission's National Patient Safety Goals (see http://www.jointcommission.org).

## National Academy for State Health Policy

*The National Academy for State Health Policy (NASHP) is an independent group of health policymakers who focus on approaches to improving patient safety on a state level. It examines how states monitor and respond to quality and patient safety issues. NASHP conducts policy analysis and case studies, provides technical assistance to states, identifies and disseminates "best practices" among the states, and conducts policy seminars related to quality and patient safety. NASHP aims to assist state officials in efforts to ensure that the health care delivery system meets patients' needs and is based on the best scientific knowledge so that care is safe, effective, patient-centered, timely, efficient, and equitable. (www.nashp.org/_catdisp_page.cfm?LID=124)*

Current areas of focus include the states' roles in addressing patient safety, adverse event reporting systems, patient safety centers and coalitions, medical malpractice, high performance health systems, and others (see www.nashp.org).

## The Leapfrog Group

The Leapfrog Group is a voluntary consortium of many of the nation's largest publicly and privately held corporations, business coalitions, and public agencies that purchase health care benefits, as well as products and services that support value-base purchasing.

> *In 1998 a group of large employers came together to discuss how they could work together to use the way they purchased health care to have an influence on its quality and affordability. They recognized that there was a dysfunction in the health care market place. Employers were spending billions of dollars on health care for their employees with no way of assessing its quality or comparing health care providers. (www.leapfroggroup.org/about_us/how_and_why)*

The 1999 report by the Institute of Medicine gave the Leapfrog founders their initial focus—to reduce preventable medical mistakes. The founders realized that they could take "leaps" forward with their employees, retirees, and families by rewarding hospitals that implement significant improvements in quality and safety. The Leapfrog Group was officially launched in November 2000 with funding from the Business Roundtable (BRT) and has since been supported by the BRT, The Robert Wood Johnson Foundation, Leapfrog members, and others.

The Leapfrog Group began collecting hospital data in June 2001 by surveying urban and suburban hospitals in the United States. The Leapfrog Hospital Survey is divided into four areas or "Leaps" of hospital quality and safety practices, which are:

1. Computerized physician-order entry (how well the system alerts users to common, serious prescribing errors)
2. High-risk treatments (coronary artery bypass graft, etc.)
3. Intensive care unit (ICU) staffing by physicians experienced in critical care medicine
4. Leapfrog Safe Practices (e.g., leadership, creating and sustaining a culture of safety, improving information transfer, medication management, hospital-acquired infections, and care processes).

In 2008, AMI (acute myocardial infarction) and pneumonia (both common, acute conditions that represent a large outlay of health care expenditures for private health care plans) were added in addition to pressure ulcers and "injuries occurring during the stay"—two hospital-acquired conditions on the list of conditions for which the Centers for Medicare & Medicaid Services (CMS) has said it will no longer pay.

In 2005, The Leapfrog Group launched its first rewards program. The Leapfrog Hospital Rewards Program (LHRP) measures hospital performance on five conditions based on quality and efficiency using data submitted by hospitals via the Leapfrog Hospital Survey and their data vendors. Hospitals that demonstrate excellence or show improvement along both dimensions are rewarded. The Leapfrog Group, based on its experience with the current LHRP program and lessons learned through other pay-for-performance projects, has worked to develop a next-generation hospital incentives and rewards program.

In 2007, the Leapfrog Group decided to give public recognition to hospitals that were willing to take all the right steps in the rare event that a serious reportable adverse event occurs in their facility. Their attention was to "applaud hospitals that make aggressive attempts to learn from their mistakes, publicly disclose them, and make every effort to prevent the mistakes from ever happening again" (http://www.leapfroggroup.org/for_hospitals/leapfrog_hospital_quality_and_safety_survey

_copy/never_event/, p. 1). Thus, the Quality and Safety Survey evolved and identified the following steps when an adverse event occurred:

1. Apologize to the patient and/or family affected by the never event.
2. Report the event to at least one of the following agencies: Joint Commission on Accreditation of Healthcare Organizations (JCAHO), as part of its Sentinel Events policy; state reporting program for medical errors; or a Patient Safety Organization (e.g., Maryland Patient Safety Center).
3. Agree to perform a root-cause analysis, consistent with instructions from the chosen reporting agency.
4. Waive all costs directly related to a serious reportable adverse event (http://www.leapfroggroup.org/for_hospitals/leapfrog_hospital_quality_and_safety_survey_copy/never_events/, p. 1).

Finally, "Leapfrog provides ongoing technical support to Rewarding Results, an $8.8 million national initiative to help purchasers and health plans align incentives for high-quality health care. Rewarding Results helps employers, states, health plans, and other purchasers and payors develop financial and nonfinancial incentives to reward physicians and hospitals for higher quality, consistent with recommendations of the Institute of Medicine. The Robert Wood Johnson Foundation and the California HealthCare Foundation sponsor Rewarding Results, which provides grants, technical assistance, workshops, and how-to publications to help purchasers and health plans. Additional support is provided by the Commonwealth Fund" (www.leapfroggroup.org/for hospitals/incentives and rewards/rewarding results/, p. 1).

## The Joint Commission

The Joint Commission (TJC) is "an independent, not-for-profit organization which accredits and certifies more than 15,000 health care organizations and programs in the United States. Its mission is to continuously improve the safety and quality of care provided to the public through the provision of health care accreditation and related services that support performance improvement in health care organizations" (http://www.jointcommission.org/about us/, p. 1). The Joint Commission strives to minimize error as it develops and annually updates standards and elements of performance. It reviews sentinel event data and highlights problem areas in health care.

*A sentinel event is an unexpected occurrence involving death or serious physical or psychological injury, or the risk thereof. Serious injury specifically includes loss of limb or function. The phrase, "or the risk thereof" includes any process variation for which a recurrence would carry a significant chance of a serious adverse outcome. Such events are called "sentinel" because they signal the need for immediate investigation and response. (http://www.jointcommission.org/sentinel events/, p. 1)*

Evidence-based solutions are captured in the national patient safety goals (NPSG). Examples of NPSG include improving the accuracy of patient identification, improving the safety of using medications, standardizing and limiting the number of drug concentrations, reducing the risk of health care-associated infections, reconciling medications across the continuum of care, reducing the risk of patient harm resulting from falls, encouraging patients' active involvement in their own care for patient safety, and identifying safety risks inherent in the organization's patient population (http://www.jointcommission.org/patientsafety/national patient safety goals).

In 1994, The Joint Commission initiated a public reporting system on the performance of JC-accredited organizations (organization-specific performance reports). An enhanced version was introduced in 2004 and renamed the "Quality Report" of the organization. This summary can then be compared against national and state information (http://www.jointcommission.org/qualitycheck).

## Centers for Medicare and Medicaid Services

The Centers for Medicare and Medicaid Services (CMS) is an agency of the U.S. Department of Health and Human Services (USDHHS). The Medicare program had paid for services "under fee-for-service payment systems without any regard to quality, outcomes, or overall costs of care" (retrieved May 18, 2009, from www.cms.hhs.gov/mediareleasedatabase/p. 2.) In an effort to reallocate those monies toward prevention, CMS began to work with provider groups to identify quality standards that will be a basis for public reporting and payment. In the past few years, several demonstration projects (e.g., Physician Group Practice Demonstration, the Premier Hospital Quality Incentive Demonstration, the Health Care Quality Demonstration, and the Care Management Performance Demonstration) have been launched to support payment adjustment to quality and efficiency. Because cases with a hospital-acquired condition consume significantly more resources than those cases that don't, CMS announced that they will stop payments for hospital-acquired infections (HAIs), beginning in the fall of 2008. This is part of the Deficit Reduction Act. Hospital-acquired complications include pressure ulcers, urinary tract infections (UTIs), deep vein thrombosis/pulmonary embolisms (DVT/PE), peptic ulcers, other postoperative infections (surgical site infections), and coronary artery bypass grafts with mediastinitis. Hospital-acquired complications that are anticipated in the next few years include sepsis, ventilator-acquired pneumonia, central line-associated bloodstream infections (CLAB), clostridium difficile, and methicillin-resistant *Staphylococcus aureus* (MRSA).

CMS also partnered with the NQF to identify "never events," for which payment would be reduced or eliminated and monies subsequently reallocated toward prevention. These were previously described under the NQF section.

The Hospital Compare consumer Website (http://www.hospitalcompare.hhs.gov/) was initiated in March 2005 to give the consumer access to quality and reliability of care (e.g., patient experience data, Medicare payment and volume information, and hospital mortality scores). There are currently a total of 26 process-of-care measures, three outcome-of-care measures, two children's asthma-care measures, and 10 patient experience-of-care measures. Hospital Compare also contains information about the number of certain elective hospital procedures provided to patients and what Medicare pays for those services.

As measures are publicly reported, access by the consumer has been notably increased and CMS has subsequently seen improvement nationally in specific areas (e.g., AMI). "CMS believes that all hospitals, regardless of their mortality rates, should use the data available in these free, detailed reports to find ways to continually improve the care they deliver" (http://www.cms.hhs.gov/apps/media/press/release.asp?Counter=1863/, p. 3).

## The Institute for Healthcare Improvement

The IHI does not charge members for joining, but requires the participating organization to make changes at a fast pace, share ideas with others, and report progress. The IHI provides participants with detailed information about each intervention, supporting evidence, and implementation tools (http://www.ihi.org/ihi/about).

The 100,000 Lives Campaign is a nationwide initiative launched by the IHI in December 2004 and supported by numerous national and local health care organizations to significantly reduce morbidity and mortality in the United States. The IHI believes that by introducing proven best practices from across the county and enlisting the collective help of thousands of hospitals, 100,000 lives could be saved over an 18-month period (January 2005–June 2006) and every year after. The campaign started with the following six changes:

1. **Deploy rapid response teams** consisting of physician, ICU nurse, and a respiratory therapist at the first sign of patient decline using objective criteria for early recognition of warning signs as defined.
2. **Deliver reliable, evidence-based care for acute myocardial infarction** to prevent deaths from heart attack. Ensure rapid EKG on admission with chest pain and minimize time to cardiac catheterization laboratory.
3. **Prevent adverse drug events (ADEs)** by implementing medication reconciliation upon admission, which is updated throughout the patient stay.
4. **Prevent central line infections** by implementing a series of interdependent, scientifically grounded steps called the "Central Line Bundle."
5. **Prevent surgical site infections** by reliably delivering the correct perioperative care including first dose of antibiotic, prepping of skin by clipping instead of shaving.
6. **Prevent ventilator-associated pneumonia** by implementing a series of interdependent, scientifically grounded steps called the "Ventilator Bundle" (http://www.ihi.org/ihi/programs/campaignoverviewarchive.htm).

As described in *Good to Great*, "tremendous power exists in the fact of continued improvement and the delivery of results. When you do this in such a way that people see and feel the buildup of momentum, they will line up with enthusiasm (the flywheel effect)" (Collins, 2001, pp. 174–175). As tangible accomplishments were highlighted with the "100K Lives Campaign" and reduction in infections and adverse effects were identified, there was an increasing confidence that these steps would work. Nursing has been instrumental in spearheading these interventions by collaborating with physicians, being empowered to "stop the procedure" if all the steps are not taken as they were structured, and sustaining the initiatives through careful vigilance and care.

Because the 100,000 Lives Campaign was such a major success in 2006, six new interventions were added to reinforce the fundamental principle of harm prevention in the "5 Million Lives Campaign" (scheduled through December 2008).

These new interventions are:

1. Prevent harm from high-alert medications starting with a focus on anticoagulants, sedatives, narcotics, and insulin.
2. Reduce surgical complications by reliably implementing all of the changes in care recommended by SCIP, the Surgical Care Improvement Project.

3. Prevent pressure ulcers by reliably using science-based guidelines for their prevention.
4. Reduce methicillin-resistant *Staphylococcus aureus* (MRSA) infection by reliably implementing scientifically proven infection-control practices.
5. Deliver reliable, evidence-based care for congestive heart failure to avoid readmissions.
6. Get Boards onboard by defining and spreading the best-known leveraged processes for hospital boards of directors so that they can become far more effective in accelerating organizational progress toward safe care (http://ihi.org/IHI/Programs/Campaign/Campaign.htm?Table1).

## The Society of Critical Care Medicine

The Society of Critical Care Medicine (SCCM) is the only organization that represents all professional individuals of the critical care team (physicians, nurses, respiratory therapists, pharmacists). It is "composed of 14,000 members in 80 countries. It offers a variety of activities that promote excellence in patient care, education, research, and advocacy" (www.sccm.org/home/p. 1).

To support its vision of Right Care, Right Now™, SCCM has partnered with other groups to participate in patient safety initiatives. These include, but are not limited to, the American Medical Association (AMA) Physician Consortium for Performance Improvement (developing evidence-based clinical performance measures that enhance quality and foster accountability), the High Reliability Organization Task Force (which developed a tool with the Anesthesia Patient Safety Foundation [APSF] to evaluate reliability concerning delivery of patient care to ensure safety and improve outcomes), the Hospital Quality Alliance (developed Hospital Compare), the National Quality Forum (ensured measures are relevant to critical care), and the American Association of Critical Care Nurses (developed essentials of a healthy work environment) (http://www.sccm.org/Pages/default.aspx).

As of this writing the Society of Cardiovascular Anesthesiologists Foundation is embarking on the FOCUS (flawless operative cardiovascular unified systems) Initiative, with Peter Pronovost, MD, as principal investigator, to reduce human error in cardiovascular surgery.

## American Association of Critical Care Nurses

The American Association of Critical Care Nurses (AACN) is a national organization consisting of a powerful community of over 70,000 members of "dedicated professionals who strengthen the voice of acute and critical care nursing, shape best practices and influence the quality of care for patients and patients' families" (http://www.aacn.org/DM/MainPages/AACNHomePage.aspx/, p. 1). The primary purpose is to promote and enhance consumer health and safety by establishing and maintaining high standards of professional practice excellence through certifying and recertifying nurses in the care of acutely and critically ill patients and their families. In recognizing the links among quality of the work environment, excellent nursing practice, and patient care outcomes, "the AACN established six standards to define and establish a healthy work environment. These are:

1. Skilled communication—Nurses must be as proficient in communication skills as they are in clinical skills.
2. True collaboration—Nurses must be relentless in pursuing and fostering true collaboration.
3. Effective decision making—Nurses must be valued and committed partners in making policy, directing and evaluating clinical care, and leading organizational operations.
4. Appropriate staffing—Staffing must ensure an effective match between patient needs and nurse competencies.
5. Meaningful recognition—Nurses must be recognized and must recognize others for the value each brings to the work of the organization.
6. Authentic leadership—Nurse leaders must fully embrace the imperative of a healthy work environment, authentically live it, and engage others in its achievement" (American Association of Critical Care Nurses, 2005, pp. 187–197).

## American Organization of Nurse Executives

The American Organization of Nurse Executives (AONE) is a subsidiary of the American Hospital Association and is a national organization of over 6,000 nurse leaders who design, facilitate, and manage care. The organization provides leadership, professional development, advocacy, and research so as to advance nursing practice and patient care, promote nursing leadership excellence, and shape health care public policy. In April 2006, the Board of Directors of AONE approved the Guiding Principles for "the role of the nurse executive in patient safety, to help lead best practices and establish the right culture across multiple disciplines within the organization" (www.aone.org/resource/home/, p. 1).

In 2008, supported by a grant from the Robert Wood Johnson Foundation (RWJF), AONE led the dissemination of the Transforming Care at the Bedside (TCAB) initiative with 68 hospitals. The focus of the TCAB model, started in 2003 (created by RWJF and IHI) is built around improvements in safe and reliable care, vitality and teamwork, patient-centered care and value-added care processes for medical–surgical units. Examples include rapid response teams to "rescue" patients before a crisis occurs, communication models, preceptorships and educational opportunities, liberalized diet plans and meal schedules for patients, and redesigned workspace to enhance efficiency and reduce waste. Through nurses' creativity, teamwork, and focus on the patient, this project is fulfilling one of AONE's important strategic goals of creating care delivery models of the future (www.aone.org).

## American Nurse Credentialing Center

The American Nurse Credentialing Center (ANCC) is the world's largest and most prestigious nurse credentialing organization and a subsidiary of the American Nurses Association (ANA). Its Magnet Recognition program® was developed by the ANCC "to recognize health care organizations that provide nursing excellence and provide a vehicle for disseminating successful nursing practices and strategies" (www.nurse-credentialing/org/Magnet/programoverview.aspz/, p. 1). In 1983, the original Magnet research study first identified 14 characteristics (which later became the Forces of Magnetism) that differentiated organizations that were best able to recruit and retain nurses during the nursing shortages of the 1970s and 1980s. These provide the conceptual framework for the Magnet appraisal process. Patient safety is a major component of the specific force of Magnetism entitled "Quality of Care." "Recognizing quality patient care, nursing excellence, and innovations in professional nursing practice, the Magnet Recognition Program provides consumers with the ultimate benchmark to measure the quality of care that they can expect to receive. When U.S. News & World Report publishes its annual list of "America's Best Hospitals," being a Nurse Magnet™ facility contributes to the total score for quality of inpatient care." Of the medical centers listed on the 2009 Honor Roll rankings (July 10, 2009), 15 of the top 21 were Magnet hospitals (www.nursecredentialing.org/headlines/, p. 1).

Although no single solution or policy group can eliminate iatrogenic events, many organizations continue to come together for the purpose of improving safety and quality of patient care. Organizational outcomes are summarized in Table 4.1.

## Conclusions

Clearly, the involvement of multiple organizations and professional societies on all levels has escalated and become more robust over the past decade. Why is it then that we have not been able to reduce adverse effects in hospitals to the same degree as the efforts that have been invested? Some common factors that may impede progress toward continuous and sustained improvement and potential solutions are described here:

1. The workload may be too great as a result of inadequate staffing. Staff shortages, higher acuity or complex patients, system inefficiencies, and nurse inexperience all contribute to a stressful work environment. The nurse may acquire additional responsibilities when there is a shortage of other health care members (respiratory, dietary, social worker, etc.). Oftentimes, the critical care nurse, as a member of the rapid response team or code team, responds to medical emergencies outside the ICU. The critical care team often addresses patient care issues, "at the moment," (such as treating delirium with sedation) and it is generally the nurse who remembers to consider the long-term effects (when the patient goes home, level of support from family, etc.), and the impact interventions may have overall. Professional nursing associations have been dedicated to supporting healthy work environments in which professional autonomy and decision making are fostered, collaborative physician–nurse relationships are encouraged, and professional practice is promoted. Although there is much emphasis on collaboration and team participation, it is often the critical care nurse who leads these efforts—coordinating the patient's care, ensuring guidelines are followed, assessing the patient's progress, and anticipating problems. As individual contributions are respected, nurses feel greater control over their environment. Additional resources such as personnel and technology may be required to ensure these goals are met.
2. Lack of knowledge and experience of the staff may be exaggerated by systems that are too complex to implement. Guidelines should be easy to access, simple, and easy to use. It should also be noted that guidelines may need to be tailored to age-specific populations and potential different responses to

## 4.1  Organizational Outcomes

|  | Mission | Structure | Process | Outcomes |
|---|---|---|---|---|
| IOM | Advisor to federal government regarding medical care, research, educational issues | 1. Increase knowledge in safety<br>2. Identify/learn from errors through mandatory and voluntary reporting<br>3. Increase standards for improvement<br>4. Create safety systems at the delivery level | Motivators used:<br>1. Internal (personal motivation, ethics)<br>2. External (provide knowledge and tools, visibility of leadership, legislative and regulatory initiatives, actions of purchasers)<br>3. Organizational (strong leadership, an effective program, organizational culture encouraging learning from errors) | Landmark study & recommendations prompted national attention and spearheaded widespread efforts to promote patient safety. Congress appropriated $50 M funds to AHRQ |
| NQF | Not-for-profit organization to develop/implement national strategy for health care quality measurement and reporting.<br><br>Goal to reduce risk of error and patient harm by identifying safe practices that could be universally implemented. | Focused on faulty "systems" vs. individual, which:<br>1. decrease likelihood of harming patient<br>2. are generalizable/ applicable to multiple settings<br>3. are likely to have significant benefit to patient safety<br>4. provide usable knowledge for consumers, purchasers, providers, and researchers | Identified 30 Safe Practices with support of CMS and JC (NPSGs):<br>1. Creating and Sustaining Safety Culture<br>2. Communication among caregivers, patients (hand-off, disclosure)<br>3. Medication Management (high alert medications, med reconciliation)<br>4. HAI Prevention (CLABS, SSI)<br>5. Condition- and site-specific practices (DVT, pressure ulcer prevention) | Knowledge for consumers, purchasers, providers, and researchers |
| IHI | Nationwide initiative to reduce morbidity and mortality in the United States. | With six improvement aims of safety, effectiveness, patient centeredness, timeliness, efficiency and equity the 100,000 Lives Campaign (6/05–6/06) and 5 Million Lives Campaign (6/06–12/08) launched. | Bundles of Care were developed to reduce HAIs (i.e., CLABS and VAPS bundles). Checklists were developed to ensure that all components of bundles were followed. | Standardization of Care Reduced infections |

*(continued)*

**Table 4.1** *(continued)*

|  | Mission | Structure | Process | Outcomes |
|---|---|---|---|---|
| Leapfrog | Voluntary consortium of largest corporations, business coalitions and public agencies that purchase health care benefits and seek to select and reward hospitals that prevent medical mistakes by implementing safety practices. | Identified quality & safety practices required for hospitals to be eligible for Leapfrog status:<br>1. CPOE<br>2. Provision of many high-risk treatments (CABG, etc.)<br>3. ICU staffing by intensivists<br>4. Leapfrog Safe Practices:<br>Leadership<br>Create/sustain culture of safety<br>Improve information transfer<br>Medical management<br>HAIs<br>Care processes<br>Additional indicators (added in 2008):<br>■ AMI<br>■ Pneumonia<br>■ Pressure ulcers<br>■ Injuries occurring during hospitalization | Hospital self-reporting of inclusion of safe practices in their delivery of patient care.<br><br>Outlined steps to initiate when an adverse event occurs.<br><br>Provides technical support to Rewarding Results (development of financial/ nonfinancial incentives to reward MDs and hospitals for higher quality). | Leapfrog Hospital Rewards Program (LHRP) Rewarding Results (Pay for Performance) Recommended ICU staffing with intensivists 24/7. |

*(continued)*

**Table 4.1** *(continued)*

|  | Mission | Structure | Process | Outcomes |
|---|---|---|---|---|
| AHRQ | Federal agency to improve quality, safety, efficiency, and effectiveness of health care for all Americans. | 1. Develop test/ technology to reduce medication errors 2. Conduct large-scale demonstration projects to test safety/error reporting 3. Support multidisciplinary teams of researchers to determine cause of errors and develop new knowledge 4. Fund researchers/ organizations to develop/ demonstrate/ evaluate new approaches | Supports research with funding, i.e., studies resulted in identification of 14 Patient Safety Indicators (PSIs) to define errors. Provides education for individual consumers on how to improve the quality of care services they receive. Contracted with NQF to produce list of "never events." | 14 Patient Safety Indicators to define errors and thus promote cost-effective interventions. "Never events" identified with NQF and CMS and used as a basis for a mandatory reporting system. Education booklet for consumers was created |
| NASHP | Independent group with state-level focus | Assist state officials in efforts to ensure best scientific knowledge is used to provide safe, effective, patient-centered, timely, efficient, and equitable care. | Conducts policy analysis and case studies, technical assistance, disseminates "best practices" and conducts policy seminars related to quality and safety. | Current areas of focus include state's roles in addressing patient safety, adverse event reporting, medical malpractice, and others. |
| JC | Independent, not-for-profit organization. Improve safety/ quality Accredits and certifies health care organizations and programs | Establish standards of performance Provide annual updates Evidence-based solutions captured in national patient safety goals (NPSGs) | Unannounced facility site visits Facility self-reported monitoring of compliance with standards and NPSGs Sentinel event review | Performance improvement initiatives result from JC standards Accreditation Public Reporting: Quality Report |

*(continued)*

**Table 4.1** *(continued)*

|  | Mission | Structure | Process | Outcomes |
|---|---|---|---|---|
| CMS | Agency of U.S. Dept. of Health and Human Services. Works with provider groups to ensure quality standards are followed. | Identify quality standards as a basis for public reporting and payment | Developed "never events" with NQF for which payment would be reduced or eliminated. Initiated Hospital Compare Website to give consumers access to quality and reliability of care. Demonstration Projects supported payment adjustment to quality and efficiency . | Stop payments for HAIs; Reallocate monies to prevention. Consumer access to Hospital Compare-patient experience data, hospital mortality rates |
| SCCM | Professional organization whose members represent the critical care team | Promotes excellence in patient care, education, research, advocacy | Partnered with other groups to participate in patient safety initiatives. Evidence-based clinical performance measures that enhance quality and foster accountability were endorsed by SCCM to promote consistency in ICUs throughout the Unied States. | "Right Care, Right Now" was created to ensure timeliness of implementing the appropriate intervention in the ICU setting. Fosters interdisciplinary collaboration through its membership and its projects. |

*(continued)*

**Table 4.1** *(continued)*

| | Mission | Structure | Process | Outcomes |
|---|---|---|---|---|
| AONE | National professional organization that is a subsidiary of the American Hospital Association. | Provides leadership, professional development, advocacy, & research to advance nursing practice and patient care. "Guiding Principles for Nurse Executive in Patient Safety" are:<br>1. Lead cultural change<br>2. Provide shared leadership<br>3. Build external partnerships<br>4. Develop leadership competencies | Create future care delivery models, i.e., "Transforming Care at the Bedside" (TCAB) initiative sought to improve:<br>1. Safe, reliable care<br>2. Vitality and teamwork<br>3. Patient centered care<br>4. Value added processes for medical surgical units:<br>Rapid response teams<br>Communication models<br>Preceptorships & education opportunities<br>Liberalized diet plans/ meal schedules<br>Redesigned work space | Partnership with RWJ: TCAB Provides evidence-based standards for nurse executives to lead nurses in the delivery of excellent patient care. |
| AACN | National organization of critical care nurses that defines best practices, which result in quality care. | Promote consumer safety by establishing high standards of professional practice excellence through certification. | The AACN established six standards of a "Healthy Work Environment," that are:<br>Skilled communication<br>True collaboration<br>Effective decision making<br>Appropriate staffing<br>Meaningful recognition<br>Authentic leadership | CCRN (Critical Care Registered Nurse) certification requirements encompass elements of providing a quality work environment, excellent nursing practice, and patient care outcomes. The "Beacon Award" provides a mechanism by which units can measure systems, outcomes and environments against national evidence-based criteria for excellence. |

*(continued)*

**Table 4.1 (continued)**

|  | Mission | Structure | Process | Outcomes |
|---|---|---|---|---|
| ANCC-Magnet Hospitals | Largest and most prestigious credentialing organization. Provide vehicle for disseminating successful nursing practices/strategies | AACN has defined criteria to measure the quality of nursing care provided and identify those institutions that are best able to recruit and retain excellent nurses. Eligibility for the magnet recognition award are based on the following:<br><br>Transformational leadership<br><br>Structural empowerment<br><br>Professional organization involvement<br><br>Exemplary professional practice<br><br>New knowledge, innovation and improvement in patient care | Application for magnet designation/re-designation requires evidence to support enculturation of the forces of magnetism and patient outcome data of the institution.<br><br>Patient outcomes are measured by "Nurse-sensitive indicators," which include, but are not limited to:<br><br>Bloodstream infections<br><br>UTIs<br><br>VAPS<br><br>Restraint use<br><br>Pediatric IV infiltrates | *US. News and World Report* publishes magnet facilities in its "Best Hospitals" edition. Magnet recognition provides consumers with the ultimate benchmark of the quality of care provided by the nurses of the institution. |

therapy. Perhaps we may need to rethink age and consider degree of organ function, activity, and sensory deficits (hearing, vision) that may affect recovery. Standardized protocols provide an opportunity to create redundancies and reduce error. Simulation and team training are based on principles successfully used in aviation to improve technical skill and communication among providers. Communication techniques such as SBAR (situation, background, assessment, response) and patient handoffs are methods used to provide information in a clear and succinct way from one caregiver to another and thus reduce the risk of patient injury and improve patient outcomes.

3. The IOM report suggested that fatigue can contribute to slowed reaction time, omission errors, impaired problem-solving abilities, and attention lapses. Many state organizations have recommended acceptable working hours for the RN and suggested protocols for providing "periods of rest" during work hours. The banning of mandatory overtime, except in emergency situations

has been legalized in many states to prevent overwork. More investigation is needed to see if these interventions reduce fatigue. The impact of an aging workforce and differing sleep requirements may also need to be considered (Bahr et al., 2008).

4. Regulatory requirements and associated documentation continue to be more stringent and take away the nurse's time from providing direct patient care. Lack of technical resources makes it difficult to see the return on the investment and long-term benefits. Technology aids in optimizing data entry and retrieval to track outcomes. Better systems to capture the multiple medications required as the patient ages and methods to improve communication to all providers of care could improve compliance with medical reconciliation, for instance. Computerized physician-order entry (CPOE) and bar coding are technological solutions available to minimize error. Evidence of improvements in length of stay, decreased complications, and associated cost reductions take time, but are rewarding when realized.

5. With the overall effectiveness of these initiatives still unknown, there may be a general resistance to change. Experienced staff of all levels may rely less on evidence-based practice and more on a "we always did it that way" mentality. Providing data and compelling evidence that demonstrates improvement in clinical outcomes can be used to support change in practice. Likewise, it is important to achieve individual accountability of all staff by engaging those who will be affected by the change as much as possible to achieve results.

6. Lack of leadership from the top down and slow administrative processes may impede progress toward improvement and create frustration and apathy. Most organizations now include patient safety in their mission statements and have hired directors of patient safety who can lead the efforts to standardize these practices. Leadership may agree with the concepts of patient safety, but frontline staff require resources and support to successfully implement and sustain the patient-safety imperatives.

7. Lack of financial incentives is beginning to be addressed as hospitals are required to report conditions that are present on admission. This will help identify conditions that are hospital-acquired, which are associated with higher costs, and will no longer be partially offset by reimbursement from Medicare, Medicaid, and other payors. Hospitals will need to invest in prevention and early treatment as opposed to responding to adverse events.

8. Power struggles between hospital staff and physicians and intimidating and disruptive behaviors can undermine team effectiveness and collaboration. This creates an unhealthy and potentially hostile work environment. The Joint Commission introduced a new Leadership standard that requires a code of conduct and the implementation of a process to address disruptive and inappropriate behaviors. Similarly, fear of disclosing error within the institution impedes the ability to improve systems. Disclosing errors or near misses can be better captured if they can be reported anonymously. This helps create a culture of safety in which the focus is placed on improving the system, rather than on the individual error.

9. Finally, involving the patient and family in the care is an essential element to promoting patient safety. This includes educating the staff on how to partner with family members to learn how to best care for the patient (identify routines, etc.), encouraging the family to ask more questions about safety issues (families are able to call a rapid response team if they feel the patient is unsafe), and actively participate in candid conversations about the care (truthful disclosure). Joint Commission patient safety and medical/health care error reduction standards for hospital practitioners stipulate that "patients and, when appropriate, their families are informed about the outcomes of care, including unanticipated outcomes" (www.jointcommission.org/PatientSafety/SpeakUp). Patient–family centered care has expanded to include family participation in meetings, open visiting hours, and presence during codes (Berntsen, 2006).

10. Finally, failure to provide effective communication contributes to a lack of teamwork and a propensity for errors. There are many reasons for poor communication. It can be related to inexperience and inability to recognize that there is a problem. A junior member of the team may feel insecure with his clinical judgment and may postpone communication, particularly if it involves waking up someone in the middle of the night. A lack of clear guidelines on who to notify if the patient deteriorates can result in delayed notification of the appropriate person and subsequently a delay in an important intervention. This could ultimately affect the patient's outcome. Lack of support from senior leaders can escalate the problem and, if the caregiver is not satisfied with the response, can also delay intervention. Crew Resource Management (CRW) and team training programs have been successfully used in the aviation industry to address failures in decision-making skills, teamwork, and crisis management skills of cockpit crews. These concepts can similarly be applied to the health care setting. Simulation training provides a forum for interdisciplinary teams to experience principles of role allocation, repetition, and situational evaluation through videotaped scenarios in a controlled, nonthreatening environment. The goal is to help participants effectively communicate, sharpen technical skills (e.g., CPR, intubation, etc.), anticipate problems (through scenarios), manage resources (how to delegate and to whom), manage crises, and ultimately foster teamwork, improved patient care, and outcomes (Lighthall et al., 2003).

In summary, there are a number of system factors that affect safety, including institutional procedures and regulations, hospital staffing and expectations for quality, the culture of the institutions and the way in which teams work together, individual provider factors, and patient characteristics. Each and any of these factors has a profound impact on safety on any given day. As we move into the next decade, it will be crucial to create a seamless safety net for older individuals in our care and in particular those who are most vulnerable: the elderly patient in the critical care environment. The challenges are exciting in that so much can be done to analyze ways to improve the systems currently in place. Using the cutting-edge initiatives sought by both governmental and private agencies and organizations, we can look with confidence toward a health care system that is known as a safe place for all patients.

## Selected Web Resources for Patient Safety

American Association of Critical-Care Nurses.
  http://www.aacn.org, accessed 03.31.09
American Nurses Association.
  http://www.nursingworld.org, accessed 03.31.09
Centers for Disease Control and Prevention.
  http://www.cdc.gov/mmwr, accessed 03.31.09
Department of Health and Human Services, Agency for Healthcare Research and Quality.
  http://www.ahrq.gov/about, accessed 03.31.09
Department of Health and Human Services, Centers for Medicare and Medicaid Services.
*National Health Expenditures for 1995.*
  http://www.cms.hhs.gov/apps/media/press/release.asp?Counter+1863
  accessed 03.31.09
Institute of Medicine.
  http://www.iom.edu/CMS/3239.aspx, accessed 03.31.09
Institute for Healthcare Improvement.
  http://www.ihi.org/ihi/about, accessed 03.31.09
Medicare Quality Improvement Community.
  http://www.medqic.org, accessed 03.31.09
Modern Healthcare.
  http://www.modernhealthcare.com, accessed 03.31.09
National Academy for State Health Policy.
  http://www.nashp.org/, accessed 03.31.09
National Quality Forum.
  http://www.qualityforum.org/about/, accessed 03.31.09
Society of Critical Care Medicine.
  http://www.sccm.org/Pages/default.aspx, accessed 03.31.09
The American Organization of Nurse Executives.
  http://www.aone.org, accessed 03.31.09
The Joint Commission.
  http://www.jointcommission.org, accessed 03.31.09
The Leapfrog Group.
  http://www.leapfroggroup.org, accessed 03.31.09

## References

American Association of Critical Care Nurses. (2005). AACN standards for establishing and sustaining healthy work environments: A journey to excellence. *American Journal of Critical Care, 14*(3), 187–197.

Amin, A. (2008, June 15). Strategies for glucose control in the intensive care unit. *ACP Hospitalist*, pp. 6–10.

Bahr, S., Buth, C., Martin, R., Peters, N., Swanson, K., Warhanek, J., & Ryan, P. (2008). *Nurse scheduling and fatigue in the acute care 24 hour setting*. White paper. Wisconsin Organization of Nurse Executives, Retrieved March 31, 2009, from www.w-one.org/uploads/FatiguePaper1-10-08.pdf

Beaver, M. (2008). Catheters give life but sometimes take it: Hospitals experiment with best methods to reduce infection. *Infection Control Today, 5,* 62–66.

Berntsen, K. J. (2006). Implementation of patient centeredness to enhance patient safety. *Journal of Nursing Care Quality, 21*(1), 15–19.

Brennan, T., Leape, L., & Laird, N. (1991). Incidence of adverse events and negligence in hospitalized patients: Results of the Harvard medical practice study I. *New England Journal of Medicine, 324,* 370–376.

Brody, J. (2008, Jan. 22). A basic hospital to-do list saves lives. *The New York Times,* p. D7.

Case, N., Townsend, T., Twibell, R., Simons, S., Osborne, K., Hurst, D. S., et al. (2008). Oral care protocol combined with ventilator bundle reduces VAP rates. *Infection Control Today.* Retrieved March 31, 2009, from http://www.infectioncontroltoday.com/articles/402/oral-care-protocol-ventilator-bundle-vap.html#

Collins, J. (2001). *Good to great: Why some companies make the leap and others don't.* New York: Harper Business.

The Commonwealth Fund Commission on a High Performance Health System. (2008, July). *Why not the best? Results from the National Scorecard on U.S. Health System Performance, 2008.* New York: Author.

Fulmer, T. (1991). Grow your own experts in hospital elder care. *Geriatric Nursing, 12*(2), 64–65.

Fulmer, T. (2007). How to try this: Fulmer SPICES. *American Journal of Nursing, 107*(10), 40–48.

Gawande, A. (2007, Dec. 10). The checklist. *New Yorker,* pp. 86–95.

Glick, D. B., Girard, T. D., & Bergese, S. (2008, June 8). Practical considerations in sedation management to improve outcomes. *SCCM Congress Review,* p. 8.

Haugh, R. (2003). Reinventing the VA: Civilian providers find valuable lessons in a once-maligned health care system. *Hospitals & Health Networks, 77*(12), 50–55.

Holzinger, U., Feldbacher, M., Bachlechner, A., Kitzberger, R., Fuhrmann, V., & Madl, C. (2008). Improvement of glucose control in the intensive care unit: An interdisciplinary collaboration study. *American Journal of Critical Care, 17*(2), 150–158.

Institute of Medicine. (2000). *To err is human: Building a safer health system.* Washington, DC: National Academy Press.

Kollef, M. H. (2004). Prevention of hospital-associated pneumonia and ventilator-associated pneumonia. *Critical Care Medicine, 32*(6), 1396–1405.

Lehmann, L., Puopolo, A., Shaykevich, S., & Brennan, T. (2005). Iatrogenic events resulting in intensive care admission: Frequency, cause, and disclosure to patients and institutions. *American Journal of Medicine, 118,* 409–413.

Lighthall, G. K., Barr, J., Howard, S. K., Geller, E., Sowb, Y., Bertacini, E., et al. (2003). Use of a fully simulated intensive care unit environment for critical event management training for internal medicine residents. *Critical Care Medicine, 31*(10), 2437–2443.

Martindale, R., Wischmeyer, P., & Heyland, D. (2008, June) The impact of enteral nutrition on outcomes in critical care. *SCCM Congress Review,* pp. 17–19.

Maruyama, T., Niederman, M. S., Koboyashi, T., Koboyashi, H., Takagi, T., D'Alessandro-Gabazza, C. N., et al. (2008). A prospective comparison of nursing home-acquired pneumonia with hospital-acquired pneumonia in non-intubated elderly. *Respiratory Medicine, 102*(9), 1287–1295.

Montuclard, L., Garrouste-Orgeas, M., Timsit, J. F., Misset, B., De Jonghe, B., & Carlet, J. (2000). Outcome, functional autonomy, and quality of life of elderly patients with a long-term intensive care unit stay. *Critical Care Medicine, 28*(10), 3389–3395.

National Quality Forum. (2007). *Safe practices for better healthcare-2006 update: A consensus report* (pp. v–viii). Washington, DC: Author.

O'Grady, N. P., Masur, H., Alexander, M., Dellinger, E. P., Gerberding, J. L., Heard, S. O., et al. (2002). Guidelines for the prevention of intravascular catheter-related infections. *MMWR: Morbidity & Mortality Weekly Report, 51*(31 Suppl.), 1–29.

Pisani, M. A., Araujo, K. L., Van Ness, P. H., Zhang, Y., Ely, E. W., & Inouye, S. K. (2006). A research algorithm to improve the detection of delirium in the intensive care unit. *Critical Care, 10*(4), R121.

Provonost, P. J., Wu, A. W., & Sexton, J. B. (2004). Acute decompensation after removing a central line: Practical approaches to increasing safety in the intensive care unit. *Annals of Internal Medicine, 140*(12), 1025–1033.

Ryan, D., Conlon, N., Phelan, D., & Marsh, B. (2008). The very elderly in intensive care: Admissions characteristics and mortality. *Critical Care Resuscitation, 10*(2), 106–110.

Stone, K. L., Ancoli-Israel, S., Blackwell, T., Ensrud, K. E., Cauley, J. A., Redline, S., et al. (2008). Actigraphy-measured sleep characteristics and risk of falls in older women. *Archives of Internal Medicine, 168*, 1768–1775.

# Part II

# Social Aspects of Critical Care Nursing of Older Adults

# Ethical Decision Making

# 5

Ethel L. Mitty

## Introduction

Nurses caring for critically ill older adults are in the unique, but not necessarily enviable, position of managing the interaction of medical technology; social policy; ethical principles; cultural diversity—and a patient's health care wishes, interests, and goals. The context of acute care for older adults is suffused with differing opinions about age indicators for aggressive interventions (including antibiotics, blood transfusions), the goals of medicine, definitions of quality of life, determination of capacity to make health care decisions, and the use of advance directives. In the midst of these crosscurrents, the nurse is a moral agent of and in society; practice is guided by the combination of principle-based ethics and the ethics of care.

Principle-based ethics or *principlism* consist of four principles: respect for autonomy, beneficence, nonmaleficence, and justice (described below). Some ethicists combine them differently such that "respect for person" is a stand-alone ethical principle. The principles originated in the "common morality" associated with the practice of medicine (Beauchamp & Childress, 2001, p. 37). For some philosophers and ethicists, the four principles are "rights," "virtues," "values," or even specific rules that guide action. Nevertheless, the moral framework compellingly articulated by Beauchamp and Childress is part of nursing's *moral agency* and accountability.

The notion of "ethics of care," based on a study of the moral development of women, argued that the moral imperative for women was grounded in relationship and mutual responsibility (Gilligan, 1982). In contrast to the conceptualization of morality as justice, equality, and reciprocity (associated with male moral development), Gilligan's formulation was that women constructed morality in terms of caring. The issue is not an either-or construction of morality but, rather, the fact that women start off from the care perspective, whereas men do not. The ethics of care are associated with emotional and cognitive maturation and proceed through three stages: (a) concern for survival, (b) focus on goodness, and (c) the imperative of care. This linear progression starts from self-preservation needs and dependency, moves to recognition that the choices one makes will affect others, to a notion of goodness as self-sacrifice (that is, putting other's needs ahead of one's own needs), and ends with the recognition of connectedness as constituting responsibility for self and others. Just as one would not do harm to one's own person, one is morally obligated to do no harm to "an other."

Ethical decision making is a process by which to arrive at a "principled solution" that identifies all concerned parties: their needs, interests, feelings, and values. It includes getting the facts (medical condition, nursing needs, etc.); discussion of the goals of care *and* the medical uncertainties, a benefit–burden (gain/loss) formulation; knowledge of how decisions were made in the past and by whom; and recognition of the influence of law, culture, and religion. A principled solution is transparent and is characterized by the fairness of the process. This chapter describes the bioethical principles in the context of care of the critically ill older adult; the bedside dilemmas that confound them; and the moral, principled approaches to resolve them.

## Bioethical Approaches

Moral principles are rather like rules; they make a statement about what is right or wrong, or good or bad; they speak to shoulds and should nots; oughts and ought nots. Ethics is a branch of philosophy. Bioethics is the study of the issues and controversies that do not lend themselves to easy solutions and that are brought about by advances in medical technologies, the increase in treatment options, and the alternatives in accessing care and services. Grounded in fundamental ethical principles, bioethics or *applied ethics* is concerned with the patient's comfort, dignity, choices and decision making, access to health services, and justice in health policy and resource allocation.

## Autonomy

Autonomy means self-determination (i.e., self-governance) and, by extension, the right to make an informed choice (i.e., informed consent). It is the right to say "no" as well as the right to say "yes." Autonomy implies having personal power to direct one's care—what is done to one's body—and control of one's personal information (Post, Blustein, & Dubler, 2007). Patients with diminished or fluctuating cognitive capacity may rely on or even delegate decision making to others whom they trust. In some cultures, decision making is delegated to the family or another person—often, a spiritual advisor. The right to leave a written document of health care treatment preferences and those interventions that are not desired was codified by the Patient Self-Determination Act (PSDA, 1991). In practice, a nurse can ask herself, "What can I do to preserve or increase my patient's right to self-determination? To decide what will or will not be done with his person?"

## Informed Consent

Informed consent is a process engaged in by patients with capacity or surrogates acting on behalf of patients without capacity. It includes the following elements:

- Decisional capacity
- Disclosure of sufficient information relevant to the decision in question
- Understanding of the information provided
- The ability to choose options voluntarily and, on the basis of these choices, providing consent or refusal of the proposed intervention.

To ascertain understanding, the patient should not be asked if he or she understood what he or she was just told. Any self-respecting adult would be loathe to say, "I didn't understand"; much too embarrassing. Instead, the patient should be instructed to "Tell me in your own words what the doctor said to you/told you about the procedure, etc." True informed consent is not possible absent sufficient information and the cognitive capacity to evaluate benefits and burdens, as well as risks and consequences of each treatment option.

Exceptions to the consent requirement can occur in three circumstances that are, by intention, narrowly defined (Post et al., 2007). First, it is not required in emergency care situations when the patient's wishes are unknown, or the patient is unable to participate in the decision, or when delaying treatment to obtain an "informed consent" places the patient's very life at risk. The second exception, "therapeutic exception," pertains if the physician believes that providing the patient with information about his or her illness or prognosis will cause him or her to suffer major and immediate harm (Post et al.). The third exception—waiver of consent—honors a patient's right not to be burdened with information or the demand to make a health care decision. The patient can delegate decision making to another but this voluntary relinquishing of his/her right to make his/her own health care decisions has to be documented, as does the description of the patient's understanding of the consequences associated with giving up decisional authority.

## Respect for Person

Respect for person is held by some ethicists to be a component of, superordinate to, or of equal importance to autonomy. It includes *veracity* or *truth telling, confidentiality,* and *fidelity* or keeping promises, all of which are basic to the trusting relationship between caregiver and patient. The notion of *disclosure* implies respect for a patient's (or family, surrogate) right to information necessary for decision making; it has both ethical and legal ramifications. Worldviews on truth telling and disclosure vary from that of individual responsibility and the right to know everything to the notion that giving bad news directly to patients causes pain and suffering, increases their burdens, and might even hasten death (Braun, Pietsch, & Blanchette, 2000; Crow, Matheson, & Steed, 2000).

## Beneficence and Nonmaleficence

*Beneficence* and *nonmaleficence* mean doing good and preventing or relieving harm and suffering. Nonmaleficence "First, do no harm" is a core health care principle to avoid unintentionally causing pain, harm, distress, or suffering. As with beneficence, the calculus of burdens, benefits, risks, and consequences must be disclosed and discussed. Individual or idiosyncratic perceptions of benefit and burden and best interest can vary among caregivers as well as patient and family, and drives the desire to include the patient's voice in health care decision making. The critical care nurse asks himself or herself, "Is this treatment doing good?" "Is it forwarding the patient's wishes and treatment goals?" "What harm (burden) is this treatment creating?"

## Justice

Justice is a complex ethical principle that traditionally consisted of a group of norms regarding the fair distribution of benefits, burdens, risks, and costs in a population. More recent conceptualizaions include concerns about access to health care services and rationing. Given our aging society in the United States (as well as worldwide), concerns and fears about the solvency of the Medicare and Social Security entitlement programs and the use of costly advanced medical technology to sustain life are generating debate about distributive justice: the principle that "defensible" reasons must be used to justify why a particular individual or group receives benefits (or avoids burdens) that are not available to (or denied) another individual or group (Post et al., 2007).

Callahan (1999) argues that the elderly are not served by suggesting that the lack of resources or political power stands between them and living longer. The question is not whether we have succeeded in giving longer life to the aged but rather, whether medicine has helped make old age a decent and honorable time of life. Callahan suggests that government (and medical science) should help people live out a "natural life span" beyond which society's obligation is to relieve suffering, not to provide life-extending interventions. Needless to say, there is considerable debate about what constitutes a natural life span and this debate is a source of moral distress. Among the questions the nurse asks is, "Are the treatment burdens proportionate to the risks?" When the preservation of autonomy leads to a patient decision that exposes him to potential harm or increased risk, what ethical principles are invoked by failure to address the patient's informational needs (disclosure)? The patient's decisional capacity?

## Rationing and Triage

Rationing is a method used to control spending: A limited resource is allocated among competing service or care areas; meaning in effect that beneficial services are denied to some patients. A variation of rationing is when an *expensive* resource, such as an

ICU (intensive care unit) bed, becomes a *scarce* resource by placing a limit on the number of ICU beds available overall (Post et al., 2007).

Triage, a method used in ICUs and EDs (emergency departments), decides the order in which care is provided and patients are attended to. The criteria invoked address urgency and likely benefit. Critical care physicians must make these often lightening-quick decisions but critical care nurses are instrumental in those decisions by describing current ICU patient status and their nursing needs. Organizational ethics and institutional responsibilities require that patients must receive care in the most appropriate setting. Hence, critical care does not have to be provided in an ICU setting—"critical care is a resource and a set of skills, not a location" (Post et al., 2007, p. 197).

Disaster preparedness is necessitated by man-made and natural disasters: 9/11, Katrina, California fires. The Task Force for Mass Critical Care, meeting in Chicago in 2007, proactively developed recommendations for the allocation of scare critical care resources in the event of an influenza pandemic (Devereaux et al., 2008). In their scenario, critical care resources are simultaneously limited across the country; patients can no longer expect to receive standard care, let alone life-sustaining interventions; rationing could be inevitable. The Sequential Organ Failure Assessment (SOFA) scoring system can be used to begin an equitable triage process that will ultimately require decisions regarding the allocation of critical care resources. The SOFA score is drawn from six organ systems (respiratory, cardiovascular, hepatic, renal, neurological, and coagulation) on a scale of 0–4, where 4 represents extreme failure or dysfunction. Among cardiovascular patients, a total SOFA score (TSM) greater than 6 is not predictive of survival (Janssens et al., 2001).

Exclusion criteria regarding access to or use of critical care resources would apply to patients with a high risk of death, little likelihood of benefit from the use of critical care resources, severe chronic illness (of various types) with a short life expectancy, and being age 85 or older (Devereaux et al., 2008). Without question, the legal and ethical constructs that justify the allocation of scarce resources and a mechanism to review the triage process in the light of experience and research must be part of a triage plan. There is a compelling need to hear the voice, the narrative, of critical care nurses from those parts of the world where health care resources are continuously depleted or overwhelmed by man-made and natural disasters: the Middle East (terrorist violence), Africa (famine and genocide), and Southeast Asia (earthquake and tsunami), for example.

# An Ethics of Aging

An *ethics of aging* is grounded in respect for the autonomous right of older adults to exercise control over their own lives even in the face of confusion and forgetfulness. Among the most difficult situations are those in which medicine and nursing have different perspectives about the goals of care for the patient, his or her previously stated wishes and present capacity to make health care decisions, the benefits and burdens associated with treatment options, varying conceptions of quality of life, and the manner and time of death. "Old people are old only incidentally, people's rights, protections and responsibilities do not wither at age sixty-five. First among those rights is the prerogative to chart the course of their own lives, they have the right to make their own mistakes" (Dubler & Nimmons, 1993, p. 193). Under the guise of beneficence and nonmaleficence, elderly patients are tethered to tubes and wires and sometimes restrained. Yet, guided by those same principles but consistent with the older adult's past opinions and decisions, life-support tubes and wires are removed; the patient is empowered. These are ethical dilemmas generated by rule-driven adherence to the ethical principles. The moral distress associated with this dilemma is that we feel that we are abandoning this patient because his/her decision or stated treatment preference, possibly made years before, failed to adequately consider the potential risks of nontreatment. It is an ethical tightrope.

The hectic pace and constantly changing faces of bedside caregivers conspire against having or taking—the time to learn about the elderly patient's preferences, personality, and peculiarities. It is difficult to assess mental status or cognition when personality factors and the likelihood of vision and hearing impairment interfere with understanding and expression. Talk to the patient first, before talking to the spouse, children, or others. The patient can "make known in myriad ways who they are and what they want" (Dubler & Nimmons, 1993, p. 215). Arguably, old people have the right to take risks; they have a lifetime of learning from experience.

Nursing's *Professional Code of Ethics*, first issued in 1976 and revised in 2001, speaks to respect for human dignity; safeguarding the right to privacy, health care and safe practice; maintaining competence; and improving standards of practice (American Nurses Association [ANA], 2001). Nursing care of the older adult should be that of support, protection, and nurturance while meeting basic human needs, provision of useful and understandable information, reduction of fear of isolation and abandonment, effective and culturally sensitive communication, and advocacy for reflective and compassionate patient-centered decision making. Nursing's responsibility lies in assisting the older adult with identifying and expressing her or his values and beliefs relevant to the situation or choices to be made; acknowledging the validity of his or her beliefs and values; providing the patient with sufficient information to choose among alternatives; helping him or her to express personal choices; *and* advocating for the patient when she or he lacks the ability, power, or resources to have his or her voice heard and values and choices honored.

## Capacity to Make a Health Care Decision

The fact that a patient chooses to refuse care or rejects an option highly recommended by the health care team is not, in and of itself, evidence that the person lacks decision-making capacity. The elements of decisional capacity include the ability to:

- Understand and process information about diagnosis, prognosis, and treatment options;
- Weigh the relative benefits, burdens, risks, and consequences of accepting or refusing the care options;
- Apply a set of personal values to the analysis (and if asked, explain or describe those values);
- Arrive at a decision that is consistent over time (i.e., ask the patient to explain and state his decision a few hours or a day later); and
- Communicate the decision.

There is no gold standard instrument or "capacimeter" that assesses decisional capacity (Kapp & Mossman, 1996). The Mini-Mental Status Examination (MMSE; Folstein,

Folstein, & McHugh, 1975) estimates orientation, long- and short-term memory, and mathematical and language dexterity. It is not a test of executive function—but is an assessment more likely to evaluate reasoning and recall—and is, therefore, not helpful in estimating a patient's ability to understand the consequences of a decision (Allen et al., 2003). However, an MMSE score below 19 or above 23 might differentiate between those who lack capacity and those who have the capacity for health care decision making (Karlawish, Casarett, James, Xie, & Kim, 2005). Persons with mild to moderate dementia can make, or least participate in, treatment decisions but impaired recall might be a barrier to their demonstrating understanding of treatment options (Moye, Karel, Gurrera, & Azar, 2006). Among a group of respondents including geriatricians, psychologists, and ethics committee members, the standard of decision-making capacity most highly valued was the ability to appreciate the consequences of a decision (Volicer & Ganzini, 2003). The least supported standard was that the decision had to be reasonable. Despite the fact that there is no consistent standardized definition of decisional capacity, there is sufficient evidence that safe and appropriate decision making is retained in early-stage dementia (Cain, Kim, & Karlawish, 2002).

A "sliding scale" to approximate decision-making capacity is useful insofar as the risk of harm associated with the seriousness of the decision is taken into account. In practice, recourse to a sliding-scale determination of decisional capacity requires attention to whether or not the patient fully appreciates the consequences of his decision. It is vitally important to evaluate the decision-making process in which the patient engaged and not just focus on the outcome. Capacity is questioned only when the patient disagrees with the recommendation of the clinicians and/or family. The patient risks being disempowered in precisely that circumstance in which he makes an idiosyncratic or highly personal decision. "Think about it—when was the last time you saw a capacity consult called to evaluate a patient who had just agreed with the doctor?" (Post et al., 2007, p. 29).

## Ethical Dilemmas in Critical Care for Older Adults

An *ethical dilemma* is a conflict between two equally unfavorable alternatives or a difficult problem seemingly incapable of a satisfactory (and satisfying) solution. *Moral distress* occurs when an ethicomoral choice—"it's the right thing to do"—is blocked from becoming a (moral) action. It also occurs when a person acts in a way other than their personal or professional values require, or their conscience dictates. This contrary action challenges the person's authenticity and integrity; his or her sense of accountability as a moral agent. Hardly an uncommon experience among nurses, unrelieved moral distress can lead to personal suffering and burnout; it is associated with nurses leaving the profession (Rushton, 2006). Among those who remain, recurrent moral distress is associated with loss of trust, impaired communication, defensiveness, increased turnover, and poor collaboration with colleagues; in short, the patient suffers (AACN, 2004a).

Ethical dilemmas in the practice of medicine become, almost always, ethical issues for nurses. Pain management and relief, the distinction between withholding and withdrawing treatment, euthanasia and assisted suicide, ordinary and extraordinary treatment, notions of medical futility, the principle of double or unintended effect, and the implementation of do-not-resuscitate (DNR) orders engage nurses' time, concerns, values, and guts. (The limitations of this chapter do not allow full discussion of these enormously significant subjects; the reader is urged to learn more not only for at-the-bedside understanding but also to contribute to the discourse in ethics committees and public policy decisions.)

## Pain Management and Relief

Pain relief is a moral imperative as well as a clinical necessity and obligation. For the patient who is unable to express his/her wishes and is clearly in pain, pain management can bypass the requirement of informed consent for treatment (i.e., the autonomy principle). It goes straight to the heart of beneficence. Compassionate care is respect for, and protection of, the patient. "No expressed informed consent is required precisely because relieving pain is central to the very notion of healing, and, for that reason alone, it requires no additional justification (Post et al., 2007, p. 114).

## Withholding and Withdrawing Life-Sustaining Treatment

Culpability for *acting and failing to act* is based on common law doctrine which holds that there is no general "duty to rescue." However, the act/nonact distinction does not have a comfortable fit with regard to medical decisions to withhold or withdraw life-sustaining treatment (LST). (Note: The issue is not withholding or withdrawal of "care," yet families often tend to view it that way.) The courts sometimes permit withholding and characterize it as an "omission" but hold withdrawal impermissible and characterize it as an "act." These distinctions are difficult to explain but the notion that withholding treatment is an act of omission and hence more defensible than withdrawal challenges medicine's and nursing's obligation to provide beneficial interventions to patients.

The President's Commission (1982) held that distinctions between withholding and withdrawing are a "slippery slope." Continuing a treatment long after its benefit to the patient has disappeared out of fear that discontinuing it will require special justification is as wrong as not starting a treatment with some potential for therapeutic benefit out of fear that the treatment cannot be stopped if its effect was less than hoped for (Hall, Ellman, & Strouse, 1999). As such, most legal scholars and bioethicists consider treatment withholding and withdrawal the same thing; they make no distinction between them.

The two seminal issues here are whether or not the treatment (intervention) is benefiting the patient or causing/contributing to suffering and prolonging dying, and whether or not the patient or family/surrogate believes that the treatment should be withheld or withdrawn (Post et al., 2007). Artificial nutrition and hydration (ANH) is associated with nurturing, with family. It is also beset with misinformation as well as with embedded cultural and religious beliefs. For the family, limiting a life-sustaining treatment like ANH can feel like abandonment. The research shows that ANH at the end of life increases discomfort (Huang & Ahronheim, 2000)—but are we sharing this information with the family in a timely way?

An extensive review of the literature regarding nurses' attitudes toward ANH for terminally ill patients or those with end-stage dementia revealed that nurses' opinions reflected not only the popular opinion but the prevailing misinformation as well (Bryon, de Casterlé, & Gastmans, 2007). Both proponents and opponents of

ANH argued from the same moral perspective: quality of life and a dignified death. Arguments in favor of ANH were grounded in notions of autonomy and the sanctity of life (i.e., an ethical–legal position), that it was basic nursing that provided hydration, nutrition, and/or medication (i.e., the clinical position), and that it honored family request, medical orders, and the health care team's consensus support of the intervention (i.e., the social–professional position). For some nurses, withdrawal of ANH caused patients extreme discomfort associated with dehydration and was the same as killing the patient (Bryon et al.).

Argument in opposition to ANH included beneficence/nonmaleficence, that is, to avoid patient discomfort (based on the research, to date), assuring a natural death, and that nurses could provide good nursing care that would alleviate any distressing symptoms such as dry mouth. Few nurses mentioned cost-effectiveness, family request, medical orders, or team consensus in support of withholding/withdrawing ANH, or advanced age as justification for not providing ANH. Given nurses' respect for the sanctity of life, their ignorance or denial of the scientific evidence that ANH does not lengthen the life span of a patient dying in a terminal stage of illness (including dementia), is both interesting and dismaying—it speaks to the need for dissemination of evidence-based practice guidelines.

## Palliative Care Nursing

The goal of LST is to preserve organ or system function: to sustain life. Foregoing LST and moving to the provision of aggressive palliative care is a shift of goals from curing to caring; the intent is to maximize comfort, reduce suffering, and not prolong the dying process. The ethical issue is not that the patient is being deprived of care but, rather, is being protected from burdensome interventions that are not beneficial. Death is a result of the underlying disease; it is not an outcome of assisted suicide or euthanasia (Post et al., 2007).

Physicians are under no moral obligation to provide a medical benefit if no medical benefit exists, despite patient or family demand for it. A medical opinion that a treatment option is *medically futile* removes the intervention from the range of options available to the patient (family, surrogate). Typically, the statement made is not that the treatment/intervention will harm the patient but, rather, that it will not produce the sought-after benefit (i.e., the *physiologic impossibility* of treatment effect); it will fall below a therapeutic standard (Post et al., 2007). Describing a treatment with questionable benefit as "futile" simultaneously addresses the patient's best interests as well as economic interests. Patients and families should not be offered futile treatment and "false choices" (Tomlinson & Brody, 1990). Only a small number of cases involve absolute medical futility from a physiological perspective. The much larger number of cases involve value judgments about the patient and the allocation of health care resources. For a critical care nurse, this means being mindful that futility claims could be denying options to patients who might be willing to live with a compromised or changed quality of life (Truog, Brett, & Frader, 1992).

## Euthanasia and Assisted Suicide

Commonly known as "mercy killing," euthanasia evokes legal, ethical, medical, social, and emotional reactions. Euthanasia is defined as "the intentional termination of life by someone other than the person concerned, at the latter's request" (De Bal, Gastmans, & Dierckx de Casterlé, 2008). Active euthanasia is illegal in all 50 states (but is legal in Belgium and the Netherlands under strict constraints and rules). "The agent of death is the clinician," acting to relieve a patient's unrelenting pain or suffering; it is an act motivated by compassion (Post et al., 2007, p. 116).

Passive euthanasia encompasses intentional nontreatment, from withdrawing or withholding, to, in some cases, the principle of double effect (discussed below) and is not illegal in the strict sense of the phrase.

Nurses are frequently asked by patients for assistance with dying and, in fact, are often the first health care professionals to receive the request (De Bal et al., 2008). This is hardly surprising; nurses are with their patients 24/7 and are expected, by the patient, to advocate for their needs and wishes. (Indeed, it is so stated in nursing's professional code.) Contextual issues include the nurse–physician relationship, setting of care, time, and the legalities. Emotional issues described by nurses confronted with these requests include grief, fear, anxiety, uncertainty, guilt, and extreme moral distress (DeBal et al., 2008).

Assisted suicide is the act of a clinician who facilitates a patient's death by the provision of information, instruction, medication, or means (e.g., a prescription). The patient is the "agent" of death but the clinician has acted with the knowledge that the patient intends to end his life using the information and means provided by the clinician. Assisted suicide is illegal in all states except Oregon, where it can occur only under specific circumstances and following specific steps.

The principle or doctrine of *double effect* holds that the "intent" behind administration of morphine, for example, is to relieve pain and suffering and increase comfort. The death of the patient pursuant to this act is not intended; therefore, the act is not wrong. The "motive" is compassionate care, not to kill, and reflects the beneficent ethic of palliation. It is legally, ethically, and medically justified and is not an instance of euthanasia or assisted suicide (Post el al., 2007). Morally, it is permissible if four conditions are met. (Imagine the administration of morphine sulfate while reading this.) The first condition is that the action (or administration) is good or indifferent in and of itself. Two: The person acting (i.e., administering the morphine) has no evil intentions; the action is sincerely meant to be beneficial for the receiver/patient. The third condition is concerned with "immediacy" of the effect. In other words, the good effect must occur as soon as the evil effect: simultaneously, the patient no longer experiences respiratory anxiety, "pulling," or horrific pain but his or her respiratory rate is slowed and depth of respiration is diminished. The fourth condition holds that there must be a "proportionally grave reason" that allowed the evil to occur (Fry & Veatch, 2006, p. 207).

## Ordinary and Extraordinary Treatment

The distinction between ordinary and extraordinary treatment was explicated by the Catholic Church and has support in Judaism, Islam, and other religions. What is ordinary in one case might be extraordinary in another; treatment context and therapeutic goals must be understood and evaluated. *Ordinary* is defined as all medicine, surgeries, and treatments that offer a reasonable hope of benefit that are obtained without excessive pain and suffering, expense, or other hardship. *Extraordinary* means are those medicines, surgeries, and treatments that cannot be obtained without excessive pain or cost (etc.) *or,* if used, do not have a reasonable potential for benefit (Hall et al., 1999). Sometimes called an "expendable" treatment, or one that is unusual or complex, extraordinary is further differentiated from ordinary by virtue of the latter being "simple" or "statistically common" (Fry & Veatch, 2006, p. 200). Assessment of the burden of treatment on the patient or family, consideration of the patient's interest in treatment termination, and "disproportionate" investment in equipment or personnel are things that also have to be considered.

The notion of "extraordinary burden" might be applied when considering whether or not cardiopulmonary resuscitation (CPR) would cause more harm than benefit given a patient's stage of illness, frailty, and so on. The Presidents Commission (1982) adopted the precepts articulated by Roman Catholic theology: A treatment was expendable if it was useless *or* if the burden exceeded the benefit. Each treatment option has to be evaluated separately, on both criteria. Interestingly, the President's Commission (1982) suggested that the distinction between "ordinary" and "extraordinary" was better made at the end of an ethical discussion of options, rather than at the outset.

## Do Not Resuscitate and Cardiopulmonary Resuscitation

The influences on do not resuscitate (DNR) and cardiopulmonary resuscitation (CPR) orders include assessment of futile care, beneficence and nonmaleficence, self-determination, and disclosure. Consent to resuscitation is presumed; a DNR order requires consent to withhold this particular procedure. It can be argued, however, that if resuscitation would not provide a medical benefit and might even harm the patient, then physicians should not be required to even discuss this option with the patient or family. Critical care nurses have likely been in situations in which the patient and/or family was informed about CPR and then received information that it would produce no benefit; that is, preservation of life but with profound neurological damage, broken ribs, ruptured spleen, bruised liver, and so on. Rather than enhancing autonomy by implying that a meaningful choice is possible, mixed messages about CPR minimize the value of informed decision making; indeed, it makes a mockery of it.

In caring for the critically ill older adult, especially those whose quality of life by every value-free objective measure seems minimal or absent, critical care nurses need to be aware whether or not an advance directive (or clear and convincing evidence) requesting or refusing CPR is being honored. Similarly, critical care nurses must be vigilant about any coercive influence on an elderly patient or her or his family to forgo aggressive treatment/interventions. Patients and their families (or surrogates) need time to think about these directives—and medical orders. They should not be asked to make a decision when the patient is at death's door; that is not respect for person. Among the pervasive ethical concerns among acute and long-term-care nurses (and families) about DNR orders is that such an order is, ipso facto, permission to "do not treat." Clearly, research is needed in this regard especially as more is learned about the benefits and outcomes of palliative care.

## Managing Moral Distress

Critical care nurses have recourse to two models that can help the practitioner identify the source(s) of moral distress, the ethical dilemma(s) that pertain, and the best action to take from an ethical perspective: Rest's four-component model (1986) and the AACN Model to Rise Above Moral Distress (AACN, 2004b). A third model for analyzing an ethical dilemma includes a process for constructing the "fact pattern," making the ethical diagnosis, goal setting and implementation, and evaluation (Fletcher, Hite, Lombardo, & Marshall, 1997).

## Rest's Four-Component Model

This model focuses on the practitioner: from the time she/he first recognizes that an ethicomoral dilemma exists to implementation of the plan of action that is most justifiable morally. The model has four components: (a) *moral sensitivity*, (b) *moral judgment*, (c) *moral motivation*, and (d) *moral action* (Rest, 1986). Ethicists sometimes include an additional component: moral character or integrity. Other than ethical dilemmas about disclosure to the patient or family about treatment risks, disagreement about what is in the patient's best interests and who has decisional authority, everyday ethical issues in critical care nursing practice are those of *recognition* that an ethical situation is present (i.e., moral sensitivity) (Rushton & Penticuff, 2007). A nurse's feelings of obligation to safeguard the patient (i.e., moral motivation) are sometimes restrained by the possibility of an undesirable outcome as a result of her moral action. For example, assertiveness in protecting and assuring that the authentic voice of the patient is heard could result in honoring the wishes of a patient whose decision is medically unwise but who is an older adult with capacity whose decision is an expression of lifelong values and beliefs.

### Moral Sensitivity

Moral sensitivity is awareness of others' perspectives, values, beliefs, interests, and understanding of facts and events. It means being empathic and aware of different options and the possible outcomes of each action. Recognition is "framed" by personal history, culture, religion, scientific data, emotions, education, relationships, and so on. Nurse ethicists hold that moral sensitivity has a good fit with a caring ethic. It is holistic because it considers the context of the ethical issue as well as the embedded relationships and interactions (Rushton & Penticuff, 2007).

### Moral Judgment

Moral judgment relies on dispassionate reasoning to reach a justifiable course of action. Grounded in ethical principles, decisions have to be based on more than emotion, intuition, and having good feelings about the decisions. The process of moral reasoning (i.e., judgment) requires collection of and clarity about the relevant facts from all involved parties, articulation of the ethical issue(s), including the patient's values and views on what is beneficial and what is not (or even harmful), formulation of possible options and the consequences of each, and justification of what is presumably an ethical course of action. Ethical obligations of the caregivers must also be factored in. Elements of the situation carry moral "weight," such as the patient's diagnosis and prognosis, treatment options, location of care, patient and family understanding of the medical situation and likely trajectory of the illness, and the patient's sense of duty to the family (a very complex relationship).

## Moral Motivation

Moral motivation is a combination of knowing the right thing to do *and* acting on it. Feeling unable to do the right thing is a precursor to moral distress. Moving forward requires clarity of purpose and assertiveness (Rushton & Penticuff, 2007). *Moral character* influences actions. It is like "applied wisdom" that considers all aspects of the situation and is based on the total "fact pattern" of values and beliefs of all the parties *and* the clinical realities.

## Moral Action

Moral action moves the ethically constructed plan from the table to a sphere of action that has, itself, ethical parameters. As noted earlier, this is where the "principled solution" is unveiled. The transparency and fairness of the process is vital in order to deal with resistance to the plan, particularly when there is high emotional content embedded in the situation.

The Rest model could be useful in continuing education, with use of case studies, to facilitate understanding of ethical dilemmas. For practical purposes, however, it might be too complex or even unwieldy in delineating the ethical dilemma and construction of a plan.

# 4-A Model to Rise Above Moral Distress: Ask, Affirm, Assess, Act

The "4-A" model, articulated by the American Association of Critical Care Nurses (AACN, 2004b), is a systematic way for an individual nurse as well as an organization to identify and reduce or ameliorate moral distress. Not incidentally, the model is a 4-step "process tool" to provide quality care by nurses actively engaged in creating an environment that supports critical examination of the workplace. Each step has a goal.

## Ask

As the first step, ask what is generating (my) anger, anxiety; that is, my feelings of distress. What does my moral distress look and sound like? (In other words, "How do I know I am distressed?"). Am I, or other nurses, talking in terms of feeling helpless; impotent to make a difference? The AACN grouped common responses to suffering moral distress as those that are physical (e.g., lethargy, overactivity, somatic complaints, appetite and sleep changes); emotional (e.g., sarcasm, depression); behavioral (e.g., apathetic, avoiding, controlling); and spiritual (e.g., altered religious practices and changes in meaning).

Looking at the source(s) of moral distress can help shape the approach. Is it a department or organizational policy, a particular practice, lack of clarity about treatment goals among all parties? Is the treatment prolonging living or prolonging dying? What ethical principles appear to be compromised? The goal of this step is to become alerted to the fact that you are morally distressed.

## Affirm

This second step seeks to affirm moral distress by validating it with others and with the obligations set forth in nursing's professional code (ANA, 2001). Nurses' primary obligations are to the patients; respect is demonstrated by attending to the patients' (and family) needs. In extreme circumstances, such as when a nurse feels that a family's persistent requests to preserve a terminally ill patient's life is prolonging dying and not in the patient's best interests, moral distress can be profound. The goal of this second step is to set aside time and effort to deal with your moral distress. Citing Provision 5 of the ANA Code, that nurses are obligated to care for themselves as for others when their physical or mental integrity is at risk, Rushton (2006) states that "without a compassionate response to their own distress, nurses may have a diminished capacity to respond to the suffering and distress of others" (p. 164).

## Assess

The third step is identification of the specific source and severity of the moral distress, such as a specific patient care situation, a unit-based practice, and/or poor interactions with the care team (AACN, 2004b). Distress can be rated on a scale from 0 to 5, where 0 is no distress and 5 is high distress (AACN). Evaluation of readiness and willingness to act, given the risks and benefits, can be facilitated by self-assessment of readiness (which has some similarity to assessment of assertiveness readiness). The readiness items ask about the importance to you of acting to change a situation for you, your colleagues, and the patient and/or family, and your confidence and determination in bringing about the change. Another exercise is construction of a list of the likely benefits and risks associated with the change (AACN).

This step also includes awareness of the skills needed to create a plan of action and how to acquire those skills that are lacking; for example, the ability to verbalize and document the ethical and clinical issue. The goal of this step is readiness to construct a plan of action. If uncertain about whether or not to proceed, "4 Rs" are suggested: **R**elevance (or likely outcome of the action), **R**isk(s) of not acting and likely outcomes affecting the patient and yourself, **R**ewards (imagine feeling good after the change has occurred), and **R**oadblocks (make a specific list and strategy for managing each one) (AACN, 2004b). After this exercise, it is suggested that the self-assessment for readiness to act is repeated.

## Act

The last step is delineation of the strategy that will be used to address the source and substance of the moral distress. The goal of this step is the preservation of integrity and personhood. Preparation of the plan contains two vital elements that are similar to preparation for acting assertively: (a) Create a realistic self-care plan, (b) identify internal and external supports (whom you might want to contact to discuss or describe your plan and get their feedback). The AACN document (2004b) that was the source for this discussion of the 4-As outlines specific strategies that can be taken with regard to patient care, unit-based, and interdisciplinary situations.

Long-term actions should be instituted to monitor the frequency, duration, and types of moral distress experienced by critical care nurses (Rushton, 2006). Data collection should include classification of the ethical principles invoked by the distress or conflict situation; the parties involved; the physical, verbal, and behavioral expression(s) of moral distress; whether and how moral distress affected patient (and family) care, as well as collaborative and collegial practice.

## Root Cause Analysis

Root cause analysis could be useful for understanding the why and how and causal relationships of moral distress with the goal of preventing or reducing its recurrence for the same or similar situations (Rushton, 2006). It is a type of problem solving that goes for the "root cause" of the problem or situation, rather than just attending to its presentation (i.e., symptoms). There are several root cause analysis techniques but all seek solution to the problem, not simply its cause. The basic steps of root cause analysis begin with statement of the problem; followed by data collection; identification of the associated causal factors and relationships; determination of which cause, if removed or altered, is most likely to prevent recurrence of the problem; selection of the solution most likely to be effective and that does not cause other problems; implementation; and observation ("Root Cause," 2008).

## A Model to Analyze an Ethical Dilemma

The 4-component model developed by Fletcher and colleagues (1997) is useful in contributing to the information needs alluded to in the Rest model and more specifically addressed in the AACN model.

- ■ *Fact Pattern:* Collect a broad range of data beginning with the patient's medical condition, prognosis, uncertainties, treatment goals, and recommendations. Contextual factors include the patient's culture, language spoken, lifestyle, education, spiritual beliefs, socieconomics, and family relationship(s). The patient's preferences regarding treatment goals and quality of life, and the patient's capacity for decision making are important, as is the role of the family: for example, their interests and their sense of burden in caring for the patient. Source and content of conflict need to be identified. Interestingly, this section of the model asks if there are any other parties who have not been heard from and if there are institutional or organizational issues that might contribute to the ethical problems (e.g., workload, malpractice fears, treatment withdrawal, etc).
- ■ *Moral Diagnosis:* Reach for an understanding of how the ethical issue (i.e., "moral problem") has been framed by the various parties. It is suggested that the various moral issues should not only be identified but ranked in order of their importance or relevance. Consult the literature for similar cases that might be instrumental in proffering other views and analysis. Acceptable options for resolving the ethical dilemma prepare for the next stage.
- ■ *Goal Setting and Implementation:* This is a time of deliberation, negotiation, and conflict resolution, which, if unsuccessful, could warrant ethics committee review, an ethics consultation, or as a last recourse, judicial review.
- ■ *Evaluation* is both current and retrospective. If the plan is not working, why not? Does the plan need to be modified, based on the observed conditions? Were factors omitted in constructing the plan? Does the patient's care reflect best practices and standards? Retrospectively, the process itself is evaluated with a view to the types of data collected and

how they were used, whether the care the patient received was less than optimal, and whether an opportunity to resolve the ethical issue had been missed. This last stage is somewhat of a jumping-off point for addressing necessary or desirable changes in organizational policy, ethics education, and the practice environment.

## Critical Thinking and Ethical Decision Making

Critical thinking is inseparable from nursing practice. It is a type of problem solving that is purposeful, logical, reflective, and essential for the management of complex dilemmas. As with ethical decision making, it is both a process and an outcome that relies on facts, knowledge, cognitive skills, and creativity. There is a remarkable convergence of critical thinking and ethical decision-making characteristics: being open-minded, truthfulness and transparency, analytic ability, being focused yet open to other ways of knowing, confidence in one's in ability to reflect and reason and to present a cogent explanation and argument (Facione, Sanchez, Facione, & Gainen, 1995; Fletcher et al., 1997; Post et al., 2007; Scheffer & Rubenfeld, 2000).

Critical-thinking skills can be taught, as can ethical decision-making skills, using case study exemplars. For example, "terminal sedation" is inextricable from considerations of the sanctity of life, beneficence, and nonmaleficence. The principle of double effect holds that death pursuant to morphine injection was not killing and was not wrong if death was not intended. The critical argument is that the death of the patient was not the means to the good effect of pain relief. Even if a nurse is quite sure that a terminally ill patient will die shortly after morphine administration, death is not the intention of the medication administration. Argument is sometimes made that "the morality of the action can be distinguished from the blameworthiness of the actor" (Fry & Veatch, 2006, p. 209). The ANA professional code of ethics for nurses (2001) addressed this issue by stating that a nurse is obligated to relieve pain in a dying patient even if the intervention risks quickening death but a nurse cannot—even out of compassion—act with the explicit intent of ending a patient's life. Hence, the ANA "appears" to differentiate between indirect and direct killing and the risk of killing a patient when the intention is to relieve suffering. "The ANA thus supports the double effect position as well as the principle of the sanctity of human life" (Fry & Veatch, p. 210).

## Summary

Preparation and readiness for ethical decision making and the continuous development and sharpening of critical-thinking skills are joint hallmarks of professional competency. Both processes are iterative and evolving as additional information is brought to the dialogue. There are a variety of ethical decision-making models but all share certain elements:

- Facts: obtain and clarify the medical facts and ensure that all parties understand them;
- Options: identify the consequences of each alternative, including doing nothing;

■ Values: identify the values inherent in each option *and* the meaning of those values for *each* participant in the decision.

■ Start with the patient, then move to advance directives (i.e., the patient's authentic voice), then to other decision makers (i.e., substitute judgment, best interest), and as a last resort, the courts (Dubler & Nimmons, 1993).

Because they are with the patient 24/7, critical care nurses are best positioned to describe—and perhaps defend—the patient's capacity to make a health care decision. Critical care nurses can speak to whether or not the patient understands or appreciates the situation, which is a basic tenet of informed consent; whether or not the patient is using his personal framework to process the decision; and whether or not the patient has the ability to communicate his wishes.

The best resolutions to ethical dilemmas are those that begin with patient values, preferences, and wishes, and emerge from dialogue with the patient, proxy, family, and the professionals who care for them. The courts should not become the center and source of ethical decision making and the fact that they often assume this role reflects the failure of health care professionals to anticipate, appreciate, and analyze actual and potential ethical dilemmas. Empowered and educated to articulate and actuate ethical principles, critical care nurses can inform and significantly influence health care practice at the bedside and in the conference room, in the boardroom, and in policy-making venues for critical care of older adults.

# References

American Association of Critical Care Nurses (AACN). (2004a). *Position statement: Moral distress.* Retrieved May 22, 2008, from www.aacn.org/WD/Practice/Docs/Moral_Distress.pdf

American Association of Critical Care Nurses (AACN). (2004b). *The 4As to rise above moral distress.* Retrieved May 22, 2008, from www.aacn.org/WD/Practice/Docs/4As_to_Rise_Above_Moral_Distress.pdf

American Nurses Association (ANA). (2001). *Code of ethics for nurses with interpretive statements.* Washington, DC: Author.

Allen, R. S., DeLaine, S. R., Chaplin, W. F., Marson, D. C., Bourgeois, M. S., Dijkstra, K., et al. (2003). Advance care planning in nursing homes: Correlates of capacity and possession of advance directives. *The Gerontologist, 43*(3), 309–317.

Beauchamp, T. L., & Childress, J. F. (2001). *Principles of bioethics* (5th ed.). New York: Oxford University Press.

Braun, K. L., Pietsch, J. H., & Blanchette, P. L. (2000). *Cultural issues in end-of-life decision making.* Thousand Oaks, CA: Sage.

Bryon, E., de Casterlé, B. D., & Gastmans, C. (2007). Nurses' attitudes towards artificial food or fluid administration in patients with dementia and in terminally ill patients: A review of the literature. *Journal of Medical Ethics, 34,* 431–438.

Cain, E. D., Kim, S. Y., & Karlawish, J. H. (2002). Current state of research on decision-making competence of cognitively impaired elderly persons. *American Journal of Geriatric Psychiatry, 10*(2), 157–165.

Callahan, D. (1999). A miscellany of hard choices. Rationing health care according to age. In J. D. Arras & B. Steinbock (Eds.), *Ethical issues in modern medicine* (5th ed.). Mountain View, CA: Mayfield.

Crow, K., Matheson, L., & Steed, A. (2000). Informed consent and truth-telling. Cultural directions for healthcare providers. *Journal of Nursing Administration, 30,* 148–152.

De Bal, N., Gastmans, C., & Dierckx de Casterlé, B. (2008). Nurses' involvement in the care of patients requesting euthanasia: A review of the literature. *International Journal of Nursing Studies, 45,* 626–644.

Devereaux, A. V., Dichter, J. R., Christian, M. D., Dubler, N. N., Sandrock, C. E., Hick, J. L., et al. (2008). Definitive care for the critically ill during a disaster: A framework for the allocation of scarce resources in mass critical care. *Chest, 133,* 51–66.

Dubler, N. N., & Nimmons, D. (1993). *Ethics on call. Taking charge of life-and-death choices in today's health care system.* New York: Vintage Books.

Facione, P. A., Sanchez, C. A., Facione, N. C., & Gainen, J. (1995). The disposition towards critical thinking. *Journal of General Education, 44*(1), 1–25.

Fletcher, J. C., Hite, C. A., Lombardo, P. A., & Marshall, M. F. (1997). *Introduction to clinical ethics* (2nd ed.). Frederick, MO: University Publishing Group.

Folstein, M., Folstein, S., & McHugh, P. (1975). Mini-Mental State Examination: A practical guide for grading the cognitive state of patients for clinicians. *Journal of Psychiatric Research, 12*(3), 189–198.

Fry, S. V., & Veatch, R. M. (2006). *Case studies in nursing ethics.* Sudbury, MA: Jones and Bartlett.

Gilligan, C. (1982). *In a different voice.* Cambridge, MA: Harvard University Press

Hall, M. A., Ellman, I. M., & Strouse, D. S. (1999). *Health care law and ethics.* St. Paul, MN: West Group.

Huang, Z. B., & Ahronheim, J. C. (2000). Nutrition and hydration in terminally ill patients: An update. *Clinics in Geriatric Medicine, 16*(2), 313–325.

Janssens, U., Dujardin, R., Graf, J., Lepper, W., Ortlepp, J., Merx, M., et al. (2001). Value of SOFA (Sequential Organ Failure Assessment) score and total maximum SOFA score in 812 patients with acute cardiovascular disorders. *Critical Care, 5* (Suppl. 1), 225.

Kapp, M. B., & Mossman, D. (1996). Measuring decisional capacity: Cautions on the construction of a "capacimeter." *Psychology and Public Policy Law, 2,* 73–95.

Karlawish, J. H., Casarett, D. J., James, B. D., Xie, S. X., & Kim, S. Y. (2005). The ability of persons with Alzheimer's Disease (AD) to make a decision about taking an AD treatment. *Neurology, 64*(9), 1514–1519.

Moye, J., Karel, M. J., Gurrera, R. J., & Azar, A. R. (2006). Neuropsychological predictors of decision-making capacity over 9 months in mild-to-moderate dementia. *Journal of General Internal Medicine, 21,* 78–83.

Post, L. F., Blustein, J., & Dubler, N. N. (2007). *Handbook for health care ethics committees.* Baltimore, MD: Johns Hopkins University Press.

Patient Self-Determination Act. (1991). Sec. 4206, 4751 of the Omnibus Reconciliation Act of 1990. Pub L No. 101-508.

President's Commission for the Study of Ethical Problems in Medicine and Biomedical and Behavioral Research. (1982). *Making health care decisions.* Washington, DC: U.S. Government Printing Office.

Rest, J. R. (1986). *Moral development: Advances in research and theory.* New York: Praeger.

Root cause analysis. (2008). Wikipedia. Retrieved August 1, 2008, from http://en.wikipedia.org/wiki/Root_cause_analysis

Rushton, C. H. (2006). Defining and addressing moral distress. Tools for critical care nursing leaders. *AACN Advanced Critical Care, 17*(2), 161–168.

Rushton, C. H., & Penticuff, J. H. (2007). A framework for analysis of ethical dilemmas in critical care nursing. *AACN Advanced Critical Care, 18*(3), 323–328.

Scheffer B. K., & Rubenfeld, M. G. (2000). A consensus statement on critical thinking in nursing. *Journal of Nursing Education, 39,* 352–359.

Tomlinson, J. B., & Brody, H. (1990). Futility and the ethics of resuscitation. *Journal of the American Medical Association, 264,* 1276–1280.

Truog, R. D., Brett, A. S., & Frader, J. (1992). Sounding board: The problem with futility. *New England Journal of Medicine, 362,* 1560–1564.

Volicer, L., & Ganzini, L. (2003). Health professionals: Views on standards for decision-making capacity regarding refusal of medical treatment in mild Alzheimer's disease. *Journal of the American Geriatrics Society, 51*(5), 1270-1274.

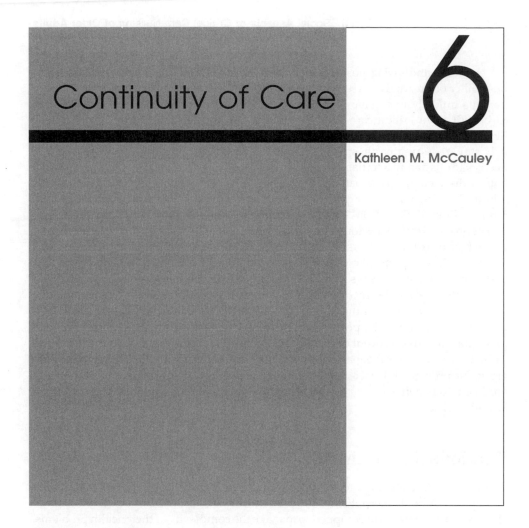

# Continuity of Care

Kathleen M. McCauley

## Introduction

Elders over the age of 65 comprise approximately 50% of patients receiving care in intensive care units (ICUs) (Rockwood et al., 1993; Vosylius, Sipylaite, & Ivaskevicius, 2005) and those over 80 years of age make up 15% of ICU admissions (Rady & Johnson, 2004). Several studies suggest that survival seems to be related to the severity of the underlying illness, length of stay in the ICU, prior need for critical care services, number of comorbidities, and catastrophic conditions such as respiratory failure, rather than age (Fried, 2000; Rockwood et al.; Williams, Dobb, Finn, & Webb, 2005). In other studies, older age, particularly over 75 years of age, carried a significantly greater risk of dying, predominantly as a result of organ dysfunction (Vosylius et al.). For a cohort of older (> 80 years) patients, degree of impairment in functional status prior to admission, defined as "no limitation" through being bedridden on the APACHE II scale (acute physiological chronic health evaluation; Knaus, Zimmerman, Wagner, Draper, & Lawrence, 1981) and the absence of an underlying fatal condition, proved to be the strongest predictors of survival. When contacted on average nearly 2 years following discharge, 80% of these very elderly ICU survivors were living at home and more than 50% reported good functional status (Boumendil et al., 2004).

A factor underlying positive survival data for older critical care patients is the possibility of preadmission selection bias and withholding intensive care services from patients unlikely to survive despite aggressive treatment. Similarly, patients judged to benefit from critical care services in their 80s and 90s may have fewer chronic illnesses (Demoule et al., 2005). In contrast, patients who survive a long, complicated ICU stay, requiring posthospital care in an extended care facility, are more likely to need readmission to a tertiary care hospital. Whether or not readmission is required, half of these complicated patients will die within 1 year of discharge and two thirds within 2 years, with older patients fairing more poorly (Nasraway, Button, Rand, Hudson-Jinks, & Gustafson, 2000). These findings were supported by a study by Rady and Johnson (2004), who found that octogenarians who were able to be discharged home had nearly twice the survival of those requiring extended care.

For elders in particular, clinical deterioration prompting readmission to the ICU and adverse events present serious barriers to return to preillness function. The profile of patients likely to be readmitted, the common types of adverse events, and the outcomes that occur with these patients will be discussed in this chapter. Improved continuity of care has the potential to prevent or detect early the situations likely to precipitate an adverse event or an ICU readmission. Careful attention to the transition from hospital to home is equally important if complications and causes of deterioration are to be prevented. Hence, improvements in care processes to promote continuity are likely to benefit elderly patients who are doing well in addition to those who are at higher risk.

## Readmission to the ICU

In an era of close attention to reducing costs of care, pressure to shorten ICU length of stay (LOS) holds the potential for premature transfer of highly acute patients to care areas where staff is ill equipped to manage the complexity of their health problems. Although premature ICU discharge was felt to be highly related to ICU readmission in 22 to 42% of patients (Rosenberg & Watts, 2000), the problem is much more complex.

It has been well established that ICU readmission is associated with significant increases in overall mortality, compared with outcomes for those who were successfully discharged from the ICU without need for readmission (Campbell, Cook, Adey, & Cuthbertson, 2008; Rosenberg, Hofer, Hayward, Strachan, & Watts, 2001). Although only 6 to 7% of patients on average (range 2.7 to 14%) require readmission, they have a risk of dying while in the hospital that is 2 to 17 times higher than the single ICU admission patients (Alban, Nisim, Ho, Nishi, & Shabot, 2006; Bardell, Legare, Buth, Hirsch, & Ali, 2003; Campbell et al.; Kogan et al., 2003; Metnitz et al., 2003; Rosenberg et al.; Rosenberg & Watts, 2000;). Patients requiring multiple ICU readmissions have the highest mortality rate (Metnitz et al.)

Readmitted patients tend to require much more intense clinical services, including vasoactive medication, mechanical ventilation, and complex intravascular access and monitoring, both during their initial ICU stay and on readmission. The ICU patient particularly at risk for readmission is older, with serious underlying disease, some degree of organ failure requiring greater organ support even on the last day of the initial ICU admission (Metnitz et al.), and was hospitalized for a longer time prior to needing critical care services (Rosenberg & Watts, 2000). These complex and severely ill patients tend to spend more time intubated in the ICU (50 versus 33%), be extubated for a shorter length of time prior to initial ICU discharge (1 versus 2 days on average) than their nonreadmitted counterparts (Metnitz et al., 2003), and have unstable vital signs and low hematocrit at the time of the initial ICU discharge (Rosenberg & Watts, 2000). In studies where severity of overall illness and complexity of physiologic status were measured, the readmitted patients tended to score more poorly on physiologic measures such as the Acute Physiology and Chronic Health Evaluation (APACHE II) (Campbell et al., 2008; Rosenberg & Watts).

The most common causes of readmission are respiratory failure/pneumonia, neurological decompensation, upper gastrointestinal bleeding, sepsis, medication toxicities, and cardiac problems, including arrhythmias and cardiac arrest (Alban et al., 2006; Campbell et al., 2008; Kogan et al., 2003; Rosenberg et al., 2001; Rosenberg & Watts, 2000). These patients are at high risk for hospital-acquired pneumonia because of their inability to clear secretions, have limited ventilatory reserve, and a prolonged hospitalization complicated by multiple comorbid conditions. Length of stay for the entire hospitalization tends to be twice as long for readmitted patients (35–47 days compared with 16 to 21 days) and the LOS for the initial ICU care was on average 0.7 days longer (Rosenberg & Watts).

Nursing and collaborative medical actions to prevent hospital-acquired infections leading to sepsis and pneumonia; careful attention to elders' ability to tolerate pharmacological interventions, including modified dosages and monitoring for interactions; and early detection and management of potentially catastrophic complications are critical in this vulnerable population. A compartmentalized, single-body-system approach to management is especially problematic for these vulnerable elders, who, because of age and multiple comorbid conditions, are far less able to recover from complicated, multiproblem illnesses.

## Adverse Events

Given the severity of underlying disease and risk imposed by poor prehospital functional status and coexisting conditions, identifying deterioration and preventing adverse events becomes even more important in an elder's survival and retention of function. Patients experiencing adverse events tended to be older with worse APACHE II scores on admission to the ICU (Chaboyer, Thalib, Foster, Ball, & Richards, 2008) or within the first 24 hours following ICU discharge (McLaughlin, Leslie, Williams, & Dobbs, 2007). Ineffective fluid management (over- or underhydration), respiratory deterioration, altered neurological status (McLaughlin et al.), hospital-acquired infection, sepsis or injury, and complications such as deep vein thrombosis, myocardial infarction, or cardiac arrest (Chaboyer et al.) were the most common causes of adverse events. Clinical findings found to be highly predictive of an impending event include abnormal serum potassium levels, tachycardia, respiratory rate less than 10 or more than 25 per minute, oxygen saturation less than 90%, decrease in Glasgow coma scale greater than 2, and care needs requiring 1 to 1 nursing presence (Chaboyer et al.).

Events were more likely to occur during the evening or night and in patients discharged from the ICU during those hours; 64% of events were likely to be judged by a review panel as preventable. Examples of preventable events included volume overload and dehydration, blocked tracheostomy tubes, stage III pressure sores, and hypoglycemia (McLaughlin et al., 2007). Factors that contribute to care problems are inadequate monitoring or failure to increase monitoring with early signs of deterioration; discontinued, interrupted care or failure to institute needed care on the general care unit; and failure to summon expert help. It is interesting that McLaughlin et al.'s study was done in a setting with a well-established medical emergency team (MET) and 24-hour coverage by clinical nurse specialists who were charged with identifying patients at risk for deterioration and with advising the nursing staff on proper management. Adverse events may be even more frequent in facilities lacking these supports. Clearly, gaps in continuity of care caused by the provider's lack of knowledge of the patient's specific needs or insufficient clinical judgment skills place elders, in particular, at high risk for preventable deterioration.

Care strategies that support vigilance, continuity, and familiarity with the patient's unique responses are therefore critical to prevention, early detection, and prompt management of complications in their early stages. In particular, critical care nurses must anticipate problems and intervene before they occur. Families must be integrated into care so that their familiarity with the patient's unique responses can inform the nurse's assessment. Communication with all members of the health care team concerning the patient's particular areas of vulnerability should result in a coordinated plan to prevent and/or rapidly manage deterioration. Each day, the team should ask the question, "If this particular patient were to experience significant complications or clinical deterioration, what would be the cause, how would it be manifested, and how can we prevent it?"

## Patient Responses to Transfer From the ICU

Relocation stress, an approved nursing diagnosis, refers to a state in which the person experiences physiological or psychological unrest related to transferring from one care environment to another (Carpenito-Moyer, 2008). The personal impact of this stress is thought to be related to coping resources, the degree of environmental change, level of pain and fatigue that may reduce coping, and disruption in relationships and trust in the health care staff. Transfer from the ICU has been viewed by patients as a positive step toward normalcy or as a loss of needed care and monitoring (McKinney & Deeny, 2002). In a phenomenology study of pre- and post-ICU transfer, interviews with patients aged 42 to 75 who had spent between 4 and 10 days in an ICU revealed that prior to transfer, patients tended to view the move to a general care unit positively (McKinney & Deeny). Patients reflected on their progress toward recovery, desire to move to a more normal life, and praise for the staff. Following transfer, some patients retained positive feelings but physical and psychological symptoms, differences in staffing and attention, and recollection of dreams and memories of events in the ICU placed them at greater need for support.

Odell's (2000) qualitative study of patients following transfer from the ICU supported these concerns. Posttransfer, patients reported feeling helpless, afraid, depressed, and had little recollection of information given to them in the ICU and at the time of transfer. They were content to hand over control to the staff and acceptance of their need to trust the staff was a common feeling. Whether this was the result of patients being poorly prepared for transfer or, despite intensive preparation, they were too ill and frail to take an active role in their recovery could not be determined from this study. Daffurn, Bishop, Hillman, and Bauman (1994) noted that on interview 3 months following an ICU stay, patients were most likely to report residual pain (44%), emotional problems (33%) and feeling tired (26%) (Daffurn et al.).

This vulnerability, coupled with the devastating impact of clinical deterioration leading to readmission to the ICU, presents challenges and opportunities for the health care team. Prevention of adverse events, promoting healing, and preserving function are critical to the elder's survival of a serious illness and require careful attention to continuity of care.

# Enhancing Continuity of Care in the Inpatient Setting

Noting that a systematic transition plan for managing a patient's discharge from the ICU to a general care area is uncommon, Chaboyer, James, and Kendall (2005) suggest that fragmented ICU transition processes stem from lack of feedback to the ICU staff about their patients' progress and needs after transfer, lack of policies governing an effective transition, and inadequate staff education. An example of an effective strategy to improve outcomes by enhanced continuity of care is the multidimensional process-improvement program implemented at Inova Fairfax Hospital in Virginia. Cardiac surgery patients, including elders, were able to be transferred from the ICU to a specialized telemetry unit on the day of surgery without loss of quality through a program that involved all stakeholders in the planning and was pilot tested prior to full implementation. In this program a nurse coordinated care processes between the physicians and staff on both units and detailed, evidence-based clinical protocols guided care. All staff, particularly the telemetry unit nurses, were educated about patients' care needs, quality data were continuously measured and communicated, and problems were promptly identified and resolved. Examples of strategies to ensure quality included use of a critical pathway that outlined key components of care such as extubation timelines, line and catheter discontinuation, ambulation, pain management and antibiotic protocols, pulmonary hygiene, and patient and family education. Deviations from the pathway were documented and addressed. A patient-focused pathway was also used to orient patients to upcoming experiences and integrate their preferences into care (Sakallaris, Halpin, Knapp, & Sheridan, 2000).

This intervention incorporated the actions performed by an ICU liaison or discharge nurse who is charged with supporting patients and families during the transition and serves as a clinical resource for staff on the receiving unit. The nurse in this role tends to have ICU experience, strong skills in collaboration to bring together critical care medicine and nursing expertise, and focuses on empowering the receiving unit staff to manage the patient effectively. Additional research is needed to evaluate the outcomes and cost-effectiveness of this role, but some evidence exists that these nurses have reduced readmissions to the ICU (Chaboyer et al., 2005).

Many organizations have implemented Rapid Response Teams to bring qualified resources to a non-ICU patient's bedside to manage early signs of deterioration; prevent cardiopulmonary arrest; and collaboratively, with the patient's team, get the patient the care needed at the time. The Institute for Health Care Improvement notes that initiatives such as these have been enormously effective in saving lives (www.ihi. org/Programs/Campaign/. Any care provider is encouraged to activate the system when deterioration is detected thereby minimizing failure-to-rescue scenarios and enhancing communication between critical care experts and general care unit providers (Thomas, Force, Rasmussen, Dodd, & Whilden, 2007). Implementation of a critical care outreach team, designed to advise the general care unit staff on the patient's needs for monitoring, laboratory testing, as well as revised medical and nursing management has been shown to decrease readmissions to the ICU and survival to hospital discharge (Ball, Kirkby, & Williams, 2003). These strategies can enhance continuity of care by providing needed care management advice, fill in gaps in knowledge and service, and prevent deterioration.

The success of these programs is grounded in careful planning, diverse strategies to enhance communication, and a commitment to meeting the patient's individual needs. Effective communication and teamwork have also been linked to improved mortality outcomes. In a study comparing perceived quality of team effectiveness in 17 ICUs, it was found that predicted versus actual patient mortality varied according to the quality of team interaction. Comparing actual mortality rates with those predicted by APACHE III scores revealed that outcomes were better than predicted in ICUs where team members perceived the quality of their teamwork to be high. The opposite was true in units with poor perceived teamwork (Wheelan, Burchill, & Tilin, 2003). These findings support prior studies showing similar linkages between quality of team interaction and patient mortality (Baggs, Ryan, Phelps, Richeson, & Johnson, 1992; Knaus, Draper, Wagner, & Zimmerman, 1986).

These findings influenced the strategic action of the American Association of Critical-Care Nurses (AACN) in their development of their Standards for Establishing and Sustaining Healthy Work Environments (AACN, 2005). These six standards and their accompanying critical elements charge nurses and others with transforming their work environments to support and foster excellence in patient care. Four of the standards relate directly to promoting continuity of care and achieving the kind of teamwork that can save lives. In achieving the standards of skilled communication, true collaboration, effective decision making, and authentic leadership an interdisciplinary team will ensure that critical patient information is shared, the input of all providers and the patient and family are heard, and that the authority to make decisions about patient care rests with those with the relevant knowledge and skill. Authentic leaders both at the bedside and in management strive to produce a work environment that promotes accountability and excellent practice. The Standards are listed in Exhibit 6.1. The reader is urged to access the standards at http://www.aacn.org/WD/HWE/Docs/HWEStandards.pdf.

## Enhancing Continuity of Care in the Transition From Hospital to Home

All of these findings support the premise that as health care providers we must manage not only the care in each setting, but also the transition between settings, with much more vigilance. Patients are unprepared for how poorly they will feel physically and psychologically and have limited ability to advocate for themselves. A myriad of connected, complex, yet often preventable problems position elders to experience poor outcomes in the transition from hospital to home. Their primary health problem, coupled with multiple comorbid conditions, preexisting or hospital-generated functional decline, and possible cognitive impairment present a significant challenge to the patient and family support system. A prior pattern of poor health practices and insufficient and ineffective education about postdischarge health management contribute to motivational and knowledge barriers. The inadequacies of the health care system, including communication breakdowns among providers, patient

# Exhibit 6.1

## AACN Standards for Establishing and Sustaining Healthy Work Environments

1. Skilled Communication: Nurses must be as proficient in communication skills as they are in clinical skills.
2. True Collaboration: Nurses must be relentless in pursuing and fostering true collaboration.
3. Effective Decision Making: Nurses must be valued and committed partners in making policy, directing and evaluating clinical care, and leading organizational operations.
4. Appropriate Staffing: Staffing must ensure the effective match between patient needs and nurse competencies.
5. Meaningful Recognition: Nurses must be recognized and must recognize others for the value each brings to the work of the organization.
6. Authentic Leadership: Nurse leaders must fully embrace the imperative of a healthy work environment, authentically live it, and engage others in its achievement.

*Note:* From AACN (2005).

inability to access providers when needed, and limited access to services that would support the patient's self management in the home, further exacerbate an already devastating situation. It is known that without attention to this transition and without appropriate home follow-up elders may fail to report changes in their condition, be unable to manage their treatment plan, and need frequent preventable inpatient care (Naylor, 2003).

## Effective Transitional Care Strategies

A series of randomized controlled trails have consistently demonstrated that advanced practice nurses (APN) coordinating care in the transition from hospital to home improved outcomes at lower cost compared with usual care. The 2-week to 3-month intervention consisted of inpatient team collaboration/discharge planning and postdischarge home visit and/or telephone follow-up. Outcomes included longer time to first readmission or death, reduced number of readmissions and total hospital days, and reduced overall cost for up to 52 weeks of follow-up (Naylor et al., 1994, 1999, 2004; Naylor & McCauley, 1999).

A disease management model in which APNs coordinated follow-up services to improve communication between patients' families and the health care team and support family caregiving processes was tested by Douglas, Daly, Kelley, O'Toole, and Montenegro (2007) in a population of chronically critically ill patients with multiple comorbid conditions. Elders were significantly more likely to require care in extended care facilities after discharge. As compared to the control group, more intervention patients had improved physical-health-related quality of life when patients who died or were lost to follow-up were excluded from the analysis and intervention patients incurred lower care costs related to readmissions. There were no other significant differences between groups (Douglas et al.).

## Specific Interventions to Promote Continuity of Care

Successful ICU transition is likely to be enhanced by actively engaging patients and families in the process, encouraging their input and correcting knowledge deficits, promoting the positive aspects of this transition while being realistic about expectations, and transferring patients during the day whenever possible (Chaboyer et al., 2005). This can be accomplished through ongoing explanations and education, identification of patient's and family's preferences, and encouraging them to express needs and notify staff of new or bothersome symptoms.

Content analysis of clinical notes documenting the care of nurse specialists providing home follow-up to patients after a hospital admission for heart failure revealed that nursing actions focused on assessing and monitoring of patients' physical, psychosocial, and adaptive progress; intervening to manage symptoms via support of patient self-management and provider intervention; and patient-specific strategies to avoid institutionalization, manage their own care, and deal with social isolation and end-of-life issues (Davidson, Paull, Rees, Daly, & Cockburn, 2005). Although the duration of this intervention was unlimited based on patient need and the impact on readmission, cost and patient satisfaction are not reported, the activities of the nurse specialists are similar to those reported by Naylor, Bowles, and Brooten (2000).

Specifically, our research team has found that managing symptoms and comorbid conditions, strengthening the patient/provider relationship, and marshalling family and community resources are critical to a successful transition. Because this model is built on a temporary (up to 3 months) intervention, the APN must focus on strategies to enable the patient, family, and provider to work together effectively to comanage complex health problems. Identification of the patient's specific goals and using those to guide the breadth and intensity of care interventions and to motivate the patient to make needed lifestyle changes has been enormously helpful. In addition, an end-of-intervention summary letter that describes the patient's progress and ongoing problems, identifies caregiver and social support resources, builds on their goals and integrates wishes related to advance directives, was sent to the patient's physician. A summary letter, in language understandable to patients that outlines their ongoing responsibilities and symptoms to report was provided for patients and caregivers (McCauley, Bixby, & Naylor, 2006). Douglas et al. (2007) supplied similar end-of-intervention summary letters to providers.

APNs functioning as transition coaches rather than as health care providers achieved significantly fewer rehospitalizations with lower hospitalization costs for patients with heart failure compared with those patients receiving usual care. Patients and their coaches focused on correcting problems causing the index hospitalization, developed effective strategies for medication use, increased ownership by the patient of health information, and appropriate and ongoing health care provider contact. In particular, patients were taught about signs and symptoms indicating illness exacerbation and actions to take. They used a study-provided personal health record to organize and communicate health care information, improve their ability to manage their illness and to note questions for providers. Through telephone calls and home visits beginning in the hospital and extending through 28 days postdischarge, the coach helped the patient and caregiver build confidence in living with heart failure, actively managing their care, and becoming a partner with their providers (Coleman, Parry, Chalmers, & Min, 2006).

Specialized outpatient clinics and provider practices have been established to provide ongoing management of the patient's physical, psychosocial, and functional health on an ongoing basis. For patients with heart failure, care in an APN-coordinated, multidisciplinary outpatient clinic resulted in significantly fewer hospitalizations and reduced hospital days compared with their hospital usage prior to use of the clinic (Paul, 2000). This same investigator outlined a comprehensive evidence-based educational program for patients with heart failure (Paul, 2008).

Similar themes occur in all of these interventions: correction of patient and caregiver knowledge deficits, overcoming barriers to effective self-management and provider access, practical strategies to empower patients to self-manage their conditions, timely partnering with providers to deal with exacerbations in symptoms, accurate record keeping and communication of patient information, and individualized and patient-centered approaches to management.

## Conclusions and Recommendations

The stakes are high for elders facing an illness requiring acute and critical care services. They are more vulnerable, more likely to have significant comorbid conditions and chronic health problems, and more likely to suffer devastating consequences when adverse events or clinical deterioration interrupt their recovery. Although the transition from the ICU to the general care unit is frequently perceived as positive, many patients continue to experience significant residual symptoms and fatigue that tax their coping abilities (McKinney & Deeny, 2002; Odell, 2000). Without the support of highly experienced nurses to manage the transition and guide clinical judgment decisions, the current reality of general care unit staffing contributes to breaks in continuity of care that result in late detection and missed opportunities for prevention of problems. Similarly, when patients and families are unable to manage the transition back to home, preventable gaps in continuity of care drive patients back to needing acute care services (Naylor et al., 1999, 2004).

Fortunately, evidence-based solutions designed to promote continued implementation of the correct treatment plan, to detect and manage worsening health problems, and to maximize the patient's functional abilities have been identified. Although deterioration is unlikely to be completely preventable, systems such as ICU Liaison Nurses and Rapid Response Teams can be deployed to support local care providers (Chaboyer et al., 2005; Thomas et al., 2007). A variety of effective transitional care models, including nurse-coordinated specialty-based clinics (Paul, 2000) and APNs functioning as providers and coaches have demonstrated their clinical and cost-effective worth (Coleman et al., 2006; Naylor et al., 1999, 2004). What remains to be done is the widespread implementation of these models. This will require partnership with health systems and payers.

Our own research team, under the leadership of Mary Naylor, PhD, RN, FAAN, has successfully partnered with a national insurance company, a national health plan, and a major health system to answer the following questions:

1. Are similar quality and cost outcomes that were possible under the strict confines of research projects achievable in a real-world translation?
2. What are the facilitators and barriers to translating the Naylor Transitional Care Model into the real world of both managed health care and clinical practice?
3. Is an APN required for the intervention? Would an experienced baccalaureate-prepared nurse, perhaps in consultation with an APN, be as effective?

These projects are underway, supported by funds and/or partnerships with the Commonwealth Fund; the Jacob and Valeria Langeloth Foundation; the Aetna Corporation; the Marian S. Ware Alzheimer's' Program; the John A. Hartford Foundation, Inc.; the California HealthCare Foundation; the Gordon and Betty Moore Foundation; and Kaiser Permanente. The University of Pennsylvania Health System has adopted the model in partnership with Independence Blue Cross to improve health outcomes and reduce costs for groups of patients known to be at high risk for rehospitalization. Also, we are in the process of examining the effectiveness of the Naylor Transitional Care Model for elders with cognitive impairment through the support of the National Institute on Aging at the National Institutes of Health (R01AG023116).

All of these partners understand the clinical and economic imperative. Usual care doesn't work. Our population of elders is growing and becoming more complex as we live longer with more chronic health problems, and often with fewer family-caregiving resources. Our health system, focused on providing acute, episodic, often silo-driven care, is not designed to manage complexity, or to support the exquisite communication that our current population of chronically ill elders requires. There is an immediate need to shift the way we think about transitions and to recognize that continuity of care during transitions is cost-effective, high-quality care. The convergence of financial imperatives such as Pay for Performance, enhanced focus on quality and interdisciplinary collaboration, and the emerging demand of an aging population provide important opportunities for nurses to do what we do best.

## Case Study

The following case is an illustration of care coordinated by an Advanced Practice Nurse implementing the Naylor Transitional Care Model (TCM) for an elder with complex medical problems and mild cognitive impairment.

Mrs. V. is an 80-year-old Caucasian female who was admitted to a tertiary care hospital for an exacerbation of heart failure complicated by sudden onset of atrial fibrillation. Her past medical history was significant for a history of hypertension for 40 years, well controlled for the past 5 years, hypercholesterolemia, distant smoking history (30-year pack history, quitting at age 50), myocardial infarction at age 77, with onset of heart failure at age 78. She has had four admissions for heart failure in the past year but this was her first episode of atrial fibrillation. Her medications on admission were furosemide 40 mg bid, enalapril 5 mg bid, simvastatin 20 mg at bedtime, aspirin 82 mg OD, and carvedilol 6.25 mg bid. This medication regimen had been prescribed during her most recent hospitalization, 6 weeks prior to this episode. Although a formal diagnosis of dementia had not been established, she experienced periods of disorientation in the hospital.

She reported feeling more tired than usual and more short of breath with minimal activity for 2–3 days prior to awakening in the early morning, with a feeling that her heart was racing as well as dyspnea. She called her son who lives 20 minutes away. When he arrived she was extremely dyspneic and complaining of chest tightness. He called 911 for emergency assistance and she was transported by ambulance to the emergency department, where presence of atrial fibrillation was confirmed with a ventricular rate of 120–130 beats per minute and her blood pressure was 100/60 mmHg. She received intravenous furosemide and digitalis and was transferred to the Cardiac Care Unit. Anticoagulation therapy with heparin was initiated and amiodarone therapy was begun. Given her probable recent onset of atrial fibrillation and her persistent dyspnea and hypotension an electrical cardioversion with sedation was performed and sinus rhythm restored with heart rate in the 70s. A myocardial infarction was ruled out and after diuresis and further stabilization she was transferred to a telemetry unit. No additional episodes of atrial fibrillation occurred and she was discharged on her admission medications plus amiodarone 200 mg per day. She was instructed to follow up with her cardiologist within a week. Her son noted that she has been unable to pay her bills accurately and on time for the past year and is often forgetful of recent events. He said that she reported taking her medications correctly but admitted that he had never checked further to determine if this was the case.

The Transitional Care Model advanced practice nurse (APN) became involved on day 2 of hospitalization, after the patient had converted back to normal sinus rhythm. His assessment revealed the following problems and needs:

1. Residual heart failure requiring further diuresis and stabilization;
2. Management of the transition from the CCU to the telemetry unit and then to home;
3. Resumption of ambulation and patient participation in self-care activities;
4. Assessment of home situation, sources of support, and patient's and family's ability to manage care responsibilities on discharge, including self-care deficits that may have contributed to hospitalization;
5. Identification of the plan of care for ongoing management of patient's health problems.

The TCM emphasizes the importance of using the patient's goals as a key driver of lifestyle change to support wellness. The APN established a relationship with Mrs. V. and learned that her goals were to remain in her home, caring for herself, and to avoid hospitalizations. She also wanted to be well enough to attend church services.

The APN focused on the following strategies to support achievement of the patient's goals, manage transitions during hospitalization and to home, and prevent adverse events:

1. Establish a collaborative relationship with health care team during hospitalization and with cardiologist and primary care provider postdischarge.
2. Ensure that all pertinent patient information, preferences, and goals were accurately communicated to the health care team on the telemetry unit and to the cardiologist and primary care physician postdischarge.
3. Evaluate the patient's response to diuresis with gradual reduction in symptoms.
4. Work with the patient's primary nurse on the telemetry unit to enable the patient to resume self-care activity, including ambulation and activities of daily living.
5. Assess cognitive function, collaborate with health care team to minimize causes of delirium such as dehydration, electrolyte imbalance, and sleep deprivation.

6. Establish a relationship with the patient's son and develop a plan for home visits postdischarge. The nurse discussed the home environment with the son and determined that with APN home visits and the son's support, the patient could safely return home.
7. Ensure that patient was discharged with correct prescriptions and appointments for follow-up care.

There were no further episodes of atrial fibrillation or disorientation once the patient was transferred to the telemetry unit. The patient was discharged home 5 days after admission. The APN visited her at home within 24 hours of discharge and performed a home assessment focusing on safety factors, medication adherence, and sodium restriction. From the volume of medications in the home and the fill date of the prescriptions, the APN determined that the patient had not been taking medications as prescribed. She admitted that she frequently forgot to take her medications and thought that when she felt well she could stop taking them. The APN related medication adherence to symptom reduction and being able to live successfully in her home alone, with her son's frequent support. The patient's son obtained her prescriptions from the pharmacy and the APN determined that they coincided with the plan of care on discharge. The APN gave the patient a medication organizer and taught the son to fill it. The son agreed to call his mother in the morning and evening to remind her to take her medications. The APN also assessed food in the home, taught Mrs. V. and her son about sodium restriction, reading labels, and discussed meal-preparation strategies and nutrition. The APN related all of these lifestyle changes to reduced symptoms and the goal of staying in her home.

A key component of the TCM is the APN, with the patient's permission, accompanying the patient to physician office visits. The patient, her son, and the APN met with the cardiologist and reviewed her health status, the purpose of current therapy, and plans for future treatment. The cardiologist planned to increase the dose of carvedilol once the patient stabilized further and welcomed the APN's support in managing that transition. They also discussed implementing a home exercise program consisting of walking within her house and eventually outside. They all acknowledged her goal of going to church and recognized the need to increase her walking tolerance to accomplish this.

The APN also worked with the patient and her son to recognize symptom status change and to report deterioration promptly. They developed a written general health plan, including medications, exercise, rest periods, and diet. They also agreed on a "911" plan to guide the patient in identifying and reporting changes in symptomatology. The goal was to prevent rehospitalization by intervening at the beginning of deterioration.

The patient was discharged from the TCM care model after 8 weeks of home visits. Total visits: hospital = 3; home = 7 plus 5 telephone calls; MD office visit = 1. The APN wrote a letter to the patient summarizing her health problems, treatment, and self-care activities. He also wrote to the cardiologist summarizing the TCM intervention, the patient's status in self-care and symptom management at the time of TCM discharge, and recommendations for ongoing management.

## Outcomes Achieved

1. Patient's son learned to fill the medication organizer accurately and worked with a local pharmacy to ensure supply of medications. He called her twice per day and visited once or twice a week.
2. Her carvedilol was successfully increased to 12.5 mg bid and amiodarone was discontinued with no recurrence of atrial fibrillation.
3. She stopped cooking with salt, learned to avoid salty foods, and substituted frozen for canned vegetables.
4. Her exercise tolerance increased so that she was able to do light housekeeping, cooking, and walk outside daily. By 8 weeks postdischarge, she accompanied her son and his family to church.
5. Her cognitive function stabilized with no further episodes of disorientation, but she still needed assistance with bill paying, financial decisions, and managing her home.
6. There were no further hospitalizations at 52 weeks of follow-up.

# References

Alban, R. F., Nisim, A. A., Ho, J., Nishi, G. K., & Shabot, M. M. (2006). Readmission to surgical intensive care increases severity-adjusted patient mortality. *Journal of Trauma, 60*(5), 1027–1031.

American Association of Critical-Care Nurses. (2005). AACN Standards for establishing and sustaining healthy work environments: A journey to excellence. *American Journal of Critical Care, 14*(3), 187–197.

Ball, C., Kirkby, M., & Williams, S. (2003). Effect of the critical care outreach team on patient survival to discharge from hospital and readmission to critical care: Non-randomized population based study. *BMJ, 327*(7422), 1014–1017.

Baggs, J. G., Ryan, S. A., Phelps, C. E., Richeson, J. F., & Johnson, J. E. (1992). The association between interdisciplinary collaboration and patient outcomes in a medical intensive care unit. *Heart & Lung, 21*(1), 18–24.

Bardell, T., Legare, J. F., Buth, K .J., Hirsch, G. M., & Ali, I. S. (2003). ICU readmission after cardiac surgery. *European Journal of Cardio-thoracic Surgery, 23*, 354–359.

Boumendil, A., Maury, E., Reinhard, I., Luquel, L., Offenstadt, G., & Guidet, B. (2004). Prognosis of patients aged 80 years and over admitted in medical intensive care unit. *Intensive Care Medicine, 30*(4), 647–654.

Campbell, A. J., Cook, J. A., Adey, G., & Cuthbertson, B. H. (2008). Predicting death and readmission after intensive care discharge. *British Journal of Anaesthesia, 100*(5), 656–662.

Carpenito-Moyer, L. J. (Ed.). (2008*). Nursing diagnosis: Application to clinical practice* (12th ed., pp. 512–521). Philadelphia: Lippincott Williams & Wilkins.

Chaboyer, W., James, H., & Kendall, M. (2005). Transitional care after the intensive care unit: Current trends and future directions. *Critical Care Nurse, 25*(3), 16–28.

Chaboyer, W., Thalib, L., Foster, M., Ball, C., & Richards, B. (2008). Predictors of adverse events in patients after discharge from the intensive care unit. *American Journal of Critical Care, 17*(3), 255–263.

Coleman, E. A., Parry, C., Chalmers, S., & Min, S. J. (2006). The care transitions intervention: Results of a randomized controlled trial. *Archives of Internal Medicine, 166*(17), 1822–1828.

Daffurn, K., Bishop, G. F., Hillman, K. M., & Bauman, A. (1994). Problems following discharge after intensive care. *Intensive & Critical Care Nursing, 10*(4), 244–251.

Davidson, P., Paull, G., Rees, D., Daly, J., & Cockburn, J. (2005). Activities of home-based heart failure nurse specialists: A modified narrative analysis. *American Journal of Critical Care, 14*(5), 426–433.

Demoule, A., Cracco, C., Lefort, Y., Ray, P., Derenne, J. P., & Similowski, T. (2005). Patients aged 90 years or older in the intensive care unit. *Journal of Gerontology, 60*(1), 129–132.

Douglas, S. L., Daly, B. J., Kelley, C. G., O'Toole, E., & Montenegro, H. (2007). Chronically critically ill patients: Health-related quality of life and resource use after a disease management intervention. *American Journal of Critical Care, 16*(5), 447–457.

Fried, L. P. (2000). Epidemiology of aging. *Epidemiologic Reviews, 22*(1), 95–106.

Institue for Healthcare Improvement. (2006). *Protecting 5 million lives from harm.* Retrieved on September 9, 2009, from http://www.ihi.org/IHI/Programs/Campaign/

Knaus, W. A., Draper, E. A., Wagner, D. P., & Zimmerman, J. E. (1986). An evaluation of outcomes from intensive care in major medical centers. *Annals of Internal Medicine, 104,* 410–418.

Knaus, W. A., Zimmerman, J. E., Wagner, D. P., Draper, E. A., & Lawrence, J. E. (1981). APACHE: Acute physiology and chronic health evaluation: A physiologically based classification system. *Critical Care Medicine, 9,* 591–597.

Kogan, A., Cohen, J., Raanani, E., Sahar, G., Orlov, B., Singer, P., & Vidne, B. A. (2003). Readmission to the intensive care unit after "fast track" cardiac surgery: Risk factors and outcomes. *Annals of Thoracic Surgery, 76,* 503–507.

McCauley, K. M., Bixby, M. B., & Naylor, M. D. (2006). Advanced practice nurse strategies to improve outcomes and reduce cost in elders with heart failure. *Disease Management, 9*(5), 302–310.

McKinney, A. A., & Deeny, P. (2002). Leaving the intensive care unit: A phenomenological study of the patients' experience. *Intensive & Critical Care Nursing, 18*(6), 320–331.

McLaughlin, N., Leslie, G. D., Williams, T. A., & Dobbs, G. J. (2007). Examining the occurrence of adverse events within 72 hours of discharge from the intensive care unit. *Anaesthesia & Intensive Care, 35*(4), 486–493.

Metnitz, P. G., Fieux, F., Jordan, B., Lang, T., Moreno, R., & Gall, J. R. (2003). Critically ill patients readmitted to intensive care units lessons to learn? *Intensive Care Medicine, 29,* 241–248.

Nasraway, S. A., Button, G. J., Rand, W. M., Hudson-Jinks, T., & Gustafson, M. (2000). Survivors of catastrophic illness: Outcome after direct transfer from intensive care to extended care facilities. *Critical Care Medicine, 28*(1), 19–25.

Naylor, M. D. (2003). Transitional care of older adults. In J. J. Fitzpatrick, P. G. Archibold, & B. Stewart (Eds.), *Annual review of nursing research* (Vol. 20, pp. 127–147). New York: Springer Publishing Company.

Naylor, M. D., Bowles, K. H., & Brooten, D. (2000). Patient problems and advanced practice nurse interventions during transitional care. *Public Health Nursing, 12,* 94–102.

Naylor, M. D., Brooten, D. A., Campbell, R., Jacobsen, B. S., Mezey, M. D., Pauly, M. V., et al. (1999). Comprehensive discharge planning and home follow-up of hospitalized elders: A randomized clinical trial. *Journal of the American Medical Association, 281*(7), 613–620.

Naylor, M. D., Brooten, D. A., Campbell, R. L., Maislin, G., McCauley, K. M., & Schwartz, J. S. (2004). Transitional care of older adults hospitalized with heart failure: A randomized, controlled trial. *Journal of the American Geriatrics Society, 52*(5), 675–684.

Naylor, M. D., Brooten, D. A., Jones, R., Lavizzo-Mourey, R., Mezey, M., & Pauly, M. (1994). Comprehensive discharge planning for the hospitalized elderly: A randomized clinical trial. *Annals of Internal Medicine, 120*(12), 999–1006.

Naylor, M. D., & McCauley, K. M. (1999). The effects of a discharge planning and home follow-up intervention on elders hospitalized with common medical and surgical cardiac conditions. *Journal of Cardiovascular Nursing, 14*(1), 44–54.

Odell, M. (2000). The patient's thoughts and feelings about their transfer from intensive care to the general ward. *Journal of Advanced Nursing, 31*(2), 322–329.

Paul, S. (2000). Impact of a nurse managed heart failure clinic: A pilot study. *American Journal of Critical Care, 9*(2), 140–146.

Paul, S. (2008). Hospital discharge education for patients with heart failure: What really works and what is the evidence? *Critical Care Nurse, 28*(2), 66–82.

Rady, M. Y., & Johnson, D. J. (2004). Hospital discharge to care facility: A patient-centered outcome for the evaluation of intensive care for octogenarians. *Chest, 126*(5), 1583–1591.

Rockwood, K., Noseworthy, T. W., Gibney, R. T., Konopad, E., Shustack, A., Stollery, D., et al. (1993). One-year outcome of elderly and young patients admitted to intensive care units. *Critical Care Medicine, 21*(5), 687–691.

Rosenberg, A. L., Hofer, T. P., Hayward, R. A., Strachan, C., & Watts, C. M. (2001). Who bounces back? Physiologic and other predictors of intensive care unit readmission. *Critical Care Medicine, 29*(3), 511–518.

Rosenberg, A. L., & Watts, C. (2000). Patients readmitted to ICUs: A systematic review of risk factors and outcomes. *Chest, 118,* 492–502.

Sakallaris, B. R., Halpin, L. S., Knapp, M., & Sheridan, M. J. (2000). Sameday transfer of patients to the cardiac telemetry unit after surgery: The rapid after bypass back into telemetry (RABBIT) program. *Critical Care Nurse, 20*(2), 50–55, 59–63, 65–68.

Thomas, K., Force, M. V., Rasmussen, D., Dodd, D., & Whilden, S. (2007). Rapid response team challenges, solutions, benefits. *Critical Care Nurse, 27*(1), 20–27.

Vosylius, S., Sipylaite, J., & Ivaskevicius, J. (2005). Determinants of outcome in elderly patients admitted to the intensive care unit. *Age & Ageing, 34*(2), 157–162.

Wheelan, S. A., Burchill, C. N., & Tilin, F. (2003). The link between teamwork and patients' outcomes in intensive care units. *American Journal of Critical Care, 12*(6), 527–534.

Williams, T. A., Dobb, G. J., Finn, J. C., & Webb, S. A. (2005). Long-term survival from intensive care: A review. *Intensive Care Medicine, 31*(10), 1306–1315.

# Family Responses to Critical Care of the Older Adult

# 7

Jane S. Leske

## Case Study

The electronic doors of the regional trauma center's entrance swung open and Mrs. B., along with a neighbor who drove her, hurried in. Earlier she was telephoned by the State Police Department and informed that her 78-year old husband had survived a head-on collision with another car and was being airlifted by Flight for Life to the trauma center. Mr. B.'s fishing companion and best friend, Mr. K., was pronounced dead at the scene along with the two people in the other car, which suddenly veered into their congested lane of early-morning traffic. Mrs. B., aged 76, went to the information desk to ask the condition of her husband and when she could see him. Mrs. B. found herself overwhelmed and unable to locate her insurance information or complete the admission forms. She was directed to the waiting room where the initial minutes seemed like hours and the hours seemed like days. Soon she was joined by another friend as the health care team worked vigorously to save Mr. B.'s life. They waited 2 hours before being notified that Mr. B. was being taken to the operating room and then would be admitted to the surgical intensive care unit (SICU). The next few days would determine his chances for survival. As they waited, there were a few more Flight for Life admissions; a heart attack, another motor vehicle crash, and a fall were the worst of them. The admission of each patient brought other distraught family members to the waiting room. Mrs. B. was not alone.

## Introduction

A discussion of the situation just described will exemplify that the critical care experience takes place within the context of the family. Family-centered critical care recognizes the positive role of the family in the health and rehabilitation of the patient (Auerbach, Kiesler, Wartella, Rausch, Ward, & Ivatury, 2005; Davidson et al., 2007; Institute for Family-Centered Care, 1999; Leske & Pasquale, 2007; Medina, 2005; Webster & Johnson, 2007). Previous research suggests that positive family outcomes play an important role in enhancing patient outcomes in critical care (Azoulay et al., 2001; DeGeneffe & Lynch, 2006; Leske & Jiricka, 1998; Paparrigopoulous et al., 2006; Pochard et al., 2005). Nowhere is the need for family-centered care greater than with critically ill older adult patients (Davidson et al., 2007; Leske & Heidrich, 1996). However, existing methods of care delivery do not adequately address the complex needs of families that need to be addressed to foster positive family outcomes during the critical care period (Davidson et al., 2007; Leske & Pasquale, 2007).

## Family Members of Older Adults

The Institute of Medicine (IOM) strongly recommends a health-care system that supports family members (IOM, 2001). A major assumption of family-centered critical care is that family members, as well as patients, are affected by critical illness and in need of care. But what if the patient is an older adult? What are the unique characteristics of the aged population that need to be considered in providing nursing care to families? What are some areas for family assessment and intervention? What is the impact of critical care on the family?

The family of the older adult can function as a source of support for the patient and as a resource for the nursing staff (Eggenberger & Nelms, 2007; Jacelon, 2006; Maxwell, Stuenkel, & Saylor, 2007). The older adult spouse, adult children, aged siblings, grandchildren, great-grandchildren, and other family members and friends all play unique roles during a critical illness and ultimately in the treatment, rehabilitation, and discharge of the older adult patient. Hospitalization for a critical illness can disrupt even the most highly organized and functional family (Auerbach et al., 2005; Azoulay et al., 2005; Eggenberger & Nelms, 2007). Assessment and interventions with family members of aged patients require consideration of the questions posed earlier.

Although continuing knowledge is being obtained about the physiology of aging and treatment modalities in advanced age, little research has been conducted in the area of family members of older adults who are critically ill. Little is known about how the critical care experience is interpreted by middle-aged or aged family members. However, nurses need to understand the family of a critically ill older adult patient to provide optimal, holistic, and evidence-based care.

This chapter uses a bidirectional approach to family care. This approach advises clinicians to recognize the impact that families have on the patient and the effect older adults have on their families. The contents of this chapter will focus on ways to identify and organize the contribution of family members to optimal outcomes for geriatric patients, as well as ways to: (a) conduct family assessments, (b) provide family interventions, (c) apply selected family theories, and (d) understand the impact of critical illness on the family.

## Demographic Trends

People who are over 65 years of age are the fastest growing segment of the U.S. population (Marik, 2006). During the 20th century, the number of persons over age 65 increased by approximately 1,000%, from 3.1 million (1 in every 25 Americans) in 1990 to 35 million (one in eight) in 2000 (U.S. Census Bureau, 2000). By virtue of living longer, increasing numbers of older adults are being admitted to critical care and, more important for this chapter, these patients can be expected to have other family members involved in their care. Older adult patients account for 24–52% of intensive care unit (ICU) admissions and almost 60% of ICU days (Suresh, Kupfer, & Tessler, 1999).

Managing family responses to critical illness involves an understanding of the changing demographics of our society. The first of the baby boomers, approximately 2.9 million people, celebrated their 60th birthdays in 2006. A substantial increase in the number of older adults will occur from 2010 to 2030 after the first baby boomers turn 65 in 2011. By 2030, this age group is anticipated to represent 72 million people, or 20% of the total U.S. population (He, Sengupta, Velkoff, & Debarros, 2005).

## General Needs of Family Members After Critical Illness

Numerous studies have been conducted to identify various needs of families when one member was hospitalized in a critical care unit (Azoulay et al., 2001; Fry & Warren, 2007; Leske & Pasquale, 2007; Maxwell et al., 2007; Verhaeghe, Defloor, van Zuuren, Duijnstee, & Grypdonck, 2005; Walters, 1995). Most results are based on data obtained from the Critical Care Family Needs Inventory (CCFNI) or a researcher-modified version of this instrument. The CCFNI consists of 45 need statements that are to be rated on a scale of (1) not important to (4) very important by family members. The needs have been identified in a variety of patient populations, including cardiac surgery, terminal illness, trauma, spinal cord injury, burns, and general critical care patients. Although families have many needs, five main areas of concern repeatedly arise: families place the utmost importance on receiving assurance, remaining near the critically ill person, receiving information, being comfortable, and having support (Leske, 1991, 1992a).

All of these needs appear universal and are not associated with age, gender, relationship to patient, prior critical care experience, or patient medical diagnosis, at least, during the first few days of the critical care experience (Leske, 1992b). Research results also show some inconsistencies among perceptions of patients, families, and health care professionals about the importance of family needs. Family members tend to rate needs as more important than nurses do. Similarly, marked disagreement has been found between family members and nurses about how well needs are met. The obvious conclusion is that the family members perception of needs ought to be assessed for an effective plan of care to be developed. It is the individualizing of interventions to meet these needs that require age-specific considerations.

Assurance reflects the family's need to hope for a desired outcome, part of which is based on their confidence and trust in the health care system. Family's rate assurance needs as very important across numerous studies. Families report a need for reassurance that the best possible care is being provided to the patient. Families want to be assured that the hospital cares about the patient and that the patient will be cared for even when the family leaves. Assurance is one category of family needs that, if perceived as supplied, can alleviate family stress and promote an accurate appraisal of the situation.

Family members' need for personal contact and to remain physically and emotionally close to the critically ill person also is important. In addition, family visitation in the critical care area may facilitate psychological recovery of the patient (Davidson et al., 2007; Gonzalez, Carroll, Elliot, Fitzgerald, & Vallent, 2004; Redekopp & Leske, 2007). Family stress is often exacerbated by the physical separation from their family member (Leske, 1992a, 1998, 2000). When families are physically separated behind the closed doors of critical care areas, they often fear the worst. Open versus closed visitation remains an ongoing clinical debate but flexible, individualized, and contracted visitation is effective in meeting family needs (Davidson et al., 2007; Gonzalez et al., 2004; Mendonca & Warren, 1998; Redekopp & Leske, 2007). This debate does require further discussion. There currently is a gap in knowledge about the frequency and duration of visits by family members and the effect of such visits on patient outcomes. Recent research indicates that about 25% of patients have no visitors and most of these patients were older adults (Eriksson & Bergbom, 2007). Older adult patients may have a greater need for caring relationships and discharge planning from health care professionals.

Following initial notification of a life-threatening illness, all families need to have consistent and realistic information about the ill member. Families want information about the condition, prognosis, progress, and comfort of their family member offered at a level they can understand (Lee & Lau, 2003; Leske & Pasquale, 2007; Mendonca & Warren, 1998). They want information imparted with openness to questions, a caring attitude, honesty, acceptance, and respect (Auerbach et al., 2005; Azoulay et al., 2005; Leske & Pasquale, 2007). This tremendous need for information is most prevalent in the initial critical care period (Azoulay et al., 2005; Henneman, McKenzie, & Dewa, 1992; Lautrette et al., 2007; Leske & Pasquale, 2007). However, it is this need for information that is most often left unmet by health professionals (Leske, 1992a, 1992b; Mendonca & Warren, 1998). Unmet family needs manifest themselves in issues regarding dissatisfaction with patient care. Risk-management literature indicates that in situations in which the health care professional has provided poor information or not been available families are more apt to sue (Beckman, Markakis, Suchman, & Franken, 1994; Duclos et al., 2005). Structured family informational interventions: (a) decrease family stress, (b) increase family satisfaction, (c) help family members accurately appraise the situation and make informed decisions, (d) help family members perceive some control over the situation and plan realistic coping strategies, and (e) increase family understanding of the patient's condition (Azoulay et al., 2005; Chien, Chiu, Lam, & Ip, 2005; Lee & Lau, 2003; Leske & Pasquale, 2007).

In addition, personal comforts allow family members to remain near the ill member for extensive periods of time. Personal comforts include comfortable waiting-room facilities, telephones, bathrooms, and food (Rashid, 2007). Family members usually are not concerned about their own personal needs during the initial critical illness experiences. However, if family members are to remain a source of support for the patient, they must receive adequate rest, nutrition, hydration, and personal hygiene.

Supportive interventions have been developed to help families deal with the stress after critical illness (Leske & Pasquale, 2007; Vandell-Walker, Jensen, & Oberle, 2007). These interventions allow participants to share common experiences, express common concerns, and foster a sense of hope (Davidson et al., 2007). Early interventions in critical care to assist families in tapping their own resources, empowering them to understand the current situation, mitigating the negative effects of the critical care experience, and supporting coping mechanisms need to be based on using family strengths within a collaborative practice model (Leske & Pasquale, 2007; Vandell-Walker et al., 2007).

It is important to recognize that the needs of the older critical care patient and the needs of the family member, particularly an older adult's spouse, may conflict. For example, confusion and agitation are common but distressing sequellae of acute illness and/or admission to critical care for older patients. Estimates of the incidence of acute confusion range from 24% to 80% of all hospitalized older adult patients (Foreman, 1989). The downward trajectory into acute confusion is often viewed as a normal progression of events, and the patient is allowed to move through this decline without benefit of intervention. Prompt intervention is essential because of the increase morbidity and mortality associated with untreated acute confusional states (Francis & Kapoor, 1992).

It is recommended that history of confusion be sought in all older adult patients. One way to minimize acute confusion is to have familiar persons in the critical care environment. The older adult spouse may be asked or know from experience that staying with the patient will help reduce these symptoms. (Juneau, 1996; Tolley & Prevost, 1997). Yet that same spouse, because of his or her age, may be highly fatigued and sensitive to the same environmental stressors, such as sensory overload, as the patient and in need of rest and time away from the hospital to maintain health. The role of the nurse as patient and family advocate is important in this situation.

## Collaboration in Critical Care

Without the synchronous, ongoing collaboration among health professionals, family needs cannot be optimally satisfied within the complexities of today's health care system (AACN, 2005; Tilden, Tolle, Nelson, Thompson, & Eggman, 1999). Multidisciplinary collaboration is based on interaction among health professionals that creates an optimal environment for the exchange of knowledge in delivering quality health care (AACN, 2005; Baggs et al. 1997; Wheelan, Burchill, & Tilan, 2003). Collaboration among health professionals results in shorter patient hospital days despite higher patient acuity, lower mortality rates, greater staff and family satisfaction, and overall cost containment (Baggs et al., 1997; Wheelan, Burchill, & Tilan, 2003). Other researchers report that collaboration is important in achieving optimal patient outcomes (Baggs et al., 1997; Wheelan, Burchill, & Tilan, 2003). These studies emphasize the importance of the "process" of care.

The family is seen as the primary partner in any collaborative venture (American Association of Critical-Care Nurses [AACN], 2005; Davidson et al., 2007; Institute for Family-Centered Care, 1999). This implies sharing information, communication, and equal participation in decision-making (Tilden et al., 1999; Williams, 2005). The beneficial effects of health professional-family collaboration are documented in the literature (Tilden et al., 1999; Williams, 2005). However, lack of collaboration among health professionals increases family stress, reduces satisfaction, and perpetuates a lack of understanding, producing less than optimal family outcomes (DeGeneffe & Lynch, 2006; Williams, 2005).

## Meeting Family Needs

The obvious role of the critical care nurse is to manage the physiological crisis of the patient. Keeping up with procedures and the technological explosion is one explanation for the lack of nursing intervention with families. Several factors may serve to deter nurses from including families in the domain of care. Nurses may be rewarded for completing tasks, carrying out the medical regimen, learning new technology, and in doing so, keeping the unit running smoothly. On the other hand, care that is rendered to the family is not as easily recognizable, and thus may not be fostered. Many nurses do not perceive themselves as qualified or knowledgeable enough to provide family care. However, family assessment and intervention is a key element of holistic care. It cannot be emphasized enough that a nurse cannot talk to the family too much! To determine appropriate and supportive interventions, nurses must first accurately assess family members. Given prior evidence that meeting family needs can reduce family stress, the question arises: How do nurses intervene to meet family needs to promote optimal family health and coping during critical illness, especially when the patients are older adults?

### Understanding Family Goals

Integral to intervening to meet family needs is recognizing the goals of any family during the critical care experience (Rushton, Reina, & Reina, 2007). Families experiencing a critical illness are confronted with several tasks that may differ depending on the stage of the family life cycle, as well as needs for assurance, visitation, information, comfort, and support (Leske, 1992a). These tasks or goals pertain to aged family members as well. Goals for family life-cycle stage include dealing with the critical illness of a parent or spouse. Some family goals for meeting assurance needs include developing confidence and trust in the health care team, keeping or redefining hope, and managing discouraging or dreadful news. Family goals for visitation needs consist of maintaining familial relationships, networking with the health care team, and participating in patient care planning. Learning what needs to be known and balancing understanding with information overload, making decisions, and understanding the hospital environment are family goals for meeting information needs. An additional family goal is to balance work, home, and hospital activities while taking care of their personal needs. Family goals for meeting support needs include handling problems that arise, seeking or accepting assistance, and preparing for the role changes with an uncertain future. When the family members are older adults, there may be a tendency not to involve them fully in formulating plans of care or to adequately address their unique goals. However, standards of practice state that nurses continually evaluate family responses to interventions to determine progress toward goal attainment (American Nurses Association, 2001).

## Areas for Family Assessment

Assessment is the act of viewing the family situation from a database to identify specific areas for intervention. The focus of the nurses' initial interaction with the family is to assess the initial response to and understanding of the critical illness situation.

Getting back to our case study: The charge nurse found Mrs. B. in a state of shock, huddled together with her friends in the crowded SICU waiting room. The nurse introduced herself and said she wanted to be of help but first needed to inquire about Mr. B.'s condition. She also asked Mrs. B. if any other family members needed to be notified. The nurse escorted Mrs. B. to a more private waiting area, instructed her on how to make "outside" telephone calls, and said she would return in 30 minutes.

### Initial Family Contact

Initial contact with family members is very important because it sets the foundation for a trusting relationship between the nurses and family (Bouley, von Hofe, & Blatt, 1994; Rushton et al., 2007). Ideally nurse–family contact is initiated as soon as possible after the critical care admission. Most families need immediate and tangible information to balance their acute state of uncertainty. Allowing a family to wait without any knowledge about the situation conveys a blatant lack of respect for any family's value and dignity. Early contact has been reported to reduce family stress, anxiety, and uncertainty (Leske & Heidrich, 1996). Acknowledgment of feelings, such as "It is very difficult to wait," communicates support and conveys to the family that their situation is recognized. The knowledge that someone else is empathetic is comforting to most family members. It also is important to make explicit to the family what they can expect in regard to frequency of communication, sharing of "bad" news, and discussing aspects of treatment (Rushton et al., 2007). Unspoken expectations about the frequency of communication with health care professionals can create opportunities for distrust.

Nurses should be prepared for a variety of responses such as crying, anger, hysteria, frustration, impatience, and even withdrawal. However, initial responses from aged family members may be difficult to predict. Today's cohort of older adults was brought up in an era in which displaying emotions or asking for help or further information was considered unacceptable. The nurse may need to anticipate the concerns of older adult persons and not assume that silence or acquiescence means that there are no problems. The nurse focuses on the immediate problems related to the critical care experience and encourages the family members to do likewise. It is important to encourage verbalization of feelings and perceptions. Meeting in an area that provides privacy and is separate from the general waiting room is conducive to a productive initial family meeting.

## Case Study

When the nurse returned, Mrs. B. was provided information about Mr. B.'s condition. He was being transferred to the SICU within the next 2 hours. The nurse assured Mrs.

B. that the best possible care was being given and went on to explain what was happening. She explained what Mr. B. would "look like" and "all the tubes" in understandable terms. The nurse attempted to answer questions honestly. The one question Mrs. B. asked, "Was Mr. B. going to live?" was too premature to answer, and the nurse gave her an honest response. After an hour of discussion, questioning, worry, and seeking some explanations, Mrs. B. was beginning to realize that her husband was gravely injured. The charge nurse introduced Mrs. B. to the nurse who would be caring for Mr. B. The charge nurse told Mrs. B. that she would be back in another hour to talk to her some more.

## Gathering the Family Database

The family database provides the information on which nursing diagnoses and interventions are based. Obtaining information that includes family roles and relationships can facilitate gathering a family database. The family assessment lays the foundations for future planning. The information helps align family expectations with interventions to promote satisfaction with care. Questions to consider for the family database include: What does the family need most? Are there other health care professionals who should be consulted? In the process of gathering such data, families will ask fundamental questions that need to be addressed: "What happened?" "How did it happen? Why?" Because the admission to critical care is such a stressful time for the family, the nurse may not be able to gather all the family information during the initial interview. Information can be easily added to the family profile following each subsequent family interview.

When gathering information about aged family members, a number of factors need to be considered. These include: What is the meaning of the critical illness; how do they cope; what are the family resources; health of the older person; closeness (physical and emotional) of other family members, particularly siblings and adult children; role of the older adult in the family, particularly in the case of spouses; living arrangements of the patient; and who makes treatment decisions.

## Identify Appraisal or Meaning of Critical Illness

First, the family must formulate an initial response to the illness by defining the threat, impact, and experience. Families may need assistance in defining this threat in a realistic way, or they may need the nurse to help correct any misperceptions about the situation. On the other hand, nurses need to understand the family's perception and definition of the illness. This is the root of many of the dilemmas concerning decision making for the frail, older adult patient. Stereotypes and lack of information about the health, emotional responses, and family relationships of the older family members can interfere with adequate assessment and intervention with the family.

Health professionals often assume that older adults prefer quality of life over quantity, but that is not always the case, even for the very old. Many do prefer quality to quantity and would choose less invasive procedures if they were critically ill. Some, however, prefer quantity of life in their current state of health. Unfortunately, neither health professionals nor family members, in one study, could accurately predict the patient's preference (Tsevat et al., 1998). In addition, when faced with critical decisions in critical care, families are unsure of "what to want" besides the recovery of their loved one (Kaufman, 1998). Often it is the nurse who notes the communication problem or who is in the position of translating and ensuring understanding among family members, patients, and health care providers.

## Assess Coping

Older adults may find multiple personal and environment stressors occurring concurrently. It is important to know whether the family has experienced any recent losses, such as resources, autonomy, roles, or death. How the family coped with these previous experiences can serve as the foundation for future coping. Even though older adults exhibit less outward distress during a crisis, or have had previous experience with critical illness situations, or may consider such an experience "normative" or expected in old age, this should not be interpreted to mean that they need less support or attention from health care providers. Attention to how older adult family members are coping with the stress of the situation is essential. Families can serve as valuable patient care resources. Most aged patients will return home rather than to another institution. Furthermore, family members provide most noninstitutional care for the older adult. The care provider and the older adult patient form a dyad that is not always apparent in critical care. The interruption in family ties during critical illness has important implications for nursing care and discharge planning. With the onset of critical illness, effective coping becomes important. Because families' responses to stress have implications for the family, patient, and nursing staff, it is advantageous for everyone that nurses direct care so that optimal levels of family coping are supported.

## Evaluate Resources

The first step in building resources within a family is to identify and acknowledge their existing resources, on which the family can build. An examination of these resources can be part of the initial interview process. Families also must begin to understand how resources must be garnered to treat the critical illness. Then the family learns how to manage the illness in the context of other, ongoing aspects of daily life (such as paying bills, doing the grocery shopping, and, for older persons, getting to their own doctor's appointments). How families manage this process is not well understood. Yet, critical care nurses can be attuned to these ongoing issues and prepare families for these demands.

## Assess Health of Aged Family Member

With aged family members, special attention should be directed to their physical condition. Older adult persons, particularly women, report an average of three chronic health problems. The most common include hypertension, other cardiovascular disease, and arthritis. Often, the older person is taking multiple medications, both prescription and over-the-counter drugs (Ebersole, Touhy, Hess, Jett, & Luggen, 2008). Older persons also may experience some deficits in hearing and vision. Each of these factors needs to be considered in developing appropriate strategies for aged family members.

Another important consideration is the emotional well-being of the older family member. As noted earlier, many older persons do not report emotional distress, at least to the same extent that younger adults do. This is, in part, caused by their socialization to keep feelings private, to "keep a stiff upper lip" and not burden others with their problems, and to the stigma attached to emotional "problems." Asking an older person about feelings of anxiety, depression, or signs of emotional distress may elicit a denial of any kind of affective symptoms. When an aged person is experiencing emotional distress, however, he or she is likely to report or seek treatment for somatic symptoms and not attribute these symptoms to stress. Symptoms such as insomnia, early waking, loss of appetite, indigestion, and headaches are common symptoms experienced by older persons (Ebersole et al., 2008). These may be caused by chronic health problems, common physiological changes associated with aging, or emotional distress. Asking questions about these types of symptoms, onset, and duration will provide some basis for the nurse to assess the emotional well-being of the aged family member and suggest interventions to reduce the severity of symptoms.

## Assess Availability of Other Family Members

The majority of older adults live alone or with a spouse independently in the community (American Association of Retired Persons [AARP], 2007). Given the geographic mobility in the U.S. population, adult children and siblings may not live close by. However, even when older adults are separated physically from their immediate family, they do maintain frequent contact by telephone or Internet. Because of this, family members are an important source of emotional support to the older person, but they may not be available to provide more instrumental types of support. Necessities such as transportation to the hospital, taking care of household chores, paying the bills, and preparing meals can loom as major problems for an older adult family member during a critical care experience. The nurse needs to identify whether other family members, especially adult children, are available and what kinds of support they can offer. Friends are particularly important to aged persons as sources of both quality and quantity of support (Ebersole et al., 2008). It is often the support network of friends and neighbors who need to be called on to fill in gaps when the family member of the critically ill person is an older adult. In dealing with the aged, the family database should contain information about friends and neighbors who may be available and essential as support persons.

## Assess Aged Family Member's Role

Typically, the aged family member of a critically ill older adult is the spouse, although it may be a sibling or a child. Knowledge about generational differences in family roles is necessary to guide nurses in gathering essential information. For instance, many women who are now in their 70s and 80s who still have spouses have no knowledge of their family finances. They may not know about their sources of income or their expenses, how to pay bills, or what kind of life insurance policies their husbands have. They may not have a driver's license and may never have learned how to drive a car. Younger health professionals may not be aware of these generational differences or may attribute the wife's lack of information or knowledge of how to get things done to some age-related cognitive "decline," rather than understand the way earlier generations of women were socialized into family roles. The nurse needs to be sensitive to the fact that older women may be dealing with issues and making decisions in areas in which they have had no previous experience. This may be an added source of stress for the older family member that may not be an issue for younger or middle-aged persons.

## Assess Family Spokesperson for Treatment Plans

It is expected that the number of families involved in treatment decisions for the older adult will increase markedly in the coming decade (Hansen, Archbold, Stewart, Westfall, & Ganzini, 2005). The issue of designating a family spokesperson is of immense importance during a critical care situation, but who takes the telephone calls may be different from who makes treatment decisions with older family members. Critical care nurses need to be prepared for disagreements among family members about treatment options. Even health care professionals may disagree about treatment plans. When the critically ill patient is older, there are often family disputes about treatment options. Although many family members state that they know what the older patient would want, this information may be inaccurate or may not be used appropriately to make treatment decisions (Kapp, 1991; Sonnenblick, Friendlander, & Steinberg, 1993). The nurse needs to be prepared to deal with conflicting family wishes and emotional responses when treatment decisions are being made for older adult family members.

## Case Study

Let us consider again the example of Mr. and Mrs. B.: The charge nurse returned to the waiting room and provided an update on Mr. B.'s condition. She then proceeded to initiate the family assessment database. Information from the initial database indicated that Mr. and Mrs. B. have been married for over 50 years. Just a month ago everyone helped them celebrate another anniversary. Mr. and Mrs. B. have three daughters, all of them live out of state. Jean is a registered nurse in a pediatric intensive care unit. Linda is a kindergarten teacher and Chris is a flight attendant with frequent European assignments. All three currently are making travel plans to be with their mother and father.

Mrs. B. reported that she has hypertension, arthritis, and a minor hearing loss. She takes her medications in the morning. Mrs. B. does not drive a car and relies on friends for transportation. The daughter, Jean, who would be arriving the next day, was designated by her mother to be the family contact person for the numerous friends and other relatives who would be inquiring about Mr. B.'s condition. Family telephone numbers were obtained and documented. The nurse gave Mrs. B. the telephone number of the SICU and reminded her that she could call at any time, day or night. Mrs. B. had no experience with critical care.

Mrs. B. also received a copy of the *Family Guidelines for Visiting in the SICU*. This pamphlet, brief and in large print, was developed by the nursing staff to meet some of the informational needs of family members that related to critical care.

Mrs. B. expressed visible distress that "Mr. B. might die." The nurse paged the hospital clergy and listened carefully as she talked about the uncertain future. Mrs.

B.'s friends obviously were tired and were encouraged to go home. The nurse assured them that Mrs. B. would be well cared for.

## Suggested Family Interventions

Critical care interventions have been shown to provide significant benefits to older persons, including the very old (Rush, 1997). Mortality rates for older ICU patients are similar to those for all age ranges (Kass, Castriotta, &, Malakoff, 1992; Wu, Rubin, & Rosen, 1990). However, older adults admitted to critical care fall into two very distinct groups: those who are functionally independent but struck by an acute serious illness such as myocardial infarction, and those who are frail and have multiple degenerative illnesses whose condition becomes unstable (Kaufman, 1998). It is the second group that comprises 70 to 80% of hospital admissions and who pose the most dilemmas for families and health professionals.

One of the goals of family-centered care is to reduce stress among family members (Azoulay et al., 2005; Davidson et al., 2007; Institute for Family-Centered Care, 1999; Leske, 1998). Interventions begin on orientation to the critical care area with family members and continue throughout the critical care period. Suggested nursing interventions and activities associated with the five need categories serve as a guide for initial implementation.

### Case Study

When the initial family assessment was completed, the nurse asked Mrs. B. if she would like to see the SICU before Mr. B. arrived. She carefully observed that Mrs. B. remained quiet and stoic. Medical treatments, procedures, machines, and surroundings were explained. The pictures in the brochure also were used. The nurse returned Mrs. B. to the waiting room and said she would notify her when she could visit Mr. B.

### Orient to Critical Care Environment

Regardless of previous experience with critical care or lack of it, the critical care environment can be very intimidating to family members. The vast array of machines and technology is overwhelming (Eggenberger & Nelms, 2007). Family members report that the greater number of machines involved in patient care, the more serious the illness. They describe the sounds emitted by machines as alarms that signify a crisis; therefore, the more alarms, the greater the crisis. In addition, the "Do Not Enter" signs or locked entry doors are obstacles to family visitation.

Families not experienced with critical illness do not know what to expect. Feelings of anxiety are intensified when entering the critical care unit. Factors that contribute to family anxiety include unusual sounds and odors, complex equipment, numerous critically ill patients, and the many treatments and procedures that the patient undergoes. Families may perceive the business of critical care as chaotic and disorganized, and they may feel that they "are in the way." Aged family members are especially concerned about "not bothering anyone." However, educating families about a loved one's illness, treatments, and physical status help prepare families for what they will encounter when they visit the patient.

The hospital environment also may not be "elder friendly." The lighting may produce glare; floors may be slippery; chairs may be on wheels, unstable, or not even available at the bedside. The biggest obstacle is the cluttered environment (Fletcher, 2007). Providing a safe environment for the family visitor is a major goal given the antiquated design of some hospitals and the plethora of equipment now available at the point of care.

## Providing Assurance

Providing assurance is especially important for any family experiencing uncertainty in diagnosis, treatment, and outcome of illness, regardless of the age of family members. Establishing a calm and relaxed atmosphere that will support a trusting and empathic relationship is a necessary part of assurance. Professionals and families need to establish a relationship that is mutually respectful, trusting, and collaborative (Maxwell et al., 2007; Rushton et al., 2007). The development of any further interventions will depend on the initial rapport established between care providers and family members.

Nursing interventions that provide assurance are difficult to describe, probably because nurses provide assurance by exhibiting genuine concern for family members' welfare while listening, encouraging, and positively responding to them. Exchanging of names is an important but simple introduction that is often overlooked in nurse–family interaction. However, addressing aged family members or patients by their first names unless specifically asked to do so may be inappropriate. Using first names may convey a lack of respect or loss of dignity to the older person. Be cautious about communicating ageist attitudes, even inadvertently, such as referring to someone as a "sweet little old lady."

Results of prior research indicate that to feel hope is a very important assurance need of family members of the critically ill (Leske & Pasquale, 2007). Hope is keeping a possible positive outcome in mind in an uncertain situation (Verhaeghe, van Zuuren, Defloor, Duijnstee, & Grypdonck, 2007). Nurses need to support hope because hope can be associated with positive patient outcomes (Tracey, Fowler, & Magarelli, 1999). However, families do want wish to cherish false hope that is letting them hope for something impossible. There is some indication that older adult family members need more time than younger ones to work through the critical illness and adjust their hopes (Verhaeghe et al., 2007). Many hope-inspiring strategies focus on relationships with others. These relationships involve nurses, family, friends, and a higher power (Kaye & Heald, 1996).

## Facilitating Visitation

By seeing the critically ill patient, family members validate the seriousness of the situation. It is reported that most family members desire an unlimited number of visits per day and believe that visiting is important to the recovery of the critically ill patient (Redekopp & Leske, 2007). Family members feel that their visits affect patients by calming their fears, uplifting their spirits, promoting a positive attitude, and giving some inner strength for recovery (Maxwell et al., 2007). Balancing the needs of family members with the needs of the patient, unit, and health care personnel is no easy task. However, visitation practices should have a scientific base, rather than one governed by institutional or environmental regulations. Visitation contracts appear to be a popular compromise between rigid rules and unlimited policies (Haber & Looney, 2000). By using a visitation contract, visiting frequency, length of visit, and approved visitors are tailored to individual family situations. Family members need unit telephone numbers and the names of who to contact. In addition, beeper systems have offered family members respite from the waiting-room vigil (Menkhaus, Turner, Gueldner, & Michele, 1996).

Remember that, for a number of reasons, some older women may have difficulty getting to and from the hospital. Also, their own health problems may interfere with their ability to spend long hours in the waiting room. However, even when the spouse must remain at home, she or he can make important contributions to the patient's recovery. Specific arrangements for telephone call updates and progress reports may be a beneficial intervention.

## Providing Information

Giving information is an important intervention aimed at preparing or moving the family toward understanding and accepting the critical situation and possible outcomes. Nursing interventions are designed to foster family member's management of the vast amount of information that may be directed to them. Providing information to older adult family members requires special approaches to accommodate age-related changes that may influence the ability to understand or retain new information. Sensory overload from the strange environment of the hospital or critical care unit and sensory impairments, such as declines in vision and hearing, may interfere with an aged family member's ability to process or retain information. Aged family members are just as capable of remembering and understanding as younger family members. However, under conditions of environmental and memory overload, difficulty can occur with processing the information. For instance, many older persons have some hearing loss. An unfamiliar and stressful environment may exacerbate the problem. Be careful not to misinterpret a hearing loss as a cognitive impairment. When there is a hearing loss, it is helpful to speak in lower tones but no louder than you would with colleagues.

Modifying traditional teaching approaches to address the special needs of older adult family members will enhance the effectiveness of any teaching (Dellasega, Clark, McCreary, Helmuth, & Schan, 1994). Reducing memory "overload" by initially providing only essential information to relieve their immediate concerns will be more effective than providing too much information. Simple terminology without medical jargon will enhance the older family member's ability to understand and remember explanations. In addition, selecting an area of the unit that has minimal distraction may be beneficial for providing information.

New material is best processed if it is presented in small increments at frequent but manageable intervals. Continual identification of the aged family member's energy level is an important consideration; fatigue can influence processing ability. Complicating the issue of providing information is the fact that the educational level in the elderly is generally lower than in younger generations. About 40% of those aged 75 years plus are high school graduates; the number is lower for Blacks and Hispanics (AARP, 2007). Because of the differences in educational levels, most written materials should be prepared at about the eighth-grade reading level and, because of the vision loss that comes with age, larger print should be used.

Family conferences may be another option for providing information to families. These conferences can be used to discuss plans of care, especially when patients are not able to communicate for themselves (Lindgren, Barnett, & Bloom, 2006). Prior research results indicate that family members reported frequent problems regarding not being asked often enough about their views and not being involved in decisions as much as they would have liked (Maxwell et al., 2007; Vom Eigen, Walker, Edgeman-Levitan, Cleary, & Delbanco, 1999). Certain steps may need to be taken before a family conference. It is important to understand the family's prior knowledge, attitudes, and reactions to the critical care experience. Conferences ought to be held in a nonthreatening environment. The goals of the conference are to discuss the patient's progress, prognosis, and what the patient would want if he or she were in a position to discuss the matter. It is important to support the family's decision and confirm that there is a common understanding of the treatment goals. Taking these steps should improve the communication process of the family conference.

Knowledge of age-related differences in information processing can help the critical care nurse use special skills when providing information. Speaking at a slower pace; being visible; making sure the family members have the needed prosthetics, such as hearing aids; and allowing increased time for responses and additional questions are all measures that can enhance communication.

## Facilitating Comfort

Sitting in the waiting room produces changes in eating habits, lack of physical or mental activity, and certainly prevents people from employment (Bengtson, Karlsson, Wahrborg, Hjalmarson, & Herlitz, 1996; Eggenberger & Nelms, 2007). Family members need to have high energy levels to maintain the hospital "vigil" and care for the discharged patient. They often need to be encouraged to eat and take some time away from their relentless vigil. Families also need adequate space for consultation and education (Rashid, 2007).

These considerations take on added importance when the family member is an older adult. Aged family members often have musculoskeletal limitations and decreased mobility. Sitting for hours in the waiting room can be painful. Typical waiting room furniture contributes to problems for the older family member. For instance, no one has identified comfortable chairs for the older adult who may have arthritis, osteoporosis, or pulmonary problems. It is important to assess if waiting will be difficult. In addition, aged family members need to be encouraged to take breaks from sitting and walk around.

The lights and noise of the waiting room and surrounding areas also may interfere with adequate vision. Because of the normal changes in vision that come with age, some aged family members may find it difficult to navigate the hospital maze. Glare from lighting and small print on signs and cluttered directional maps may contribute to confusion and anxiety in the older person.

## Enhancing Support

Nurses use many mechanisms to provide support to families, but few of these methods have been evaluated. It is impractical for nurses and possibly unhealthy for families for practitioners to provide all the necessary family support. Therefore, family groups need to be used during the critical care experience (Leske & Pasquale, 2007). These groups provide the opportunity for participants to share common experiences, build mutual support, ventilate common concerns, foster a sense of hope, reduce anxiety, and obtain information common to the groups' needs.

Within the current cohort of aged people, however, there may be some for whom sharing feelings, personal issues, and private family matters are unacceptable. A support group may not be a beneficial intervention because the idea is foreign to some aged family members and not part of their upbringing or lifestyle. They have not been socialized to participate in these groups. If they would attend, special attention would need to be directed to particular issues of older persons. Support groups also may be more acceptable if the content focuses on information and tasks rather than sharing feelings and concerns. The critical care nurse will need to take direction from the group, rather than have a set agenda.

A commonly used method for assisting with support is to ask the aged family member to identify others who assist with specific tasks. Both friends and family, particularly adult children, may be available to help with day-to-day tasks and problems. Remember that friends may be more important than family members in providing emotional support and nurturance to the older person. Asking the aged family member if he or she has a close friend or confidante is one way of assessing the availability of emotional support. Encouraging older people to take some time to talk to or be with friends may give them permission to take care of themselves.

## Involving Family in Care

Older adult critically ill patients are at risk for decline in functioning and quality of life that may consist of one or more dysfunctional syndromes. These syndromes include acute confusion, incontinence, falls, nutritional problems, and pressure ulcers. Dysfunctional syndromes (DS) are primarily associated with age-related physiological changes, medical problems, and side effects of treatments (Li, Melnyk, & McCann, 2004). One strategy for decreasing the risk of DS is to involve the family caregiver in hospital care. Family members of older adults can provide social stimulation, psychological and emotional support, as well as some physical care. Family members need guidance about how they can participate in care (Li, Stewart, Imle, & Archbold, 2000).

## Encouraging Reminiscence

Family members may want to share the impact of the critical illness on the family and remember how the patient was before the injury. This story-telling experience may reflect a sense of loss as family members mourn for the person they once knew. This reexamination has therapeutic and clinical value for family-centered care. Recalling the joyous times can help families focus on positive aspects of family relationships. In addition, reminiscence with family members may provide the nurse with information on how to personalize patient care (McQuay, Schwartz, Goldblatt, & Giangrasso, 1995).

## Case Study

Members of the health care team met daily with Mr. B.'s family. Mrs. B. remained quiet and asked few questions. Her daughter, Linda, was overtly distressed. She knew her parents would never be the same. She wondered also how this injury would affect her own life. All family members understood Mr. B.'s condition but grieved for the loss of his friend and avoided the fact that he would have to be told of the death. The staff also began to notice some physical deterioration in Mrs. B. She looked tired and walked with more difficulty.

Once the initial crisis was over, and Mr. B. was expected to survive, the waiting room vigils decreased. Each family member began taking care of personal needs. They no longer needed to be reminded to eat and sleep. Daughter Chris, needed to return home. It was determined that Mrs. B. needed help with maintaining the family home and finances. The critical care experience created tensions within the family unit because roles, priorities, and expectations were altered. A family care conference was scheduled for all family and health care team members.

## Role of Nurse With Family Members

At times, the family of the patient in critical care may replace the patient in the typical nurse–patient relationship so the relationship becomes the nurse–family relationship. This partnership between nurse and family may take a while to develop or may never develop adequately, leaving families and staff working toward different goals for the patient. A key ingredient to foster family-centered care is to clarify the meaning and conditions of the family/health care professional relationship. Establishing therapeutic boundaries and identifying shared meaning of the relationship helps avoid misunderstandings. There are strategies used by families and nurses that help develop this relationship. The strategies used by nurses include demonstrating commitment, persevering, and being involved (Leske & Heidrich, 1996). Demonstrating commitment involves responding to the family member as a person, spending time with the family, encouraging family participation, showing empathy, and respecting family rituals. Persevering requires spending time with families and gathering information so the nurse gets to know the family. Being involved includes concepts of patient advocacy and bending bureaucratic rules.

Family strategies for developing the nurse–family relationship in critical care include determining who is the "good" nurse, how to be a "good" visitor, and how to be trustworthy. Families spend time trying to evaluate staff and determining which nurses are the "good" nurses (Hupcey, 1998). They watch care provided and look for signs of kindness and genuine interest on the part of the nurse toward the patient. This critique of nursing staff continues in the waiting room as families discuss who to trust and who provides competent care. Many families also invest a lot of effort into trying to please the nursing staff and be "good" visitors. They try to be friendly, cooperative, and help the nurses out. They may bring gifts and provide positive feedback. As the nurse–family relationship develops, families begin to trust certain nurses and accept the nurse's explanations without constant questioning. They begin to go home and take care of themselves.

## Stress and the Family in Critical Care

Critical illness is a potential crisis situation for family members (Auerbach et al., 2005; Kosco & Warren, 2000; Leske & Jiricka, 1998). The unexpected hospitalization after critical illness has a significant impact on family members (Auerbach et al., 2005; Azoulay et al., 2005; Eggenberger & Nelms, 2007; Kosciulek, McCubbin, & McCubbin, 1993). During this period, families must deal with many stressors, including role changes, financial concerns, uncertain prognosis, isolation from other family members, dramatic disruption in daily routines, making decisions, and unfamiliar critical care environments (Davidson et al., 2007; Eggenberger & Nelms, 2007; Fry & Warren, 2007; Gulranjani, 1995; Hallgrimsdottir, 2004; Leske, 1992a, 2000; Titler, Bombei, & Schutte, 2005). Health professionals expect families to absorb highly technical and potentially devastating information while making rapid decisions when they face the potential sudden loss of a family member (Eggenberger & Nelms, 2007; Gulranjani, 1995; Hallgrimsdottir, 2004; Kojlak, Keenan, Plotkin, Giles-Fysh, & Sibbald, 1998). However, challenges in forming and maintaining relationships with other family members and health care providers are the most frequently cited family stressors (Azoulay et al., 2001; Weigand, 2006).

Because critical illness often occurs without warning, there is little time for family members to prepare for this experience. Most families usually report feeling powerless, vulnerable, and helpless (Fry & Warren, 2007; Leske, 1998; Schlump-Urquhart, 1990). They have no clear knowledge of what to expect from health professionals caring for their family member or what to expect in regard to the illness and expected outcome. Families can act as buffers for patient stress and serve as valuable patient care resources. However, when families have high levels of stress, they may be unable to support the patient, and, in fact, may transfer their stress to the patient (Degeneffe & Lynch, 2006; Leske & Pasquale, 2007; Paparrigopoulos et al., 2006; Pochard et al., 2005). Unmitigated family stress may manifest itself in distrust of hospital staff, noncompliance with the treatment regimen, and even lawsuits. It is advantageous for everyone that care is provided so that optimal levels of family functioning are supported.

Stresses produced by critical illness vary in intensity and duration, but certainly have the potential to create a heavy burden for families. In contrast to younger persons, however, family members of older adult patients most likely have had prior experiences with critical care. Whether these experiences were positive or negative may determine their response to the stress of another critical care situation (Hansen et al. 2005; Leske & Heidrich, 1996). In addition, some family members may view critical illness of an older adult person as a normal part of aging (Peirce, Wright, & Fulmer, 1992). In fact, critical illness may trigger some anticipatory grieving. Some families may feel more prepared for death as an outcome with critically ill older family members than with younger family members and so begin to grieve before death.

Stress also may interfere with the ability of any family to use effective coping skills and maintain patterns of family functioning (Fink, 1995; Leske & Jiricka, 1998; McCubbin & McCubbin, 1996). Basic coping techniques do not seem to change with age, and it is important to remember that emotional coping styles are determined more by the personality characteristics of the person than by age. However, because older adults may anticipate serious illness in old age, they may use different coping resources for dealing with critical illness in the family. They may also show less overt emotional distress in a critical situation.

In many instances, a family member, most often an older adult wife, has cared for the older adult patient admitted to critical care. Caregiving can be a chronic and stressful event with negative effects on the caregiver's emotional and financial well-being (Li et al., 2003, 2004; Nijboer et al., 2000). Caregiver distress has been described in numerous ways by caregivers, including feelings of burnout, depression, isolation, fear, frustration, anxiety, low morale, sleeplessness, fatigue, and loneliness (Brody, 1990; Nijboer et al., 2000). It is alarming to note that caregivers have reported even higher levels of depression and psychological distress, a more negative affect, and higher use of psychotropic drugs than people in the general population (Cuellar & Butts, 1999; Kleinpell, 2006; Neundorfer, 1991; Titler et al., 1995)

Caregiving also affects the physical health of the caregiver. One large epidemiological study has shown that older adult caregivers who experience emotional strain are more likely to die than noncaregivers (Schulz & Beach, 1999). Nurses dealing with spouses who have been caregivers of the ICU patient need to be aware that these family members are at greater risk, not only for emotional distress and depression, but also for serious physical health problems. The added stress of having a spouse admitted to critical care puts that caregiver in a high-risk situation in relation to his or her own health. Therefore, any way in which the nurse can intervene to reduce the distress of the family members and to increase health-protective behaviors of that family member should be attempted. Nursing interventions also need to focus on discharge planning for the caregiver as well as the patient. Because of shortened hospital length of stays and higher acuity needs in the discharged patient, caregivers often continue to provide care after hospitalization (Clark, 1997; Li et al., 2004). The needs of caregivers, such as support for themselves as well as support services for the patient, should be part of discharge planning if family-centered care is the goal (Fournet, 1992; Kleinpell, 2006).

Communication with health care providers also can be a significant stressor, particularly when decisions about treatment must be made. Family members, particularly those who are older, may have a limited understanding of what the information that health care providers give them really means. At times, health care providers assume that family members understand if no questions are asked. Family members also may think they understand what health professionals are saying when in reality they do not. Research has pointed out that physicians and patients, physicians and family members, and patients and family members either do not communicate or, when they do, misunderstand or misperceive the communication (Eggenberger & Nelms, 2007; Jacelon, 2006; Maxwell et al., 2007). This is especially problematic when the communication is about end-of-life treatment decisions (Kaufman, 1998; Weigand, 2006). For example, family members may inform the nurse that the patient does not want to be on life support, but they do not understand that mechanical ventilation is life support. More research is needed on family decisionmaking during stressful periods or the crisis of critical illness.

Because of the enormous amount of time that a family spends at the hospital after a critical illness, a series of changes may occur within the family system. These may include reorganization of roles and tasks, changes in communication patterns, and emotional struggles. These changes may even become more complicated in geriatric family members, as there are multiple adult family members, representing a couple of generations, with varying levels of responsibility to the older patient. These levels of responsibility need to be assessed considering current and past relationships the patient has had with the family; degree of economic threat the illness poses to the family; trajectory expectations for the illness that the family holds; and the impact of the rehabilitation, discharge, and possible disability on ability to perform the caregiving role.

# Family Frameworks Useful for Critical Care

Theoretical frameworks are a systematic collection of concepts and relationships (White & Klein, 2008). Theories guide research, assist in the organization of research findings, demonstrate how ideas are connected to each other and to other theories, help make sense out of phenomena, and guide treatment. Ideas about family come from many sources. However, there are several features of families as social groups that are different from other groups. One, families last longer than other social groups. Two, families are intergenerational. In addition, families contain both biological and affinal relationships with each other. These biological (and affinal) aspects of families link them to larger organizations (such as the health care system). One has no choice about one's family membership compared to an optional membership in another social group. There are several family theoretical frameworks but systems theory, developmental theory, and family stress models may be useful to guide assessment and intervention for family-centered critical care with older adults.

## Systems Theory

One theory that is useful in understanding family and health provider interactions in critical care is family systems theory. A key concept in family systems theory is that a change in one part of the system (for example, the hospitalization of a critically ill parent) affects the entire family system, resulting in a strain on coping resources and possibly family distress. One way that systems, such as families, attempt to maintain or restore equilibrium and thereby reduce distress is by controlling "inputs and outputs"; for example, controlling what is allowed to enter or leave the system. A major input and output that is very relevant to critical care nurses is the two-way communication of information.

In family systems theory, families have been described as "open" or "closed" systems according to how much communication and support is allowed to enter or leave the family system. Some families are "closed" systems. For these families, information sharing or use of outside resources is not trusted and is perceived as disruptive and a cause of stress to the family. Such families may neither offer nor be receptive to teaching or information gathering by the nurse. These families are sometimes labeled as being "in denial" or "uncooperative," but these families are acting in ways that they perceive are in the best interest of the family. Other families are "open" systems that perceive the exchange of information or resources as adding energy and stability to the system. Open families can be very receptive and cooperative in receiving and giving information or support, or they can be viewed as "demanding" or "controlling" because of their insistence on getting the answers that they need. Again, these families are acting in ways that, in their view, are best for the family. The key to effective communication with both types of families is developing trust.

Broadly speaking, trust is confidence in others to act in accordance with accepted social, ethical, legal, and medical norms (Rushton et al., 2007). Trust is built incrementally and earned behaviorally. Critical care professionals demonstrate trust when they work closely with families to clarify their intensions and assess their preferences. Trust can be built, or rebuilt, by engaging the family in ongoing discussions (Lynn-McHale & Deatrick, 2000). These discussions can help families in their decision-making process and foster respect for the choices that are made.

## Family-Life-Course Development Theory

In addition to systems theory, an understanding of family developmental issues also can assist the nurse in dealing effectively with families of older patients. Family life course development is a powerful paradigm that has been greatly overlooked as a therapeutic framework. A family crisis may occur when a critical illness does occur. The degree of disruption to the family system is affected by the timing of the illness in the family life cycle, the nature of the illness, openness of the family system, and role of the ill person (Carter & McGoldrick, 1999; White & Klein, 2008). Therefore, it is important to consider families in the larger time frame of family development. Understanding how families respond to developmental changes can be used as a guide in identifying major family issues during critical illness.

Spouses of critical care older adult patients typically are old and perhaps frail. Siblings, who are increasingly important as sources of support in old age, also may be older and frail. Illness is a prominent concern to older adults. Fears of loss of physical and mental functioning, chronic pain, and degenerating conditions are common concerns even though older adults do maintain good health. Older individuals in our society are often stereotyped as frail, depressed, lonely, and cognitively slow or impaired. It would be a mistake for nurses working with these family members to hold these attitudes, particularly since the salient transitions of later life hold the potential for transformation and growth. In fact, research on aging shows that older persons are happier and more satisfied with life than young or middle-aged persons. Further, variability in health, cognitive ability, and emotional well-being is greater in old age than at any other time in life (Carter & McGoldrick, 1999). In addition, there is a myth that older persons are isolated from their families. Although some family members may live in distant communities, many older adults have daily or weekly contact with family members.

Adult children of the older adult patient are often in midlife. In terms of age, this stage usually extends from the midforties to the midsixties. There is currently little terminology available to describe this phase of the family life cycle. Some use the term "empty nest" but this has negative connotations. Many demographic changes in adult development have made this a lengthy stage in the family life cycle. Typically, during the empty nest time of life children are teenagers or in college, bringing both emotional and financial stresses, careers are often at their peak, the quality of marital relationships can decline, people begin to notice the first physical signs of aging or first develop a serious health problem, and often both time and money are devoted to helping care for aging parents. Having aging and ill parents, in and of itself, is a stressor. For the first time, the adult child may be confronted with his or her own mortality, as well as the parent's. A critical illness in the parent often changes the parent–child relationship so that roles reverse and the adult child is given the responsibility of making decisions, communicating family wishes, or interacting with health care providers.

Understanding developmental issues for a family may be crucial to understanding the impact of the critical illness of the older patient. Other family members may be called on to assume new roles and responsibilities. In addition, prior divorce can negatively affect the parent–child relationship even in the latter part of life, weakening economic ties, and reducing informal caregiving (Schone & Pezzin, 1999). Divorced parents may not be able to count on the economic and personal support of their children. Divorced fathers are particularly vulnerable to receiving less care in later life because of weaker ties with their children. In addition, the ties to children may be further weakened by remarriage. It appears that remarried parents received less informal care from their children and purchase more hours of formal care (Schone & Pezzin, 1999). These results raise concerns about future generations of older adult patients, who will have experienced higher rates of divorce and may place greater demands on social and economic programs for assistance.

## Resiliency Model of Family Stress, Adjustment, and Adaptation

A third conceptual approach to family care is described as the Resiliency Model of Family Stress, Adjustment, and Adaptation (McCubbin & McCubbin, 1996). This model is one of the major theoretical applications of developmental life course theory. The model has been used in research with families of older adults (Fink, 1995), disabled individuals (Frain et al., 2007; Lim & Zebrock, 2004; Tak & Lee, 1997), trauma (Ketchum, 2000; Kosciulek et al., 1993; Leske, 2000, 2003; Leske & Jiricka, 1998), organ transplantation (Nolan et al., 1992), and cardiovascular surgery (Leske, 2003). The framework depicts family stressors and strengths as key concepts influencing family outcomes. The assumptions of the model are that families: (a) develop basic strengths designed to protect the family from major disruptions in the face of stressors, (b) need to adapt to the situation after critical illness, and (c) benefit from interventions particularly during periods of family stress (Boss, 2002; McCubbin & McCubbin, 1996; Patterson, 2002). The intent of the model is to understand what families do well and to build on this base to help the family function.

Types of stressors that contribute to increased family stress include: (a) prior stressors, including both those in process and those resulting from unresolved problems;(b) severity of patient illness; and (c) stage of family life cycle. Family stressors are viewed as cumulative in the Resiliency Model. However, the uncertainty of patient prognosis or treatment outcomes in critical care may place additional stress on the family.

Family strengths include appraisal, resources, coping, and problem-solving communication. Appraisal refers to the definitions the family attaches to the situation in terms of the critical illness and the family's ability to manage the event. In the beginning, appraisal is focused on the specific critical illness, prior stressors, severity of patient's illness, and what it means to the family. Then, the family determines its capabilities for management of the stressor. Although appraisals are held individually, the family as a unit also can share them (McCubbin & McCubbin, 1996; Patterson, 2002; Walsh, 2007).

Resources of individual family members, the family unit, and the community can already exist or be developed and used for management of specific critical illness. Personal resources of family members include factors such as age, education, and prior experience with critical care. Family resources include flexibility and clear family rules. Community resources are those persons, groups, and institutions outside the family that can be called on to manage the stressors (McCubbin & McCubbin, 1996; Patterson, 2002).

Coping refers to specific cognitive and behavioral efforts used by the family to reduce or manage the stressors placed on the family and bring resources to manage the situation. Coping strategies can be grouped into patterns designed to maintain or strengthen the organization and relationships of the family unit, maintain emotional stability and satisfaction of family members, or manage a specific situation (McCubbin & McCubbin, 1996; Patterson, 2002).

Patterns of problem-solving communication, that is, communication that can either escalate conflict or be more supportive, are also part of the family's responses to stressors and represent generalized ways of responding that usually transcend different types of stressful situations (McCubbin & McCubbin, 1996; Patterson, 2002). Coping and problem-solving communication are directed at reducing or eliminating the stressor, acquiring additional resources, and shaping appraisal.

In the Resiliency Model, family adaptation is the outcome of family efforts to achieve a balance between stressors and strengths in response to the crisis of critical illness (McCubbin & McCubbin, 1996; Patterson, 2002). However, a stressor–strength imbalance can bring about inadequate family adaptation. At the individual to family level, the demands of the stressors may exceed the strengths of the family to manage the critical illness. Inadequate family adaptation is the result of family members' increased stress and low sense of family satisfaction. The fact that the Model conceptualizes adaptation to stressors is a dynamic and developmental process that can disturb the organization and process of family life.

## Impact of Critical Care on the Family

The following review focuses on the prior research on critical illness, family stressors, strengths, and outcomes to critical illness; and rational for the need for family-centered interventions.

## Critical Illness

Critical illness interferes with family structure, functions, and challenges the family's established patterns of behavior (Auerbach et al., 2005; Hallgrimsdottir, 2004; Kojlak et al., 1998; Medina, 2005; Pochard et al., 2005; Van Horn & Tesh, 2000). If the critical care event is not handled optimally, the result may be prolonged physiologic and psychologic instability of family members (Medina, 2005; Redley, Beanland, & Botti, 2003). At the time of the highest level of stress, which is the initial phase of critical illness, the least amount of attention may be given to the family (Azoulay et al., 2001; Leske, 1992a). Attention to family stressors and strengths may serve as a guide for assessment and intervention with older adults.

## Family Stressors

### Prior Stress

Because family crises evolve over time, families are seldom dealing with a single stressor. Prior family stressors contribute to increased family stress during the critical care period (Davidson et al., 2007; Leske, 1998, 2003; McCubbin & McCubbin, 1996). Most families carry residual strains that result from earlier stressors. There is strong evidence that residual strains and daily hassles have debilitating effects on family outcomes. Experiencing multiple stressors over long periods can lead to enormous strain, a situation that places the family at risk for inadequate adaptation (Fink, 1995; Leske & Jiricka, 1998). Prior research suggests that previous strains, rather then the actual stressor event, may predict psychosocial family adaptation (Auerbach et al., 2005; Fink, 1995; Leske, 2003; Pochard et al., 2005; Van Horn & Tesh, 2000). However, the stressor of severe patient illness may contribute to increased difficulty with family adaptation (Auerbach et al., 2005; Azoulay et al., 2005; McCubbin & McCubbin, 1996; Patterson, 2002). At this time a clear need exists to evaluate prior stressors and factors such as the mental health, physical health, and functional ability of the patient's potential primary caregiver, as well as the caregiver's ability to manage stress.

### Patient Illness Factors

Severity of patient illness places stressors on families that may undermine their adaptation (Gilliss & Knafl, 1999; Landsman et al., 1990). Reports of the relationship between severity of patient illness and family adaptation currently contain conflicting results. Some authors report an inverse relationship between patient severity of illness and family functioning, whereas other authors report no significant relationship (Johnson et al., 1998; Leske, 1992a; Richmond, Kauder, Hinkle, & Schults, 2003). However, both lengths of stay (LOS) and hospital charges increase as a function of illness severity. This longer LOS is associated with a prolonged period of patient recovery and major delays in achieving acceptable levels of functional competency and return to work (MacKenzie, Siegel, Shapiro, Moody, & Smith, 1988; Richmond et al., 2003). These residual self-care and physical limitations may increase family stress and debilitate family adaptation over time (Azoulay et al., 2005). Although the greatest impact of patient illness is the loss of life, function, and human distress, the financial costs are extensive. However, families consider the patient to be severely ill and at risk for dying when admitted to critical care, regardless of the mode or severity of illness (Leske, 2000, 2003; Leske & Jiricka, 1998).

## Family Strengths

### Appraisal

The definition a family places on the critical illness is one of the most important variables in understanding family stress and is directly related to family adaptation (Boss, 2002; McCubbin & McCubbin, 1996; Patterson, 2002). Families often have little or no information about the condition of their family member and this initial uncertainty is associated with poor adaptation (Kosciulek et al., 1993; Leske, 1998; Leske & Jiricka,

1998; Mishel & Braden, 1987). When the family appraises its overall capability as inadequate to the crisis of critical illness, an imbalance in the family emerges that shapes responses. Each family member attaches unique meanings to the situation. These unique meanings may positively or negatively affect family adaptation (Fink, 1995; Lim & Zebrack, 2004; McCubbin & McCubbin, 1996). From this perspective, it is important to understand an individual family members' appraisal or meaning of the critical care situation.

## Resources

Another strength used to manage a stressor event by preventing a crisis is described as family resources. Resources are an essential factor in determining family adaptation (Agaibi & Wilson, 2005; Fink, 1995). Families possessing a large repertoire of resources more effectively manage and adapt better to stressful situations such as critical illness (Leske, 2000, 2003; Leske & Jiricka, 1998; McCubbin & McCubbin, 1996). Personal, social, and economic family resources appear to mediate the relationship between stressful events and family outcomes (Kosciulek et al., 1993). These family resources are especially needed in the early stages of patient illness and are found to reduce the postcrisis stress of families (Fink, 1995; Patterson, 2002). The importance of accurate understanding of family resources is necessary for appropriate intervention and discharge planning. In addition, adequate resources may be the key ingredients for positive family outcomes.

## Coping

Family coping refers to strategies, patterns, and behaviors designed to: (a) maintain and/or strengthen the family, (b) maintain the emotional stability of family members, (c) obtain and/or use resources to manage the situation, and (d) initiate efforts to resolve the family strains created by the stressor (McCubbin & McCubbin, 1996). How families cope with stressors can adversely affect their health and well-being (Agaibi & Wilson, 2005; Boss, 2002). Emotional reactions of family members during hospitalization are found to directly influence patient coping responses (Agaibi & Wilson, 2005; Davidson et al., 2007). Others report a significant relationship between positive family coping and positive patient outcomes (Davidson et al., 2007). Much of the variance in family coping seems attributable to the crisis event more than individual differences in coping styles, but clearly an individual/event interaction exists (Agaibi & Wilson, 2005). However, prior research findings with critically ill patient's family members indicate that they are able to initially manage the critical illness (Leske, 2000, 2003; Leske & Jiricka, 1998). Therefore, coping strategies may serve as a guide for further understanding of the process of positive family outcomes after critical illness.

## Communication

The family's ability to organize a stressor into manageable components, identify alternative courses of action, and cultivate patterns of communication needed to gain control over the situation refers to problem-solving communication (McCubbin & McCubbin, 1996; Patterson, 2002). Family problem-solving communication is strongly related to positive family adaptation (DeGeneffe & Lynch, 2006; Fink, 1995; Patterson, 2002). Understanding the medical condition and having information about the patient's progress are necessary for appropriate family problem solving to occur. In addition, families with open communication patterns are found to adapt more successfully after critical illness (Leske, 1998b, 2003; Patterson, 2002).

## Family Outcomes

There is growing evidence that the stressor of critical illness exerts a powerful influence on family outcomes (Auerbach et al., 2005; DeGeneffe & Lynch, 2006; Figley & Barnes, 2005; Gilliss & Knafl, 1999; Leske, 1998). Physical and emotional health of family members suffers during patient hospitalization. Most of the empirical work on family outcomes in critical care has been with spouses of cardiac patients. Spouses report higher stress levels than patients and high anxiety, depression, and stress-related symptoms are identified up to a year after the cardiac event (Dracup et al., 2004; Gilliss & Knafl, 1999; Moser, 2007). The spouse's ability to deal in an optimal manner with the ill patient has a significant impact on the health and functioning of the family (Dracup et al., 2004; Moser, 2007; Moser & Dracup, 2000).

### State Stress

Any clinical course that runs counter to the family's expectations for a positive patient outcome is an important contributor to family stress (Auerbach et al., 2005; Azoulay et al., 2005; Chui & Chan, 2007; Figley & Barnes, 2005; Winston, Baxt, Kassam-Adams, Elliot, & Kallan, 2005). These researchers suggest that about one third of family members are at major risk for stress-related symptoms. In addition, about 10% of family members experience significant acute stress at patient discharge (Chien et al., 2005; Winston et al., 2005). Higher rates of stress are reported among family members who felt information was incomplete in the critical care setting and who felt dissatisfied with the extent to which they were informed about the patient's condition (Auerbach et al., 2005; Azoulay et al., 2005; Fox-Wasylyshyn, El-Masari, & Williamson, 2005; Winston et al., 2005). In addition, family stress levels do not lessen with longer stays in the critical care unit (Chui & Chan, 2007). Stress levels of family rise when their needs are not met (Davidson et al., 2007; Fox-Wasylyshyn et al., 2005). One role of the critical care practitioner is to make expectations explicit and clarify what can be done to treat the patient's illness. Be careful not to make suggestions that are unlikely to change the outcomes in an attempt to reduce family distress.

### Satisfaction

Family satisfaction is another important outcome measure in critical care (Leske & Pelczynski, 1999; Wall, Engelberg, Downer, Heyland, & Curtis, 2007; Wasser, Pasquale, Matchett, Bryan, & Pasquale, 2001). Dissatisfied families are less able to provide positive support to the patient and are less effective caregivers after patient discharge (Auerbach et al., 2005; Leske, 1998; Leske & Pelczynski, 1999). Dissatisfied family members also are less likely to trust health care providers and less ready to contribute if important decisions need to be made (Auerbach et al., 2005; Fox-Wasylyshyn et al., 2005). The most prominent cluster of needs that families have rated as dissatisfying is related to lack of patient information (Auerbach et al., 2005; Fox-Wasylyshyn et al., 2005; Johnson et al., 1998; Leske, 1992a). Researchers suggest that providing interventions to promote family satisfaction may improve patient care outcomes (Agaibi &

Wilson, 2005; Auerbach et al., 2005; Institute for Family-Centered Care, 1999; Lilly & Daley, 2007).

## Summary of Research

The review of prior research confirms increased risk for difficult family adaptation after critical illness but also indicates that this outcome is not inevitable. Previous studies are largely without theoretical guidance; rely on measures using only the spouse's perspective of the family; use descriptive or survey designs; have small sample sizes, include few diverse families or families in different development stages; and primarily focus on outcomes related to patient or spouse's psychosocial functioning as an influence on the recovery process. Minimal research has been reported that contributes to understanding the changes in family processes, especially in determining the difference in families that have made a smooth recovery and families that have made a difficult recovery from significant health events in family members. Little is known about how the critical care experience is interpreted by aged family members. However, nurses need to intervene with the family of a critically ill older adult patient to lower stress and promote satisfaction in critical care.

## Responses of Aged Family Members

Gerontological research consistently shows that, as people age, they become less and less like others of the same age (AARP, 2007). This evolving awareness of the increasing heterogeneity of older people suggests that an older adult's biological, cognitive, and psychological function can vary greatly, from healthy and active to severely disabled. Older adult family members differ from younger family members in important ways that potentially affect how they cope with the stress of critical illness:

- They have diminished baseline physiological reserve, lack cardiac and respiratory reserve, are at risk for dehydration; decreased daily energy has implications for older adult family members.
- They may have chronic illnesses that can exacerbate or intensify the response to stress.
- They report less emotional distress but develop somatic symptoms indicative of distress.
- They may need longer time to process information.
- They may have family members who do not live nearby who therefore can't provide needed support.
- They may have friends or neighbors, instead of relatives, who provide a support system.
- They may have different attitudes and expectations toward health care providers.

These age-related changes need to be taken into account when dealing with older family members because they may affect how well the family members can cope and adapt to the critical illness situation. These changes also need to be addressed when assessing the family, particularly as the patient may return to the care of the aging spouse.

## Summary

Is Mrs. B.'s family unusual? Is this a hypothetical situation made too dramatic? The answer to both questions is "no." This situation is real, the family is real, and a typical elderly spouse was driven to feel helpless and out of control, experiencing what no person should ever go through, and needing to rethink her future.

The ultimate goal for any family faced with a critical illness is to reorganize and stabilize function as the affected member progresses from the acute to the rehabilitative phases of recovery. Stabilization of family function is achieved to the extent that the family can mobilize the necessary resources to cope effectively with the situation.

It is well documented that families can use some intervention, especially in early stages of the patient's illness and treatment, but it remains unclear as to what specific interventions are the most effective. It is even less clear as to which interventions are effective for aged family members. The majority of families confronted with critical illness may do well, with or without specific interventions (Leske & Heidrich, 1996). On the other hand, the stresses associated with critical illness may increase family vulnerability to a wide range of emotional, behavioral, or adjustment problems. The aged family member may be at increased risk for changes in family roles and routines that alter his or her ability to fully participate in patient care. Research is needed to develop theoretically grounded and empirically based approaches for aged family member interventions. Until then, critical care nurses are encouraged to be creative and innovative in designing and evaluating interventions to meet specific needs of family members. The challenges are to identify which interventions are helpful to aged families and how they can best be used in clinical practice.

Hospitalization for a critical illness can disrupt even the most highly organized and functional family. The waiting: waiting for information, waiting to visit, waiting to know how the critical illness experience will turn out causes families intense pain and distress. The essence of this experience is one in which nurses have profound influence over the tone of critical illness for families. Family-focused care may mitigate family stress by providing support based on the unique needs of each family. Family members may suffer as much distress as the patient. They, too, deserve special attention and consideration. Professionals who are interested in the welfare and functioning of the family must ensure that the family of the patient receives adequate and appropriate care, no matter what the age of its members.

## References

Agaibi, C. E., & Wilson, J. P. (2005). Trauma, PTSD, and resilience: A review of the literature. *Trauma, Violence, & Abuse, 6*, 195–216.

American Association of Critical-Care Nurses. (2005). *AACN standards for establishing and sustaining healthy work environments: A journey to excellence.* Aliso Viejo, CA: AACN. Available at www.aacn.org

American Association of Retired Persons. (2007). *The state of Americans 50+.* Washington, DC: American Association of Retired Persons. Available at www.aarp.org

American Nurses' Association. (2001). *Standards and scope of gerontological nursing practice* (2nd ed.). Kansas City, MO: Author.

Auerbach, S. M., Kiesler, D. J., Wartella, J., Rausch S., Ward, K. R., & Ivatury, R. (2005). Optimism, satisfaction with needs met, interpersonal perceptions of the health care team, and emotional distress in patients' family members during critical care hospitalization. *American Journal of Critical Care, 14*, 202–210.

Azoulay, E., Pochard, F., Chevret, S., Lemaire, F., Mokhtari, M., LeGall, J., et al. (2001). Meeting the needs of intensive care unit patient families. *American Journal of Respiratory Critical Care Medicine,* *163,* 135–139.

Azoulay, E., Pochard, F., Kentish-Barnes, N., Chevret, S., Aboab, J., Annane, D., et al. (2005). Risk of post-traumatic stress symptoms in family members of intensive care units patients. *Respiratory and Critical Care Medicine, 171,* 987–994.

Baggs, J., Schmitt, M. H., Mushlin, A., Eldredge, D. H., Oakes, D., & Hutson, A. D. (1997). Nurse–physician collaboration and satisfaction with decision-making in three critical care units. *American Journal of Critical Care, 6,* 393–399.

Beckman, H. B., Markakis, K. M., Suchman, A. L., & Franken, R. M. (1994). The doctor–patient relationship and malpractice: Lessons from plaintiff depositions. *Archives of Internal Medicine, 154,* 1365–1370.

Bengtson, A., Karlsson, T., Wahrborg, P., Hjalmarson, A., & Herlitz, J. (1996). Cardiovascular and psychosomatic symptoms among relatives of patients waiting for possible coronary revascularization. *Heart & Lung, 25,* 438–443.

Boss, P. G. (2002). *Family stress management: A contextual approach* (2nd ed.). Thousand Oaks, CA: Sage.

Bouley, G., von Hofe, K., & Blatt, L. (1994). Holistic care of the critically ill: Meeting both patient and family needs. *Dimensions of Critical Care Nursing, 13,* 218–223.

Brody, E. M. (1990). Social factors in care: The elderly patient's family. In W. R. Hazzard, E. L. Bierman, & J. P. Blass (Eds.), *Principles of geriatric medicine and gerontology* (2nd ed., pp. 232–240). New York: McGraw-Hill.

Carter, B., & McGoldrick, M. (1999). *The expanded family life cycle: Individual, family, and social perspectives* (3rd ed.). Needham Heights, MA: Allyn & Bacon.

Chien, W. T., Chiu, Y. L., Lam, L. W., & Ip, W. Y. (2005). Effects of a needs based education programme for family carers with a relative in an intensive care unit: A quasi-experimental study. *International Journal of Nursing Studies, 43,* 39–50.

Chui, W., & Chan, S. (2007). Stress and coping of Hong Kong Chinese family members during a critical illness. *Journal of Clinical Nursing, 16,* 372–381.

Clark, M. C. (1997). A causal functional explanation of maintaining a dependent elder in the community. *Research in Nursing & Health, 20,* 515–526.

Cuellar, N., & Butts, J. B. (1999). Caregiver distress: What nurses in rural settings can do to help. *Nursing Forum, 24*(3), 24–30.

Davidson, J. E., Powers, K., Hedayat, K. M., Tieszen, M., Kon, A. A., Shephard, E., et al. (2007). Clinical practice guidelines for support of the family in the patient-centered intensive care unit: American College of Critical Care Medicine Task Force 2004–2005. *Critical Care Medicine, 35,* 605–622.

DeGeneffe, C. E., & Lynch, R. T. (2006). Correlates of depression in adult siblings of persons with traumatic brain injury. *Rehabilitation Counseling Bulletin, 49,* 130–142.

Dellasega, C., Clark, D., McCreary, D., Helmuth, A., & Schan, P. (1994). Nursing process: Teaching elderly clients. *Journal of Gerontological Nursing, 20* (1), 31–38.

Dracup, K., Evangelista, L. S., Doering, L., Tullman, D., Moser, D. K., & Hamilton, M. (2004). Emotional well-being in spouses of patients with advanced heart failure. *Heart & Lung, 33,* 354–361.

Duclos, C. W., Eichler, M., Taylor, L., Quintela, J., Main, D. S., Pace, W., et al. (2005). Patient perspectives of patient-provider communication after adverse events. *International Journal for Quality in Health Care. 17,* 479–486.

Ebersole, P., Touhy, T., Hess, P., Jett, K., & Luggen, A. S. (2008). *Toward healthy aging—Human needs and nursing response* (7th ed.). St. Louis, MO: Mosby.

Eggenberger, S. K., & Nelms, T. P. (2007). Being family: The family experience when an adult member is hospitalized with a critical illness. *Journal of Clinical Nursing, 16,* 1618–1628.

Eriksson, T., & Bergbom, I. (2007). Visits to intensive care unit-frequency, duration and impact an outcome. *Nursing in Critical Care, 12,* 20–26.

Figely, C. R., & Barnes, M. (2005) External trauma and families. In P. C. McKenry & S. J. Price (Eds.), *Families & change: Coping with stressful events and transitions* (3rd ed., pp. 379–401). Thousand Oaks, CA: Sage.

Fink, S. V. (1995). The influence of family resources and family demands on the strains and well-being of caregiving families. *Nursing Research, 44,* 139–146.

Fletcher, K. (2007). Optimizing reserve in hospitalized elderly. *Critical Care Nursing Clinics of North America, 19,* 285–302.

Foreman, M. (1989). Confusion in the hospitalized elderly: Incidence, onset, and associated factors. *Research in Nursing & Health, 12,* 21–29.

Fournet, C. (1992). Support for significant others of elderly patients. *AACN Clinical Issues in Critical Care Nursing, 3,* 73–78.

Fox-Wasylyshyn, S. M., El-Masari, M., & Williamson, K. M. (2005). Family perceptions of nurses' roles toward family members of critically ill patients: A descriptive study. *Heart & Lung, 34,* 335–344.

Frain, M. P., Berven, N. L., Tschopp, M. K., Lee, G. K., Tansey, T., & Cronister, J. (2007). Use of the resiliency model of family stress, adjustment and adaptation by rehabilitation counselors. *Journal of Rehabilitation, 73,* 18–25.

Francis, J., & Kapoor, W. (1992). Prognosis after hospital discharge of older medical patients with delirium. *Journal of the American Geriatrics Society, 40,* 601–606.

Fry, S., & Warren, N. A. (2007). Perceived needs of critical care family members: A phenomenological discourse. *Critical Care Nursing Quarterly, 30,* 181–188.

Gilliss, C. L., & Knafl, K. A. (1999). Nursing care of families in non-normative transitions: The state of science and practice. In A. S. Hinshaw, S. L. Feetham, & J. L. Shaver (Eds.), *Handbook of clinical nursing research* (pp. 231–249). Thousand Oaks, CA: Sage.

Gonzalez, C., Carroll, D. L., Elliott, J. S., Fitzgerald, P. A., & Vallent, H. J. (2004). Visitation preferences of patients in the intensive care unit and a complex care medical unit. *American Journal of Critical Care, 13,* 194–198.

Gulranjani, R. P. (1995). Physical environmental factors affecting patient's stress in the accident and emergency department. *Accident and Emergency Nursing, 3,* 22–27.

Haber, D., & Looney, C. (2000). Health contract calendars: A tool for health professionals with older adults. *The Gerontologist, 49,* 235–239.

Hallgrimsdottir, E. M. (2004). Caring for families in A & E departments: Scottish and Icelandic nurses' opinions and experiences. *Accident and Emergency Nursing, 12,* 114–120.

Hansen, L., Archbold, P., Stewart, B., Westfall, U. B., & Ganzini, L. (2005). Family caregivers making life-sustaining treatment decisions. *Journal of Gerontological Nursing, 31,* 28–35.

He, W., Sengupta, M., Velkoff, V. A., & Debarros, K. A. (2005). 65+ in the United States: 2005. In *U.S. Census Bureau, current population reports*. Washington, DC: U.S. Government Printing Office.

Henneman, E. A., McKenzie, J. B., & Dewa, C. S. (1992). An evaluation of interventions for meeting the information needs of families of critically ill patients. *American Journal of Critical Care, 3,* 85–93.

Hupcey, J. E. (1998). Establishing the nurse-patient relationship in the intensive care unit. *Western Journal of Nursing Research, 20,* 180–194.

Institute for Family-Centered Care. (1999). Family-centered care: questions and answers. *Advances in Family-Centered Care, 5*(5), 2–4.

Institue of Medicine. (2001). *Crossing the quality chasm: A new health system for the 21st century.* Washington, DC: National Academy Press.

Jacelon, C. S. (2006). Directive and supportive behaviors used by families of hospitalized older adults to affect the process of hospitalization. *Journal of Family Nursing, 12,* 234–250.

Johnson, D., Wilson, M., Cavavaugh, B., Bryden, C., Gudmundson, D., & Moodley, O. (1998). Measuring the ability to meet family needs in an intensive care unit. *Critical Care Medicine, 26,* 266–271.

Juneau, B. (1996). Special issues in critical care gerontology. *Critical Care Nursing Quarterly, 19,* 71–75.

Kapp, M. B. (1991). Health care decision making by the elderly: I get by with a little help from my family. *The Gerontologist, 31,* 619–623.

Kass, J. D., Castriotta, R. J., & Malakoff, T. (1992). Intensive care unit outcomes in the very elderly. *Critical Care Medicine, 20,* 1666.

Kaye, J., & Heald, G. (1996). Spirituality among family members of critically ill adults. *American Journal of Critical Care, 5,* 242.

Kaufman, S. R. (1998). Intensive care, old age, and problems of death in America. *The Gerontologist, 38,* 715–725.

Ketchum, K. M. (2000). Patient and family psychosocial adjustment during the first week following traumatic injury. *Dissertation Abstracts International: Section B: The Sciences and Engineering, 61*(5-B), 2472.

Kleinpell, R. M. (2006). Focusing on caregivers of the critically ill: Beyond illness into recovery. *Critical Care Medicine, 34,* 243–244.

Kojlak, J., Keenan, S. P., Plotkin, D., Giles-Fysh, H., & Sibbald, W. J. (1998). Determining the potential need for a bereavement follow-up program: How well are family and health care workers' needs currently being met? *Official Journal of the Canadian Association of Critical Care Nurses, 9,* 12–16.

Kosciulek, J. F., McCubbin, M. A., & McCubbin, H. I. (1993). A theoretical framework for family adaptation to head injury. *Journal of Rehabilitation, 59,* 40–45.

Kosco, M., & Warren, N. A. (2000). Critical care nurses' perceptions of family needs as met. *Critical Care Nursing Quarterly, 23*, 60–72.

Landsman, I. S., Baum, C. G., Arnkoff, D. B., Craig, M. J., Lynch, I., Copes, W. S., et al. (1990). The psychological consequences of traumatic injury. *Journal of Behavioral Medicine, 13*, 561–581.

Lautrette, A., Darmon, M., & Megarbane, L. M., Joly, L. M., Chevret, S., Adrie C., et al. (2007). A communication strategy and brochure for relatives of patients dying in ICU. *New England Journal of Medicine, 356*, 469–478.

Lee, L. Y., & Lau, L. L. (2003). Immediate needs of adult family members of intensive care patients in Hong Kong. *Journal of Clinical Nursing, 12*, 490–500.

Leske, J. S. (1991). Overview of family needs following critical illness: From assessment to intervention. *AACN Clinical Issues in Critical Care Nursing, 2*, 220–226.

Leske, J. S. (1992a). Needs of adult family members after critical illness: Prescriptions for interventions. *Critical Care Nursing Clinics of North America, 4*, 587–596.

Leske, J. S. (1992b). Comparison ratings of need importance after critical illness from family members with varied demographic characteristics. *Critical Care Nursing Clinics of North America, 4*, 607–613.

Leske, J. S. (1998). Treatment for family members in crisis after critical injury. *AACN Clinical Issues: Advanced Practice in Acute and Critical Care, 9*, 129–139.

Leske, J. S. (2000). Family stresses, strengths, and outcomes after critical injury. *Critical Care Nursing Clinics of North America, 12*, 237–244.

Leske, J. S. (2003). Comparison of family stresses, strengths, and outcomes after trauma and surgery. *AACN Clinical Issues: Advanced Practice in Acute and Critical Care, 14*, 33–41.

Leske, J. S., & Heidrich, S. M. (1996). Interventions for aged family members. *Critical Care Nursing Clinics of North America, 8*, 91–102.

Leske, J. S., & Jiricka, M. K. (1998). Impact of family demands and family strengths and capabilities on family well-being and adaptation after critical injury. *American Journal of Critical Care, 7*, 383–392.

Leske, J. S., & Pasquale, M. A. (2007). Family needs, interventions, and presence. In N. C. Molter (Ed.), *Creating healing environments: Protocols for practice* (2nd ed., pp. 29–64). Sudbury, MA: Jones and Bartlett.

Leske J. S., & Pelczynski, S. A. (1999). Caregiver satisfaction with preparation for discharge in a decreased-length-of-stay cardiac surgery program. *Journal of Cardiovascular Nursing, 14*, 35–43.

Li, H., Melnyk, B. B., & McCann, R. (2004). Review of intervention studies of families with hospitalized elderly relatives. *Journal of Nursing Scholarship, 36*, 54–59.

Li, H., Melnyk, B. B., McCann, R., Chatcheydang, J., Koulouglioti, C., Nichols, L.W., et al. (2003). Creating avenues for relative empowerment (CARE): A pilot test of an intervention to improve outcomes of hospitalized elders and family caregivers. *Research in Nursing & Health, 26*, 284–299.

Li, H., Stewart, B. J., Imle, M. A., & Archbold, P. G. (2000). Families and hospitalized elders: A typology of family care actions. *Research in Nursing & Health, 13*, 375–384.

Lilly, C. M., & Daley, B. J. (2007). The healing power of listening in ICU. *New England Journal of Medicine, 356*, 513–515.

Lim, J., & Zebrock, B. (2004). Caring for family members with chronic physical illness: A critical review of caregiver literature. *Health and Quality of Life Outcomes, 2*, 50–59.

Lindgren, V. A., Barnett, S. D., & Bloom, R. L. (2006). Who is dying in our critical care units? A single center's experience. *Journal of Nursing Care Quality, 21*, 78–85.

Lynn-McHale, D. J., & Deatrick, J. A. (2000). Trust between family and health care providers. *Journal of Family Nursing, 6*, 210–230.

MacKenzie, E. J., Siegel, J. H., Shapiro, S., Moody, M., & Smith, R. T. (1988). Functional recovery and medical costs of trauma: An analysis by type and severity of injury. *Journal of Trauma, 28*, 281–297.

Marik, P. E. (2006). Management of the critically ill geriatric patient. *Critical Care Medicine, 34*, (Suppl.), S176–S182.

Maxwell, K. E., Stuenkel, D., & Saylor, C. (2007). Needs of family members of critically ill patients: A comparison of nurse and family perceptions. *Heart & Lung, 36*, 367–376.

McCubbin, H. I., & McCubbin, M. A. (1996). Resiliency in families: Family stress theory and assessment: A conceptual model of family adjustment and adaptation in response to stress and crisis. In H. I. McCubbin, A. Thompson, & M. McCubbin (Eds.), *Family assessment: Resiliency, coping, and adaptation-inventories for assessment and research.* (pp. 1–64). Madison, WI: University of Wisconsin Press.

McQuay, J. E., Schwartz, R., Goldblatt, P. C., & Giangrasso, V. M. (1995). "Death-telling" research project. *Critical Care Nursing Clinics of North America, 7*, 549–555.

Medina, J. (2005). A natural synergy in creating a patient-focused care environment: The critical care family assistance program and critical care nursing. *Chest, 128,* 99–102.

Mendonca, D., & Warren, N. A. (1998). Perceived and unmet needs of critical care family members. *Critical Care Nursing Quarterly, 21,* 58–67.

Menkhaus, S., Turner, N., Gueldner, S., & Michele, Y. (1996). Effectiveness of the family beeper program (FBP) in the critical care unit. *American Journal of Critical Care, 5,* 236.

Mishel, M. H., & Braden, C. J. (1987). Uncertainty: A mediator between support and adjustment. *Western Journal of Nursing Research, 9,* 43–57.

Moser, D. K. (2007). "The rust of life": Impact on anxiety on cardiac patients. *American Journal of Critical Care, 16,* 361–369.

Moser, D. K., & Dracup, K. (2000). Impact of cardiopulmonary resuscitation training on perceived control in spouses of recovering patients. *Research in Nursing & Health, 23,* 270–278.

Neundorfer, M. (1991). Family caregivers of the frail elderly: Impact of caregiving on their health and implications for interventions. *Family & Community Health, 14,* 48–58.

Nijboer, C., Triemstra, M., Tempelaar, R., Mulder, M., Sanderman, R., & Bos, G. (2000). Patterns of caregiver experiences among patterns of cancer patients. *The Gerontologist, 40,* 738–746.

Nolan, M., T., Cupples, S. A., Brown, M. M., Pierce, L., Lepley, D., & Ohler, L. (1992). Perceived stress and coping strategies among families of cardiac transplant candidates during the organ waiting period. *Heart & Lung, 21,* 540–547.

Paparrigopoulous, T., Melissaki, A., Efthymiou, A., Tsekou, H., Vadala, C., Kribeni, G., et al. (2006). Short-term psychological impact on family members of intensive care unit patients. *Journal of Psychosomatic Research, 61,* 719–722.

Patterson, J. M. (2002). Understanding family resilience. *Journal of Clinical Psychology, 58,* 233–246.

Peirce, A. G., Wright, F., & Fulmer, T. T. (1992). Needs of the family during critical illness of elderly patient. *Critical Care Nursing Clinics of North America, 4,* 497–606.

Pochard, F., Darmon, M., Fassier T., Bollaert, P., Cheval, C., Colloigner, M., et al. (2005). Symptoms of anxiety and depression in family members of intensive care unit patients before discharge or death: A prospective, multicenter study. *Journal of Critical Care, 20,* 90–96.

Rashid, M. (2007). Developing scales to evaluate staff perception of the effects of the physical environment on patient comfort, patient safety, patient privacy, family integration with patient care, and staff working conditions in adult intensive care unit. *Critical Care Nursing Quarterly, 30,* 271–283.

Redekopp, M. A., & Leske, J. S. (2007). Family visitation and partnership. In N. C. Molter (Ed.), *Creating healing environments: Protocols for practice* (2nd ed., pp. 65–90). Sudbury, MA: Jones and Bartlett.

Redley, B., Beanland, C., & Botti, M. (2003). Accompanying critically ill relatives in emergency departments. *Journal of Advanced Nursing, 44,* 88–98.

Richmond, T. S., Kauder, D., Hinkle, J., & Shults, J. (2003). Early predictors of long-term disability after injury. *American Journal of Critical Care, 12,* 197–205.

Rush, P. (1997). Guidelines for critical care and the elderly: The search continues. *Critical Care Medicine, 25,* 1619–1620.

Rushton, C. H., Reina, M. L., & Reina, D. S. (2007). Building trustworthy relationships with critically ill patients and families. *AACN Advanced Critical Care, 16,* 19–30.

Schlump-Urquhart, S. R. (1990). Families experiencing a traumatic accident: Implications and nursing management. *AACN Clinical Issues in Critical Care Nursing, 1,* 522–534.

Schone, B., & Pezzin, L. (1999). Parental marital disruption and intergenerational transfers: An analysis of lone elderly parents and their children. *Demography, 36,* 287–297.

Schulz, R., & Beach, S. R. (1999). Caregiving as a risk factor for mortality. *Journal American Medical Association, 282,* 2215–2219.

Sonnenblick, M., Friendlander, Y., & Steinberg, A. (1993). Dissociation between the wishes of terminally ill patients and decisions by their offspring. *Journal of the American Geriatrics Society, 41,* 599–604.

Suresh, R., Kupfer, Y. Y., & Tessler, S. (1999). The greying of the intensive care unit: Demographic changes 1988–1998. *Critical Care Medicine, 27* (Suppl.) A27.

Tak, Y. R., & Lee, H. Y. (1997). Family stress, perceived social support, and coping in family who has a developmentally disabled child. *Korean Journal of Child Health Nursing, 3,* 42–51.

Tilden, V. O., Tolle, S. W., Nelson, C. A., Thompson, M., & Eggman, S. C. (1999). Family decision making in foregoing life extending treatments. *Journal of Family Nursing, 5,* 426–442.

Titler, M. G., Bombei, C., & Schutte, D. L. (1995). Developing family-focused care. *Critical Care Nursing Clinics of North America, 7,* 375–386.

Tolley, G., & Prevost, S. (1997). Case management of critically ill elders: A case study. *AACN Clinical Issues in Critical Care Nursing, 8,* 635–642.

Tracy, J., Fowler, S., & Magarelli, K. (1999). Hope and anxiety of individual family members of critically ill adults. *Applied Nursing Research, 12,* 121–127.

Tsevat, J., Dawson, N. V., Wu, A. W., Lynn, J., Soukup, J. R., Cook, E. F., et al. (1998). Health values of hospitalized patients 80 years or older. *Journal of the American Medical Association, 279,* 371–375.

U.S. Census Bureau. (2000). *Profile of general demographic characteristics.* Retrieved March 2, 2008, from http://fact-finder.census.gov.2000

Vandell-Walker, V., Jensen, L., & Oberle, K. (2007). Nursing support for family members of critically ill adults. *Qualitative Health Research, 17,* 1207–1218.

Van Horn, E., & Tesh, A. (2000). The effect of critical care hospitalization on family members: Stress and responses. *Dimensions of Critical Care Nursing, 19,* 90–96.

Verhaeghe, S. T., Defloor, T., van Zuuren, F. J., Duijnstee, M., & Grypdonck, M. (2005). The needs and experiences of family members of adult patients in an intensive care unit: A review of the literature. *Journal of Clinical Nursing, 14,* 501–509.

Verhaeghe, S. T., van Zuuren, F. J., Defloor, T., Duijnstee, M., & Grypdonck, M. (2007). The process and the meaning of hope for family members of traumatic coma patients in intensive care. *Qualitative Health Research, 17,* 730–743.

Vom Eigen, K. A., Walker, J. D., Edgeman-Levitan, S., Cleary, R. D., & Delbanco, T. L. (1999). Care partner experiences with hospital care. *Medical Care, 37,* 33–38.

Wall, R. J., Engelberg, R. A., Downer, L., Heyland, D. K., & Curtis, J. R. (2007). Refinement, scoring, and validation of the Family Satisfaction in the Intensive Care unit (FS-ICU) survey. *Critical Care Medicine, 35,* 271–279.

Walsh, F. (2007). Traumatic loss and major disasters: Strengthening family and community resilience. *Family Process, 46,* 207–227.

Walters, A. J. (1995). A hermeneutic study of the experiences of relatives of critically ill patients. *Journal of Advanced Nursing, 22,* 998–1005.

Wasser, T., Pasquale, M. A., Matchett, S. C., Bryan, Y., & Pasquale, M. (2001). Establishing reliability and validity of the critical care satisfaction survey. *Critical Care Medicine, 29,* 192–196.

Webster, P. D., & Johnson, B. H. (2007). *Developing a family-centered vision, mission, and philosophy of care statements.* Bethesda, MD: Institute for Family-Centered Care.

Wheelan, S., Burchill, C., & Tilan, F. (2003). The link between teamwork and patient outcomes in intensive care units. *American Journal of Critical Care, 12,* 527–534.

White, J. M, & Klein, D. M. (2008). *Family theories* (3rd ed.). Thousand Oaks, CA: Sage.

Weigand, D. (2006). Withdrawal of life-sustaining therapy after sudden, unexpected life-threatening illness or injury: Interactions between patients' families, healthcare providers, and the healthcare system. *American Journal of Critical Care, 15,* 178–187.

Williams, C. M. (2005). The identification of family members' contribution to patients' care in the intensive care unit: A naturalistic inquiry. *Nursing in Critical Care, 10,* 6–14.

Winston, F. K., Baxt, C., Kassam-Adams, N. L., Elliot, M. R., & Kallan, M. J. (2005). Acute traumatic stress symptoms in child occupants and their parent drivers after crash involvement. *Archives of Pediatrics and Adolescent Medicine, 159*(11), 1074–1079.

Wu, A. W., Rubin, H. R., & Rosen, M. J. (1990). Are elderly people less responsive to intensive care? *Journal of the American Geriatrics Society, 38,* 621–627.

# End-of-Life Care and Decisions About Life-Sustaining Treatments

# 8

Karen Kehl
Karin T. Kirchhoff

Mary is a 76-year-old widow who presented to the emergency room (ER) with left-sided paralysis, aphasia, and respiratory distress. She has a history of hypertension and atrial fibrillation and had a cerebrovascular accident (CVA) 3 months ago that left her with speech difficulties and left-sided weakness. After her hospitalization for that CVA she entered an assisted-living facility because her children were concerned about falling while living alone. Mary has a son and daughter who live nearby and another daughter, Sarah, who lives 900 miles away. In the ER Mary was assessed and it was determined that she had another cardioembolic CVA. Because of her respiratory distress, Mary was intubated and placed on a ventilator. Mary's son, John, is her activated durable power of attorney for health care. When John arrived at the ER he requested aggressive care so his sister Sarah could see his mother alive. Mary is transferred to the intensive care unit (ICU). In ICU Mary remains stable for the 48 hours it takes Sarah to arrive. John is not sure what his mother would choose because she has said she "doesn't want to be kept alive on machines," but she recovered from her earlier CVA enough to enjoy visits from her grandchildren and some of the activities at the assisted-living facility. Sarah is concerned about her mother "starving to death" so when the resident recommends a percutaneous endoscopic gastrostomy (PEG) tube on day 3, the family readily agrees. Initial attempts at weaning Mary from the ventilator have been unsuccessful. On day 7, Mary remains in ICU on synchronized intermittent mechanical ventilation (SIMV). She has an intermittent low-grade fever that has not responded to antibiotics. She is receiving intravenous hydration and nutrition via the PEG tube. Mary has periods of responsiveness, but does not have the capacity to participate in medical decision making. The family wants to know what to do. Sarah is asking if she should stay or return home, John is hesitant to take action, and their sister, Jane, is insistent that their mother would not want to live like this.

## Introduction

Older adults who are dying in the critical care setting need the same quality care as is given to any patient who is facing his or her final days in critical care. Where the care of older adults differs is often in decision making, the consequences of care decisions, and in modifications to symptom management to account for the physiologic changes seen with aging. Good end-of-life care in any setting requires effective communication with the patient and the family, facilitation of decision making, management of complications of the treatment and the disease, symptom control, psychosocial–spiritual care of the patient and the family, and holistic care at the time of death (Foley & Gelband, 2001).

Decision making is often a key issue in ICU. Health care professionals who may not expect young adults to have planned for future medical needs are frequently surprised when older adults, who are generally in declining health, have not addressed future medical decision making. Families of older adults may not be prepared to make medical decisions when the patient loses decision-making capacity.

For older adults facing their final days, the consequences of their health care decisions may include facing death in the hospital or ICU setting or making the transition to another setting to die. Families may be poorly prepared for these consequences and transitions. Proactive discussion of the consequences of medical decision making, along with excellent management that allows transitions to be made as smoothly and seamlessly as possible, can improve the experience for patients and families.

For older adults who receive end-of-life care in the critical care setting, often a shift occurs from curative care or care that extends life, to comfort or palliative care. The focus of palliative care is on making the person as comfortable as possible by good symptom management, attention to spiritual and psychosocial needs, and providing support to the family. Good palliative care includes preparing both the patient and family for the death. Nurses also need to notify and support families immediately after the death and facilitate decisions about autopsy and organ donation.

## Decision Making in Critically Ill Older Adults

The importance of medical decision making has been accentuated because of recent cases such as the Terri Schiavo case, the Patient Self-Determination Act, and research about whether patient preferences are followed in care decisions. A sentinel report, the Study to Understand Prognoses and Preferences for Outcomes and Risks of Treatments (SUPPORT) (SUPPORT Investigators, 1995), was a major impetus to the recent increase in research about end-of-life care. SUPPORT was conducted in the early 1990s and had two phases, an observational phase, which took place over 2 years and an interventional phase. Over 9,000 patients with one or more of nine life-threatening illnesses were enrolled from five medical centers. The intervention used was a nurse who interacted with the patient, family, and staff to provide information to the attending physicians on prognoses and patient/surrogate information and preferences for care. The mean patient age was 63 years, 44% of patients were female, and 16% were Black. Overall survival to 6 months was 53%. In risk analyses that adjusted for sex, ethnicity, income, baseline functional status, severity of illness, and aggressiveness of care, each additional year of age increased the risk of death by 1.0% for patients 18 to 70 years of age, and by 2.0% for patients older than 70 years of age. Estimates of 6-month mortality rates were 44% for 55-year-old patients, 48% for 65-year-old patients, 53% for 75-year-old patients, and 60% for 85-year-old patients. Surprisingly, age contributed less to the risk of death than aggressiveness of care, acute physiology, and diagnosis (Hamel et al., 1999). Based on this information, age should not be as important in decision making as comorbidities and the patient's clinical condition. It is important not to make decisions solely on the patient's age, but to carefully consider these other elements to determine the most appropriate treatment.

The Hospitalized Elderly Longitudinal Project (HELP) was a subset of the SUPPORT sample and consisted of adults 80 years or older. A total of 417 HELP patients died within a year of enrollment. Most of the patients (70%) said they preferred comfort care rather than care aimed at extending life (Somogyi-Zalud, Zhong, Lynn, & Hamel, 2000). A total of 72 HELP patients died during their enrollment hospitalization. Of these patients, 70% wanted comfort-focused care and 80% had a Do Not Resuscitate (DNR) order. Yet, of the 72 who died, 63% received one or more life-saving treatments, 54% were admitted to an intensive care unit, and 43% were on a ventilator before they died (Somogyi-Zalud, Zhong, Hamel, & Lynn, 2002). In general, these older patients preferred to have their families and the physician make decisions for them rather than strictly follow their communicated preferences at the end of life (Puchalski et al., 2000).

Although these patients preferred family and physicians making decisions, they frequently did not have the conversations required to inform physicians about their wishes. The SUPPORT study also revealed that even though most patients who had long (more than 14 days) ICU stays had a high likelihood of dying in the next 6 months (55% died), fewer than 40% of the patients reported that their physicians talked to them about their prognosis or preferences for life-sustaining treatment. Only 29% of the patients who preferred a palliative approach felt that the care they received was consistent with the goal of comfort care (Teno, Fisher, et al., 2000).

Although older patients were less likely to want aggressive treatments than younger patients, the majority of older patients wanted cardiopulmonary resuscitation, and many wanted care that emphasized life extension rather than comfort. Families and physicians underestimated the elders' desire for aggressive treatment. An examination of age-related differences in hospital care for SUPPORT patients revealed that after adjustment for sociodemographic factors, severity of illness, and patients' preferences for aggressive care, decisions to withhold life-sustaining treatments were more frequent for older patients (Hamel et al., 2000). These factors all contribute to a discrepancy between older adults' preferences and the care they receive at the end of life.

## Survival of Older Adults in Critical Care

There is conflicting information about the risk of death and chance of survival of older adults. The findings of the SUPPORT study indicate that as age increases, people have a greater risk of dying and a lower chance of survival. Even when adjustments were made for the use of less aggressive care in the older adult, this increased mortality risk because of age persisted (Hamel et al., 2000). Yet, for those dying following withdrawal of ventilatory support, there is no relationship between age and time to death (Campbell, 2007). Furthermore, older adult ICU patients have survival similar to younger patients when severity of illness is similar (Kleinpell & Ferrans, 1998) unless the patient is very old (85+) (Van Den Noortgate, Vogelaers, Afschrift, & Colardyn, 1999). Because the relationship of aging to mortality risk is not clear, care decisions should be made on the likelihood of survival of each individual rather than on the chronological age of the patient.

The likelihood of survival, or the prognosis in terms of approximate length of life of the older hospitalized adult, can be estimated from the clinical information in the medical chart and a brief interview with the patient or surrogate. By adding information about prognosis from the physician, and patient preferences in care, accuracy of the estimate can be improved (Teno, Harrell, et al., 2000). When physician estimates of intensive care survival are less than 10% it is more likely that life-sustaining treatment will be limited and this is more predictive of ICU death than illness severity, organ dysfunction, or the use of inotropes or vasopressors (Rocker et al., 2004).

## Advance Care Planning

Under the Patient Self-Determination Act, hospitals are mandated to ask whether a person has an Advance Directive (AD). Despite this legislation and the wide promotion of ADs, the completion rates have not met recommended levels (Ramsey & Mitty, 2003). When ADs are present, they do not consistently guide care in ICUs (Goodman, Tarnoff, & Slotman, 1998). Even when the older adults have completed a living will or health care power of attorney, they might not have understood the form (Jezewski & Meeker, 2005) or the impact of these decisions. Chronically ill older adults tend to live life a day at a time, not looking too far into the future, and plan to "cross the bridge" when they get to it (Carrese, Mullaney, Faden, & Finucane, 2002) so they may not have completed an AD or discussed their preferences with the person they have designated as a surrogate decision maker or health care agent.

One approach that has been more consistently effective is the use of orders such as Physician Orders for Life-Sustaining Treatment (POLST). In one study of the older adults in an Oregon program, POLST was followed consistently for cardiopulmonary resuscitation (CPR) (91%), antibiotics (86%), IV fluids (84%), and feeding tubes (94%) (Lee, Brummel-Smith, Meyer, Drew, & London, 2000).

One challenge in advance care planning with older adults is that their preferences often shift over time (Ditto, Jacobson, Smucker, Danks, & Fagerlin, 2006), or the patients are not clear about their preferences (Schneiderman, Pearlman, Kaplan, Anderson, & Rosenberg, 1992). Further, documented preferences may not reflect the patient's current wishes. When older adults were asked about end-of-life care situations before, soon after, and several months after a hospitalization, participants reported less desire to receive life-sustaining treatment at the posthospitalization interview than they did at the interview conducted prior to hospitalization. However, desire for life-sustaining treatment returned to near prehospitalization levels at the annual interview conducted several months after hospitalization (Lloyd, Nietert, & Silvestri, 2004). The timing of such discussions seems to be a factor in choices; recent memories of aggressive treatment tend to reduce the desire for such treatment.

Even when older adults are sure of their preferences concerning end-of-life care, they rarely have discussions with their physicians about their preferences. A recent study examined 80 patients older than 64 years to address preferences about end-of-life care and CPR as their disease progressed. Although 40% did not wish to have CPR, only two had previously discussed their CPR preferences with their physicians (Formiga et al., 2004). In another study of 115 patients with oxygen-dependent chronic obstructive pulmonary disease (COPD), less than one third reported having a discussion about end-of-life care with their physicians (Knauft, Nielsen, Engelberg, Patrick, & Curtis, 2005). It seems that neither patients nor health care professionals are raising the topic. A recent study showed that even in the oldest-old veterans, those greater that 85 years, only 50 of 149 (34%) had documented care preferences (Wu, Lorenz, & Chodosh, 2008). In this study only age and number of outpatient visits were associated with advance-directive completion, so perhaps as we age the issue is raised more often.

In addition to the POLST, there are other suggestions about improving advance directives or advance care planning. Recommendations include improving documentation of discussions, putting a short AD on Medicare cards (Pollack, 2000), simplifying completion (reducing requirements for witnessing), and emphasizing the need for discussion with the physician over completion of documents (Lo & Steinbrook, 2004). The use of gerontological advance practice nurses for advance care planning as well as coordination of care and symptom management has also been recommended (Henderson, 2004).

In the ICU, where patient conditions are unstable, it is often critical to assess patient preferences for care, but difficult to do so. The treatments and medications used in ICUs often prevent patients from participating in communication about wishes. Information provided by family members, especially when a consensus forms, is often the basis for decision making (Tonelli, 2005). This can be difficult on family members who may be elderly themselves and for adult children who have never discussed with their parents what their wishes for care would be. Another complication concerns the dynamics of the family. Older adults may have had multiple marriages and may have extended family who are scattered across the country. Reaching family consensus when the family includes the current spouse and adult children from a previous marriage can be difficult at best. State laws vary concerning who has the legal right to make decisions for an incapacitated patient without an AD.

Families may not understand the implications of the choices that they are asked to make. For example, in the case study that opened the chapter the family readily agreed to a perataneous endoscopic gastrostomy (PEG) tube for nutrition. Although the family was informed of the risks of PEG placement, they were not well informed of the risks and benefits of initiating tube feedings, including the risk of diarrhea, aspiration pneumonia, infection, ulcers, or the difficulties in stopping tube feedings. Figure 8.1 has examples of how such a scenario might occur. How information is presented can clarify or confuse the decision makers. When family members are asked questions such as, "If your family member is not able to breathe on her/his own do you want a tube put into help her/him?" or "If your family member's heart stops, do you want to us to try to restart it?" they may feel that they are choosing death for the patient if they say no. As a result, families may choose more aggressive care for even the very old patient. In doing so, however, they might be choosing a longer and more painful road to death (Kaufman, 1998).

Careful communication is needed to present true options to families without encouraging medically futile treatment. Families often have unreasonable expectations about what medical treatment can offer or the seriousness of their family member's condition (Winzelberg, Patrick, Rhodes, & Deyo, 2005). Communication about treatment options is complicated by the fact that physicians have a different view and different values than the family concerning what is best for the patient. Communication with family about the choices at the end of life requires careful consideration of patient and family values and ethical principles (Gordon, 2002). The final outcome should be a plan of care that is tailored to the patient's and family's values, beliefs, and wishes, and that offers the most appropriate treatment to meet the jointly determined goals of care. These goals may include returning to the prehospitalization state of functioning or palliation of symptoms.

Using words that are easily understandable by the family yet as clear as possible is recommended. Often families will use a euphemism for death such as "passing on" or "expire" and it is appropriate to use this term when speaking with a family. If they do not give such verbal clues, use the words "death" and "dying" to avoid misunderstandings. There are a few phrases that can be greatly clarified or improved with slight changes. For example, it is not appropriate to tell a family that you "know exactly how they feel." This takes the focus off of the family and puts it onto you. It is better to use this as an opening for the family to express their feelings by saying, "Often families are very upset when facing these changes. Are you having a hard time with this?" Another term that is often used by professionals that can be misinterpreted by families is "failed." We may say that the patient has failed chemotherapy or failed weaning from the ventilator. This implies to the family that the patient had some control over the situation. It is better to say that the treatment is no longer effective or that the ventilator was not able to be removed. Particularly disturbing to families are statements about "withdrawing care" and that there is "nothing more we can do." Kirchhoff (2005) recommends that critical care staff stop using the phrase "withdrawing care" because it implies that if life-sustaining therapies are withdrawn, the patient will not receive any care. It is more appropriate to talk about changing to a comfort or palliative focus and to be clear that when we stop life-sustaining efforts, the patient will still get the best symptom management and comfort care possible.

When a conversation with the patient is not possible, having an informed surrogate who has had a recent discussion with the patient about end-of-life wishes is the best substitute. Recent pilot work suggests that surrogates can better understand and

# 8.1

**Flow diagram of possible outcomes of treatment.**

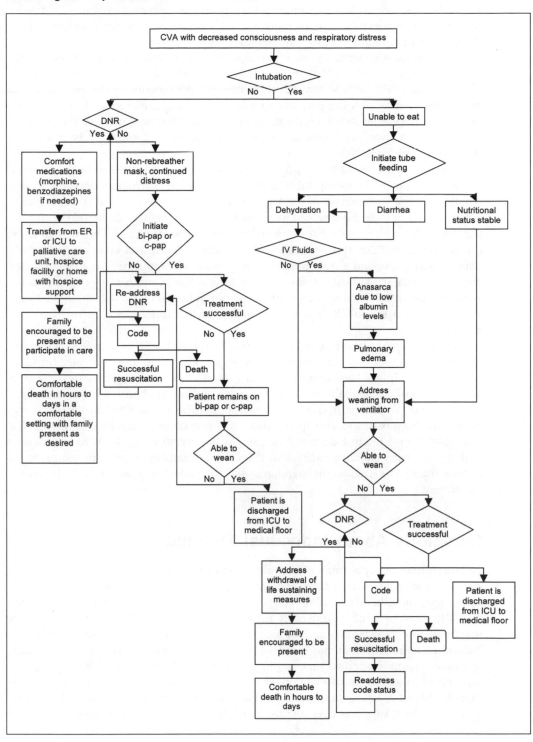

communicate the patient's wishes when a trained facilitator interviews the patient in the presence of the surrogate (Briggs, Kirchhoff, Hammes, Song, & Colvin, 2004). In this study the interview group was compared to a group receiving standard advance directive care. Greater understanding on the part of the surrogate, such as occurs with this intervention, leads to a number of positive outcomes: increased congruence between the choices made by the patient and the surrogate, greater satisfaction with the process of decision making, and less decisional conflict.

Because most patients and their surrogates will not have had a facilitated discussion, it is important to find other ways to assist the decision-making surrogate. The first is to carefully review any advance-directive documents or documentation of recent discussions with the patient about his or her care preferences. In the absence of a clear, applicable advance directive or written documentation of the patient's wishes, one of two principles is adopted: substituted judgment or best interests (Krohm & Summers, 2002).

The principle of substituted judgment is designed to guide the role of the decision-making surrogate. In using substituted judgment, the surrogate decision maker, whether or not that person is the legal power of attorney for health care, tries to determine what the patient would have wanted had he or she understood the circumstances under which treatment or procedures would be provided. One way to assist the surrogate to think this way is to ask, "If [the patient] had known what would happen and wrote you a note to read right now, what would he/she have said he/she wanted done?" Although there are some ethical issues and controversy associated with the use of substituted judgment (Brostrom, Johansson, & Nielsen, 2007; Nagasawa, 2008; Shapiro, 2007), it is still the approach that most courts favor (Krohm & Summers, 2002).

The principle of best interest is often the default of health care professionals and the principle that allows treatments to be withheld if they are medically futile. In using the principle of best interest, the surrogate decision maker must assess the risks and benefits of the available treatment options and try to choose the *best* option for the welfare of the patient. In choosing the best option, issues such as pain and suffering, as well as prognosis, and anticipated success of procedures must be considered. The principle of best interest does not necessarily recognize or conform to any desires that the patient may have expressed. If legal guardianship is sought, the principle of best interest is usually the standard used to guide the guardian's decisions for the patient.

## Decisions About Individual Treatments

Although many people think of end-of-life decision making as one grand, sweeping decision, the reality is that there are many separate decisions about individual treatments that must be made. Making decisions about individual interventions for the critically ill older adult is especially difficult as the results of one treatment choice may lead to complications and/or side effects that will prompt additional choices. Individual treatments that may be offered include the use of antibiotics for pneumonia, nutritional support such as tube feedings or parenteral nutrition, hydration support through intravenous fluids or hypodermoclysis, surgical procedures, use of medications for blood pressure support, use of pacemakers or internal cardiac defibrillators, and ventilatory support. Even family members who are well prepared to act as a health care decision agent may be confused and unsure of what the patient would choose in these complex situations.

Pneumonia in the older adult is a common reason for the use of antibiotics. Pneumonia is a frequent cause of hospital admission and death in older adults, and the risk of incidence and mortality increases with age (Kaplan et al., 2002; Loeb, McGeer, McArthur, Walter, & Simor, 1999). The symptom pattern and expression of pneumonia differs from that of younger patients, with delirium as a common sign in the older population. Aspiration is the most common cause (Marik & Kaplan, 2003) and aspiration pneumonia is often underdiagnosed (Marrie, 2000). Treatment decisions for pneumonia should not be based on age alone. For community-acquired pneumonia the Infectious Diseases Society of America and the American Thoracic Society (Mandell et al., 2007) recommended that decisions about whether to give antibiotics should be based on the assessment of the severity of the illness and the goals of care. For older adults who have no other life-limiting illness, there is no reason to withhold antibiotics. But, for the patient with late-stage Alzheimer's disease, treatment for pneumonia might only serve to prolong the dying process, and it is reasonable to discuss this with the family.

Nutrition and hydration support are issues that have emotional overtones for most families. Administration of intravenous solutions is relatively easy for the short term, but must be weighed against the physiological burden of increased fluid intake for older adults whose systems may not be able to adequately process extra fluids. Decisions of hydration should be based on thorough assessment of the patient and clarification of the goals of hydration therapy.

For patients who have difficulty swallowing or eating, whether because of disease or loss of consciousness, long-term nourishment requires assistance. For those with an intact gastrointestinal tract, tube feedings are the preferred method. The PEG tube is the most commonly used means of providing tube feedings. Because the mortality 1 year after PEG placement is approximately 60% (McMahon, Hurley, Kamath, & Mueller, 2005), there should be care consideration of the patient's overall condition prior to placement. A systematic nutritional assessment in older patients admitted to the ICU and treated by mechanical ventilation is important (Dardaine, Dequin, Ripault, Constans, & Ginies, 2001). Please refer to chapter 14, "Nutrition and Hydration" for more information.

At times, decisions need to be made about surgery options. Surgeries that were once limited to younger patients, such as coronary artery bypass grafts, are now being performed on older patients with good outcomes; however, there are a number of considerations to keep in mind. The effects of aging in the patient should be assessed and taken into account in determining surgical risk. Older adult patients frequently are using their reserve to maintain equilibrium, and when additional stress is placed on the patient, the reserves are insufficient to survive. Although good data regarding optimal perioperative management of the older adult are presently lacking, awareness of the areas of potential vulnerability allows treatment to be designed with these limitations in mind.

Decision making about cardiac-assist devices includes whether to initiate, and whether or when to discontinue such devices. Cardiac assist devices (CADs) include pacemakers, implantable cardiac defibrillators (ICDs), left ventricular assist devices (LVADs), and artificial hearts. CADs are being offered to more and more older adults (Goldstein & Lynn, 2006) and Medicare is reimbursing more often for devices such as ICDs. When considering placement of cardiac-assist devices, especially devices such as ICDs, which may affect comfort, there needs to be frank discussion with the patient about the benefits and burdens of such treatment. Devices should only be implanted in appropriate older adults, as outlined by the 2006 ACC/AHA/ESC guidelines (i.e., they should not be implanted in patients with a prognosis of less than 1 year) (Zipes et al., 2006). Discussion about the possibility of discontinuing a CAD as the patient nears the end of life should be initiated as part of the preplacement counseling (Stevenson & Desai, 2006).

Research indicates that clinicians are rarely having discussions with patient or family about deactivating ICDs at the end-of-life (Goldstein, Lampert, Bradley, Lynn, & Krumholz, 2004). When devices are deactivated, the deactivation is usually in response to distressing actions of the ICD in the hours before the death (Goldstein et al., 2004). Conversations about deactivating ICDs may be awkward, especially because many patients and family members think of the ICD as a means of preventing death. With prognosis in cardiac patients being very difficult to determine, even when death is near, the opportunity to discuss deactivation of CADs may pass before the need to have the conversation becomes obvious (Goldstein et al.).

The question of deactivating a CAD should be raised when a diagnosis of an unrelated life-limiting condition such as a malignancy or sepsis occurs, or with progression of the cardiac disease. When the person is dying, the actions of some CADs, such as the ICD, may no longer be desirable. As the patient's condition deteriorates and there is more cardiac instability, the ICD may fire more often, resulting in painful shocks and anxiety (Eckert & Jones, 2002; Glikson & Friedman, 2001). According to Goldstein and Lynn (2006, p. 15), "the dying that is in store with the device—a struggle to breathe or cognitive failure, for example—is much worse that the possible sudden death without it."

Withdrawal of pacemakers and ICDs is neither painful nor difficult. In most cases they can be reprogrammed noninvasively (Mueller, Hook, & Hayes, 2003). People do not usually die shortly after deactivating these devices, and the cause of death may be unrelated to the cardiac condition treated by the device (Goldstein & Lynn, 2006).

With LVADs, artificial hearts, or other devices, there can be complications such as bleeding, infections, and cerebrovascular accidents that are undesirable (Goldstein & Lynn, 2006). With these devices, death may occur immediately after deactivation. In these cases it is important to reinforce for the patient and the family that deactivating the device allows for a natural death.

Another treatment decision relates to the use of ventilatory support. Older adults are at an increased risk of developing respiratory failure in response to an acute illness. Age-related changes to the chest wall and lungs, a reduced ventilatory response to hypercarbia, and a reduced response to hypoxemia during REM (rapid eye movement) sleep contribute to the increased risk of respiratory failure. About half of ICU admissions have a major respiratory component (El Solh & Ramadan, 2006). The current recommendation in older adults is that ventilatory support should be used for only potentially reversible situations.

Recent research indicates that for patients who have relatively good short-term prognoses, ventilator support and aggressive care are economically worthwhile, even for patients 75 years and older (Hamel et al., 2001). In one study, survival of older ICU patients ($n = 116$) after mechanical ventilation, at discharge, and at 6 months was studied in one ICU. Mortality in the ICU and 6 months after discharge was 31% and 52%, respectively. Most of the patients (91%) who survived for 6 months were able to return to their place of residence, and 89% had similar or improved functional status compared with their preadmission functional status (Dardaine et al., 2001).

The use of CPR in older adults is thought to be of little benefit (Edin, 2007) despite the fact that it is regularly offered. There are racial differences in preference for cardiopulmonary resuscitation with Black Americans more frequently choosing CPR (Borum, Lynn, & Zhong, 2000). A decision to forgo CPR, a Do Not Resuscitate (DNR) order, has implications beyond just the avoidance of CPR. How the issue of a DNR order is raised may lead families to believe that they are choosing certain death as compared to life.

Patients and families have concerns that care may be compromised when a DNR decision has been made. There is some evidence that might support this fear. One study of residents and attending physicians showed that, in hypothetical situations, physicians chose to initiate fewer interventions unrelated to CPR when a DNR order was present versus absent (Beach & Morrison, 2002). In another study, nurses had lower levels of agreement about whether they would use monitoring interventions (vital signs, weighing the patient) when the hypothetical patient had a DNR than when he/she did not (Sherman & Branum, 1995).

Recent guidelines from the Society of Critical Care Medicine stated that when comfort is the goal for a patient in critical care, each intervention, such as monitors or tests, should be evaluated in light of whether it increases comfort (Truog et al., 2008). Some treatments that are routine in the ICU such as routine laboratory tests, chest X-rays, daily weights, and endotracheal suctioning may not contribute to the patient's comfort and should not be continued. Other treatments, such as intravenous administration of vasopressors or inotropes, may be consistent with a goal of comfort because they cause little pain, yet they increase perfusion of vital organs, which may increase the level of consciousness, hepatic and renal functions, and therefore decrease distressing symptoms (Truog et al.).

Discussions about care decision should take place with the patient and the family and should be held shortly after admission to the ICU (Lilly et al., 2000). This family meeting allows for an early discussion of the patients' goals and expectations and the plan of care. Good communication early in the ICU stay can lead to the appropriate use of advanced life-support technology for patients with a high potential for survival and may allow the earlier withdrawal of life-support measures when they are ineffective (Lilly, Sonna, Haley, & Massaro, 2003).

## Limiting Treatment

When the burdens of therapy substantially outweigh the benefits, decisions concerning continuation of life-sustaining treatments need to be reevaluated. Although ethically, withholding and withdrawing treatment are considered equivalent (Nuffield Council on Bioethics, 2006; Pawlik, 2006), the emotional impact of the two choices can be very different. Families may find it less distressing to "choose comfort" as opposed to "stopping care." In either situation, families commonly express guilt and anger. It can be helpful to remind the family that neither they nor the health care team are responsible for the patient's poor prognosis (Henig, Faul, & Raffin, 2001), but they all share the goal of determining the best course of treatment for the patient.

Because families may find it less distressing to withhold rather than withdraw life-sustaining treatments, it is critical to carefully consider decisions to initiate life-sustaining treatments such as antibiotics, tube feedings, vasopressors or inotropes,

| 8.1 Signs of Improvement or Decline for Families to Watch for in Elderly Patients in Critical Care | | |
|---|---|---|
| **System** | **Improvement** | **Decline** |
| **Respiratory** | Weaning from ventilator | Inability to wean from ventilator |
| **Circulatory** | Weaning from vasopressors | Inability to wean from vasopressors |
| | | Mottling of extremities |
| **Genitourinary** | Normal urine volume and concentration | Decrease in urine volume |
| | | Increase in BUN (blood urea nitrogen test), Creatinine |
| **Neurological** | Return to baseline level of consciousness | Continued unresponsiveness |

and ventilatory support. Often in the critical care setting decisions to initiate such treatments need to be made rapidly. With older adults rapid decision making may be difficult. Older adults are more likely to have older surrogate decision makers who may be used to deferring to the decision of the physician or who may desire a longer time to contemplate the consequences of decisions. For other older patients, decisions may be made by adult children or other relatives who want to seek the advice and agreement of additional family members before committing to a course of action. One way to reduce the time pressure in such situations is to "bring the family along" through the entire course of treatment. Letting family members, particularly family decision makers, know what the health care team is thinking in terms of what symptoms they are seeing and what those symptoms likely mean in terms of survival is important. One helpful technique is to identify clear milestones that indicate improvement or decline such as those shown in Table 8.1 (Henig et al., 2001). Families interviewed after a family member died in an ICU often expressed that they had no idea how serious things were until they were asked to make a decision regarding life-sustaining treatment (Kehl & Kirchhoff, 2004).

## Withdrawal of Life-Sustaining Treatment

When decisions are being made about whether to withdraw life-sustaining treatment, the patient is seldom able to participate. Families make these decisions with support from the health professionals (Prendergast & Puntillo, 2002). Timely information about prognosis coupled with support is helpful to the families. Ideally, a family meeting should be held that will include family members, physicians, nurses, a social worker, a chaplain if desired by family, and other consultants such as palliative care team members or ethics consultants. This meeting should provide the family with information, as well as give them an opportunity to ask questions and express emotions (Curtis et al., 2002). To be most effective the clinicians should have timely information that can be conveyed in an honest and clear manner to the family. The clinicians also need to listen to what the family says and and respond to their needs (Norton, Tilden, Tolle, Nelson, & Eggman, 2003).

Life-support devices are intended to provide temporary support for patients with potentially reversible conditions and not intended to prevent death from occurring

(Wood & Marik, 2004). When decisions need to be made about withholding or withdrawing life-sustaining measures, the presence of preexisting disease is a key consideration (Plaisier, Blostein, Hurt, & Malangoni, 2002). Older adults often have other conditions or comorbidities that make the use of life-sustaining therapies less advisable. In addition, elders are vulnerable to severe injury and have limited physiologic response to stress (Chang & Schecter, 2007). Withholding usual treatments in the presence of multiple comorbidities may be analogous to allowing natural death to occur.

Some recommendations have been suggested about how to best provide for a comfortable process when withdrawing ventilatory support. Campbell (2007) completed a systematic review of the research about how to withdraw mechanical ventilation. If the patient is brain dead, sedation or analgesia before or during withdrawal is not indicated. If premedication is needed, patient behaviors should guide the initiation and escalation of sedatives and opioids. Doses of opioids used to manage dyspnea are similar to those used during ventilator withdrawal.

Selection of a method for weaning the patient from the ventilator seems to be dependent on clinician preference rather than on patient characteristics (Campbell, 2007). Sometimes the endotracheal tube is removed immediately (extubation); sometimes the tube is removed after ceasing ventilatory support (terminal extubation). Terminal weaning is the process during which there is a gradual reduction of ventilatory support, with the tube removed at the end of the withdrawal. In general the endotracheal tube should be removed as early in the process as possible while taking into consideration the possibility of airway compromise. There are no specific recommendations for weaning from the ventilator based on age.

For older adults in the critical care setting, there are three possible outcomes: They may recover and be discharged from the ICU, aggressive therapy may be continued until it is no longer effective and the patient dies, or a shift in goals of care from cure to comfort may be chosen and the patient dies. When it is apparent that curative care is no longer possible, the options are narrowed to continuing aggressive therapy or focusing on comfort care. In either situation, patients and families will require open and honest communication, physical, psychosocial, and spiritual support, and preparation for the patient's death.

# Transition to Palliative Care

Once a decision has been made to withhold or withdraw treatment, the focus of care shifts from life-saving treatment to holistic, then palliative care (Mularski & Osborne, 2003). Good palliative care in the ICU includes symptom management, attending to the patient's spiritual and psychosocial needs, supporting the family, and preparing the patient and family for the death. The shift to palliative care begins with assessing what the patient and family believes is a good death. The concept of a good death is highly individual and dependent on cultural, spiritual, family, and personal values (Kehl, 2006). To optimally care for an older adult dying in the critical care setting, we must first understand the patient's wishes and then work with the patient and family to design care to meet the dying person's needs.

Palliative care for older adults in the ICU requires aggressive care to promote comfort. Tests or procedures that do not promote comfort, laboratory work, and painful procedures should be discontinued. The nurse must be perceptive and vigilant regarding changes in condition. Good communication with both the family and the rest of the health care team can reduce family questions and concerns, as well as keep them informed and involved. It is important to avoid offering "nonoptions" as choices to family. If the physician or care team has decided that a treatment is medically futile, it should not be offered as an option to family, nor should the benefits be discussed. This provides consistent information from all care team members and reduces family confusion. Questions about medical futility should be discussed with the physician, the care team, and if there are persistent conflicts, with an ethics team or whatever institutional guidelines specify.

Transition to palliative care may also mean a transition to another location of care such as a palliative care unit, a hospice facility, or even the patient's home. Although such transitions may be necessitated by hospital policies, economic factors, and the family's ability to provide care, they should be kept to a minimum and they should be initiated as early as possible. One recent study found that one of the most common regrets of family members was that they did not transition to hospice sooner (Kehl & Kirchhoff, 2004). Other researchers have found that transition to a different setting during the last days of life can be confusing and traumatic (Duggleby & Berry, 2005). These transitions can be complicated in older adults, especially if they have memory impairment, because they disrupt relationships the patient has come to rely on, which can increase the risk of complications (Flannery, 2002).

# Symptom Management

## Pain

Symptom management is critical in palliative care, and pain is often considered the most distressing symptom. The SUPPORT study described up to 40% of older adults as having unrelieved or poorly relieved pain in their final days (SUPPORT Investigators, 1995). Managing pain in older adults requires excellent assessment of the pain and its sources. Often older adults experience both long-term or chronic pain from conditions such as arthritis or venous insufficiency, and an acute pain from coronary disease, cancer, or other acute illnesses. Both must be managed (Stein, 2006). This may require use of multiple agents such as NSAIDs (nonsteroidal antiinflammatory drugs) for arthritic pain, opioids for acute pain, and antidepressants for neuropathic pain.

There are a number of challenges to providing pain management to older adults in their final days. Usually the patient cannot communicate verbally and assessment of pain must use other mechanisms. There are a number of good nonverbal pain assessment tools. One example is the PASLAC (pain assessment checklist for seniors with limited ability to communicate), which was developed as an observational pain assessment tool for seniors (Fuchs-Lacelle & Hadjistavropoulos, 2004). PASLAC is considered one of the best nonverbal pain assessment instruments (Zwakhalen, Hamers, Abu-Saad, & Berger, 2006) because it discriminates between pain events and nonspecific distress (Fuchs-Lacelle & Hadjistavropoulos, 2004). A brief 24-item version is useful in clinical settings (Zwakhalen, Hamers, & Berger, 2007) and could be easily adapted to critical care.

Families often have many questions regarding pain management. These include whether pain medication is needed when the patient is unresponsive, if giving pain medication will hasten death, and if all pain can be controlled. Generally, if the patient is unresponsive, has no signs of pain, and is not on a medication that would mask signs of pain (such as pancuronium), a trial of reducing the medication can be attempted. Medications should be reduced by = 50% in 24 hours (Portenoy, 1994). If the patient shows any signs of pain, such as those on the PAINAD (pain assessment in advanced dementia (Warden, Hurley, & Volicer, 2003), the medication should be returned to the previous level. If there are no signs of pain, medications may be reduced by 25% every 8 hours with careful assessment.

There is no evidence that use of opioid pain medication hastens death in most situations. A classic study by Bruera, Macmillan, Pither, and MacDonald (1990) showed that patients who received morphine for end-stage symptom management had less dyspnea and less pain, but no significant changes in respiratory rate, $pO_2$ or $pCO_2$. Other research (Campbell, Bizek, & Thill, 1999; Chan et al., 2004) has reported no association between analgesia or sedation and time to death following withdrawing ventilatory support.

Evidence of how older adults respond to dosing of opioids is scarce or inconclusive (Masica et al., 2007). Aging results in an increased fat-to-lean body-mass ratio as well as decreased renal and hepatic functioning, which leads to slower metabolism of medications and increased risk for the build up of harmful metabolites (Stein, 2006). Older people may be more sensitive to analgesic effect of opioids with higher peak effect and longer duration of action (Kaiko, Wallenstein, Rogers, Grabinski, & Houde, 1982). Drugs such as meperidine and propoxyphene should be avoided, as should opioids with longer duration of action such as levorphanol, methadone, and sustained-release fentanyl. The latter should only be used in opioid-tolerant patients, and only if the patient does not tolerate other opioids such as morphine. Sedation and nausea are common in the first 24–72 hours with opioids, and the patient and family should be warned this is a common occurrence and not a sign of drug allergy.

Another risk in pain management with older adults is managing the accompanying constipation. Many older adults have underlying issues with constipation. When the constipating effects of opioids are added to this, the result can cause pain and complications such as bowel obstruction. Patients who are starting opioid therapy should be concurrently started on laxatives, in addition to whatever usual bowel management protocol they followed prior to initiating opioid therapy.

Pain in dying patients can be controlled, but sometimes the price is awareness. In cases where pain is unrelieved by usual management, palliative sedation may be an option. Palliative sedation is the use of sedative medications to make the patient unaware, usually caused by severe, intractable symptoms at the end of life (Cherny, 2006). If there is no treatment capable of providing adequate pain relief, a discussion of the risks and benefits of palliative sedation may be initiated by the health care provider. It is important that the patient and family understand that the purpose of palliative sedation is comfort, and that resuscitation is not desirable. Patients and family members should also understand that it is likely that the person will die without regaining consciousness, so good-byes must be said prior to initiating sedation. For further information concerning pain management in older adults, please refer to chapter 18, "Pain in the Critically Ill Older Adult."

## Dyspnea

Dyspnea is distressing to both the patient and the family; it occurs in up to 70% of dying persons, regardless of diagnosis (Reuben & Mor, 1986). For older adults who choose not to accept ventilatory support, or for those being withdrawn from ventilatory support, dyspnea may be a major concern. Dyspnea can be assessed and managed at the end of life, both with medications and nonpharmacological methods. The best way to assess dyspnea is self-report. For patients who cannot speak, behavioral clues such as restlessness, grunting at end-expiration, and a look of fear may indicate dyspnea (Campbell, 2004). After assessment, the first step in management is to remove or alleviate physical causes of dyspnea such as pulmonary edema, partial obstruction caused by mucus, or metabolic acidosis. Next, nonpharmacological methods can be employed. Positioning the patient upright maximizes the lung capacity and can decrease dyspnea. Positioning the patient in front of a fan provides cool airflow to the cheek (Schwartzstein, Lahive, Pope, Weinberger, & Weiss, 1987) and nose (Burgess & Whitelaw, 1988), which can reduce the perception of breathlessness.

The effectiveness of oxygen in relieving dyspnea in dying persons has not been clearly established (Bruera et al., 2003; Qaseem et al., 2008). Generally, if the patient is hypoxic and oxygen helps subjectively, it may be used. Some research has shown hypoxic cancer patients' rating of dyspnea, respiratory rate, and respiratory efforts improve with oxygen use (Bruera, de Stoutz, Velasco-Leiva, Schoeller, & Hanson, 1993). Some patients may pull off the mask or cannula repeatedly and say the oxygen delivery system is suffocating them; for these patients, use of a fan is a better option.

Opioids, particularly morphine, have been used for more than a century to manage dyspnea. Low-dose morphine can decrease the sensation of breathlessness without decreasing the respiratory function of terminally ill patients (Bruera et al., 1990; Jennings, Davies, Higgins, & Broadley, 2001; Lorenz, Rosenfeld, & Wenger, 2007). Nebulized morphine has been tried, but there is no evidence that it is effective in treating dyspnea (Jennings et al.; Lorenz et al.). Sedatives have also been used in treating dyspnea, but the results have been mixed. Given the risk of paradoxical effects of longer acting sedatives, and the high risk that older adults will experience adverse effects (Senninger & Laxenaire, 1995), sedatives should only be used to reduce breathlessness if other alternatives have failed. Further research is needed before sedatives are widely used to reduce breathlessness at the end of life.

Audible secretions, often referred to as a "death rattle" are another troublesome symptom at the end of life. In patients on mechanical ventilation, audible secretions are often managed by increased suctioning and maintaining the endotracheal tube in place. For those who are not mechanically ventilated, or for patients who are extubated prior to death, this sound can be one of the most distressing issues for family, even though patients do not seem to be aware of it. Families need explanations that the noisy breathing does not indicate distress. The primary treatment is antisecretory agents, although there is currently no strong evidence of their effectiveness (Wee & Hillier, 2008). Hyoscyamine sulfate is the preferred medication (Back, Jenkins, Blower, & Beckhelling, 2001; Bennett et al., 2002; Wildiers & Menten, 2002). Hycoscyamine can be administered orally, buccally using oral drops, or parenterally. If audible secretions are a persistent issue, scopolamine transdermal patches can be used to dry secretions and reduce the noisy breathing. The patch lasts for approximately 3 days, but the onset is about 4 to 6 hours, so it is not a good choice if the patient's condition is changing rapidly. Suctioning should be considered only if the secretions are distressing to the patient, proximal and accessible, and there is inadequate response to antisecretory agents because suctioning is irritating and can be traumatic to the patient.

## Terminal Delirium/Restlessness

Terminal restlessness or delirium occurs in up to 88% of dying persons (Kehl, 2004). The condition has been described as "agitated delirium in a dying patient, frequently associated with impaired consciousness and multifocal myoclonus" (Burke, 1997, p. 39). Indicators of terminal delirium include frequent nonpurposeful motor activity (e.g., picking at bed sheets), the inability to concentrate or relax, disturbances in sleep–rest patterns, fluctuating levels of consciousness, cognitive failure and/or anxiety, and potential progression to agitation.

Management of terminal delirium begins with a thorough assessment. Issues such as pain, full bladder or bowels, and alcohol or tobacco withdrawal may cause restlessness and delirium. Other areas for assessment include existential distress and spiritual distress. Conditions that might contribute to restlessness should be resolved before pharmacologic measures are taken.

First-line pharmacological treatment for terminal restlessness or delirium is either haloperidol or chlorpromazine (see Table 8.2). Caution should be used in administering lorazepam because of the high risk of side effects in older adults. Further information on management of delirium can be found in chapter 26, "Delirium in Critical Illness."

Nearing-death awareness (NDA) often appears similar to restlessness and delirium. NDA is an experience that occurs in many people who are close to death. It almost always includes seeing or speaking to deceased loved ones (Callanan & Kelley, 1992) and may include other visions. NDA differs from hallucinations in a number of ways. A person experiencing NDA does not find the experience disturbing. If the patient is frightened or disturbed by what he or she is hearing or seeing, medication such as haloperidol, which is appropriate for hallucinations, should be given. NDA generally does not respond to antipsychotic medications. In some cases, the dying person may have a message for the family that is conveyed as part of the nearing-death experience. This message is often very symbolic. Much nearing-death communication is conveyed in travel terms or in ways that are appropriate to the lifestyle of the patient. Patients or family members may be unsure of how to respond to NDA. Calm reassurance that these are normal experiences for someone who is nearing death can greatly comfort both the patient and the family.

## Skin Care

There are numerous aspects of the dying process that affect skin care in older adults. Older adults have lost much of the elasticity of their skin. Skin is often friable and needs protection from pressure and shear. Near the end of life, decreased nutritional and fluid intake are common. Decreased mobility and changes in the circulatory system also affect the skin, which makes decubiti a common occurrence.

The primary goals of wound care in older adults at the end of life are maintaining optimal skin integrity and minimizing discomfort (Schim & Cullen, 2005). These goals may not both be achievable in the final days and patient comfort should always take top priority. Good skin hygiene can assist in meeting both goals, as well as to reassure both the patient and the family that the patient is receiving good nursing care. Daily cleansing and use of appropriate moisturizers can increase comfort and prevent painful infection (De Conno, Ventafridda, & Saita, 1991). The advantages of turning the patient

## 8.2   Recommended Pharmacological Treatment of Terminal Restlessness

| | Preferred Medication | Dose Adjusted for Older Adults | Considerations | Alternative Medication | Dose Adjusted for Older Adults | Considerations |
|---|---|---|---|---|---|---|
| **First-line treatment** | Haloperidol IV, IM, or PO* | **Initial dose—** 0.125–0.5 mg IV or IM, repeat dose q 30 minutes to titrated response. Maximum dose up to 100 mg per day. | Watch for extrapyramidal reactions, neuroleptic malignant syndrome, and tardive dyskinesia at high doses. | Chlorpromazine IM, IV, PR, PO* | **Initial dose—** 6.25–25 mg IM, PO, PR 6.25–25 mg IV diluted and given at rate of no more than .5 mg per minute. Repeat dose in 1 to 4 hours as needed. Titrate to response (up to 400 mg q 4 hours). | Watch for significant cardiovascular side effects (hypotension, arrhythmias, angina), extrapyramidal reactions, neuroleptic malignant syndrome, tardive dyskinesias. |
| **Second-line treatment** | Midazolam SC or IV | **Initial dose—** 0.5 mg bolus then start drip at 0.5–1.5 mg per hour. Titrate dose to response. Usual maintenance dose 1-20 mg per hour. | Patients usually become sedated at high doses. Monitor respiratory status closely. May experience pain at injection site. | Propofol IV | **Initial dose—**5–10 mg bolus. Start drip at 10 mg per hour. Titrate dose to response. Usual maintenance dose 5-200 mg per hour. | Sedation is expected outcome. Monitor respiratory status closely. May experience pain at injection site. |

*Note:* Oral route is usually not effective for terminal restlessness and delirium because of difficulties with administration and severity of symptoms.

Adapted from Kehl (2004), Jackson and Lipman (2000), and Trzepacz (1999).

to decrease further pressure sores should be carefully weighed against any discomfort caused by turning and the patient's wishes (Langemo, 2006). If the patient has significant skin breakdown and terminal skin failure, use of a low-pressure system is recommended to eliminate the need to turn the patient frequently and to decrease the pressure and pain on the skin surface.

The Kennedy terminal ulcer is a pressure sore that is unique to patients who are nearing death. It usually appears on the sacrum and is pear-shaped with irregular borders (Kennedy, 1989). Initially it often appears as if the skin is bruised or scraped. Tissue deterioration with the Kennedy terminal ulcer is rapid, and an ulcer that is barely noticeable may have progressed to stage III or IV within 8 hours. Because this type of ulcer usually occurs within 48 hours of the patient's death, it is often left untreated other than covering the ulcer to prevent infection and managing any discomfort associated with it.

## Preparation for Death

Although there is widespread agreement that patients and families need to be prepared for the death, there is little empiric evidence of how to do so. When the patient is an older adult, the family may include a spouse who is also older, siblings, adult children, and grandchildren. It is difficult to find materials to assist in preparing such a wide range of ages and education levels for death. The best starting point is to assess what they know, what they expect will happen, and what they want to know. Although many patients and families want detailed information about what the dying person will experience, others may prefer limited information.

In preparing patients, it is important to assess which issues would make their death "good" or "bad" (Kehl, 2006). Knowing the patient's idea of a good death provides guidance both for future decision making and for planning care surrounding the death. For patients, offer to talk about the signs and symptoms that are likely for them and that would indicate imminent dying. It is very important to dispel myths regarding dying. The patient should be reassured that they should NOT expect uncontrolled pain, dyspnea, or loss of control. Assess the patient's wishes concerning palliative sedation for these symptoms if other management is not effective.

Preparing the family for death is as important as preparing the patient. Unprepared family members are more likely to have complicated grief or depression (Barry, Kasl, & Prigerson, 2002; Houts, Lipton, Harold, Simmons, & Barthlolomew, 1989). If the patient is having life-support measures withdrawn, preparation should begin at the family meeting when this decision is made. A pilot study testing a theoretically developed informational intervention showed some promise for helping families know what to expect at the time and possibly reducing later negative moods at 2 to 4 weeks (Kirchhoff, Palzkill, Kowalkowski, Mork, & Gretarsdottir, 2008). The intervention is based on Johnson's self-regulation theory (Johnson, 1999) and includes information on what the family members are likely to experience; the reasons or causes for what they will experience; the time frame and usual sequence of events; the environment, equipment, and personnel present; and information on what they can do or say during the withdrawal experience.

Although many nurses give information on signs and symptoms the patient may experience (Kirchhoff, Beckstrand, & Anumandla, 2003), families also need information on what they will see and hear and the timeframe to expect. When families know what to expect they can make a more informed decision about whether to be present during the withdrawal process. Clinical experience indicates that although some families may want this preparatory information before the withdrawal begins, others may need the information to be given as the withdrawal unfolds. Families need to know that health care professionals will aggressively treat symptoms and manage the patient's comfort.

Telling families common signs and symptoms helps them know what to expect. Common signs and symptoms in the final hours include dyspnea, pain, restlessness or delirium, fatigue, breathing-pattern changes, audible secretions, cold extremities, and mottling or cyanosis. Some of these signs or symptoms, like breathing-pattern change, do not require intervention if the goal of care is comfort, but families should be prepared for what they will see and be reassured that the breathing-pattern changes such as apnea are normal and not distressing to the patient. Families also need to be told what to do. They often need permission to touch or speak to the patient at this time. Although not age related, this appears to be a common issue. Current research by Kehl is exploring the best ways to prepare families for the final hours (Kehl, 2008).

Some patients will undergo an unsuccessful resuscitation attempt prior to death. Institutional policy will dictate whether family may be present during resuscitation efforts. If family is not allowed to be present, a family support person should offer to stay with the family. Another individual should be designated to bring information from the health care team to the family. Families are very frightened during such events and need both support and information. Families of older adults should be prepared for the possibility that resuscitation may not be successful, especially if the patient has multiple comorbidities or is frail. After the patient has died and the room has been quickly straightened, the family should be invited to spend time with the patient.

# Care After Death

## Organ Donation

Although there are no upper age limits on organ donation (Health Resources and Services Administration, 2008) there are often conditions that make the organs of older adults less desirable or ineligible for organ donation (Carter et al., 2000). Under the 2006 Universal Anatomical Gift Act (UAGA), organs of those who have indicated prior to death that they want to donate organs (such as on a driver's license) must be considered for donation. If the individual signed a refusal for donation prior, then family members cannot override that refusal and should not be asked about donation. If there is no indication of the patient's wishes, then it may be necessary to approach the family. If there is a discrepancy between the patient's previous written wish to make an anatomical gift and an advance directive that requests withholding or withdrawing of life-sustaining measures, the health professionals may first determine the medical suitability of a patient's organs. This way, if an older adult is not considered a suitable donor, questions about donation or a conflict between the desire to donate and desire for a natural death do not need to be raised (National Conference of Commissioners on Uniform State Laws, 2008).

## Family Care After the Death

After the death, the patient's family requires care and support. Family members who are present may need to hear it said that the patient has died. If the family is not present, they should be notified that the patient has died and offered the opportunity to come to the unit to see the patient.

Deceased patients who are organ donors may need to be taken to the operating room immediately after the heart stops to facilitate a controlled donation. This event can be especially hard on families, particularly if they are not present at the time of death. These family members may wish to visit the unit or view the room to assist them in accepting the patient's death.

Families should be given as much control as possible after the death. They should be asked whether they would like a support person (social worker, chaplain, or personal spiritual leader) or would like any personal, family, cultural, or spiritual practices observed. If the family is present, they should be invited to assist in cleaning up the patient. If they prefer not to participate, they should be asked if they would like to be present for the final cares, or if they would prefer to wait in a private room while the body is prepared.

Patients should receive final cares according to hospital policy and their preferences. Usually, if there is a possibility that an autopsy may be required or requested, all tubes and lines must be left in place. Obvious soiling should be removed and the patient should be covered modestly. If an autopsy is not needed and institutional policy permits, the family should be asked if they would prefer having the endotracheal tube, intravenous lines, oxygen tubing, and other devices removed.

In their good-byes some families will wish for private time, and others want a professional present. Even if they wish to be alone with the patient, staff should be available if they change their minds. Although institutional policy may limit the time family can spend with the deceased, it is important to provide as much time as the family needs.

After-death bereavement programs are present in some critical care units and range from presence at the time of death, to bereavement calls and cards, or bereavement support groups (Williams, Harris, Randall, Nichols, & Brown, 2003). Bereavement support groups and grief counselors are often available through local hospices if the hospital does not offer these services. Families sometimes contact the critical care unit after the death to express thanks or to seek assistance with their grieving.

## Summary

Caring for older adults who are facing end-of-life issues in the critical care setting can be challenging. Skill in communication, facilitation of decision making by the patient and family, excellent assessment skills, good symptom management, attention to the psychosocial–spiritual needs of the patient and family, and preparation for the time of death are all key elements to good end-of-life care. Assessment of the patient's wishes for end-of-life care is a necessary starting point. For patients who have not provided information on their preferences through an advance directive or other communication, it is important to work with family to determine the goals of care. It is especially important to keep family members aware of the current condition of the patient as things may change rapidly in the critical care setting.

Withholding or withdrawing life-sustaining therapies are valid options for patients whose primary goal is quality of life. In these situations as the goals of care shift from a curative focus to a comfort focus, families should be reassured that the patient will continue to receive excellent care. Aggressive symptom management can provide physical comfort in the final days.

Whether death follows a failed resuscitation attempt, withdrawal of life-sustaining therapy, or occurs after a deliberate choice for comfort care, families need to be supported and given as much control as possible. Critical care units may choose to provide bereavement support to families after the death or they may refer individuals to local support groups or bereavement counselors. Throughout the process, from the first indications that death may be the outcome of the critical care stay, until after the death, open and honest communication and skill at facilitating patient and family discussions can make the end-of-life experience easier for older adults and their families.

# References

Back, I. N., Jenkins, K., Blower, A., & Beckhelling, J. (2001). A study comparing hyoscine hydrobromide and glycopyrrolate in the treatment of death rattle. *Palliative Medicine, 15*(4), 329–336.

Barry, L. C., Kasl, S. V., & Prigerson, H. G. (2002). Psychiatric disorders among bereaved persons: The role of perceived circumstances of death and preparedness for death. *American Journal of Geriatric Psychiatry, 10*(4), 447–457.

Beach, M. C., & Morrison, R. S. (2002). The effect of do-not-resuscitate orders on physician decision-making. *Journal of the American Geriatrics Society, 50*(12), 2057–2061.

Bennett, M., Lucas, V., Brennan, M., Hughes, A., O'Donnell, V., & Wee, B. (2002). Using anti-muscarinic drugs in the management of death rattle: Evidence-based guidelines for palliative care. *Palliative Medicine, 16*(5), 369–374.

Borum, M. L., Lynn, J., & Zhong, Z. (2000). The effects of patient race on outcomes in seriously ill patients in SUPPORT: An overview of economic impact, medical intervention, and end-of-life decisions. Study to Understand Prognoses and Preferences for Outcomes and Risks of Treatments. *Journal of the American Geriatrics Society, 48*(5 Suppl.), S194–198.

Briggs, L. A., Kirchhoff, K. T., Hammes, B. J., Song, M. K., & Colvin, E. R. (2004). Patient-centered advance care planning in special patient populations: A pilot study. *Journal of Professional Nursing, 20*(1), 47–58.

Brostrom, L., Johansson, M., & Nielsen, M. K. (2007). "What the patient would have decided": A fundamental problem with the substituted judgment standard. *Medicine, Health Care and Philosophy, 10*(3), 265–278.

Bruera, E., de Stoutz, N., Velasco-Leiva, A., Schoeller, T., & Hanson, J. (1993). Effects of oxygen on dyspnoea in hypoxaemic terminal-cancer patients. *Lancet, 342*(8862), 13–14.

Bruera, E., Macmillan, K., Pither, J., & MacDonald, R. N. (1990). Effects of morphine on the dyspnea of terminal cancer patients. *Journal of Pain and Symptom Management, 5*(6), 341–344.

Bruera, E., Sweeney, C., Willey, J., Palmer, J. L., Strasser, F., Morice, R. C., et al. (2003). A randomized controlled trial of supplemental oxygen versus air in cancer patients with dyspnea. *Palliative Medicine, 17*(8), 659–663.

Burgess, K. R., & Whitelaw, W. A. (1988). Effects of nasal cold receptors on pattern of breathing. *Journal of Applied Physiology, 64*(1), 371–376.

Burke, A. L. (1997). Palliative care: An update on "terminal restlessness." *Medical Journal of Australia, 166*(1), 39–42.

Callanan, C., & Kelley, P. (1992). *Final gifts*. New York: Poseidon Press.

Campbell, M. L. (2004). Terminal dyspnea and respiratory distress. *Critical Care Clinics, 20*(3), viii–ix, 403–417.

Campbell, M. L. (2007). How to withdraw mechanical ventilation: A systematic review of the literature. *AACN Advanced Critical Care, 18*(4), 397–403.

Campbell, M. L., Bizek, K. S., & Thill, M. (1999). Patient responses during rapid terminal weaning from mechanical ventilation: A prospective study. *Critical Care Medicine, 27*(1), 73–77.

Carrese, J. A., Mullaney, J. L., Faden, R. R., & Finucane, T. E. (2002). Planning for death but not serious future illness: Qualitative study of housebound elderly patients. *BMJ, 325*(7356), 125.

Carter, J. T., Lee, C. M., Weinstein, R. J., Lu, A. D., Dafoe, D. C., & Alfrey, E. J. (2000). Evaluation of the older cadaveric kidney donor: The impact of donor hypertension and creatinine clearance on graft performance and survival. *Transplantation, 70*(5), 765–771.

Chan, J. D., Treece, P. D., Engelberg, R. A., Crowley, L., Rubenfeld, G. D., Steinberg, K. P., et al. (2004). Narcotic and benzodiazepine use after withdrawal of life support: Association with time to death? *Chest, 126*(1), 286–293.

Chang, T. T., & Schecter, W. P. (2007). Injury in the elderly and end-of-life decisions. *Surgical Clinics of North America, 87*(1), viii, 229–245.

Cherny, N. I. (2006). Palliative sedation. In E. Breura, I. J. Higginson, C. Ripamonti, & C. von Gunten (Eds.), *Textbook of palliative medicine* (pp. 976–988). London: Hodder Arnold.

Curtis, J. R., Engelberg, R. A., Wenrich, M. D., Nielsen, E. L., Shannon, S. E., Treece, P. D., et al. (2002). Studying communication about end-of-life care during the ICU family conference: Development of a framework. *Journal of Critical Care, 17*(3), 147–160.

Dardaine, V., Dequin, P. F., Ripault, H., Constans, T., & Ginies, G. (2001). Outcome of older patients requiring ventilatory support in intensive care: Impact of nutritional status. *Journal of the American Geriatrics Society, 49*(5), 564–570.

De Conno, F., Ventafridda, V., & Saita, L. (1991). Skin problems in advanced and terminal cancer patients. *Journal of Pain and Symptom Management, 6*(4), 247–256.

Ditto, P. H., Jacobson, J. A., Smucker, W. D., Danks, J. H., & Fagerlin, A. (2006). Context changes choices: A prospective study of the effects of hospitalization on life-sustaining treatment preferences. *Medical Decision Making, 26*(4), 313–322.

Duggleby, W., & Berry, P. (2005). Transitions and shifting goals of care for palliative patients and their families. *Clinical Journal of Oncology Nursing, 9*(4), 425–428.

Eckert, M., & Jones, T. (2002). How does an implantable cardioverter defibrillator (ICD) affect the lives of patients and their families? *International Journal of Nursing Practice, 8*(3), 152–157.

Edin, M. G. (2007). Cardiopulmonary resuscitation in the frail elderly: Clinical, ethical and halakhic issues. *Israeli Medical Association Journal, 9*(3), 177–179.

El Solh, A. A., & Ramadan, F. H. (2006). Overview of respiratory failure in older adults. *Journal of Intensive Care Medicine, 21*(6), 345–351.

Flannery, R. B., Jr. (2002). Disrupted caring attachments: Implications for long-term care. *American Journal of Alzheimer's Disease and Other Dementias, 17*(4), 227–231.

Foley, K. M., & Gelband, H. (2001). Executive summary. In K. M. Foley & H. Gelband (Eds.), *Improving palliative care for cancer* (pp. 1–8). Washington, DC: National Academy Press.

Formiga, F., Chivite, D., Ortega, C., Casas, S., Ramon, J. M., & Pujol, R. (2004). End-of-life preferences in elderly patients admitted for heart failure. *QJM: An International Journal of Medicine, 97*(12), 803–808.

Fuchs-Lacelle, S., & Hadjistavropoulos, T. (2004). Development and preliminary validation of the pain assessment checklist for seniors with limited ability to communicate (PACSLAC). *Pain Management Nursing, 5*(1), 37–49.

Glikson, M., & Friedman, P. A. (2001). The implantable cardioverter defibrillator. *Lancet, 357*(9262), 1107–1117.

Goldstein, N. E., Lampert, R., Bradley, E., Lynn, J., & Krumholz, H. M. (2004). Management of implantable cardioverter defibrillators in end-of-life care. *Annals of Internal Medicine, 141*(11), 835–838.

Goldstein, N. E., & Lynn, J. (2006). Trajectory of end-stage heart failure: The influence of technology and implications for policy change. *Perspectives in Biology and Medicine, 49*(1), 10–18.

Goodman, M. D., Tarnoff, M., & Slotman, G. J. (1998). Effect of advance directives on the management of elderly critically ill patients. *Critical Care Medicine, 26*(4), 701–704.

Gordon, M. (2002). Ethical challenges in end-of-life therapies in the elderly. *Drugs & Aging, 19*(5), 321–329.

Hamel, M. B., Davis, R. B., Teno, J. M., Knaus, W. A., Lynn, J., Harrell, F., Jr., et al. (1999). Older age, aggressiveness of care, and survival for seriously ill, hospitalized adults. *Annals of Internal Medicine, 131*(10), 721–728.

Hamel, M. B., Lynn, J., Teno, J. M., Covinsky, K. E., Wu, A. W., Galanos, A., et al. (2000). Age-related differences in care preferences, treatment decisions, and clinical outcomes of seriously ill hospitalized adults: Lessons from SUPPORT. *Journal of the American Geriatrics Society, 48*(5 Suppl.), S176–182.

Hamel, M. B., Phillips, R. S., Davis, R. B., Teno, J., Desbiens, N., Lynn, J., et al. (2001). Are aggressive treatment strategies less cost-effective for older patients? The case of ventilator support and aggressive care for patients with acute respiratory failure. *Journal of the American Geriatrics Society, 49*(4), 382–390.

Health Resources and Services Administration. (2008). *Organ donation & transplantation questions.* Retrieved February 20, 2008, from http://answers.hrsa.gov

Henderson, M. L. (2004). Gerontological advance practice nurses: As end-of-life care facilitators. *Geriatric Nursing, 25*(4), 233–237.

Henig, N. R., Faul, J. L., & Raffin, T. A. (2001). Biomedical ethics and the withdrawal of advanced life support. *Annual Review of Medicine, 52*, 79–92.

Houts, P., Lipton, A., Harold, A., Simmons, M., & Barthlolomew, M. (1989). Predictors of grief among spouses of deceased cancer patients. *Journal of Psychosocial Oncology, 7,* 113–126.

Jennings, A., Davies, A., Higgins, J., & Broadley, K. (2001). Opioids for the palliation of breathlessness in terminal illness. *Cochrane Database Systematic Review, 4.*

Jezewski, M. A., & Meeker, M. A. (2005). Constituting advance directives from the perspective of people with chronic illnesses. *Journal of Hospice and Palliative Nursing, 7*(6), 319–327.

Johnson, J. E. (1999). Self-regulation theory and coping with physical illness. *Research in Nursing and Health, 22*(6), 435–448.

Kaiko, R. F., Wallenstein, S. L., Rogers, A. G., Grabinski, P. Y., & Houde, R. W. (1982). Narcotics in the elderly. *Medical Clinics of North America, 66*(5), 1079–1089.

Kaplan, V., Angus, D. C., Griffin, M. F., Clermont, G., Scott Watson, R., & Linde-Zwirble, W. T. (2002). Hospitalized community-acquired pneumonia in the elderly: Age- and sex-related patterns of care and outcome in the United States. *American Journal of Respiratory Critical Care Medicine, 165*(6), 766–772.

Kaufman, S. R. (1998). Intensive care, old age, and the problem of death in America. *The Gerontologist, 38*(6), 715–725.

Kehl, K. A. (2004). Treatment of terminal restlessness: A review of the evidence. *Journal of Pain & Palliative Care Pharmacotherapy, 18*(1), 5–30.

Kehl, K. A. (2006). Moving toward peace: An analysis of the concept of a good death. *American Journal of Hospice and Palliative Care., 23*(4), 277–286.

Kehl, K. A. (2008). Caring for the patient and the family in the last hours of life. *Home Health Care Management Practice, 20*(5), 408–413.

Kehl, K. A., & Kirchhoff, K. T. (2004, October). *Family Perceptions of Qualtiy of Care at the End of Life in ICU and Hospice Facility.* Paper presented at the 2004 National State of the Science Conference, Washington, DC.

Kennedy, K. L. (1989). The prevalence of pressure ulcers in an intermediate care facility. *Decubitus, 2*(2), 44–45.

Kirchhoff, K. T. (2005). Getting our ICU language straight. *Critical Connections, 4,* 1, 11.

Kirchhoff, K. T., Beckstrand, R. L., & Anumandla, P. R. (2003). Analysis of end-of-life content in critical care nursing textbooks. *Journal of Professional Nursing, 19*(6), 372–381.

Kirchhoff, K. T., Palzkill, J., Kowalkowski, J., Mork, A., & Gretarsdottir, E. (2008). Preparing ICU families for withdrawal of life support: A pilot study. *American Journal of Critical Care, 17*(2), 113–121.

Kleinpell, R. M., & Ferrans, C. E. (1998). Factors influencing intensive care unit survival for critically ill elderly patients. *Heart & Lung, 27*(5), 337–343.

Knauft, E., Nielsen, E. L., Engelberg, R. A., Patrick, D. L., & Curtis, J. R. (2005). Barriers and facilitators to end-of-life care communication for patients with COPD. *Chest, 127*(6), 2188–2196.

Krohm, C., & Summers, S. K. (2002). The ethics of advance health care directives. In *Advance health care directives: A handbook for professionals* (pp. 23–32). Chicago: American Bar Association.

Langemo, D. K. (2006). When the goal is palliative care. *Advances in Skin & Wound Care, 19*(3), 148–154.

Lee, M. A., Brummel-Smith, K., Meyer, J., Drew, N., & London, M. R. (2000). Physician orders for life-sustaining treatment (POLST): Outcomes in a PACE program. Program of All-Inclusive Care for the Elderly. *Journal of the American Geriatrics Society, 48*(10), 1219–1225.

Lilly, C. M., De Meo, D. L., Sonna, L. A., Haley, K. J., Massaro, A. F., Wallace, R. F., et al. (2000). An intensive communication intervention for the critically ill. *American Journal of Medicine, 109*(6), 469–475.

Lilly, C. M., Sonna, L. A., Haley, K. J., & Massaro, A. F. (2003). Intensive communication: Four-year follow-up from a clinical practice study. *Critical Care Medicine, 31*(5 Suppl.), S394–S399.

Lloyd, C. B., Nietert, P. J., & Silvestri, G. A. (2004). Intensive care decision making in the seriously ill and elderly. *Critical Care Medicine, 32*(3), 649–654.

Lo, B., & Steinbrook, R. (2004). Resuscitating advance directives. *Archives of Internal Medicine, 164*(14), 1501–1506.

Loeb, M., McGeer, A., McArthur, M., Walter, S., & Simor, A. E. (1999). Risk factors for pneumonia and other lower respiratory tract infections in elderly residents of long-term care facilities. *Archives of Internal Medicine, 159*(17), 2058–2064.

Lorenz, K. A., Rosenfeld, K., & Wenger, N. (2007). Quality indicators for palliative and end-of-life care in vulnerable elders. *Journal of the American Geriatrics Society, 55*(Suppl. 2), S318–S326.

Mandell, L. A., Wunderink, R. G., Anzueto, A., Bartlett, J. G., Campbell, D., Dean, N. C., et al. (2007). IDSA/ATS Guidelines for CAP in Adults. *Clinical Infectious Diseases, 44*(Suppl. 2), 27–72.

Marik, P. E., & Kaplan, D. (2003). Aspiration pneumonia and dysphagia in the elderly. *Chest, 124*(1), 328–336.

Marrie, T. J. (2000). Community-acquired pneumonia in the elderly. *Clinical Infectious Diseases, 31*(4), 1066–1078.

Masica, A. L., Girard, T. D., Wilkinson, G. R., Thomason, J. W. W., Truman Pun, B., Nair, U. B., et al. (2007). Clinical sedation scores as indicators of sedative and analgesic drug exposure in intensive care unit patients. *American Journal of Geriatric Pharmacotherapy, 5*(3), 218–231.

McMahon, M. M., Hurley, D. L., Kamath, P. S., & Mueller, P. S. (2005). Medical and ethical aspects of long-term enteral tube feeding. *Mayo Clinic Proceedings, 80*(11), 1461–1476.

Mueller, P. S., Hook, C. C., & Hayes, D. L. (2003). Ethical analysis of withdrawal of pacemaker or implantable cardioverter-defibrillator support at the end of life. *Mayo Clinic Proceedings, 78*(8), 959–963.

Mularski, R. A., & Osborne, M. L. (2003). End-of-life care in the critically ill geriatric population. *Critical Care Clinics, 19*(4), viii, 789–810.

Nagasawa, Y. (2008). Proxy consent and counterfactuals. *Bioethics, 22*(1), 16–24.

National Conference of Commissiorners on Uniform State Laws. (2008). *UAGA summary.* Retrieved August 15, 2008, from http://www.anatomicalgiftact.org/DesktopDefault.aspx?tabindex=1&t abid=67

Norton, S. A., Tilden, V. P., Tolle, S. W., Nelson, C. A., & Eggman, S. T. (2003). Life support withdrawal: Communication and conflict. *American Journal of Critical Care, 12*(6), 548–555.

Nuffield Council on Bioethics. (2006). *Critical care decisions in fetal and neonatal medicine: Ethical issues.* Retrieved August 15, 2008, from http://www.nuffieldbioethics.org/go/browseablepublications/critic alCareDecisionFetalNeonatalMedicine/report_510.html

Pawlik, T. M. (2006). Withholding and withdrawing life-sustaining treatment: A surgeon's perspective. *Journal of the American College of Surgeons, 202*(6), 990–994.

Plaisier, B. R., Blostein, P. A., Hurt, K. J., & Malangoni, M. A. (2002). Withholding/withdrawal of life support in trauma patients: Is there an age bias? *American Surgeon, 68*(2), 159–162.

Pollack, S. (2000). A new approach to Advance Directives. *Critical Care Medicine, 28*(9), 3146–3148.

Portenoy, R. K. (1994). Management of common opioid side effects during long-term therapy of cancer pain. *Annals of the Academy of Medicine, Singapore, 23*(2), 160–170.

Prendergast, T. J., & Puntillo, K. A. (2002). Withdrawal of life support: Intensive caring at the end of life. *Journal of the American Medical Association, 288*(21), 2732–2740.

Puchalski, C. M., Zhong, Z., Jacobs, M. M., Fox, E., Lynn, J., Harrold, J., et al. (2000). Patients who want their family and physician to make resuscitation decisions for them: Observations from SUPPORT and HELP. Study to Understand Prognoses and Preferences for Outcomes and Risks of Treatment. Hospitalized Elderly Longitudinal Project. *Journal of the American Geriatrics Society, 48*(5 Suppl.), S84–S90.

Qaseem, A., Snow, V., Shekelle, P., Casey, D. E., Jr., Cross, J. T., Jr., Owens, D. K., et al. (2008). Evidence-based interventions to improve the palliative care of pain, dyspnea, and depression at the end of life: A clinical practice guideline from the American College of Physicians. *Annals of Internal Medicine, 148*(2), 141–146.

Ramsey, G., & Mitty, E. (2003). *Advance directives: Protecting patient's rights.* Retrieved November 7, 2007, from http://guideline.gov

Reuben, D. B., & Mor, V. (1986). Dyspnea in terminally ill cancer patients. *Chest, 89*(2), 234–236.

Rocker, G., Cook, D., Sjokvist, P., Weaver, B., Finfer, S., McDonald, E., et al. (2004). Clinician predictions of intensive care unit mortality. *Critical Care Medicine, 32*(5), 1149–1154.

Schim, S. M., & Cullen, B. (2005). Wound care at end of life. *Nursing Clinics of North America, 40*(2), 281–294.

Schneiderman, L. J., Pearlman, R. A., Kaplan, R. M., Anderson, J. P., & Rosenberg, E. M. (1992). Relationship of general advance directive instructions to specific life-sustaining treatment preferences in patients with serious illness. *Archives of Internal Medicine, 152*(10), 2114–2122.

Schwartzstein, R. M., Lahive, K., Pope, A., Weinberger, S. E., & Weiss, J. W. (1987). Cold facial stimulation reduces breathlessness induced in normal subjects. *American Review of Respiratory Disease, 136*(1), 58–61.

Senninger, J. L., & Laxenaire, M. (1995). Violent paradoxal reactions secondary to the use of benzodiazepines. *Annales Medico-Psychologiques (Paris), 153*(4), 278–281; discussion 281–282.

Shapiro, S. P. (2007). When life imitates art: Surrogate decision making at the end of life. *Topics in Stroke Rehabilitation, 14*(4), 80–92.

Sherman, D. A., & Branum, K. (1995). Critical care nurses' perceptions of appropriate care of the patient with orders not to resuscitate. *Heart and Lung: Journal of Critical Care, 24*(4), 321–329.

Somogyi-Zalud, E., Zhong, Z., Hamel, M. B., & Lynn, J. (2002). The use of life-sustaining treatments in hospitalized persons aged 80 and older. *Journal of the American Geriatrics Society, 50*(5), 930–934.

Somogyi-Zalud, E., Zhong, Z., Lynn, J., & Hamel, M. B. (2000). Elderly persons' last six months of life: Findings from the Hospitalized Elderly Longitudinal Project. *Journal of the American Geriatrics Society, 48*(5 Suppl.), S131–S139.

Stein, W. M. (2006). Pain in older people. In E. Bruera, I. J. Higginson, C. Ripamonti, & C. von Gunten (Eds.), *Textbook of palliative medicine* (pp. 467–481). London: Hodder Arnold.

Stevenson, L. W., & Desai, A. S. (2006). Selecting patients for discussion of the ICD as primary prevention for sudden death in heart failure. *Journal Cardiac Failure, 12*(6), 407–412.

SUPPORT Investigators. (1995). A controlled trial to improve care for seriously ill hospitalized patients. The study to understand prognoses and preferences for outcomes and risks of treatments (SUPPORT). *Journal of the American Medical Association, 274*(20), 1591–1598.

Teno, J. M., Fisher, E., Hamel, M. B., Wu, A. W., Murphy, D. J., Wenger, N. S., et al. (2000). Decision-making and outcomes of prolonged ICU stays in seriously ill patients. *Journal of the American Geriatrics Society, 48*(5 Suppl.), S70–S74.

Teno, J. M., Harrell, F. E., Jr., Knaus, W., Phillips, R. S., Wu, A. W., Connors, A., Jr., et al. (2000). Prediction of survival for older hospitalized patients: The HELP survival model. Hospitalized Elderly Longitudinal Project. *Journal of the American Geriatrics Society, 48*(5 Suppl.), S16–S24.

Tonelli, M. R. (2005). Waking the dying: Must we always attempt to involve critically ill patients in end-of-life decisions? *Chest, 127*(2), 637–642.

Truog, R. D., Campbell, M. L., Curtis, J. R., Haas, C. E., Luce, J. M., Rubenfeld, G. D., et al. (2008). Recommendations for end-of-life care in the intensive care unit: A consensus statement by the American Academy of Critical Care Medicine. *Critical Care Medicine, 36*(3), 953–963.

Van Den Noortgate, N., Vogelaers, D., Afschrift, M., & Colardyn, F. (1999). Intensive care for very elderly patients: Outcome and risk factors for in-hospital mortality. *Age & Ageing, 28*(3), 253–256.

Warden, V., Hurley, A. C., & Volicer, L. (2003). Development and psychometric evaluation of the Pain Assessment in Advanced Dementia (PAINAD) scale. *Journal of the American Medical Directors Association, 4*(1), 9–15.

Wee, B., & Hillier, R. (2008). Interventions for noisy breathing in patients near to death. *Cochrane Database System Review,* (1), CD005177.

Wildiers, H., & Menten, J. (2002). Death rattle: Prevalence, prevention and treatment. *Journal of Pain and Symptom Management, 23*(4), 310–317.

Williams, R., Harris, S., Randall, L., Nichols, R., & Brown, S. (2003). A bereavement after-care service for intensive care relatives and staff: The story so far. *Nursing in Critical Care, 8*(3), 109–115.

Winzelberg, G. S., Patrick, D. L., Rhodes, L. A., & Deyo, R. A. (2005). Opportunities and challenges to improving end-of-life care for seriously ill elderly patients: A qualitative study of generalist physicians. *Journal of Palliative Medicine, 8*(2), 291–299.

Wood, K. A., & Marik, P. E. (2004). ICU care at the end of life. *Chest, 126*(5), 1403–1406.

Wu, P., Lorenz, K. A., & Chodosh, J. (2008). Advance care planning among the oldest old. *Journal of Palliative Medicine, 11*(2), 152–157.

Zipes, D. P., Camm, A. J., Borggrefe, M., Buxton, A. E., Chaitman, B., Fromer, M., et al. (2006). ACC/AHA/ESC 2006 Guidelines for management of patients with ventricular arrhythmias and the prevention of sudden cardiac death. *Circulation, 114*(10), e385–e484.

Zwakhalen, S. M., Hamers, J. P., Abu-Saad, H. H., & Berger, M. P. (2006). Pain in elderly people with severe dementia: A systematic review of behavioural pain assessment tools. *BMC Geriatrics, 6*, 3.

Zwakhalen, S. M., Hamers, J. P., & Berger, M. P. (2007). Improving the clinical usefulness of a behavioural pain scale for older people with dementia. *Journal of Advances in Nursing, 58*(5), 493–502.

# Becoming Frail

# 9

Graham J. McDougall, Jr.
Carol L. Delville

Frailty is one of the greatest geriatric challenges (Levers, Estabrook, & Ross Kerr, 2006) compounding the complexity of critical illness in older adults. Although associated with older age and comorbidity, frailty is not an inevitable consequence of aging, nor is it caused by comorbidity (Conroy, 2009; Lally & Crome, 2007; Rothman, Leo-Summers, & Gill, 2008). And, frailty is considered similar to but different from disability (Lally & Crome; Rothman et al.).

Frailty is described as a dynamic condition with biomedical (e.g., multisystem decline involving neuromuscular, endocrine, and immune systems) and psychosocial (e.g., cognitive, sensory, and mood) aspects, leading to a decline in homeostatic reserve and resiliency (Bergman et al., 2007). There is considerable disagreement among investigators as to the exact stages comprising the process of frailty, and whether or not it is responsive to treatment (Conroy, 2009). Generally, there is agreement that frailty is a multistage spiral of decline consisting of three stages that begin with a lack of physical exercise, inadequate nutrition, unhealthy environment, injuries, and disease (Bergman et al.); however, the exact mechanisms underlying the pathogenesis of frailty remain unknown (Walston et al., 2006). The stages of frailty include:

■ Stage 1: Prefrailty, is clinically silent; physiologic reserves remain sufficient to respond to stressors (Walston et al., 2006), with the potential for complete recovery (Lang, Michel, & Zekry, 2009). Unfortunately, because this stage is latent and clinically silent, there is limited opportunity for early detection and prevention. There have been numerous attempts to identify a biomarker(s) for this stage that would enable prompt and early implementation of preventive interventions (Walston et al.). People in the prefrail stage of the cycle manifest 2 or fewer risk factors (Lang et al.).

■ Stage 2: Frailty, is manifested by progressive functional decline; physiologic reserves are insufficient to lead to complete recovery with any new acute disease; recovery is slow and incomplete (Walston et al., 2006). Multiple aspects of decline must be present to consider the person frail, with individuals manifesting at least three or more risk factors (Fried et al., 2001; Lang et al., 2009). About 7% of the general U.S. population is thought to be frail, an incidence that is apt to be higher in those experiencing a critical illness. It also is known that frailty is two-fold higher in women than in men by age (Fried et al.), and is higher in lower socioeconomic levels. Frailty is more prevalent in southern Europe, for example, Italy and Spain, than in northern Europe (Santos-Eggimann, Cuenoud, Spagnoli, & Junod, 2009). It also has been reported that individuals who are sedentary have an even greater likelihood of transition to a greater severity of frailty (Peterson et al., 2009).

■ Stage 3: Frailty complications. Some describe the third and final stage of frailty as disability (Daniels, van Rossum, de Witte, Kempen, & van den Heuvel, 2008), whereas others refer to this stage as failure to thrive (Berkman, Foster, & Campion, 1989; Messert, Kurlanzik, & Thorning, 1976; Pope & Tarlov, 1991). Complications of frailty are reported to be related to repeated episodes of physiologic vulnerability and a progressively reduced capacity to withstand stress, leading to disability and eventually to death (Lang et al., 2009).

Older adults are particularly vulnerable to adverse outcomes, especially those being mechanically ventilated (Timmerman, 2007). The syndrome of frailty is not uniquely found in the elderly, and may be found in younger patients with multiple medical conditions (Espinoza & Walston, 2005). The spectrum of frailty may be measured through decline in physical strength, mobility, and a reduced tolerance to physical and/or psychological stressors (Watson et al., 2002). Frailty may be easily overlooked in community-dwelling older adults, however, the stress of elective procedures or minor infections may be enough to overwhelm the functional reserves of these patients.

Frailty confers high risk for adverse health outcomes from greater morbidity, prolonged hospitalization, institutionalization, to death (Fried et al., 2001). With critical illness, frailty is associated with atelectasis, pneumonia, orthostatic hypotension, DVTs (deep vein thrombosis) decubitus ulcers, deconditioning, and a spiral toward death (Timmerman, 2007).

Frailty is receiving greater interest of late because many think that interventions that target the processes underling frailty might help the development of more efficacious interventions to prevent or treat patients experiencing one or more geriatric syndromes, for example, delirium, falls, incontinence, than existing interventions that target one of these syndromes (Rockwood, 2004). In this chapter we discuss risk factors for frailty, assessment methods, and interventions to prevent or treat frailty within the context of critical illness.

## Risk Factors/Markers for Frailty

Frailty is considered to be present when at least three of the following characteristics are observed in an individual: slow walking speed, low grip strength, low physical activity, self-reported exhaustion, and a greater than 5% unintentional weight loss in the past year (Fried et al., 2001; Lang et al., 2009). Continued weight loss and exhaustion are key indicators of the progression of frailty (Espinoza & Hazuda, 2009). However, these same characteristics are typically present in older people with a critical illness. The clinical challenge is determining the degree to which these characteristics are a function of the critical illness or frailty, a challenge virtually impossible to overcome in the intensive care unit (ICU).

In addition to the characteristics described previously that are considered diagnostic for frailty, researchers have found the following:

■ Women are more likely than men to become frail (Lally & Crome, 2007); one seeming contradiction to this relationship is that widowed men living alone are more likely to be depressed and these men are more likely than women to become frail (Levers et al., 2006).

■ Individuals of lower socioeconomic status (Santos-Eggimann et al., 2009) and those with less education (Santos-Eggimann et al.) have a greater likelihood of being frail.

■ Individuals with greater comorbidity are at greater risk for becoming frail (Lally & Crome).

■ Chronic inflammation has been linked with frailty as reflected by C-reactive protein, cytokine IL-6, and greater numbers of monocytes and total white blood cells (Cohen, 2000; Pawelec, 2005; Walston et al., 2006).

■ Frailty has been linked with insulin resistance by other researchers (Abbatecola & Paolisso, 2008).

■ Frailty has been associated with slowed or impaired cognitive functioning (Hubbard, O'Mahoney, & Woodhouse, 2009; Rothman et al., 2008; Sarkisian, Gruenewald, Boscardin, & Seeman, 2008).

Each predictor has been reported to be independently associated with a moderate risk of morbidity and mortality. When three or more of these predictors were identified in a client, the risk of increased falls, worsening mobility, disability with activities of daily living (ADLs), hospitalization, and mortality increases (Lally & Crome, 2007). However, it remains unclear from these facts as to what the underlying pathogenic mechanism is and how these factors contribute to the genesis of frailty (Walston et al., 2006). Given the serious nature and consequences of frailty, the manifestation of these characteristics should arouse suspicion that the individual is frail or at risk for becoming frail and to institute preventive measures as soon as the patient is capable.

## Cases

The following cases illustrate the spectrum of susceptibility to, and severity of, frailty and how clinical outcomes are affected.

### Case Study 1

An 84-year-old widowed Hispanic university professor was found at home on the floor with a fractured left hip. He lived alone, ambulated with a cane, and was brought to the hospital by a family member who stopped by after the patient failed to make his daily call about the manuscript on which they were collaborating. He was admitted to the surgical intensive care after a total-hip replacement. Past medical history included arthritis, osteoporosis, Chron's disease, and hypertension. He weighed 138 pounds and was 71 inches tall. On admission to the intensive care unit he was alert and oriented, heart rate was 90 per minute and regular, blood pressure was 110/68, respiratory rate was 18 to 20 respirations per minute, and he was afebrile. His emergent hip-replacement surgery was without complication, and after 5 days hospitalization he returned home for home physical therapy.

### Case Study 2

Brought in by her husband, a 76-year-old African American woman presented to the emergency department with an upper respiratory infection. Her vital signs were temperature, 96.7 degrees Fahrenheit orally; heart rate 88 beats per minute and irregular, electrocardiogram indicated atrial fibrillation; blood pressure was 158/88; and respiratory rate was 22 per minutes. Her past medical history included 50 pack years of smoking, rheumatoid arthritis, osteopenia, and prerenal failure related to nonsteroidal antiinflammatory use. After retiring from her secretarial position, she and her husband moved in with their daughter's family to assist with child care. However, she currently needs assistance with most activities of daily living. She reported a decrease in appetite and weight loss of 15 pounds over the past 3 months (current height 62 inches, weight 116 pounds). She was admitted to the intensive care unit, intubated, and on a ventilator with diagnoses of dehydration, pneumonia, and acute renal failure. Two days later she became delirious and uncooperative with her care. Her respiratory status slowly improved and within 3 days she was successfully weaned, extubated, and transferred out of the ICU. Within another 3 days her delirium slowly resolved. She was discharged a couple of days later to a skilled nursing facility for 2 weeks before returning to her daughter's.

### Case Study 3

A 68-year-old single Caucasian female had a history of diabetes, congestive heart failure, peripheral vascular disease, and arthritis. A retired librarian, she lived alone, and had been active in the community, but over the past couple of months her physical activity declined as a result of increased fatigue and leg pain. She reported falling twice in the past year, and attributed this to getting up from bed too quickly during the night to go to the bathroom. She was admitted to the emergency room with a diagnosis of sepsis related to an infected stasis ulcer on her lower left leg. She was admitted to the intensive care unit because of her sepsis-related hypotension, poor cardiac status, and antibiotic treatment. She weighted 265 pounds with a height of 65 inches. On admission to the ICU, her temperature was 99.4 degrees Fahrenheit orally, heart rate was 112 beats per minute, blood pressure was 85/50, and respirations 24 per minute and shallow and labored. Laboratory values were significant for elevated white blood count, hemoglobin and hematocrit, and a glucose level of 460. Her cardiac and respiratory status continued to decline; she was intubated and ventilated, and placed on vasopressors. She was slow to respond to this therapy, taking 5 days to stabilize with another 3 days before she was successfully weaned and extubated. Her hospitalization continued for another 2 weeks before she was placed in a subacute hospital, where she died 3 months later.

These three cases illustrate the spectrum of susceptibility to and severity of frailty and how clinical outcomes are affected. The patients in cases 1 and 2 appear equally robust at the onset, but patient 1 experiences a quick and complete recovery to preillness health status; recovery for patient 2 is slower and less complete. The patient in the third case is clearly frail, experiencing multiple set backs that contribute to a continued decline leading to death.

## Assessment

Older critically ill adults are at great risk for frailty and require screening to identify potentially reversible risk factors contributing to its genesis, progression, and with treatment, resolution. Multiple approaches to assessment are employed to obtain information about the myriad factors that place an individual at risk for becoming frail; these methods vary greatly and consist of self-report of selected functions (function, self-care, fatigue/exhaustion), reports from informed others (family, friends, caregivers), observation of performance (walking), paper-and-pencil tests (cognition), and physical functional task demonstration (grip strength).

This section identifies methods of assessment of the frailty phenotype that form the foundation for admission assessments in the critical care unit.

■ **Demographic factors.** Demographic and social economic factors influence disease response, length of recovery time, functional decline, and death (Saliba & Waite, 2000; Stuck et al., 1999). Advanced age is associated with frailty. Marital status effects health status, especially for men; and race and ethnicity have been associated with disparity in health outcomes, as well as differences in health beliefs, health behaviors, and self-reports regarding health and physical function (Kaplan, Bhalodkar, Brown, White, Brown Jr., 2006; Nau et al., 2005). Finally, the years of formal education are known to influence heath outcomes and access to services, as well as to provide insight into the patient's ability to comprehend questions and follow instructions (Crum, Anthony, Bassett, & Folstein, 1993).

■ **Functional ability.**

■ *Self-reports of functional ability* are considered reliable by many researchers (Rathouz et al., 1998). Yet, self-assessment of functional capacity is often overestimated and family members' evaluations underestimate physical function when compared to objective measures (Ferrucci et al., 2004; McDougall, Becker, Vaughan, Acee, & Delville, 2008).

■ *Self-reports of exhaustion.* Having the patient self-rate his/her fatigue on a 1-to-10 scale before and after activities is useful in the determination of his/her reserve capacity and changes in energy levels during the acute phase of treatment.

■ *Observation of performance of physical functional tasks.* Balance and strength are informally tested during client transfers from stretcher to bed, and bed to chair, yet these assessments are rarely documented in a manner that details the functional capacity of the client (Wells, Seabrook, Stolee, Borrie, & Knoefel, 2003). Grip strength is often used to assess strength either informally by having the client squeeze a hand, or more objectively using a dynamometer, which measures the grips in terms of pounds or kilograms (Purser et al.). This procedure may be contraindicated as a measure of strength if the client has increase intracranial pressure. The 6-minute walk test, a standard of balance, endurance, speed, and fatigue in the outpatient setting, is often beyond the functional capacity of a critically ill client, but can be approximated in the critical care setting by calculating the time it takes a client to walk 15 feet (Purser et al.). If walking is not possible, the simple sit-to-stand test (number of times a client can stand from a sitting position in 30 seconds without using the arms of the chair) can provide an excellent assessment of large muscle group strength and functional capacity, but again may be beyond the capability of the critically ill, or impractical because of the risk of increased heart rate and oxygen demand. The simplest alternative is an assessment of the number of falls over the past 6 months through self- or caregiver report, which has been demonstrated to predict further falls and declines in the ability to complete both ADL and instrumental activities of daily living (IADL) tasks in the next 6 months (Soriano, 2007).

■ *Objective evidence of fatigue/exhaustion.* The patient's functioning level of energy and reserve capacity for activity is difficult to determine in the critical care setting because of the acute nature of the medical condition. The presence of fatigue and lack of energy after minimal exertion (bed-to-chair transfer, for example) is a useful assessment. Having the patient self-rate her/his fatigue on a 1-to-10 scale pre- and postactivity is useful in the determination of her/his reserve capacity and changes in energy levels during the acute phase of treatment. The speed at which a patient is able to complete a physical task provides insight as to his/her fatigue, strength, and physical ability. However, pain and the effects of medications will influence the patient's fatigue and mobility, and should be assessed at the same time.

■ *Changes in body composition,* especially unintentional weight loss of 5% or more in the prior 12 months is especially noteworthy. Changes in weight can easily be assessed through chart review, or obtaining records from the primary provider. Care providers and family are often able to provide general information about weight changes. Obesity, defined as a body mass index of >30, is predictive of frailty in older adults, because of the decreased activity levels found in these individuals as well as increased levels of serum inflammatory markers (Strandberg & Pitkälä, 2007); unfortunately frailty is not readily apparent in obese elderly. Furthermore, fluid shifts found in many acute diseases may make body mass index an unreliable measure of the patient's "dry weight." In these instances the use of serum albumin and prealbumin levels, which are associated with increased morbidity and mortality in critically ill older adults, may serve as useful screening tools for at-risk patients and provide immediate to 6-month morbidity and mortality risk assessments based on physiological reserves of the client (Delville, 2008).

■ *Cognitive function* has been clearly demonstrated to be predictive of the ability to perform activities of daily living, instrumental activities of daily living, morbidity, and mortality in 3 to 6 months after hospital discharge (Sands et al., 2003). Unfortunately, cognitive function is rarely documented beyond the orientation of the client to person, place, and time, thus information regarding the client's baseline cognitive status may not be available (please see chapter 26 in this text). Many older adults in critical care have altered mental status because of infections or sepsis, dehydration, medication reaction, and the loss of their normal environmental clues for time and place. Caregiver report may be required to establish a baseline for the assessment of cognitive functional status in the unresponsive critical care client.

■ *Comorbidity* and concomitant medications are reported to be predictive of the onset of frailty, morbidity, and mortality during the critical care stay, and at 3 and 12 months after discharge (Wells et al., 2003). Depression and osteoporosis have been identified as independent predictors for frailty, and require specific screening when taking a medical history (Lally & Crome, 2007). The hospital record may contain the recommended screening information about osteoporosis, but there are no standards for the screening for depressive symptoms. There are many screening instruments for depressive symptoms; one of the simplest is the Geriatric Depression Scale (GDS; Yesavage, Brink, Rose, & Adey, 1983), a 15-item, yes/no questionnaire, which requires only a few minutes to complete. Depression reduces motivation, delays seeking treatment, and often prolongs a hospitalization (Wells et al., 2003). Patients with depressive symptoms, fatigue more rapidly, and are less mobile than nondepressed comparison- age-match patients, thus reducing their ability to perform ADL and IADL activities (Nourhashémi et al., 2001). The number of medical conditions, as well as the types and amounts of medications required to treat these conditions, influence a patient's recovery (Corsinovi et al., 2008). Medication interactions and errors continue to be a leading cause for hospital admissions (Holland et al., 2008). Medical history and medication list may often be obtained from the patient's primary provider or pharmacist.

The aforementioned methods developed to assess for frailty or its risk factors have been developed primarily for research purposes and tend to be impractical for clinical use (Lang et al., 2009), especially for use with critically ill elders (Purser et al., 2006). Moreover, the assessment of frailty becomes further complicated in the critical care setting because patients are often unable to communicate their baseline level of function, or the acuity of their illness may prohibit immediate formal objective testing of specific domains such as gait speed, balance, or cognition. As a result, nurses in the critical care setting need to examine the patients' functional history for the period prior to admission, including falls, weight change, caregiver reports of memory function, and comorbid conditions. Documentation of functional and cognitive capacity at the time of admission provides baseline standards to measure progress or decline throughout treatment, and assist in the discharge planning needs for the patient.

## Prevention and Treatment of Frailty

Prevention is the desired and ultimate goal of intervention; however, prevention may not always be feasible. In that case, the primary goal of treatment is to minimize further losses that would result in disability (Fried, Ferrucci, Darer, Williamson, & Anderson, 2004). Improved walking speed is a key indicator of the regression of frailty (Espinoza & Hazuda, 2009). However, less is known about efficacious interventions to treat frailty (Lally & Crome, 2007). And, although there are no data to suggest otherwise, frailty is considered reversible (Walston et al., 2006).

Efforts to prevent frailty target risk-factor reduction (Daniels et al., 2008) by providing adequate diet, regular physical exercise [especially strength, balance, and endurance training (Fried et al., 2004; Walston et al., 2006)], preventing infections, anticipating and preparing for stressful events, rapid reconditioning, and regular monitoring of risk-factor parameters (Lang et al., 2009). Consequently, therapeutic interventions need to be tailored to the specifics of the individual (Lally & Crome, 2007). Although risk factors include unintentional weight loss, sarcopenia, muscle weakness, self-reported exhaustion, slow walking speed, and low level of physical activity, interventions have primarily focused on physical exercise and nutritional supplementation (see Exhibit 9.1).

Level I activities should be initiated immediately on admission to the ICU and continue throughout hospitalization. Level I activities should even be initiated in patients who are comatose or heavily sedated (Morris et al., 2008). Activities above Level I, such as active-resistance physical therapy, require patients to be able to respond appropriately to directions from care providers (Bailey et al., 2007; Morris et al., 2008).

Mechanical ventilation is not a contraindication to getting out of bed (Bailey et al., 2007; Morris et al., 2008; Thomsen, Snow, Rodriquez, & Hopkins, 2008; Timmerman, 2007), early ambulation is an essential step toward wending (Timmerman). Clinical indications for witholding activity include physiologic instability as evidenced by hypotension, hypoxia, or dysrrhythmias among others (Morris et al.; Needham, 2008) or the presence of an unstable fracture (Needham).

Nutritional therapy to modulate the stress response in critically ill adults includes early enteral nutrition consisting of appropriate macro and micronutrients and glycemic control (Martindale et al., 2009). Components of interventions targeting nutritional factors include nutritional supplementation using commercially available, high-energy, high-protein supplements (Fairhall et al., 2008) or supplementation of micronutrients (Chin A Paw, de Jong, Schouten, Hiddink, & Kok, 2001). Treatment, such as

# Exhibit 9.1

## Progressive Early Mobility Guidelines for Critically Ill Older Adults

- Level I

    - Repositioning in bed every 2 hours
    - Passive range-of-motion exercises, three times per day
    - Level II [includes Level I activities]
    - Active resistance physical therapy
    - Sitting position in bed, 20 minutes, three times per day
    - Level III [includes Level I–II activities]
    - Sitting on edge of the bed
    - Level IV [includes Level III activities]
    - Active transfer to chair at least 20 minutes per day
    - Assists with various aspects of care activities (e.g., bathing)
    - Level V [includes Level I–IV activities]
    - Ambulation with assistance
    - Level VI [includes Level I–V activities]
    - Ambulation and care activities without assistance

Adapted from Bailey et al. (2007), Morris et al. (2008), Needlham (2008), Timmerman (2007).

resistance exercises or increased calorie-dense foods, should be targeted to minimize and reverse these changes when tolerated (Fried et al., 2004).

Given that this clinical syndrome also has psychosocial aspects, interventions must target these as well, thus it is suggested that in addition to early mobilization and nutrition, intervention to prevent or treat frailty should include cognitively stimulating activities as well as environmental modification or enrichment strategies. However, to date, the efficacy of these components as essential parts of a multicomponent intervention to prevent or treat frailty has not been tested in this patient population or any other. Strategies to target the psychosocial aspects of frailty follow:

- Cognitive stimulation protocol: Discussion of daily events, structured reminiscence, and communication to provide orientation (Borthwick, Bourne, Craig, Egan, & Oxley, 2006; Inouye et al., 1999; Lundstrom et al., 2005; Marcantonio et al., 2001; Michaud et al., 2007; Pitkala, Laurila, Strandberg, & Tilvis, 2006.; Young et al., 2008); these "conversations" can occur even when the patient is heavily sedated or comatose.
- Environmental enrichment/modification: Unit-wide noise-reduction strategies; rescheduling procedures to maximize sleep times; diurnal variation in lighting and activity; sleep-promoting activities, for example, relaxation tapes, music, or back massage can help promote a more normal environment (Inouye et al.; Marcantonio et al.; Meagher et al., 1996; Michaud et al.; Mistraletti et al. 2008; Young et al., 2008).

To date, interventions have proved efficacious only in those individuals who are moderately frail (Daniels et al., 2008); interventions have been ineffective in those with severe frailty (Lang et al., 2009) moreover, only physical exercise has demonstrated beneficial effects (Chin A Paw et al., 2001); nutritional supplementation of any kind has failed to generate any beneficial effect, possibly because the nutritional component was of insufficient dose, duration, frequency, or consisted of the wrong mix of micronutrients.

Early ambulation in critically ill patients, including those being mechanically ventilated, has been associated with the following outcomes: no change in cost of care, a reduction of ICU and total hospital days (Morris et al., 2008), others have found early ambulation to be feasible and safe (Bailey et al., 2007). Many have voiced concern regarding patient expectation and attitude about exercise while hospitalized; however, the majority of patients see exercise while in the hospital as appropriate and beneficial (So & Pierluissi, 2009).

## Summary and Conclusions

Frailty is one of the greatest geriatric challenges (Levers et al., 2006) compounding the complexity of critical illness in older adults. Although risk factors include unintentional weight loss, sarcopenia, muscle weakness, self-reported exhaustion, slow walking speed, and low level of physical activity, interventions to prevent or treat frailty have focused primarily on early ambulation in critically ill adults. However, for interventions to truly prevent or reverse frailty much work remains to uncover its underlying pathogenesis.

## References

Abbatecola, A. M., & Paolisso, G. (2008). Is there a relationship between insulin resistance and frailty syndrome? *Current Pharmaceutical Design, 14,* 405–410.

Bailey, P., Thomsen, G. E., Spuhler, V. J., Blair, R., Jewkes, J., Bezdjian, L., et al. (2007). Early activity is feasible and safe in respiratory failure patients. *Critical Care Medicine, 35*(1), 139–145.

Bergman, H., Ferrucci, L., Guralnik, J., Hogan, D. B., Hummel, S., Karunananthan, S., et al. (2007). Frailty: An emerging research and clinical paradigm issues and controversies. *Journal of Gerontology: Medical Sciences, 62A,* 731–737.

Berkman, B., Foster, L. W., & Campion, E. (1989). Failure to thrive: Paradigm for the frail elder. *The Gerontologist, 29*(5), 654–659.

Borthwick, M., Bourne, R., Craig, M., Egan, A., & Oxley, J. (2006, June). *Detection, prevention, and treatment of delirium in critically ill patients.* United Kingdom Clinical Pharmacy Association. Available at http://www.ics.ac.uk/icmprof/downloads/UKCPA%20Delirium%20Resource%20 June%202006%20v1%202.pdf

Chin A Paw, M. J. M., de Jong, N., Schouten, E. G., Hiddink, G. J., & Kok, F. J. (2001). Physical exercise and/or enriched foods for functional improvement in frail, independently living elderly: A randomized controlled trial. *Archives of Physical Medicine and Rehabilitation, 82,* 811–817.

Cohen, H. J. (2000). In search of the underlying mechanisms of frailty. *Journal of Gerontology A, Biological Sciences and Medical Sciences, 55,* M706–8.

Conroy, S. (2009). Defining frailty the holy grail of geriatric medicine [editorial]. *Journal of Nutrition, Health, and Aging, 13*(4), 389.

Corsinovi, L., Bo, M., Aimonino, N. R., Marinello, R., Gariglio, F., Marchetto, C., et al. (2008). Predictors of falls and hospitalization outcomes in elderly patients admitted to an acute geriatric unit. *Archives of Gerontology and Geriatrics.* DOI:10.1016/j.archger.2008.06.004. Retrieved September 3, 2008, from http://linkinghub.elsevier.com/retrieve/pii/S0167-4943(08)00123-4

Crum, R. M., Anthony, J. C., Bassett, S. S., & Folstein, M. F. (1993). Population-based norms for the Mini-Mental State Examination by age and educational level. *Journal of the American Medical Association, 269*(18), 2386–2391.

Daniels, R., van Rossum, E., de Witte, L., Kempen, G. I. J. M., & van den Heuvel, W. (2008). Interventions to prevent disability in frail community-dwelling elderly: A systematic review. *BMC Health Services Research, 8,* 278.

Delville, C. L. (2008). Are your patients at nutritional risk? *Nurse Practitioner, 33*(2), 36–39.

Espinoza, S., & Walston, J. D. (2005). Frailty in older adults: Insights and interventions. *Cleveland Clinic Journal of Medicine, 72*(12), 1105–1112.

Espinoza, S. E., & Hazuda, H. P. (2009). Frailty transitions in the San Antonio Longitudinal Study of Aging [abstract]. *Journal of the American Geriatrics Society, 57*(5), S142.

Fairhall, N., Aggar, C., Kurrle, S. E., Sherrington, C., Lord, S., Lockwood, K., et al. (2008). Frailty Intervention Trial (FIT). *BMC Geriatrics, 8,* 27.

Ferrucci, L., Guralnik, J. M., Studenski, S., Fried, L. P., Culter, Jr., G. B., & Walston, J. D. (2004). Designing randomized controlled trials aimed at preventing or delaying functional decline and disability in frail, older persons: A consensus report. *Journal of the American Geriatrics Society, 52,* 625–634.

Fried, L. P., Ferrucci, L., Darer, J., Williamson, I. S., & Anderson, G. (2004). Untangling the concept of disability, frailty, and comorbidity: Implications for improved targeting and care. *Journals of Gerontology Series A: Biological Sciences and Medical Sciences, 59,* M255–263.

Fried, L. P., Tangem, C. M., Walston, J., Newman, A. B., Hirsch, C., Gottdiener, J., et al. (2001). Frailty in older adults: Evidence for a phenotype. *Journal of Gerontology: Medical Sciences, 56*A(3), M146–156.

Holland, R., Desborough, J., Goodyer, L., Hall, S., Wright, D., & Loke, Y. K. (2008). Does pharmacist-led medication review help to reduce hospital admissions and deaths in older people? A systematic review and meta-analysis. *British Journal of Clinical Pharmacology, 65*(3) 303-316.

Hubbard, R. E., O'Mahoney, M. S., & Woodhouse, K. W. (2009). Characterising frailty in the clinical setting a comparison of different approaches. *Age & Ageing, 38,* 115–119.

Inouye, S. K., Bogardus, S. T., Jr., Charpentier, P. A., Leo-Summers, L., Acampora, D., Holford, T. R., et al. (1999). A multicomponent intervention to prevent delirium in hospitalized older patients. *New England Journal of Medicine, 340,* 669–676.

Kaplan, R. C., Bhalodkar, N. C., Brown, D. L., White, J., Brown, Jr., E. J. (2006). Differences by age and race/ethnicity in knowledge about hypercholesterolemia. *Cardiology Reviews, 14*(1), 1–6.

Lally, F., & Crome, P. (2007). Understanding frailty. *Postgraduate Medical Journal, 83,* 16–20.

Lang, P.-O., Michel, J.-P., & Zekry, D. (2009). Frailty syndromes: A transitional state in a dynamic process. *Gerontology,* DOI: 10.1159/000211949.

Levers, M. J., Estabrook, C. A., & Ross Kerr, J. C., (2006). Factors contributing to frailty: Literature review. *Journal of Advanced Nursing, 56*(3), 282–291.

Lundstrom, M., Edlund, A., Karlsson, S., Brannstrom, B., Bucht, G., & Gustafson, Y. (2005). A multifactorial intervention program reduces the duration of delirium, length of hospitalization, and mortality in delirious patients. *Journal of the American Geriatrics Society, 53,* 622–628.

Marcantonio, E. R., Flacker, J. M., Wright, J., & Resnick, N. M. (2001). Reducing delirium after hip-fracture: A randomized trial. *Journal of the American Geriatrics Society, 49,* 516–522.

Martindale, R. G., McClave, S. A., Vanek, V. W., McCarthy, M., Roberts, P., Taylor, B., et al. (2009). Guidelines for the provision and assessment of nutritional support therapy in the adult critically ill patient: Society of Critical Care Medicine and American Society for Parenteral and Enteral Nutrition: Executive Summary. *Critical Care Medicine, 37*(5), 1757–1761.

McDougall, G. J., Becker, H., Vaughan, P., Acee, T., & Delville, C. (in press). Revising the direct assessment of functional status for independent older adults. *The Gerontologist.*

Meagher, D. J., O'Hanlon, O'Mahoney, E., & Casey, P. R. (1996). The use of enviornmental stratgies and psychotropic medication in the management of delirium. *British Journal of Psychiatry, 168,* 512–518.

Messert, B., Kurlanzik, A. E., & Thorning, D. R. (1976). Adult "failure-to-thrive" syndrome. *Journal of Nervous & Mental Disease, 162*(6), 401–409.

Michaud, L., Bula, C., Berney, A., Camus, V., Voellinger, R., Stiefel, F., et al. (2007). Delirium: Guidelines for general hospitals. *Journal of Psychosomatic Research, 62,* 371–383.

Mistraletti, G., Corloni, E. Cigada, M., Zambrelli, E., Taverna, M., Sabbatici, G., et al. (2008). Sleep and delirium in the intensive care unit. *Minerva Anaesthesiology, 74,* 329–333,

Morris, P. E., Goad, A., Thompson, C., Taylor, K., Harry, B., Passmore, L., et al. (2008). Early intensive care unit mobility therapy in the treatment of acute respiratory therapy. *Critical Care Medicine, 36*(8), 2238–2243.

Nau, D. P., Ellis, J. J., Kline-Rogers, E. M., Mallya, U., Eagle, K. A., & Erickson, S. R. (2005). Gender and perceived severity of cardiac disease: Evidence that women are "tougher." *American Journal of Medicine, 118*(11), 1256–1261.

Needham, D. M. (2008). Mobilizing patients in the intensive care unit. Improving neuromuscular weakness and physical function. *Journal of the American Medical Association, 300*(14), 1685–1690.

Nourhashémi, F, Andrieu, S., Gillette-Guyonnet, S., Vellas, B., Albarède, J. L., & Grandjean, H. (2001). Instrumental activities of daily living as a potential marker of frailty: A study of 7364 community-dwelling elderly women (the EPIDOS study). *Journals of Gerontology. Series A, Biological Sciences and Medical Sciences, 56*(7), M448–453.

Pawelec, G. (2005). Immunosenescence and vaccination. *Immunity and Aging, 2*, 16.

Peterson, M. J., Giuliana, C., Morey, M. C., Pieper, C. F., Evenson, K. R., Mercer, V., et al. (2009). Physical activity as a preventative factor for frailty: The Health, Aging, and Body Composition Study. *Journal of Gerontology, 64A*, 61–68.

Pitkala, K. H., Laurila, J. V., Strandberg, T. E., & Tilvis, R. S. (2006). Multicomponent geriatric intervention for elderly inpatients with delirium: A randomized, controlled trial. *Journal of Gerontology: Medical Sciences, 61A*, 176–181.

Pope, A., & Tarlov, A. (1991). *Disability in America: Toward a national agenda for prevention*. Institute of Medicine (U.S.) Committee on a National Agenda for the Prevention of Disabilities. Washington, DC: National Academy Press.

Purser, J. L., Kuchibhatla, M. N., Fillenbaum, G. G., Harding, T., Peterson, E. D., & Alexander, K. P. (2006). Identifying Frailty in hospitalized older adults with significant coronary artery disease. *Journal of the American Geriatrics Society, 54*, 1674–1681.

Rathouz, P. J., Kasper, J. D., Zerger, S. L., Ferrucci, L., Bandeen-Roche, K., Miglioretti, D. L., et al. (1998). Short-term consistency in self-reported physical functioning among elderly women. *American Journal of Epidemiology, 147*(8), 764–773.

Rockwood, K. (2004). Delirium and frailty. *Primary Psychiatry, 11*(11), 36–39.

Rothman, M. D., Leo-Summers, L., & Gill, T. M. (2008). Prognostic significance of potential frailty criteria. *Journal of the American Geriatrics Society, 56*, 2211–2216.

Saliba, D., & Waite, M. S. (2000). Risk assessment and identification. In M. D. Mezey, B. J. Beerkman, C. M. Callahan, T. T. Fulmer, E. L. Mitty, G. J. Paveza, et al. (Eds.), *The encyclopedia of elder care: The comprehensive resource on geriatric and social care*. New York: Springer Publishing Company.

Sands, L. P., Yaffe, K., Covinsky, K., Chren, M. M., Counsell, S., Palmer, R., et al. (2003). Cognitive screening predicts magnitude of functional recovery from admission to 3 months after discharge in hospitalized elders. *Journal of Gerontology, 58A*, 37–45.

Santos-Eggimann, B., Cuenoud, P., Spagnoli, J., & Junod, J. (2009). Prevalence of frailty in middle-aged and older community-dwelling Europeans living in 10 countries. *Journal of Gerontology: Medical Sciences, 64*(6), 675–681.

Sarkisian, C. A., Gruenewald, T. L., Boscardin, W. J., & Seeman, T. E. (2008). Preliminary evidence for subdimensions of geriatric frailty: The MacArthur Study of Successful Aging. *Journal of the American Geriatrics Society, 56*, 2292–2297.

So, C., & Pierluissi, E. (2009). Attitudes and expectation of hospitalized older adults about exercise in the hospital. *Journal of the American Geriatrics Society, 57*(5), S97.

Soriano, T. A. (2007). Falls in the community-dwelling older adult: A review for primary-care providers. *Clinical Interventions In Aging, 2*(4), 545–554.

Strandberg, T. E., & Pitkälä, K. H. (2007). Frailty in elderly people. *Lancet, 369*(5970), 1328–1329.

Stuck, A. E., Walthert, J. M., Nikolaus, T., Bèula, C. J., Hohmann, C., & Beck, J. C. (1999). Risk factors for functional status decline in community-living elderly people: A systematic literature review. *Social Science and Medicine, 48*(4), 445–469.

Thomsen, G. E., Snow, G. L., Rodriguez, L., & Hopkins, R. O. (2008). Patients with respiratory failure increase ambulation after transfer to an intensive care unit where early activity is a priority. *Critical Care Medicine, 36*(4), 1119–1124.

Timmerman, R. A. (2007). A mobility protocol for critically ill adults. *Dimensions of Critical Care Nursing, 26*(5), 175–179.

Walston, J., Hadley, E. C., Ferrucci, L., Guralnik, J. M., Newman, A. B., Studenski, S. A., et al. (2006). Research agenda for frailty in older adults: Toward a better understanding of physiology and etiology: Summary from the American Geriatrics Society/National Institute on Aging Research Conference on Frailty in Older Adults. *Journal of the American Geriatrics Society, 54*(6), 991–1001.

Watson, J., McBurnie, M. A., Newman, A., Tracy, R. P., Kop, W. J., Hirsch, C. H., et al. (2002). Frailty and activation of the inflammation and coagulation system with and without clinical comorbidities: Results from the Cardiovascular Health Study. *Archives of Internal Medicine, 162*(20), 2333–2341.

Wells, J. L., Seabrook, J. A., Stolee, P., Borrie, M. J., & Knoefel, F. (2003). State of the art in geriatric rehabilitation. Part I: Review of frailty and comprehensive geriatric assessment. *Archives of Physical Medicine and Rehabilitation, 84,* 890–897.

Yesavage, J. A., Brink, T. L., Rose, T. L., & Adey, M. (1983). The Geriatric Depression Rating Scale: Comparison with other self-report and psychiatric rating scales. In T. Crook, S. Ferris, & R. Bartus Eds.), *Assessment in geriatric psychopharmacology* (pp. 153–167). New Canaan, CT: Mark Powley.

Young, J., Leentjens, A. F., George, J., Olofsson, B., & Gustafson, Y. (2008). Systematic approaches to the prevention and management of patients with delirium. *Journal of Psychosomatic Research, 65,* 267–272.

# The Chronically Critically Ill

# 10

Clareen Wiencek
Ronald Hickman, Jr.

## Introduction

The syndrome of chronic critical illness is an unintended consequence of modern critical care (Nierman, 2002). Increased demand for critical care and advances in life-sustaining therapies have resulted in a growing number of patients who survive the acute life-threatening event but then progress into a prolonged and chronic condition. Chronic critical illness, as distinguished from critical illness, is a complex syndrome of physiologic abnormalities, neuroendocrine and immunologic dysfunction (Carson & Bach, 2002; Nelson et al., 2004; Van den Berghe, 2002). It is characterized by prolonged medical and nursing dependence; need for life-sustaining treatments such as mechanical ventilation (MV) and hemodialysis; multiple organ dysfunction and failure; and uncertain trajectory associated with a high risk of disability, distress, and death. Except for the devastating and life-altering course these patients endure and the need for prolonged mechanical ventilation, a hallmark of the syndrome (Nierman, 2002) there is no common etiology or consistently predictable disease trajectory (Carson, 2006). The poorly differentiated characteristics of chronic critical illness not only contribute to poor outcomes but may also explain why case management programs, like those in heart failure or oncology, have not been widely used in this population (Daly,

Douglas, Kelley, O'Toole, & Montenegro, 2005). This chapter describes the pathophysiology, prevalence, outcomes of chronic critical illness, and the characteristics of the chronically critically ill (CCI) and their families. A comprehensive care model proposed to improve the care and outcomes of the CCI is also discussed.

## Case Study

H.D., a 70-year-old male, was admitted to the intensive care unit (ICU) status post coronary artery bypass graft surgery and a Maze procedure. His preexisting conditions included morbid obesity, coronary artery disease (CAD), previous acute myocardial infarction, ischemic cardiomyopathy with an ejection fraction of 25%, permanent pacemaker, atrial fibrillation, Type II diabetes, hypertension, and gout. He experienced a rocky postoperative course complicated by bleeding and reexploration on postop day 1, prolonged respiratory failure necessitating elective tracheostomy on postop day 12, low cardiac output needing prolonged vasopressor support, renal insufficiency with continuous veno-venous hemofiltration (CVVH), sepsis, and cardiac arrhythmias. Discharge planning was initiated as H.D. became hemodynamically stabile allowing transition off CVVH and ventilator weaning with 12 hours on tracheostomy collar and night ventilator support on assist/control. A percutaneous endoscopic gastrostomy (PEG) tube was placed for enteral nutritional support. H.D. was transferred to a long-term acute care hospital (LTACH) after 23 days in the ICU.

H.D. and his wife had been married for 45 years and had one son. Though driving a long distance, she faithfully visited H.D. every day. She stated that although H.D.'s health had not been perfect, he was functioning independently at home and loved being with the family, watching car racing, and loved everything about Christmas. Regularly scheduled, formal meetings away from the bedside were held with his wife to ensure goal-directed care. Because H.D. lacked decision-making capacity, she acted as H.D.'s proxy in all decision making but this role caused anxiety for her. Though treatment limitations were discussed multiple times, H.D.'s wife was conflicted and burdened over making such decisions for her husband. H.D. did not have an advanced directive. In addition to updates and clarification of patient's goals and preferences, milestones were identified at each of the four meetings. The goal was to provide full support enabling H.D. to eventually meet the milestones of hemodynamic stability, transition off of CVVH, and partial ventilator weaning and subsequent transfer to the LTACH for ongoing weaning and reconditioning.

H.D. was rehospitalized twice in a 3-month period from the LTACH back to the ICU. The first episode for fluid overload lasted 7 days. The second readmission lasted 30 days during which he was treated for sepsis and bacteremia resulting from multiple drug-resistant organisms, pulmonary edema, acute renal failure, respiratory failure requiring 24-hour ventilatory support, diastolic dysfunction, and ventilator-associated pneumonia. He complained of general discomfort and was severely deconditioned. H.D. had a depressed mood so antidepressant therapy was begun. Meetings were resumed with his wife. Slowly, H.D. progressed after being treated with five antimicrobials. However, he would repeatedly report hunger and discomfort and express the desire to go home. Because he was in the ICU during Christmas time, the unit's Christmas tree was placed directly outside his room. He was discharged back to the LTACH on the life-sustaining therapies of night ventilation, hemodialysis, and PEG tube for enteral feeding. He had progressed to using a Passy-Muir speaking valve for short intervals.

Multiple discussions were held with H.D.'s wife to discuss his chronically critically ill status and the poor prognosis for his return to preadmission status of being at home and living independently. The shared decision was made to place treatment limitations and not attempt resuscitation in the event of cardiopulmonary arrest. However, treatment was continued to optimize his cardiopulmonary status and chance for physical rehabilitation.

H.D. was cared for in the LTACH for 2 more months. Because he was making no or little progress, transfer to a long-term-care facility was planned. H.D.'s wife would call the ICU team during this period for counseling and support with this process and was in an overwhelmed state of burden, anxiety, and sadness. H.D. expired 1 week after being transferred to the long-term-care facility, surviving an approximate 6-month course of chronic critical illness. H.D. never realized his one goal of going home.

## Definition

Since Girard and Raffin (1985) first used the term *chronically critically ill* there remains no universal definition. Historically, chronic critical illness has often been used synonymously with prolonged mechanical ventilation (PMV) or long-term ICU patients. More recently, performance of an elective tracheostomy for failure to wean from the ventilator and transfer to a weaning center or long-term acute care hospital (LTACH) has been used as the markers for chronic critical illness (Nelson et al., 2004). Table 10.1 includes the definitions of CCI and PMV patients used in research studies.

Performance of an elective tracheostomy for failure to wean from mechanical ventilation has been recommended by some investigators as the defining criterion of CCI (Nelson et al., 2004, 2006, 2007). The incidence of early tracheostomy is increasing in the ICU setting (Combes et al., 2007) with one study reporting a 190% increase from 8.3 per 100,000 persons in 1993 to 24.2 per 100,000 in 2002 (Carson, Cox, Holmes, Howard, & Carey, 2006). However, Carson (2006) argued that the identification of the CCI based solely on tracheostomy placement may not fully represent this population, resulting in underestimation of outcomes such as mortality.

Though length of ventilatory support varies in the CCI, the need for a ventilator, at some point, is the only universal feature of the syndrome. Approximately 40% of adult ICU patients require mechanical ventilation (Hopkins & Jackson, 2006) with an average length of 3 to 5 days (Dasta, Mclaughlin, Mody, & Piech, 2005; Kahn, Goss, Heagerty, O'Brien, & Rubenfeld, 2006; Seneff, Zimmerman, Knaus, Wagner, & Draper, 1996; Zilberberg, Luippold, Sulsky, & Shorr, 2008) . Because the target for weaning a patient from the ventilator is 48 to 72 hours, failure to wean reflects underlying pathology (MacIntyre et al., 2005) and predicts higher mortality and need for institutionalization at ICU discharge (Epstein, Ciubotaru, & Wong, 1997). As H.D.'s case

## 10.1    Definitions of Chronic Critical Illness (CCI) or Prolonged Mechanical Ventilation

| Author(s) | Definition |
| --- | --- |
| Zilberberg et al. (2008) | Prolonged acute mechanical ventilation (PAMV) of = 96 hours |
| Scheinhorn et al. (2007) | Chronic critical illness is prolonged ventilator-dependent respiratory failure; describes outcomes in ventilator-dependent survivors of catastrophic illness transferred to LTACHs for weaning from PMV |
| MacIntyre et al. (2005) | PMV is the need for mechanical ventilation for 21 consecutive days and = 6 hours/ day |
| Daly et al. (2005) | The chronically critically ill are those patients requiring MV = 72 hours who survive to discharge from the index hospitalization |
| Nelson et al. (2004) | Chronic critical illness is a syndrome of significant derangements of metabolism and of neuroendocrine, neuropsychiatric, and immunologic function; onset of CCI defined by performance of tracheotomy for failure to wean from MV |
| Nierman (2002) | Patients who survive a critical illness but are left with significant impairments of function and quality of life and shortened life spans; dependent on intense nursing care and advanced technology |
| Carson and Bach (2002) | CCI are those patients who require continued care in an ICU for weeks to months; associated with need for PMV; 21 day ICU stay indicator that most easily reversible conditions have been addressed; PMV signals chronic or persistent condition |
| Nasraway et al. (2000) | A small subset of the ICU population who, because of underlying illness or complications, suffer a prolonged and difficult ICU course; severely weakened survivors of acute illness often ventilator dependent or renal-dialysis dependent |
| Nierman and Mechanick (1998) | Primarily elderly patients who have survived life-threatening episode of sepsis but remain debilitated and ventilator dependent |
| Douglas et al. (1997) | Patients who require LTV are also CCI; still require intensive nursing care after receiving medical therapy for primary disease; generally ICU stay > 2 weeks |
| Daly et al. (1991) | Long-term ICU patients; typically older persons who have recovered from the life-threatening crises but remain critically ill; suffer exacerbations and complications; slow to progress |
| Girard and Raffin (1985) | ICU patients who do not survive despite extraordinary life support for weeks to months |

clearly illustrates, critically ill patients who fail to reach this benchmark typically are older with higher severity of illness and more preexisting conditions (Epstein et al.).

The criteria used to define PMV vary and include mechanical ventilation greater than 2, 3, 4, 7, 21, and 28 days; diagnostic related group (DRG) 541 and 542, performance of elective tracheostomy with mechanical ventilation = 96 hours and the Health Care Financing Administration (HCFA) criterion of PMV greater than 21 days (Carson, 2006; Carson & Bach, 2002; Carson et al., 2006; Daly et al., 2005; Nelson et al., 2004). The National Association for Medical Direction of Respiratory Care (NAMDRC) in

2004 defined PMV as the need for mechanical ventilation for 21 consecutive days, 6 hours per day (MacIntyre et al., 2005).

Regardless of the precise definition, prolonged ventilator dependence is strongly related to patient outcomes. Twenty-one consecutive days of mechanical ventilation are associated with the need for ventilator support after hospital discharge (Zilberberg et al., 2008). Length of mechanical ventilation in the ICU correlates with the need for postdischarge care. A significant difference was reported in the length of mechanical ventilation between those CCI patients discharged to home (5.0 days of ventilation) versus those discharged to a postacute care facility (13 days) (Wiencek, 2008). Failure to wean from the initial PMV episode has been associated with a sevenfold likelihood of death within 1 year (Bigatello, Stelfox, Berra, Schmidt, & Gettings, 2007). Thus, PMV plays a role in the course of chronic critical illness but it is unclear whether this is causative or contributory.

ICU length of stay has also been used to define the CCI. The average length of ICU stay is 4 to 5 days (Rosenberg, Zimmerman, Alzola, Draper, & Knaus, 2000), compared to the 15 to 25 days for the CCI (Daly et al., 2005; Douglas, Daly, Gordon, & Brennan, 2002; Scheinhorn et al., 2007). The ICU length of stay has decreased over the last 2 decades with changes in weaning protocols and earlier discharges to LTACHs. Prolonged exposure to acute care environments (ICU and LTACH) not only reflects the severity of the patient's underlying illness but also the prevalence of complications. It is often this "roller coaster" of repeated complications that partially defines the CCI. In addition, age, severity of illness and preexisting conditions have been found to predict who will become CCI (Carson et al., 2006; MacIntyre et al., 2005; Nierman, 2002; Seneff et al., 1996). Thus, a universally accepted definition of the CCI remains elusive but is a combination of prolonged illness and organ dysfunction, prolonged dependency on life-sustaining treatments, and prolonged acute care needs.

The case study of H.D. fits most of these defining criteria of chronic critical illness. He was elderly with multiple preexisting conditions. The initial length of ICU stay was 23 days. In addition, H.D. required prolonged mechanical ventilation and performance of a tracheostomy. Because H.D. lacked decision-making capacity, components of a comprehensive care model, specifically regular meetings, were instituted. The components of a comprehensive care model for the CCI are described in the next section.

# Comprehensive Care Model

The characteristics, poor prognosis, and extremely poor outcomes of the CCI necessitate a different model of care than the acute care, episodic model used for the typical ICU patient. Multiple experts in the field have called for a comprehensive, patient–family focused approach to caring for this vulnerable population (Daly et al., 2005; MacIntyre et al., 2005; Scheinhorn et al., 2007; Nelson, 2002; Nelson et al., 2007; Nierman, 2002). A new approach, a comprehensive care model, includes early identification of those patients at risk for chronic critical illness; integration of patient–family-centered care principles and palliative care; a structure for communication with patients and families; goal-driven care using milestones rather than specialist or technology-driven care; case management including protocols, care maps, or benchmarking; and formalized family support. Ideally, such a model would provide each patient with the right treatment driven by patient goals and appropriate timing (Nierman).

## Early Identification of the CCI

A comprehensive care model for the CCI includes early identification of those critically ill patients at risk of progressing into chronic critical illness. Known or primary risk factors include advanced age, number of preexisting conditions, severity of illness, poor premorbid functional status, and failure to wean from the ventilator within 48 to 72 hours (Carson & Bach, 2002; Carson et al., 2006; Daly et al., 2005; MacIntyre et al., 2005; Nierman, 2002; Seneff et al., 1996) Though no one predictive model has been endorsed in the care of the CCI (MacIntyre et al., 2005), review of these known factors should be a part of multidisciplinary or case management rounds in all ICUs. If patients meet some or all of these criteria within the first week of the ICU stay, other aspects of the model should be implemented. A recently reported model (Carson et al., 2008) for predicting 1-year mortality in PMV patients found vasopressor dependency, hemodialysis, thrombocytopenia, and age = 50 years to be independent predictors of mortality in patients requiring 21 days or more of MV. These additional risk factors should be considered.

## Case Management

After early identification of ICU patients at risk of chronic critical illness, case management tools and principles should be applied to the care of the individual patient and family. Care pathways, weaning protocols, benchmarks, and other quality-improvement tools have the potential to improve outcomes and the quality of care. Optimizing nutritional status and using early-mobility strategies to maintain functional status must be included, as early as possible, in the plan of care. Patients and families should be involved in the identification and monitoring of goals and progress along the trajectory of chronic critical illness. Early identification of the CCI, proactive case management strategies, fully integrated rehabilitation, and early and effective discharge planning can help to prepare the patient and, especially, the family for posthospital needs and resources.

## Patient–Family-Centered Care

Patient- and family-centered care is being promoted by multiple regulatory bodies and associations including the Institute of Medicine (2001), the American Association of Critical-Care Nurses (AACN), and Society of Critical Care Medicine (SCCM). Nowhere is this model more essential than in the critical care setting where patients are at risk for personal preferences to be superseded by the technological imperative and families to be marginalized as surrogate decision makers. Family-centered critical care aims to recognize the needs of the patient as well as the unique psychological and informational needs of the patient's family during this stressful life event. Family members are not just visitors in the ICU, they are caregivers and decision makers managing with the psychological stress of uncertainty, potential loss of their loved one, and loss of control, and they need a supportive environment. The model of family-centered critical care approaches the family as an extension of the critically ill individual, who also experience the process of care (Alvarez & Kirby, 2006). Additionally, this progressive model of care delivery should fully integrate the principles of palliative care to reduce the burden of illness on the patient and the family (Nelson, 2002).

Key elements of the clinical practice guidelines for patient- and family-centered care in the ICU recently developed by a multidisciplinary task force (Davidson et al., 2007) and particularly relevant to the care of the CCI are as follows:

1. Family meetings are held with the multidisciplinary team within 24 to 48 hours of ICU admission and include discussion of patient preferences for life-sustaining treatments.
2. A shared decision-making model consisting of the team, patient, and family or surrogate decision maker is used to identify treatment goals and ensure consistent communication of patient status and prognosis.
3. Family support is provided by multiprofessional teams.
4. Culturally competent care is provided to the patient and family.
5. Open visitation is allowed to support family involvement in care.
6. ICU staff is trained in elements of palliative care and communication skills.

## Communication Structure

A structure for communication is an essential component of the comprehensive care model for the CCI. The prolonged course and repeated complications necessitate open and frequent goal-oriented discussions among the patient, if he or she is cognitively intact, the family and/or surrogate decision maker, and the multidisciplinary ICU team. This structure should include, at the very least, a bedside discussion of goals and the treatment plan within 24 to 48 hours of ICU admission and then regularly scheduled meetings at least weekly, or more often, depending on the patient's status and/or family's need for information. Discussion points should include patient goals and preferences, medical condition or update, the patient goal-directed treatment plan, identification of milestones, and the date for the next meeting. Outcomes of the meeting should be documented in the patient chart and communicated to the team. Because of the significant distress that families of the CCI endure and the extremely poor outcomes and prognosis for the CCI, unlike the acute or short-stay ICU patient, the burden and benefit of individual treatments must be discussed and predictors of mortality and functional status provided (Nelson et al., 2007). Compassionate and regular communication with the patient and family is central to the comprehensive care model of the CCI.

This communication structure was provided for the wife of H.D. and was successful in directing his care and providing her support as evidenced by her frequent contacts with the ICU team in the post-ICU phase of his course. However, H.D.'s wife consistently verbalized feeling overwhelmed and stressed about her husband's condition compounded by anxiety resulting from her role as decision maker.

## Family Support

The recent emphasis on family-centered care in the ICU assumes the patient and family as a focus of concern to nurses providing care to this vulnerable dyad (American

Association of Critical Care Nurses, 2006). A central role for critical care nurses is the provision of psychological support and the facilitation of quality communication to families and patients during critical illness. Recommendations have been made that nurses address the needs of families in critical care by promoting nursing research that supports effective clinical practices. In particular, AACN recommends that future inquiry into nursing interventions focus on family members of the critically ill, their involvement in caregiving activities, coaching family members on how to communicate with health care providers, and interventions to provide emotional support (AACN, 2006).

## Pathophysiology

At some critical juncture, yet to be clearly defined, persistent pathophysiologic mechanisms produce the state of chronic critical illness (Van den Berghe, 2002). These mechanisms include alterations in fatty acid and protein use, immobility and inflammatory processes, and neuroendocrine and hormonal changes.

A model of allostatic overload and proinflammatory cytokines has been proposed to explain the syndrome of chronic critical illness (Mechanick & Brett, 2005). Allostasis, in contrast to homeostasis, is defined as the process by which several homeostatic set-points are adjusted in conjunction with or in response to environmental changes (Mechanick & Brett). An allostatic load is a cumulative state of mediators like norepinephrine and epinephrine that perpetuate lipid peroxidation and oxidative stress causing cellular and end-organ dysfunction. Allostatic overload is consistent with free radical theory, which assumes aging and chronic disease states are mediated by oxidative stress and lipid peroxidation. This model further proposes that cytokine-mediated effects redirect substrates, from synthesis of (anabolic) reverse-phase reactants to (catabolic) acute phase reactants. Typically this process enhances survival; however, prolonged exposure leads to allostatic overload resulting in oxidative end-organ dysfunction (Mechanick & Brett). The clinical profile of the CCI includes multiple end-organ dysfunctions, which are assumed to be related to the chronic exposure to mediators of systemic inflammation and oxidative stress.

Immobility in the CCI is common and inflammation is a normal consequence of infection or injury. Prolonged immobility can lead to acquired muscle dysfunction that contributes to prolonged ventilator dependency and lengthy recovery. The supine position has been found to be an independent risk factor for mortality in patients requiring MV (Rauen, Chulay, Bridges, Vollman, & Arbour, 2008). Evidence suggests that immobility is prevalent in this population and less than 50% of critically ill patients are turned every 2 hours, which is the recommended frequency (Rauen et al.).

Chronic stress and chronic illness have been associated with elevated serum levels of various interleukins. The proinflammatory cytokines of Interleukin-1 (Il-1), Il-6, and tumor necrosis factor alpha (TNF-a) have been implicated in muscle degradation (Opal & DePalo, 2000; Winkelman, 2004, 2007; Winkelman, Higgins, Chen, & Levine, 2007). Also, it has been proposed that the imbalance between proinflammatory and antiinflammatory cytokines may contribute to chronic critical illness (Winkelman et al.).

Finally, imbalances in other neuroendocrine levels may contribute to the chronic phase of critical illness. Growth hormone deficiency, anterior pituitary alterations, low hypothalamus output, high prevalence of bone hyperresorption with high parathyroid hormone levels, and high prevalence of hypotestosteronemia have all been studied (Nierman & Mechanick, 1998, 1999; Van den Berghe, 2002) . More research is needed to understand the multiple derangements in hormonal, endocrine, and inflammatory physiology that demarcate chronic critical illness from critical illness. Specific factors explaining not just when, but why, critical illness becomes chronic remain unknown.

## Prevalence and Economic Implications

One third of all U.S. health care dollars are spent on in-hospital care (Levit et al., 2003). Intensive care represents a major portion of these costs and mechanically ventilated patients are additionally responsible for a substantial portion of daily ICU resource costs (Levit et al.). One study reported that the costs associated with mechanically ventilated patients were more than double the cost of critically ill patients not mechanically ventilated (Zilberberg et al., 2008).

In the United States, there are approximately 5.7 million adults admitted to the ICU each year. Approximately 40% of these patients will require mechanical ventilation (Hopkins & Jackson, 2006). Patients who require ventilatory support tend to be elderly, with increased hospital costs and higher mortality. In an analysis of 20% of U.S. hospitals, PMV of greater than 96 hours represented 39% of all mechanical ventilation and 64% of total MV costs (Zilberberg et al., 2008).

The prevalence of patients requiring mechanical ventilation has steadily increased, as has the incidence of the CCI (Nelson et al., 2006). The CCI account for approximately 6 to 10% of all patients treated in the ICU annually. The proportion of mechanically ventilated patients requiring support for more than 4 days has increased to 35% (Hopkins & Jackson, 2006). The annualized increase in PMV has been estimated at 5.5% with projected increase from 250,000 cases to over 600,000 cases by the year 2020 (Zilberberg, et al.). This increase is most likely to the result of aging demographics, increase in chronic illnesses, and the technological imperative so prevalent throughout the American health care system. These trends are also reflective of the improved ability of critical care medicine to rescue the critically ill, although return to an acceptable functional status and quality of life remains elusive for some, including the CCI.

The economic impact of caring for the CCI cannot be overstated. Patients who are chronically critically ill comprise 6 to 10% of the ICU population but consume a disproportionate 30 to 50% of ICU resources. The annual cost of caring for the CCI is estimated to be $24 billion in ICU costs per year (Carson & Bach, 2002). Though early discharge from the CCI to LTACHs has reduced the average ICU length of stay from 37 days or more (Scheinhorn, Chao, Stearn-Hassenpflug, LaBree, & Heltsley, 1997) to the current 10 to 15 days (Daly et al., 2005; Rosenberg et al., 2000), the total costs of care remain extremely high because of the prolonged use of acute care services. Mechanical ventilation increases these costs; the diagnostic group of PMV ranks third in total charges ($5 billion in 2005) and first in charges per patient (www.cms.hhs.gov; last accessed October 2008). The care of the CCI substantially contributes to this economic burden.

## Characteristics and Outcomes

Poor outcomes in the CCI include high short-term and long-term mortality rates, long length of ICU or hospital stays, high readmission rates, high symptom burden, poor functional status, reduced quality of life, and high caregiver burden and depression (Carson, Bach, Brzozowski, & Leff, 1999; Chelluri et al., 2004; Daly et al., 2005; Douglas & Daly, 2003; Douglas, Daly, Brennan, Gordon, & Uthis, 2001; Nelson et al., 2004; Wiencek, 2008). Despite resource-intensive care and major intervention studies to improve the course of chronic critical illness (Daly et al., 1991, 2005; Nasraway et al., 2000), these poor outcomes remain generally unchanged.

Hospital mortality rates in the CCI are as high as 47% and cumulative 1-year mortality rates range from 37 to 72% (Carson et al., 1999; Chelluri et al., 2004; Combes et al., 2003; Daly et al., 2005; Douglas et al., 1997, 2001; Engoren, Arslanian-Engoren, & Fenn-Buderer, 2004). Advanced age and poor premorbid functional status are strong predictors of mortality in the CCI (Carson & Bach, 2002). In one study, patients older than 75 years or 65 years old and with poor functional status had only a 5% chance of being alive 1 year after an episode of chronic critical illness (Carson et al.). NAMDRC has suggested that 1-year survival rates in PMV be used as the most meaningful indicator of outcomes in PMV patients (MacIntyre et al., 2005).

Compared to the average ICU stay of 4.7 days (Rosenberg et al., 2000), the average hospital LOS for the CCI is significantly longer at 21.9 days (Daly et al., 2005), though it has decreased from the 53 days Spicher and White (1987) reported. Readmission rates can be as high as 40% in the first 6-month posthospital discharge period (Daly et al., 2005; Douglas et al., 2001; Nasraway et al., 2000), with significant implications for patient and family burden and financial costs. Premorbid functional status, age, and comorbid conditions are strong predictors of poor outcomes in the CCI (Carson et al., 1999; Daly et al., 2002; Garland et al., 2004; MacIntyre et al., 2005).

## Symptom Burden in the Chronically Critically Ill

There are multiple sources of symptom burden in the CCI, including the underlying acute illness, complications, diagnostic and therapeutic procedures, and inflammatory processes. Research indicates that the acutely and seriously ill, who share common characteristics with the CCI, experience significant levels of pain, dyspnea, psychological distress, depression, thirst, fatigue, and delirium (Desbiens et al., 1996; Desbiens, Mueller-Rizner, Connors, Wenger, & Lynn, 1999; Nelson et al., 2001; Puntillo, 1990). Several studies report bothersome symptoms in 90 to 95% of the CCI and 44 to 48% pain prevalence (Nelson et al., 2004, 2006; Wiencek, 2008). Other prevalent symptoms include dyspnea, severe psychological symptoms, and severe distress related to impaired communication (Nelson et al.; Wiencek). Coma or delirium are also common during the ICU and postacute course and can be persistent (Nelson et al., 2006).

Because cognitive impairment is high in the CCI, families as proxies may be used to elicit symptom reports. The meaning of symptom burden may be different for CCI patients as compared to their proxies. In one study, patients reported the most bothersome symptoms to be pain, respiratory distress, and fatigue, whereas proxies perceived pain and role changes such as loss of independence, inability to communicate, and impaired cognition to be the most bothersome to the patient (Wiencek, 2008). Because a substantial number of CCI cannot self-report symptoms, necessitating the use of proxy reports, this discrepancy in the meaning of symptom burden presents a challenge to the effective management of distressing symptoms.

## Decision-Making Capacity

A characteristic of the CCI is their inability to make their own medical decisions. Cognitive impairment in the CCI consists of derangement in neuropsychiatric function (Nelson et al., 2004). It is estimated that fewer than 5% of ICU patients are able to communicate with health care providers regarding treatment preferences, including withholding or withdrawing life-sustaining therapies (Prendergrast, Claessens, & Luce, 1998). Although not all CCI may require end-of-life decision making, a majority (71%) of the CCI in one study who received a tracheostomy were cognitively impaired and unable to actively participate in the decision-making process (Nelson et al., 2007).

## Functional Status and Quality of Life

The CCI experience a substantial decline in functional status from their preadmission state (Carson et al., 1999; Chelluri et al., 2004; Daly et al., 2005; Douglas et al., 1997; Nasraway et al., 2000). Though more than 80% of CCI patients are cognitively intact and/or home dwelling prior to the acute event (Daly et al., 2005; Nelson et al., 2007), a majority of the CCI will be cognitively impaired and dependent in activities of daily living at discharge and for months after the acute event. As many as 32 to 75% need caregiver support at 2 to 3 months (Nelson et al., 2004; Spicher & White, 1987), and half need assistance at 1 year (Carson et al.). PMV patients, when compared to the typical ICU or short-term mechanically ventilated patient, are more likely to be discharged to a nursing home and experience lower quality of life up to 1 year postdischarge (Carson & Bach, 2001).

Returning to H.D.'s case, most of these typical CCI characteristics and outcomes were evident. H.D. presented with advanced age and multiple preexisting conditions predicting a high risk of mortality that proved to be true in his case (death at 6 months). Though not active, he was independent prior to admission and suffered a severe decline in functional status requiring transfer to a long-term-care facility. His symptom burden was high as he repeatedly complained of generalized discomfort, thirst, hunger, and depressed mood. For multiple reasons, H.D. did not have decision-making capacity though he was often awake and able to respond to commands or report symptoms. Additionally, H.D. suffered repeated complications in his 6-month course because of his multiple infections and fluid imbalances and required prolonged support on life-sustaining therapies.

# Chronic Critical Illness: The Family's Perspective

## General ICU Population

The admission to an ICU is often an acute, nonelective, and pivotal transition that elicits uncertainty for both patients and families. The physiological needs of the patient are the principal concerns for health care providers in this practice environment, yet psychological, social, and spiritual needs also exist. Prioritizing the needs of the critically ill, as well as the needs of the family, is essential during an episode of acute or chronic critical illness. Health care providers are recognizing the need to support the informational and psychological needs of the patient and the family at the onset of critical illness.

The ICU experience is a stressful life event for family members and is associated with symptoms of posttraumatic stress disorder (PTSD), anxiety, and depression (Hughes, Bryan, & Robbins, 2005; Pochard et al., 2001). Several studies have validated the association between stress appraisal and indicators of mood such as depressive symptoms, anxiety, and posttraumatic stress disorder in family members of the critically ill (Douglas & Daly, 2003; Hughes et al., 2005; Diong & Bishop, 1999). A French multicenter investigation of ICU family members involved in treatment limitation or withdrawal decisions reported that 66% had symptoms of either anxiety or depression (Pochard et al., 2001). Impaired psychological well-being has been confirmed to be highly prevalent in family members of patients who died while in an ICU. Siegel and colleagues (2008) found that the most prevalent psychiatric disorder was major depression (27%) and spouses of acutely ill patients were the most vulnerable for impaired psychological well-being.

Family members of the CCI are at risk for impaired psychological well-being because of chronic exposure to situational stressors, uncertainty, and the chronic instability or "roller coaster ride" associated with chronic critical illness. The needs of family members of the CCI have been generally inferred from the literature in the general ICU population; however, some evidence is available in the areas of surrogate decision making, depression, and informational needs.

## Surrogate Decision Making

Severity of illness and technological barriers often render the CCI unable to express their own treatment preferences. Estimates of cognitive impairment in CCI patients has ranged from 38% for patients requiring 3 days of acute prolonged mechanical ventilation to 82% for those who required an elective tracheostomy for respiratory failure (Daly et al., 2005; Nelson et al., 2007). Clinicians often turn to family members as surrogate decision makers in an effort to gain insight into the patient's treatment preferences and appropriate goals of care. H.D.'s case was a classic example of this situation as the health care team relied on his wife to direct his care and make major decisions for the 6-month period of his course of chronic critical illness.

The designation of a family member as the patient's surrogate decision maker is a common and practical approach to shared decision making for a cognitively impaired patient. Despite being a familiar practice in the ICU, surrogate decision making is a stress-inducing cognitive role that will exacerbate the risk for impairment of psychological well-being of the surrogate decision maker. The act of surrogate decision making by family members is just one source of psychological stress plaguing these family members. Additional sources of psychological distress for the family decision maker (FDM) include the uncertainty of adequate role performance, concerns about lack of concordance with the patient's preferences regarding medical treatments, insufficient information from critical care providers, and the long-term consequences of medical decisions.

The concept of role stress, the perceived psychological stress related to the cognitive role of being a surrogate decision maker, is associated with a reduction in psychological well-being. Tilden and colleagues (1999) confirmed psychological stress among family decision makers who were faced with making treatment-limiting or withdrawal decisions. Smerglia and Deimling (1997) studied caregivers who were surrogate decision makers and found an association between depressive symptoms and the stress-inducing act of surrogate decision making. In the FDMs of cognitively impaired CCI, Hickman (2008) found role stress to be the most significant predictor of depressive symptoms within the first week of an episode of chronic critical illness.

## Psychological Well-Being of Families of the CCI

To date, there are four studies that have examined the psychological effects of chronic critical illness on the psychological well-being of family members. In each study, depressive mood was reported based on a score > 16 using the Center for Epidemiological Studies Depression (CES-D) scale (Hertzog, Van Alstine, & Usala, 1990). The frequency of depression symptoms in caregivers of the CCI decreases as the patient transitions from an acute to chronic phase of critical illness.

Although the report of depressive symptoms is likely to decrease over time, family members who provide direct caregiving remain at risk for depression. In their study of the posthospital outcomes of caregivers and the CCI, Douglas and Daly (2003) found that these caregivers had higher depression scores than other caregiver populations. Despite the overall reduction in depression scores by 6 months after discharge, 36% of these caregivers still reported mild to severe depressive symptoms at 6 months after hospital discharge. Similar findings in caregivers of patients with PMV have been reported (Daly et al., 2005; Im, Belle, Schulz, Mendelsohn, & Chelluri, 2004; Van Pelt et al., 2007).

Several risk factors were found to be associated with the clinical risk for depression in caregivers of the CCI. In their Long-term Ventilator and Disease Management studies, Douglas and Daly (2001, 2005) found that caregivers of institutionalized patients reported higher depression scores compared to caregivers of patients who were at home at 6 months after hospital discharge. The appraisal of caregiving burden and general health status were significant contributors to caregiver depression. Hours of caregiving were found to be associated with caregiver depression scores (Im et al., 2004), but high caregiver burden was not associated with the patient's premorbid functional status in the Quality of Life after Mechanical Ventilation (QOL-MV) Study (Van Pelt et al., 2007).

To date, much of our understanding of the psychological impact of chronic critical illness on family members has been extrapolated from research on the acutely critically ill. Further research is warranted to examine the impact of chronic critical illness on the psychological well-being of the families of the CCI and to identify effective interventions.

## Informational Needs

Family members of the CCI have distinct informational needs (Nelson et al., 2004, 2007). Information is a valuable commodity for stressed family members faced with making decisions for their cognitively impaired loved one. Family members, especially those who assume the role of the surrogate decision maker, require frequent high-quality communication and psychological support to facilitate comprehension of the information (Azoulay et al., 2000; Henneman & Cardin, 2002; Nelson et al., 2007). The poor comprehension of distressed family members of the critically ill is not associated with the patient's prognosis, physician characteristics, or the method of communication

(Azoulay et al., 2000). Failure to comprehend information by families of the critically ill warrants improvements in the process of communication that are sensitive to the informational preferences and psychological distress of the individual(s).

The lack of attention to the informational preferences and psychological needs of the family decision makers during critical illness is a significant problem. Families of the CCI are faced with a multitude of psychological stressors, often without optimal support from critical care providers. Family members of the CCI are often asked to be the voice of the patient during critical illness, despite being psychologically distressed. Poor comprehension of health care information might contribute to excessive resource consumption and postdecision regret.

Communication practices require an individualized, tailored approach to meet both the informational needs and informational-processing preferences of these vulnerable individuals so they can provide more effective decision making. Nelson and colleagues (2006) suggested that health care providers employ a method of communication that entails discussions with families regarding the CCI patient's diagnosis, treatment, severity of illness, prognosis for survival, and quality of life. In addition, it is recommended that family meetings follow a structured process that includes goal setting and the use of objective clinical measures or "milestones" that allow the family to assess the patient's progress (Lilly & Daly, 2007; Lilly, Sonna, Haley, & Massaro, 2003).

## Summary

The universal definition of chronic critical illness remains elusive after more than 25 years of research and clinical experience. However, *as H.D.'s case illustrated*, prominent features of the syndrome include ongoing ventilator dependence, severe debility, metabolic abnormalities, failure of organ systems, recurring infections and complications, and high symptom burden (Nelson et al., 2007). Though not universally defined, the CCI population is increasing in the context of an aging society, increasing chronicity, and growing use of technology (Carson, 2006; Carson & Bach, 2002; Daly et al., 2005). This incidence will increase as critical care continues to be effective at rescue but ineffective at returning the CCI to full functional status and acceptable quality of life. Because of the poor outcomes in the CCI and the high burden of illness for patients and families, a fully integrated comprehensive care model must replace the episodic acute care model applied to the care of the typical critically ill patient. This model includes structured communication, patient-driven goal setting, integration of patient–family-centered principles of care, integration of palliative care, early and effective discharge planning, case management, and structured family support. The rising incidence of the CCI, projected shortages in critical care professionals, and the economic burden will not support care, as usual, of those suffering from the syndrome of chronic critical illness.

## References

Alvarez, G., & Kirby, A. (2006). The perspective of families of the critically ill patient: Their needs. *Current Opinion Critical Care, 12,* 614–618.

American Association of Critical-Care Nurses. (2006). In J. Medina & K. Puntillo (Eds.), *AACN protocols for practice: Palliative care and end-of-life issues in critical care.* Boston: Jones and Bartlett.

Azoulay, E., Chevret, S., Leleu, G., Pochard, F., Barboteu, M., Adrie, C., et al. (2000). Half the families of intensive care unit patients experience inadequate communication with physicians. *Critical Care Medicine, 28*, 3044–3049.

Bigatello, L., Stelfox, H., Berra, L., Schmidt, U., & Gettings, E. (2007). Outcome of patients undergoing prolonged mechanical ventilation after critical illness. *Critical Care Medicine, 35*, 2491–2497.

Carson, S. (2006). Outcomes of prolonged mechanical ventilation. *Current Opinion in Critical Care, 12*, 405–411.

Carson, S., & Bach, P. (2001). Predicting mortality in patients suffering from prolonged critical illness: An assessment of four severity-of-illness measures. *Chest, 120*, 928–933.

Carson, S., & Bach, P. (2002). The epidemiology and costs of chronic critical illness. *Critical Care Clinics, 18*, 461–476.

Carson, S., Bach, P., Brzozowski, L., & Leff, A. (1999). Outcomes after long-term acute care. An analysis of 133 mechanically ventilated patients. *American Journal of Respiratory and Critical Care Medicine, 159*, 1568–1573.

Carson, S., Cox, C., Holmes, G., Howard, A., & Carey, T. (2006). The changing epidemiology of mechanical ventilation: A population-based study. *Journal of Intensive Care Medicine, 21*, 173–182.

Carson, S., Garrett, J., Hanson, L., Lanier, J., Govert, J. Brake, M., et al. (2008). A prognostic model for one-year mortality in patients requiring prolonged mechanical ventilation. *Critical Care Medicine, 36*, 2061–2069.

Chelluri, L., Im, K., Belle, S., Schulz, R., Rotondi, A., Donohoe, M., et al. (2004). Long-term mortality and quality of life after prolonged mechanical ventilation. *Critical Care Medicine, 32*, 61–69.

Combes, A., Costa, M., Trouillet, J., Baudot, J., Mokhtari, M., Gibert, C., et al. (2003). Morbidity, mortality, and quality-of-life outcomes of patients requiring = 14 days of mechanical ventilation. *Critical Care Medicine, 31*, 1373–1381.

Combes, A., Luyt, C., Nieszkowska, A., Trouillet, J., Gibert, C., & Chastre, J. (2007). Is tracheostomy associated with better outcomes for patients requiring long-term mechanical ventilation? *Critical Care Medicine, 35*, 802–807.

Daly, B., Douglas, S., Kelley, C., O'Toole, E., & Montenegro, H. (2005). Trial of a disease management program to reduce hospital readmissions of the chronically critically ill. *Chest, 128*, 507–517.

Daly, B., Phelps, W., & Rudy, E. (1991). A nurse-managed special care unit. *Journal of Nursing Administration, 21*, 31–38.

Dasta, J., McLaughlin, T., Mody, S., & Piech, C. (2005). Daily cost of an intensive care unit day: The contribution of mechanical ventilation. *Critical Care Medicine, 33*, 1266–1271.

Davidson, J., Powers, K., Hedayat, K., Tieszen, M., Kon, A., Shepard, E., et al. (2007). Clinical practice guidelines for support of the family in the patient-centered intensive care unit: American College of Critical Care Medicine Task Force. *Critical Care Medicine, 35*, 605–622.

Desbiens, N., Mueller-Rizner, N., Connors, A., Wenger, N., & Lynn, J. (1999). The symptom burden of seriously ill hospitalized patients. *Journal of Pain and Symptom Management, 17*, 248–255.

Desbiens, N., Wu, A., Broste, S., Wenger, N., Connors, A., Lynn, J., et al. (1996). Pain and satisfaction with pain control in seriously ill hospitalized adults: Findings from the SUPPORT research investigations. For the SUPPORT investigators. Study to Understand Prognoses and Preferences for Outcomes and Risks of Treatment. *Critical Care Medicine, 24*, 1953–1961.

Diong, S., & Bishop, G. (1999). Anger expression, coping styles and well-being. *Journal of Health Psychology, 4*, 81–96.

Douglas, S., & Daly, B. (2003). Caregivers of long-term ventilator patients: Physical and psychological outcomes. *Chest, 123*, 1073–1081.

Douglas, S., Daly, B., Brennan, P., Gordon, N., & Uthis, P. (2001). Hospital readmission among long-term ventilator patients. *Chest, 120*, 1278–1286.

Douglas, S., Daly, B., Brennan, P., Harris, S., Nochomovitz, M., & Dyer, M.A. (1997). Outcomes of long-term ventilator patients: A descriptive study. *American Journal of Critical Care, 6*, 99–105.

Douglas, S., Daly, B., Gordon, N., & Brennan, P. (2002). Survival and quality of life: Short-term versus long-term ventilator patients. *Critical Care Medicine, 30*, 2655–2662.

Engoren, M., Arslanian-Engoren, C., & Fenn-Buderer, N. (2004). Hospital and long-term outcome after tracheostomy for respiratory failure. *Chest, 125*, 7–9.

Epstein, S., Ciubotaru, R., & Wong, J. (1997). Effect of failed extubation on the outcome of mechanical ventilation. *Chest, 112*, 186–192.

Garland, A., Dawson, N., Thomas, C., Phillips, R., Tsevat, J., Desbiens, N., et al. (2004). Outcomes up to 5 years after severe, acute respiratory failure. *Chest, 126*, 1897–1904.

Girard, K., & Raffin, T. (1985). The chronically critically ill: To save or let die? *Respiratory Care, 30*, 339–347.

Henneman, E., & Cardin, S. (2002). Family-centered critical care: A practical approach to making it happen. *Critical Care Nurse, 22*, 12–19.

Hertzog, C., Van Alstine, J., & Usala, P. (1990). Measurement properties of the Center for Epidemiological Studies Depression Scale (CES-D) in older populations. *Psychological Assessment: A Journal of Consulting and Clinical Psychology, 2*, 64–72.

Hickman, R. L., Jr. (2008). *Predictors of the psychological well-being of family medical decision makers of the chronically critically ill.* Doctoral dissertation, Case Western Reserve University, Cleveland. Retrieved August 10, 2008, from Dissertations & Theses @ Case Western Reserve University database (Publication No. AAT 3301861).

Hopkins, R., & Jackson, J. (2006). Long-term neurocognitive function after critical illness. *Chest, 130*, 869–878.

Hughes, F., Bryan, K., & Robbins, I. (2005). Relatives' experiences of critical care. *British Association of Critical Care Nurses, Nursing in Critical Care, 10*, 23–30.

Im, K., Belle, S., Schulz, R., Mendelsohn, A., & Chelluri, L. (2004). Prevalence and outcomes of caregiving after prolonged (> 48 hours) mechanical ventilation in the ICU. *Chest, 125*, 597–606.

Institute of Medicine. (2001). *Crossing the quality chasm: A new health system for the 21st century.* Washington, DC: National Academies Press.

Kahn, J., Goss, C., Heagerty, P., O'Brien, C., & Rubenfeld, G. (2006). Hospital volume and the outcomes of mechanical ventilation. *New England Journal of Medicine, 355*, 41–50.

Levit, K., Smith, C., Cowan, C., Lazenby, H., Sensenig, A., & Catlin, A. (2003). Trends in US healthcare spending, 2001. *Health Affairs (Millwood), 22*, 154–164.

Lilly, C., & Daly, B. (2007). The healing power of listening in the ICU. *New England Journal of Medicine, 356*, 513–514.

Lilly, C., Sonna, L., Haley, K., & Massaro, A. (2003). Intensive communication: Four-year follow-up from a clinical practice study. *Critical Care Medicine, 31*, S394–S399.

MacIntyre, N., Epstein, S., Carson, S., Scheinhorn, D., Christopher, K., & Muldoon, S. (2005). Management of patients requiring prolonged mechanical ventilation: Report of a NAMDRC consensus conference. *Chest, 2005*, 3937–3954.

Mechanick, J., & Brett, E. (2005). Nutrition and the chronically critically ill patient. *Current Opinion Clinics Nutritional Metabolic Care, 8*, 33–39.

Nasraway, S., Button, G., Rand, W., Hudson-Jinks, T., & Gustafson, M. (2000). Survivors of catastrophic illness: Outcome after direct transfer from intensive care to extended care facilities. *Critical Care Medicine, 28*, 19–25.

Nelson, J. (2002). Palliative care of the chronically critically ill patient. *Critical Care Clinics, 18*, 659–681.

Nelson, J., Meier, D., Litke, A., Natale, D., Siegel, R., & Morrison, R. (2004). The symptom burden of chronic critical illness. *Critical Care Medicine, 32*, 1527–1534.

Nelson, J., Meier, D., Oei, E., Nierman, D., Senzel, R., Manfredi, P., et al. (2001). Self-reported symptom experience of critically ill cancer patients receiving intensive care. *Critical Care Medicine, 29*, 277–282.

Nelson, J., Mercado, A., Camhi, S., Tandon, N., Wallenstein, S., August, G., et al. (2007). Communication about chronic critical illness. *Archives of Internal Medicine, 167*, 2509–2515.

Nelson, J., Tandon, N., Mercado, A., Camhi, S., Wesley, E., & Morrison, R. (2006). Brain dysfunction: Another burden for the chronically critically ill. *Archives of Internal Medicine, 166*, 1993–1999.

Nierman, D. (2002). A structure of care for the chronically critically ill. *Critical Care Clinics, 18*, 477–491.

Nierman, D., & Mechanick, J. (1998). Bone hyperresorption is prevalent in chronically critically ill patients. *Chest, 14*, 954–955.

Nierman, D., & Mechanick, J. (1999). Hypotestosteronemia in chronically critically ill men. *Critical Care Medicine, 27*, 2418–2422.

Opal, S., & DePalo, V. (2000). Anti-inflammatory cytokines. *Chest, 117*, 1162–1172.

Pochard, F., Azoulay, E., Chevret, S., Lemaire, F., Hubert, P., Canoui, P., et al. (2001). Symptoms of anxiety and depression in family members of intensive care units: Ethical hypothesis regarding decision-making capacity. *Critical Care Medicine, 29*, 1893–1897.

Prendergrast T., Claessens M., & Luce, J. (1998). A national survey of end-of-life care for critically ill patients. *American Journal of Respiratory Critical Care Medicine, 158*, 1163–1167.

Puntillo, K. (1990). Pain experiences of intensive care unit patients. *Heart Lung, 19*, 526–533.

Puntillo, K., White, C., Morris, A., Perdue, S., Stanik-Hutt, J., Thompson, C., et al. (2001). Patients' perceptions and responses to procedural pain: Results from Thunder Project II. *American Journal of Critical Care, 10*, 238–251.

Rauen, C., Chulay, M., Bridges, E., Vollman, K., & Arbour, R. (2008). Seven evidence-based practice habits: Putting some sacred cows out to pasture. *Critical Care Nurse, 28*, 98–123.

Rosenberg, A., Zimmerman, J., Alzola, C., Draper, E., & Knaus, W. (2000). Intensive care length of stay: Recent changes and future challenges. *Critical Care Medicine, 28*, 3465–3473.

Scheinhorn, D., Chao, D., Stearn-Hassenpflug, M., LaBree, L., & Heltsley, D. (1997). Treatment of 1,123 patients at a regional weaning center. *Chest, 111*, 1654–1659.

Scheinhorn, D., Stearn-Hassenpflug, M., Votto, J., Chao, D., Epstein, S., Doig, G., et al. (2007). Ventilator-dependent survivors of catastrophic illness transferred to 23 long-term-care hospitals for weaning from prolonged mechanical ventilation. *Chest, 131*, 76–84.

Seneff, M., Zimmerman, J., Knaus, W., Wagner, D., & Draper, E. (1996). Predicting the duration of mechanical ventilation: The importance of disease and patient characteristics. *Chest, 110*, 469–479.

Siegel, M., Hayes, E., Vanderwerker, L., Loseth, D., & Prigerson, H. (2008). Psychiatric illness in the next of kin of patients who die in the intensive care unit. *Critical Care Medicine, 36*, 1722–1728.

Smerglia, V., Deimling, G. (1997). Care-related decision-making satisfaction and caregiver well-being in families caring for older members. *The Gerontologist, 37*, 658–665.

Spicher, J., & White, D. (1987). Outcome and function following prolonged mechanical ventilation. *Archives of Internal Medicine, 147*, 421–425.

Tilden, V., Tolle, S., Nelson, C., Thompson, M., & Eggman, S. (1999). Family decision making in foregoing life-extending treatments. *Journal of Family Nursing, 5*, 426–442.

Van den Berghe, G. (2002). Neuroendocrine pathobiology of chronic critical illness. *Critical Care Clinics, 18*, 509–528.

Van Pelt, D., Milbrandt, E., Qin, L., Weissfeld, L., Rotondi, A. J., Schulz, R., et al. (2007). Informal caregiver burden among survivors of prolong mechanical ventilation. *American Journal of Respiratory Critical Care Medicine, 175*, 167–173.

Wiencek, C. (2008). *Symptom burden and its relationship to functional status in the chronically critically ill.* Doctoral dissertation, Case Western Reserve University, Cleveland, OH. Retrieved August 10, 2008, from Dissertations & Theses @ Case Western Reserve University database (Publication No. AAT 3301860).

Winkelman, C. (2004). Inactivity and inflammation: Selected cytokines as biologic mediators in muscle dysfunction during critical illness. *AACN Clinical Issues, 15*, 74–82.

Winkelman, C. (2007). Inactivity and inflammation in the critically ill patient. *Critical Care Clinics, 23*, 21–34.

Winkelman, C., Higgins, P., Chen, Y., & Levine, A. (2007). Cytokines in chronically critically ill patients after activity and rest. *Biological Research for Nursing, 8*, 261–271.

Zilberberg, M., deWit, M., Pirone, J., & Shorr, A. (2008). Growth in adult prolonged acute mechanical ventilation: Implications for healthcare delivery. *Critical Care Medicine, 36*, 1451–1455.

Zilberberg, M., Luippold, R., Sulsky, S., & Shorr, A. (2008). Prolonged acute mechanical ventilation, hospital resource utilization, and mortality in the United States. *Critical Care Medicine, 36*, 724–730.

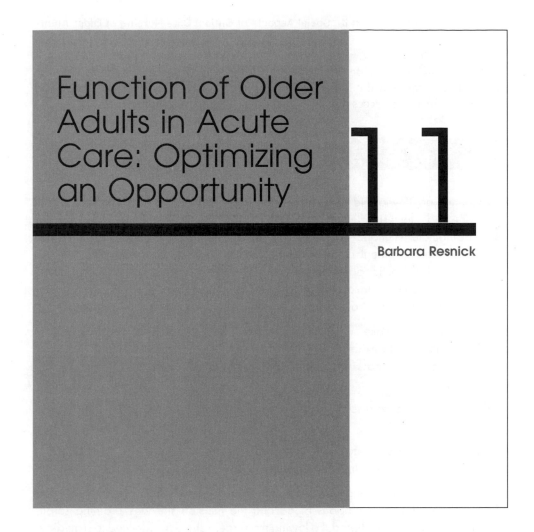

# Function of Older Adults in Acute Care: Optimizing an Opportunity

# 11

Barbara Resnick

## Introduction

Increasingly there are some models of care that attempt to keep older adults in their homes or in long-term care to manage acute medical problems that previously were only managed in acute care settings. Hospitals continue, however, to be sites in which the majority of admissions are older adults with these individuals being admitted at rates as high as three times those of younger individuals (Landefeld, 2003). Those older than 65 years of age comprise about 13.8% of the population and account for 40% of hospital admissions and 44% of the total days of care (DeFrances & Podgornik, 2006). The focus of these admissions is appropriately geared toward addressing the acute medical problem such as infection fractures; acute cardiac, pulmonary, or neurological events; or metabolic disorders. Medical stabilization may be challenging with treatment for the admission problem causing an exacerbation of comorbid problems in the individual. For example, surgical interventions or intubation in an older adult may result in secondary infections and/or exacerbate underlying comorbid conditions (e.g., congestive heart failure). It is well known that acute care admissions, and associated treatments (e.g., anesthesia and pain medications) result in a high incidence of delirium among older adults (Margiotta, Bianchetti, Ranieri, & Trabucchi, 2006; Rigney,

2006). These factors provide a logical backdrop for a possible decline in function in older adults because of the limits placed on them with regard to being immobilized and having decreased access to and awareness of their environments.

## Case Study

Mrs. Conner, an 89-year-old White female, was admitted for a left total hip replacement (THR). She had a long-standing history of degenerative joint disease and was no longer able to ambulate functional distances without significant pain. She lived alone in a continuing care retirement community and her goal was to be able to walk to the dining room and functional distances in the community so that she could go out to dinner and engage in social activities with friends and her family. She had one daughter and two grandchildren all of whom were local. Her past medical history included:

- Irritable bowel disease
- Degenerative joint disease
- Breast cancer (15 years postlumpectomy and treatment with tamoxifen)
- Hypertension

Medications prior to admission included:

- Lasix 20 mg po qd
- Metroprolol 25 mg po qd
- Loperamide prn for the irritable bowel disease

The THR was done using an epidural and she tolerated the procedure well. She was transfused 1 unit autologous blood and the incision site was draining serous drainage and was well adhered. Following the surgery she was admitted to a medical-surgical floor. Her postoperative instructions were to continue prior medications and she was started on Percocet 2.5/325 one to two tablets every 4 hours as needed, Coumadin 2.5 mg po qd, and ferrous sulfate 325 mg po tid. She was to start physical and occupational therapy in the morning and could increase activity and diet as tolerated and have the Foley removed that evening.

Her first postoperative evening she complained of pain at the incision site and in the hip and refused to sit up in the bed or transfer to the commode. The Foley catheter was removed and she was voiding in small amounts and insisted on wearing a diaper or using a bedpan when she did feel the urge to void. Her daughter supported these decisions worrying about her mother's pain and inability to tolerate the hip discomfort. She was given two Percocet by the evening nurse, repositioned with the hip abductor pillow in place, and was able to sleep with a need for repeat Percocet at intervals during the night.

Her daughter returned in the morning, planning to attend therapy with her mother and found her to be agitated and confused. Mrs. Conner insisted that they had all brought her here and were trying to lock her in and tie her down, putting sharp needles into her side and tying her legs. She also complained of discomfort when anything was over her abdomen—the blankets or the bedside table. Her blood pressure was stable 124/70, heart rate 108 and regular, and her temp was elevated now to 100.1. On exam the nurse noted distention and pain with palpation and a bladder scan revealed 720 cc of urine and the Foley was reinserted. A rectal exam had revealed hard stool high in the rectal vault and a Dulcolax suppository was given.

Her daughter was able to stay with Mrs. Conner, which had a calming effect. The daughter helped her with breakfast, which she was willing to eat. After medical follow up there were orders to obtain stat lab work, stop the Percocet, and switch her to acetaminophen 650 mg po every 6 hours for pain management and tramadol 50 mg po bid if that was insufficient. Her electrolytes, BUN (blood urea nitrogen test) and creatinine were all within normal limits with the exception of an elevated white count to 14.5, a hemoglobin of 11.2, and hematocrit of 34.7. The urinalysis was positive for bacteria, blood, and leukocytes and she was started empirically on ciprofloxacin for a urinary tract infection.

Therapy evaluated her that afternoon at the bedside and she was adamant that she could not possibly get up because of pain and fatigue. With much encouragement the physical therapist was able to do a basic evaluation and have her transfer to a chair and sit for a few minutes. Following the brief period of therapy she returned to bed and was able to manage the pain with position-limited movement and refusal even to turn on her side. Cognitively she was getting back to baseline and was aware that the medication had in fact made her confused and did not want to restart that for pain management. Nursing continued to facilitate positioning to manage pain, managed her wound care and medications.

Postop day 2 she complained of increased pain in her nonoperative leg and it was noted that she had 2+ edema up to the knee and the calf was tight, warm, and tender to touch. A venous Doppler was done and a deep vein thrombosis confirmed and stat labs of her prothrombin time and international ratio (INR) showed she was not well anticoagulated with an INR of 1.3. Consequently, she was started on Lovenox and Coumadin was increased to 5 mg po qd. She was not seen by therapy. She refused transfers to the commode due to pain, now both in the hip and the calf of her unoperative leg. Nursing responded by trying to optimize comfort with positioning, pain medication, and monitoring of the wound.

Postop day 3 therapy was held because of the deep vein thrombosis and it was not until postop day 4 that she was seen again by therapy, only following significant encouragement from the therapist. She engaged in therapy while in the therapy department but once back on the unit demanded to return to bed because of pain and fatigue. She continued to be incontinent of urine although her bladder scans were decreasing.

---

In the earlier studies the incidence of functional decline among older hospitalized patients has been reported to range from a decline in 65% (Hirsch, Sommers, Olsen, Mullen & Winograd, 1990) in a group of old adults (age 74 and above) by the second day of admission to 100% in a study of older veterans who were followed from admission to discharge (Winograd et al., 1997). More recent work (Covinsky et al., 2003; Volpato et al., 2007; Wakefield & Holman, 2007) has shown lower incidences of decline ranging from approximately 7% (Volpato et al.) to 35% (Covinsky et al.), with evidence of variability among study participants. That is, although a percentage of individuals did show a decline in function there were small percentages that also demonstrated an improvement in function over the course of the acute care admission.

Many factors have been identified as risk factors for functional decline in hospitalized older adults including age, sociodemographic characteristics, preexisting disability, cognitive decline/delirium, and specific comorbid conditions (Boyd, Zue, Guralnik, & Fried, 2005; McCusker, Kakuma, & Abrahamowicz, 2002; Sager, Rugberg, & Jalaluddin, 1996). In addition, nursing-home residency, low body mass index (BMI), elevated erythrocyte sedimentation rate, acute stroke, multiple comorbid conditions, polypharmacotherapy, cognitive decline, and a history of a fall in the previous year were all independent predictors of a decline in function during hospital stay (Volpato et al., 2007). Conversely, a recent study of veterans (Wakefield & Holman, 2007) noted that demographic factors, BMI, admission function, lab values, hospital length of stay, cognitive status, mood, social support, or evidence of a pressure ulcer did not have a significant relationship with changes in function over the course of hospitalization. Some of these differences may be sample specific or as the result of variations in the measurement of function as well as the measurement of the covariates.

## Differentiating Between Functional Decline and Disability

According to the original classification scheme proposed by Nagi (1976, p. 13) functional limitations are defined as "limitations in performance at the level of the whole organism or person." In contrast, disability is defined as "limitation in performance of socially defined roles and tasks within a socio-cultural and physical environment." Nagi conceptualized a pathway that went from pathology (disease or injury) to impairment (dysfunction and structural abnormalities) to functional limitations (restrictions in physical or mental actions) to disability (difficulty doing ADLs [activities of daily living] in real-world settings).

Chronic illnesses such as degenerative joint disease can cause pathology and impairments (e.g., torn rotator cuffs or decreased ejection fraction), which then causes functional limitations (decreased range of motion). Disability may or may not occur at this point depending on how the individual compensates for and responds to these functional limitations. Despite a decreased range in motion, for example, some individuals will adapt and perform all bathing and dressing, whereas others will ask for assistance. Intervening at the level of functional limitations and implementing interventions to increase PA can prevent disability from occurring. The inactivity associated with bedrest and hospitalization contributes to muscle shortening and change in the periarticular and cartilaginous joint structures, with a subsequent decrease in range of motion, contractures, and further loss of strength and impairment in proprioception and balance (Gill, Allore, & Guo, 2004; McCusker et al., 2002). Functional changes can occur as early as 2 days posthospitalization (Covinsky et al., 2003; McCusker et al.).

Some older adults who decline functionally during their acute care admission regain function and return to baseline by the time of discharge (McCusker et al., 2002; Volpato et al., 2007; Wakefield & Holman, 2007). There are many, particularly those who are older, who do not ever return to their prehospitalization functional performance (Volpato et al., 2007). This has a major impact on the quality of life of these individuals as well as being associated with increased risk of mortality, rehospitalization, and discharge to a more restrictive level of care (Boyd et al., 2005; Brown, Friedkin & Inouye, 2004; Covinsky et al., 2003). For these reasons it is critical to address function among older hospitalized individuals to optimize their clinical outcomes as well as decrease the cost of care associated with such things as rehospitalization.

## Additional Factors That May Influence Function Among Hospitalized Older Adults

As noted previously, although many risk factors have been identified to be associated with functional performance among older adults in the acute care setting, details of how care was provided, particularly with regard to nursing, have not been addressed. Prior research has shown that interventions designed to improve patient participation in activities of daily living can stabilize or improve function among older adults (Beck et al., 1995; Bonn, 1999; Field, 2004; Fleishell & Resnick, 1999; Galik & Resnick, 2007; Johnson et al., 2004; Marrelli, 2003; Resnick, Allen & Ruane, 2002; Resnick, Simpson, Bercovitz et al., 2006; Resnick, Simpson, Galik et al., 2006; Resnick et al., 2009; Shanti et al., 2005). Care patterns, such as providing too much assistance or an inappropriate type of assistance, can increase dependency in older adults. In addition, discrepancies between what the individual is able to do and what he or she actually performs is commonly seen in all care settings (Resnick et al., 2008; Rogers et al., 1999). Nurses, families, and other members of the health care team (e.g., physicians, therapists, and social workers/care managers) can contribute to excess disability. A variety of factors including a desire to be helpful, misconceptions and biases about aging, a focus on getting treatments completed can result in increased dependency among individuals (Resnick et al., 2008).

Mrs. Conner is an example of how care interventions and resistance of a patient to engage in functional activities resulted in multiple complications associated with immobility and subsequent deconditioning. Mrs. Conner was challenging, given her pain management, delirium, and persistent refusal to engage in activities that might cause some discomfort. Moreover, her daughter further facilitated the deconditioning process and the management of the acute medical problems further complicated her ability and willingness to engage in functional and physical tasks.

## Impact of Intrapersonal Factors on Function and Physical Activity

A number of intraindividual factors can likewise contribute to functional limitations, disability, and low physical activity (PA) in older adults (Singh, Chin A Paw, Bosscher, & van Mechlen, 2006). These factors include comorbidities, acute medical problems, and psychological factors (e.g., mood and motivation). There are also non-modifiable factors including age, gender, and race. Although it is useful to acknowledge the presence of these nonmodifiable factors, it is challenging to relate them directly to function as there is a good deal of interindividual variability. Moreover, it is impossible to separate out the multiple comorbidities common in older individuals. Appreciating the potential impact of these variables can help guide interventions; for example, knowing that someone has Parkinson's disease would affect the type of interventions used to optimize function (Pretzer-Aboff, Galik, & Resnick, 2009).

## Cognitive and Behavioral Intraindividual Challenges

Older adults in acute care settings who have a history of dementia, and/or an associated delirium with a change in behavior, are particularly challenging patients and this affects care interactions and functional outcomes (Wakefield, 2002). Changes in behavior may include hypo or hyperactive states, with the majority being associated with hypoactivity. Specifically, these individuals may have associated symptoms such as aphasia, motor apraxia, perceptual impairments, and apathy, making it difficult to engage them in functional activities (Galik & Resnick, 2007; Kolanowski, Buettner, & Moeller, 2006). Moreover, it has been noted that functional and motivational challenges, problematic behavioral symptoms such as verbal and physical aggression, insomnia, depression, and resistance to care occur in 50 to 80% of individuals diagnosed with dementia (Lyketsos et al., 1999).

Unfortunately, nurses in acute care who are challenged by the agitated and uncooperative behaviors of cognitively impaired older adults tend to focus on completing necessary task as quickly as possible so as to avoid exacerbating behavioral problems. Unfortunately, taking a "just get it done" approach to any type of care interaction limits opportunities for these patients to engage in physical and functional activity. There is a tendency for the nurse to complete the functional task rather than including the older individual in the process and working to optimize his or her function. For example, consider a patient who needs repositioning to administer medication. Nurses tend to automatically reposition the patient without trying to engage the patient in some activity, albeit limited, to optimize their function and encourage some physical activity. Alternatively these patients could be cued to push up in the bed with the lower extremities. Likewise, opportunities to optimize function with patients include giving the patient a washcloth for bathing and modeling the desired behavior (washing one's face or body), using a hand-over-hand technique for bathing patients who are totally dependent, or transferring a patient to a commode chair or walking him or her to the bathroom rather than using a bedpan.

Functional decline, contractures, and pain caused by immobility can occur more rapidly when the acute care environment and philosophy of care focuses on task completion. Specifically an acute care environment that focuses on and rewards care that gets a patient discharged as quickly as possible with the admitting medical problem stabilized (e.g., atrial fibrillation, hip fracture) may miss opportunities to address function. For example, when transferring a patient from one unit to the next nurses focused on the patients' medical problems may only provide data about the patient relevant to the clinical admitting problem and postadmission interventions related to that diagnosis. No information about patient function and optimizing function will be shared. Likewise, nurses who are rewarded for conforming with and not challenging care interventions that exacerbate functional decline (e.g., keeping a patient in bed because of a deep vein thrombosis) further exacerbate functional decline. Moreover, nurses may elect to keep a patient in bed as they feel this will decrease his or her risk of falling.

# Exhibit 11.1

## Cognitive Assessment: The Mini-Cog*

The test consists of a three item recall and a clock drawing test.

1. First the patient is asked to repeat three unrelated words.
2. The patient is then asked to draw a clock. This is the same as the Clock Drawing Test (CDT).
3. The patient is then asked to recall the three words.

The person undergoing testing is asked to:

Draw a clock.

Put in all the numbers.

Set the hands at ten past eleven.

Scoring system for Clock Drawing test (CDT)
1 point for the clock circle
1 point for all the numbers being in the correct order
1 point for the numbers being in the proper special order
1 point for the two hands of the clock
1 point for the correct time.

A normal score is four or five points.

Results of the Mini-Cog:
If the patient is unable to recall any of the three words OR if he/she scores less than a 4 or a 5 on the Clock Drawing Test then he /she is categorized as having some level of cognitive impairment.

*From Borson, S., Scanlan, J. M., Chen, P., & Ganguli, M. (2003). The Mini-Cog as a screen for dementia: Validation in a population-based sample. *Journal of the American Geriatrics Society, 51*, 1451–1454.

## Physiological Factors

Serum albumin (particularly a decline over time) (Schalk et al., 2005), endocrine immune dysregulation, sarcopenia, osteoporosis, D-dimer, and inflammatory markers (Ferrucci et al., 2000), testosterone levels (Morley, Haren, Kim, Kevorkian, & Perry, 2005), mitochondrial dysfunction (Nair, 2005), and muscle mass changes (Hicks et al., 2005) are all associated with functional decline. Anemia, defined as a hemoglobin (Hgb) of less than 12 g/dL in women and less than 13 g/dL in men, affects 40 to 44% of older adults (Garg et al., 2004; Robinson et al., 2007). Repeatedly, anemia has been associated with physical performance, mood, and quality of life (Ershler et al., 2005; Penninx et al., 2004). As with anemia, Vitamin D deficiency has been associated with muscle weakness, poor physical performance, balance problems, and falls (Franen, Lemkens, Van Laer & Van Camp, 2003; Houston et al., 2007) (see Exhibit 11.1). These two physiological factors are more modifiable than others and appropriate interventions at the intraindividual level include evaluating and managing anemia and encouraging vitamin D supplementation.

## Psychosocial Factors

Fear of falling (Fletcher & Hirdes, 2004) and depressive symptoms (Dunlop et al., 2005) have been noted to influence function in older adults. There is also evidence of a reciprocal relationship between depression and PA. Depression can decrease the individual's willingness to engage in functional activities, although participating in these activities decreases depression and improves mood (Tsauo, Leu, Chen, & Yang, 2005). Resilience is another psychosocial factor that influences function and participation in functional activities. Resilience is an individual's capacity to make a "psychosocial comeback in adversity" (Kadner, 1989, p. 20), and is defined as the ability to achieve, retain, or regain a level of physical or emotional health after illness or loss (Felten & Hall, 2001). Resilient individuals tend to manifest adaptive behavior, especially with regard to social functioning, morale, and somatic health (Wagnild, 2003) and are less likely to succumb to illness. Resilience, as a component of the individual's personality, develops and changes over time through ongoing experiences with the physical and social environment (Glantz & Johnson, 1999). Older women who have successfully recovered from orthopedic or other stressful events describe themselves as resilient and determined (Felten & Hall, 2001; Wagnild, 2003) and tend to have better function, mood, and quality of life than those who were less resilient.

## Acute Pathophysiological Events

Cardiovascular and neurological events including cerebral vascular events and myocardial infarcts have been associated with a decline in function (van Wijk, Algra, van de Port, Bevaart, & Lindeman, 2006) as have orthopedic events, particularly hip fractures (Handoll, Sherrington, & Parker, 2004). After older adults are admitted to an acute care facility with a stroke or pneumonia there is a tendency among nurses to simply perform basic tasks for the individual rather than help them optimize their remaining function (Resnick et al., 2008). Moreover, the nurse may not know, or get to know, what the individual was able to do prior to admission and what he or she will need to do to return to his/her living location prior to admission. It is particularly important during hospital admissions for acute events to consider function and help older individuals reset functional goals and focus on recovery of remaining function rather than on the nurse simply performing the functional tasks that they can no longer complete independently.

## Interpersonal Factors That Influence Function

Motivation is a component of personality but is also influenced by variables extrinsic to the individual. Bandura (1997) conceptualized motivation within the broader spectrum of the theory of self-efficacy (SE). The theory of SE suggests that the stronger the individual's SE and outcome expectations (OE), the more likely it is that he or she will initiate and persist with a given activity. SE expectations are the individual's beliefs in his or her capabilities to perform a course of action to attain a desired outcome; and OE are the beliefs that a certain consequence will be produced by personal action. Efficacy expectations are dynamic and appraised and enhanced by four mechanisms: (a) enactive mastery experience, or successful performance of the activity; (b) verbal persuasion, or verbal encouragement given by a credible source that the individual is capable of performing the activity of interest; (c) vicarious experience or seeing like individuals perform a specific activity; and (d) physiological and affective states such as pain or anxiety associated with an activity.

## Motivation to Perform Functional Activities and Exercise in Older Adults

Both SE and OE play an influential role in the performance of functional activities (Fortinsky et al., 2002; Resnick 2002). SE expectations were associated with functional recovery following a stroke (Robinson-Smith, Johnston, & Allen, 2000), cardiac (Bootsma van der Wiel et al., 2001), and orthopedic events (Resnick, Magaziner, et al., 2007). OE is particularly relevant to older adults. Older adults may have high SE expectations related to performance of functional activities but if they do not believe in the outcomes associated with performing functional activities when acutely ill, then it is unlikely that they will be willing to perform them.

### Social Support

At the interpersonal level, social support networks, including family, friends, peers, and health care providers are also important determinants of behavior. Repeatedly, motivation to perform functional activities has been found to be influenced by the social milieu of the care setting (Casado et al., 2009; Sandman, Norberg, Adolfsson, Axelsson, & Hedly, 1985). These social interactions can influence SE and OE and can alter the trajectory proposed by Nagi. The reason for admission and course of hospitalization may have less of an impact on functional activities (e.g., participating in dressing) for individuals who are encouraged by a family member to independently bathe or sit up following a surgical intervention versus a family member who bathes the individual or insists that he or she be allowed to remain in bed. The influence of any member of the patient's social network can be positive or negative depending on his/her philosophy and beliefs related to engaging in functional activities. Some families, for example, tend to advocate that maximal nursing care be provided for their loved one. This situation, coupled with the tendency of nurses, in an attempt to be more efficient and caring, to complete functional tasks for older individuals (Beck et al., 1995; Resnick et al., 2008) means that the patient might be fed, bathed, transferred, and turned by the nurses. This propagates sedentary behavior and decreases SE related to function (Resnick et al., 2008). There is a need to establish a culture and philosophy of care in which patients are motivated to engage in functional tasks and achieve realistic goals even in the face of acute medical problems.

### Environmental Support

Environments that facilitate function can help older adults achieve their optimal capability in terms of function (Rodiek, 2006; Sallis 2003; Sallis & Glanz, 2006). When environments are evaluated in the acute care setting it is generally for safety rather than optimizing functional activity. Simple and cost-efficient modifications such as improving lighting, clearing pathways, or altering the height of beds or chairs have been shown to be effective in terms of improving function (Gill, Robinson, Williams &

Tinetti, 1999; Gitlin, Mann, Tomit, & Marcus, 2001; Gitlin et al., 2006) by facilitating transfers and providing opportunity for the activity. In addition to consideration of the objective physical environment, the degree of person–environment fit (P–E fit) is critical to evaluate, especially as function declines (Iwarsson, 2005; Iwarsson & Slaug, 2001a, 2001b). Adaptation, or P–E fit, occurs when there is a match between the person and the environment. P–E fit is particularly important for individuals with lower competence in that they spend a great deal of energy overcoming and adapting to environments and consequently are unable to optimally engage in functional activities.

The Housing Enabler Instrument (Iwarsson & Slaug, 2001a,2001b) provides a way in which to comprehensively evaluate the environment and includes three steps: (a) assessment of functional limitations and dependence of the patient on mobility devices; (b) detailed assessment of the physical environmental barriers including outdoor, entrances, indoor, and communication features; and (c) a calculation of the P–E Fit. For patients in the acute care setting, the indoor-environment component is useful to consider as the fit of the patient to this environment can help to optimize function (http://www.enabler.nu/). For each environmental barrier item, the instrument comprises predefined severity ratings and is scored from 1 (potential accessibility problem) to 4 (very severe accessibility problem). The assessment of the individuals' limitations is matched with the environment and a score is calculated using Housing Enabler software. Content validity and interrater reliability have been established with better fit being associated with better function and more physical activity in older adults; there was evidence of 2-week test–retest reliability (Pomeroy & Resnick, 2007).

## Policy

The policies, procedures, and philosophy of care within each organization are critical to the way in which care is provided and in driving the focus of clinical outcomes. In the United States, policy initiatives have been successful in changing behaviors in areas such as wearing seat belts (Houston & Richardson, 2006) and use of physical restraints (Castle, 1998). There are, however, no policies that specifically address functional decline in the acute care setting. Recently, the Center for Medicare and Medicaid Services (CMS) established payment changes for acute care settings based on an outgrowth of the Inpatient Prospective Payment System (IPPS). Initiated in 2005, in an effort to align financial incentives with improvement in health care quality, Congress began the process of identifying "preventable" hospital-acquired conditions for which CMS would no longer pay. Congress instructed the Secretary for Health and Human Services to select at least two conditions that were: (a) high cost and/or high volume, (b) likely to result in assignment to a diagnostic-related group (DRG) that had a higher payment when present as a secondary diagnosis, and (c) could be reasonably prevented using evidence-based care (Davis et al., 2007).

After collaborative work with public health and infectious disease experts from the Centers for Disease Control and Prevention (CDC) 13 candidate conditions, including hospital falls, were selected. From these 13, 8 were chosen to be included in the initial reforms. The hospital-acquired conditions that will no longer be covered services by CMS include: (a) objects left in place during surgery, (b) air embolism, (c) blood incompatibility, (d) catheter-associated urinary tract infection, (e) pressure ulcer, (f) vascular catheter-associated infection, (g) mediastinitis after coronary-artery bypass grafting, and (h) injuries from falls. Falls were included, despite challenges associated with identification and prevention, because it was believed that these types of injuries and trauma should not occur in the hospital. It is likely that this will be refined and expanded to include other hospital-acquired injuries in future years.

It is not clear, however, how this new regulation will affect clinical care. It is possible, for example, that a focus on safety may actually restrict function in patients for fear that the patient may fall during the activity.

At an international level there are policies associated with national health insurance that can affect function. For example, coverage of assistive devices or therapy services can directly affect an older adults' ability to transfer and ambulate after an acute event. In Israel, for example, the national health insurance that is provided for all patients covers these services as well as services that support prevention of acute exacerbation of diseases and early intervention so that patients are admitted prior to becoming significantly deconditioned (Israel Ministry of Foreign Affairs, 2008). In other countries the coverage may not be as broad as it is in Israel and this can affect the care provided prior to and following the acute care admission and likewise has the potential to influence function.

## Interventions to Address Function Among Older Hospitalized Patients

Some work has been done to specifically address function among hospitalized older adults. This has varied from nonspecific interventions using an interdisciplinary approach (Mudge, Laracy, Richter, & Denaro, 2006; Stuck, Siu, Wieland, Adams, & Rubenstein, 1993) with a focus on such things as discharge planning (Parkes & Shepperd, 2004) and communication among health care providers (Mudge et al.), to attempts to implement more aggressive exercise interventions during the course of the hospital stay (Brown, Peel, Bamman, & Allman, 2006; de Morton, Keating, & Jeffs, 2007). In a recent *Cochrane Review* only seven randomized controlled trials and two controlled clinical trials were found to have tested exercise interventions in acute care sites. None of these had a notable impact on functional outcomes and there was no effect of the exercise programs on adverse events during hospitalization. Pooled analysis of multidisciplinary interventions suggested that there was a small significant increase in the proportion of patients discharged from the acute care to the home setting (Relative Risk = 1.08, 95% confidence interval [CI] = 1.03 to 1.14), a small reduction in acute hospital length of stay (approximately 1 day with a 95% CI −1.93 to −0.22), and a slight decrease in total hospital costs (95% CI = −491.85 to −65.44) compared to usual care. From a feasibility perspective, there was little evidence to suggest that these types of aggressive interventions can be successfully implemented in the acute care setting (Brown et al., 2006). The lack of feasibility and evidence of treatment fidelity may have contributed to why such programs had no impact on clinical outcomes.

## Restorative Care

In contrast to the unrealistic expectation of engaging acutely ill older individuals in intensive exercise programs during acute care admissions, a restorative-care approach provides a logical and practical intervention that can be incorporated into all care interactions. Moreover, a philosophy of care that integrates restorative care throughout activities can help ameliorate the decline that all too commonly occurs in hospitalized patients. Restorative care focuses on the restoration and/or maintenance of physical function, and helps the older adult to compensate for functional impairments so that the highest level of function is obtained. This type of care is focused on maximizing the individuals' abilities and assuring that they work toward achieving their highest level of capability with regard to function and physical activity. For some this may include participating in basic activities of daily living at a variety of levels of independence, for others it can incorporate specific muscle strengthening or balance activities, and for others still it might incorporate functionally relevant exercises to do at the bedside.

Restorative care is not, however, the same as rehabilitation. Rehabilitation is defined as a continuing and comprehensive team effort that generally includes the specialized knowledge of physical, occupational, and speech therapists to restore an individual to his or her former functional status or to maximize remaining function. Certainly restorative care can aid in the rehabilitation process for those patients for whom therapy has been initiated as it focuses on assuring that the patient is using his or her current ability at the highest level. Restorative care, for example, would include having the patient practice what has been learned in physical or occupational therapy sessions on the nursing unit. In addition, restorative care should be and can be initiated at the time of admission rather than waiting until the acute medical problem is stabilized and a referral to rehabilitation services made.

In the United States, another major difference between restorative care services and rehabilitation is the reimbursement structure, particularly with regard to Medicare. In the acute care setting, Medicare Part A covers rehabilitation services if there is evidence that the patient requires a relatively intense, multidisciplinary rehabilitation program; the rehabilitation program is provided by a coordinated, multidisciplinary team, and if the patient has a realistic goal of functioning at a more independent level. Conversely, there is no Medicare coverage for implementation of restorative care, which is more of a philosophy of how care is provided to patients. The goals, unlike those of rehabilitation, are focused on performing a specific function such as ambulating to the bathroom, or independently bathing and dressing. Unlike rehabilitation in which services are allocated based on ability to achieve a reimbursable goal (i.e., being able to walk a functional distance), all older adults have appropriate and relevant restorative care goals and should be exposed to restorative care to achieve those goals. A chair- or bed-bound patient may benefit, for example, by participating in some strengthening activities, or simply by undergoing daily range-of-motion exercises to prevent contractures and/or practicing transfers and sitting and standing exercises.

## Designated Restorative Care Versus Integrated Restorative Care

Different types of models of restorative care have been described in the literature. The first model, which is referred to as the designated restorative care model, includes the development of restorative care programs by hiring and training designated nurses or caregivers to perform the restorative care activities. Designated restorative care programs have been developed in long-term-care settings (Remsburg, Armacost, Radu, & Bennet, 1999), home care (Tinetti et al., 2002), and on acute care units (Holy Cross Hospital, 2009). The focus of these programs is on providing specific restorative care services such as ambulating patients, providing range-of-motion exercise, or helping a patient learn how to use and practice using a specific type of assistive device.

One of the major problems in designated restorative care programs is that the designated nurse has a rigid schedule to adhere to in providing restorative care services and in response the older individual must perform the restorative care activity at a time that is convenient for the designated restorative care nurse. This may or may not be convenient or preferred by the older individual. This might mean, for example, that the older adult has to perform bathing and dressing activities at a time when she or he is fatigued, in pain, or hungry. Clearly, nurse-driven scheduling may not be the best way to facilitate the restorative care intervention. Another major problem that occurs when using a designated restorative care model is that once a decision is made to discontinue the staff from performing restorative care services, restorative care activities may no longer be performed by the nurses. The other nurses would not be focused on such services or incentivized to provide them.

Alternatively, restorative care activities can be implemented by all nurses and acute care staff who interact with the patient. This type of model is referred to as an integrated restorative care model. In contrast to designated restorative care programs, integrated restorative care models focus on implementing a philosophy of care that is geared toward helping all older adults obtain and maintain their optimal functional capability. This philosophy of care reinforces the individuals' underlying abilities and motivates them to retain their highest level of independence. Integrated restorative care is an ongoing process that uses input from all disciplines to establish the best way to optimize the individual's underlying capability and functional performance. There is a commitment on the part of all staff to promote independent function, even though it may be quicker and easier for a nurse to perform the activity him or herself. This is in contrast to the current philosophy of care in acute care, which tends to be entirely focused on resolution of the acute medical problem, at times at the cost of decreased function (e.g., use of restraints limiting movement to allow for an intravenous line to be maintained). Restorative care activities for the older individual are incorporated into daily care interactions and may be as simple as doing hand-over-hand bathing, using assistive devices to facilitate independent eating, or encouraging the patient to push up in the bed, transfer to a commode, or ambulate to the bathroom or to a chair to facilitate another nursing care interaction such as a dressing change. It is possible, for example, that taking the time to help/encourage a patient to sit up during a care interaction might shorten the time required for a care activity (e.g., an intravenous-line insertion, dressing change). Timing of the restorative care activity in an integrated model capitalizes on the individual's preferences and personal schedule. Doing some sit-to-stand exercises or performing bathing activities, for example, might be done in the evening when the older individual is not involved in testing or treatment procedures. Restorative care activities can also be incorporated into daily tests and treatments. For example, a patient could be encouraged to walk to the elevator to get radiology for testing, or walk part or all of the way to radiology. Patient transport, instead of pushing the wheelchair, could supervise this ambulation, having the patient push the wheelchair and then sit it in it when he/she becomes fatigued. This may not occur currently because of policy that prevents individuals who transport patients from allowing them to walk as a result of misguided concerns about safety, or perceptions that this would take longer. Self-propelling a wheelchair for those who are not able to ambulate, even a short distance such as to the elevator, is also an important functional activity to help maintain endurance.

Although these different models have not been tested in the acute care setting, findings from work done in long-term care comparing designated restorative care programs from integrated restorative care programs have shown that the designated models are not maintained over time (Remsburg et al., 1999; Resnick et al., 2008). Given these findings and the many advantages of integrated restorative care programs, it is recommended that this approach be used in the acute care setting.

## Motivation of Nurses/Social Supports to Perform Restorative Care Activities

The success of implementing a philosophy of restorative care depends heavily on the receptiveness of the nurses and other health care providers as well as families and other informal caregivers to learn new skills and on their motivation to use these skills regularly. SE-based interventions have been shown to be effective with regard to restorative care activities in terms of increasing knowledge and beliefs of caregivers as to the benefits of restorative care and in performing restorative care activities with older individuals (Galik, Resnick, & Pretzer-Aboff, 2008; Resnick et al., 2002, Resnick et al., 2009; Resnick, Simpson, Galik, et al., 2006), in improving oral care (Wardh, Hallberg, Berggren, Andersson, & Sorensen, 2003), managing behavior problems (Irvine, Bourgeois, Bilow, & Seeley, 2007), feeding behavior (Chang, Wykle, & Madigan, 2006), and recognition and protection against assault (Gates, Fitzwater, & Succop, 2005).

SE related to employment activities has repeatedly been associated with and can improve job satisfaction and job performance (Bono & Judge, 2003; Wolfe, Nordstrom, & Williams, 1998). Based on these findings, Bono and Judge developed the model of Core Self-Evaluations, which suggests that SE, as one aspect of core self-evaluations, can influence job satisfaction and performance. Nurses in acute care settings who perceived themselves to be better prepared for specific tasks reported more job satisfaction (Bowcutt et al., 2008; Tabari-Khomeiran, Kiger, Parsa-Yekta, & Ahmadi, 2007). In addition, SE-based interventions such as verbal persuasion and education about care-related activities improved job satisfaction and decreased turnover among nurses (Ackerman, Kenny, & Walker, 2007; Uhrenfeldt & Hall, 2007). Thus, there is reason to believe that SE-based interventions related to restorative care can increase the confidence and restorative care skills of nurses and thereby increase their job satisfaction and retention rates.

## Implementing a Restorative Care Philosophy

Implementation of a restorative care model of care in acute care is best done using a social ecological model approach. The social ecological model that guides the implementation of the a restorative care intervention developed specifically for acute care settings (this is referred to as Res-Care-AC) provides an overarching framework for understanding the interrelations among diverse personal and environmental factors in human health and illness and addresses intraindividual, interpersonal, environmental, and policy factors. There is increasing recognition that this type of multilevel perspective is needed to address health behavior and facilitate changes in current care philosophies and care practices as has been done with regard to use of physical restraints

(Wagner et al., 2007). This model has been used to promote positive health behaviors and achieve the guidelines proposed in *Healthy People 2010* (Handoll, Sherrington, & Parker, 2004; Nigg et al., 2005), understand caregivers' expectations and care receivers' competence (Isal, Montorio, Marquez, & Losada, 2005), and improve diabetes management (Fisher et al., 2005).

The goal of Res-Care-AC is to change the philosophy of care in acute care sites from one that is focused mainly on acute management of clinical problems to one that includes a focus on engaging patients in functional tasks and physical activity during their acute care stay. The intervention is focused on educating health care providers in these sites (e.g., nurses, physicians, social workers/care managers), families, and patients about the benefits of functional and physical activity. Using an SE-based approach, the nurses and other health care providers and families are taught skills to motivate patients to engage in functional and physical activity. In so doing patients will maintain or improve admission functional status and level of physical activity, have shorter lengths of stay, be discharged to the level of care from which they were admitted (e.g., home, nursing home), and experience fewer iatrogenic events (e.g., pressure ulcers, infections) during the course of their acute care stay. Guided by a social–ecological model, the intervention will address intraindividual, interpersonal, environmental, and policy-related factors that influence restorative care activities and provide mentoring of nurses and other health care providers within the unit/facility to engage in restorative care with regard to all patients.

Res-Care-AC ideally should be coordinated and implemented by a champion, a nurse, or other member of the health care team who can serve as a leader who has a strong commitment to this philosophy of care among all the other members of the interdisciplinary team. The champion will ideally enforce the four components of the successful implementation of restorative care as delineated in the Res-Care-AC intervention. These include: (a) an initial environmental assessment; (b) education/mentoring of staff, administration, families, and patients; (c) establishing restorative care goals; and (d) making it happen. An implementation plan should be established with each site. Each component is described in more detail in the text that follows.

## Component I: Environmental and Relevant Policy Assessments

A baseline environmental assessment of the unit, including any areas that would be accessible to patients, should be completed using the Indoor Environment component of the Housing Enabler Instrument (Iwarsson & Slaug, 2001a, 2001b). Based on this assessment, environmental interventions can be explored with the members of the health care team and administration. Such interventions might involve changing the height of a chair or bed to facilitate function, increasing sitting areas in open walkways for patients, or removing bedpans and replacing these with appropriate commode chairs or clear pathways in rooms to allow patients to get safely to the bathroom. Routine interventions (if not already present in the sites) might include such things as the placement of a poster, "Focus on Function and Physical Activity" in each patient's room, and other types of cues for promoting functional and physical activity throughout the unit, such as posters to delineate easy-to-do exercises, and chairs set up in the hallway to use for a sit-to-stand exercise activity, or a mural on the hallway wall to simulate a pleasant walking area.

A comprehensive evaluation of policies and procedures that have been established on a specific unit and within the acute care site related to such things as patient transfers from the unit to procedures, use of restraints (including bedrails), and use of common space (e.g., kitchen/food storage areas) on the unit are critical to restorative care. At the onset of the implementation process, careful consideration of these policies and procedures, and how they influence restorative care activities is critical. For example, there may be a policy that states that patients must be transferred in wheelchairs or that chair height in rooms needs to remain at a certain level. Appropriate discussions with administration and legal consult may be necessary to revise these policies in such a way that function and physical activity can be optimized.

## Component II: Education/Mentoring of All Nursing Staff, Other Acute Care Staff on the Unit, Families, and Patients

Education of the interdisciplinary team is recommended and can include a simple 4-week series of classes, provided in 20- to 30-minute sessions once a week. This effort has been shown to increase knowledge of and beliefs in the benefits of restorative care (Galik et al., 2008; Resnick et al., 2009; Resnick & Simpson, 2003). The classes focus on the following:

**Class 1: Establishing a philosophy of restorative care.** This involves a brief review of the impact of an acute care admission on function and associated outcomes among older patients in these settings. A description of restorative care and the importance of this philosophy of care in the acute care setting to prevent functional decline, a review of successful examples of restorative care across a variety of clinical examples, and strengthening beliefs in the benefits of restorative care.

**Class 2: Motivating older adults to engage in functional and physical activities.**

*[1] Education*: The staff will be encouraged to provide patients and families with ongoing information about the benefits of engaging in functional and physical activities while in the acute care setting. Benefits to be emphasized include such things as shorter recovery period, maintenance and regaining of function, getting back to home setting, decreasing the risk of having a fall, better endurance, decreased pain, and a general feeling of well-being and a sense of personal accomplishment.

*[2] Verbal encouragement*: Techniques for how to provide verbal encouragement to patients focused on helping the patient believe he/she can perform the recommended functional and physical activity, and positive reinforcement for any activity performed (e.g., positive encouragement for pushing up in bed, transferring to a sitting position postoperatively, or walking partway down the hall). Conversely, telling patients to remain in bed for "safety," or inappropriate bed rest requirements should be discussed and eliminated as appropriate. Likewise the negative statements that propagate a fear of falling, "don't get up you might fall," should likewise be addressed and eliminated.

With a strong focus on prevention of falls in these settings, nursing staff may limit patients from getting up independently or may not optimize these opportunities. This can have a negative impact on function directly, but also may decrease the patient's confidence regarding transfers, toileting, and/or ambulation. Use statements such as, "It is terrific for you to get up and walk but call me so I can walk with you," or simply position the patient in ways in which he/she is not alone, and/or cannot independently transfer.

*[3] Eliminating unpleasant sensations*: Nurses should be reminded to continually evaluate patients for *unpleasant sensations around participation in functional activities.* Although questioning about pain and management of pain is one of the National Quality Forum Nursing-Sensitive Measures, the focus on pain has generally concerned the admitting diagnosis or focused intervention (e.g., hip fracture and surgical intervention). It is critical that questions about pain, or other symptoms associated with physical activity, such as fatigue or shortness of breath, be focused on *the functional or physical activities* in which we are encouraging them to participate. This is in contrast to current care, which tends to focus on asking about pain and other unpleasant sensations associated with the admitting acute medical problem or treatment (e.g., hip fracture and surgical intervention) and not in the context of performance of an activity. Interventions to decrease the unpleasant sensations associated with an activity can then be recommended such as pain medication before a walk, using massage or ice/heat treatments to painful joints, or addressing fear of falling through encouragement and exercise. These interventions can be incorporated into routine interactions with the patient.

*[4] Cueing*: Cueing with self- and role modeling is another useful way in which to strengthen the patient's beliefs in his or her ability to perform functional activities and as a reminder to actually perform those activities. This educational session reviews the development of restorative care goals with the patient, which should ideally be done around the admission period. The development of goals allows the nurse to use the information gathered at the time of admission. The goals would be clearly noted (Table 11.1) for the patient, the staff, and family and serve as a reminder to all that the patient needs to practice/engage in these activities.

**Class 3: Using/optimizing the environment and integrating restorative care into the acute care routine.** This class uses role playing and case studies to address how to best use the patients' environment and daily care interactions to engage them in functional and physical activities. Examples are basic things such as having the patient push him or herself up in bed, rather than lifting the individual, having the patient stand independently with verbal cues rather than facilitating a transfer by lifting the individual, or for more functionally independent individuals having them walk, as tolerated, to procedures with a caregiver or self-propel a wheelchair with cueing.

**Class 4: Documentation of restorative care activities through use of a weekly flow sheet.** This class addresses the utility of documenting time spent in restorative care activities so that this can be used to demonstrate the work of the nursing staff with regard to optimizing function and PA in patients and in focusing on prevention of adverse events such as falls. As noted, at

## 11.1  Restorative Care Short Term Goal Form

**Passive range of motion**
_____Ask, encourage, or provide cues to the resident to bend the arm and leg joints while passive range of motion is being performed.

**Active range of motion**
_____Ask, encourage, or provide cues to the resident to stretch and bend the arm and leg joints.

**Personal assistive devices**: glasses, hearing aids, magnifying glasses, prostheses and other supportive devices.
_____Ask or encourage the resident to apply devices.
_____Give step-by-step cues on how to apply the device.
_____Place the device in the resident's hands to facilitate independent application.
_____Other:

**Communication**
_____Use a speech board to facilitate communication with the resident.
_____Use a memory book to stimulate conversation/communication with the resident.
_____Ask the resident questions during care that stimulate conversation, e.g., "Tell me about your grandchildren." "Tell me what life was like when you were growing up."
_____Encourage the resident to communicate needs, e.g., "What would you like to wear?" "How do you feel today?"
_____Other:

**Eating/swallowing**
_____Set up food tray to facilitate independent eating.
_____Provide assistive devices to facilitate independent eating.
_____Encourage independent eating by providing cues and encouragement.
_____Encourage independent eating with finger foods.
_____Use hand-over-hand assistance to feed resident.
_____Other:

**Dressing**
_____Ask and/or encourage the resident to participate in dressing.
_____Provide cues for dressing activities to be completed.
_____Set up clothing to facilitate independent dressing.
_____Other:

**Grooming:** hair care, shaving, nail care, mouth care
_____Ask or encourage the resident to participate in grooming.
_____Provide cues for grooming activities to be completed.
_____Set up supplies to facilitate independent grooming.
_____Other:

**Bathing**
_____Ask or encourage the resident to participate in bathing.
_____Provide cues for bathing activities to be completed.
_____Set-up bathing supplies to facilitate independent bathing.

**Transferring**
_____Ask or encourage resident to transfer.
_____Give cues on how to transfer, e.g., "Slide to the edge of the chair." "Push on the arm rests with your hands."
_____Place hands to facilitate independent movement, e.g., place the resident's hands on the walker.
_____Other:

*(continued)*

## Table 11.1 *(continued)*

| | |
|---|---|
| **Bed mobility/turning and repositioning** | _____Ask or encourage resident to move or turn in bed.<br>_____Give step-by-step cues on how to move in bed, e.g., "Put your right hand on the rail and pull yourself over on your left side."<br>_____Places resident's hands on the side rail to facilitate independent movement.<br>_____Other: |
| **Walking/wheelchair mobility** | _____Ask or encourage the resident to walk or wheel him or herself in the wheelchair to the bathroom, dining room, or activities room.<br>_____Give cues to get the resident to walk, e.g., "Move your left foot forward, now move your right foot."<br>_____Deliberately take the resident for a walk for exercise.<br>_____Assist, ask, and/or encourage the resident to walk using a merry walker.<br>_____Other: |
| **Scheduled toileting plan/ bladder or bowel retraining program** | _____Ask, encourage, or remind resident to toilet in A.M., after meals, and at bedtime.<br>_____Assist the resident to transfer on and off of the commode and provide assistance with hygiene at the following times:<br>_____Other: |
| **Exercise program** | _____Ask, encourage, remind, or instruct the resident to exercise.<br>_____Take the resident to exercise class.<br>_____Remind resident to perform exercises.<br>_____Other: |
| | Long-term goals: _____ |

least in the United States, there may be policy implications of having this type of data available to administrators so as to be able to describe the type of care that is being provided to patients.

Education of families/informal caregivers (referred to as families throughout the rest of this chapter) and patients at the time of admission is also critical to consider so that patient and family satisfaction with care is realistically evaluated. The expectation of nursing care by patients and families traditionally has been that nurses provide care for and meet all needs of patients. From a *patient/family perspective*, nursing care includes such things as bathing, dressing, feeding, and administering treatments for those who are ill. In addition, a patient/family expects that the nurse will reposition, transfer a patient, and transport a patient via wheelchair to engage in all treatment associated activities. These care expectations are not based on the individual's underlying capability and does not use the expert assessment skills of the nursing staff. Patients and families need to be educated that optimal nursing care involves an assessment of the patient regarding his or her underlying function and ability and identification of goals and interventions implemented to optimize function in the patient. Handouts can be used and flyers posted on the units so that patients and families gain an understanding of the philosophy of care provided on the unit and the ultimate goals focused not just on recovery of physical health but also of optimal functional ability. Handouts for patients and families can incorporate information about the benefits and barriers to patient performance of functional and physical activities while in the hospital, and provide families with techniques for how they can optimize function and physical activity for their loved ones. This may be as simple as making sure the patient holds the cup when drinking versus the family member holding it.

## Component III: Establishing Restorative Care Goals for Patients

Goal development includes short- and long-term goals and should be based on the patients' function at the time of admission and can be revised as the previous goals are achieved. Goals are developed based on input from the patient/admission records and/or family and through the analysis of baseline performance. An identified restorative care champion may be the one to take responsibility for the development of restorative care goals of patients or this can be designated to each individual admitting nurse, with input from the primary health care provider, therapist if this has been initiated, or others with relevant input. A focused evaluation of the musculoskeletal and neurological systems, in addition to an overall medical history with information on past medical problems as well as current admission disorders is particularly helpful for determining the patient's underlying ability and establishing his or her goals (Tables 11.2 & 11.3, Exhibit 11.2).

Decisions in terms of what the individual is likely to be able to do are based on these abilities as well as the history of what the individual was doing prior to admission. Understanding the level of cognitive impairment in an individual is a critical aspect to establishing capability and setting goals. For example, those who have difficulty following a verbal command might need visual cues and supervision to perform an activity and this would be clearly stated in the goals. Once established, short-term goals can be written on the Restorative Care Short-Term-Goal Form (Table 11.1) and placed in a location that will be easily accessible to the interdisciplinary members of the health care team working with the patient, as well as for the patient and the family. Goals should be reviewed daily and updated as appropriate by the champion or nurse assigned to the patient, goals should be based on observations of function and activity and feedback from staff, patient, or families. For example, if on day 2 of admission the patient has been able to walk to the bathroom with verbal cues during the day a new goal might expand to include walking in the hallway to the nurses station a certain number of times daily, or walking to the elevator.

As part of the review of the physical history, the champion, or the nurse admitting the patient and establishing goals should also evaluate the patients' admission labs for evidence of anemia based on the World Health Organization definition of anemia (< 13g Hb/dL for men and < 12 g Hb/dL for women), and risk factors for vitamin D deficiency (Exhibit 11.2), and discuss this with the patient's admitting provider. These factors, if not addressed during the evaluation and management of the patient's admission diagnosis and treatment, should be considered because of the possible impact that they can have on function (Campbell & Allain, 2006; Chaves, Ashar, Guralnik & Fried, 2002; Dhesi et al., 2002). Treatment options can be easily addressed in the acute care setting and may involve, for example, initiation of appropriate replacement therapy for iron or vitamin D.

# 11.2  Evaluation for Contractures

Contractures should be evaluated by putting the joint through active or passive range of motion. Active range of motion should be tried first and if the patient is unable, then passive range of motion is used. Adequate space for the patient to move each muscle group and joint through its full range is necessary. Instruct the patient to move each joint through its range of motion as described below. If full range is not completed by the patient actively, put the joint through the remaining range, stopping at the point of pain.

| Area of Focus | Normal Range: Yes (Y) No (N) | Strength 0–5* | Normal Range Guidelines |
|---|---|---|---|
| 1. Right wrist | | | Flexion: 80–90 degrees |
| | | | Bend wrist so palm nears lower arm. |
| | | | Extension: 70 degrees |
| | | | Bend wrist in opposite direction. |
| | | | Radial deviation: 20 degrees |
| | | | Bend wrist so thumb nears radius. |
| | | | Ulnar deviation: 30–50 degrees |
| | | | Bend wrist so pinky finger nears ulna. |
| 2. Left wrist | | | |
| 3. Right shoulder | | | Abduction: 180 degrees |
| | | | Bring arm up sideways. |
| | | | Adduction: 45 degrees |
| | | | Bring arm toward the midline of the body. |
| | | | Horizontal extension: 45 degrees |
| | | | Swing arm horizontally backward. |
| | | | Horizontal flexion: 130 degrees |
| | | | Swing arm horizontally forward. |
| | | | Vertical extension: 60 degrees |
| | | | Raise arm straight backward. |
| | | | Vertical flexion: 180 degrees |
| | | | Raise arm straight forward. |
| 4. Left shoulder | | | |
| 5. Right ankle | | | Flexion: 45 degrees |
| | | | Bend ankle so toes point up. |
| | | | Extension: 20 degrees |
| | | | Bend ankle so toes point down. |
| | | | Pronation: 30 degrees |
| | | | Turn foot so the sole faces in. |
| | | | Supination: 20 degrees |
| | | | Turn foot so the sole faces out. |
| 6. Left ankle | | | |
| 7. Right knee | | | Flexion: 130 degrees |
| | | | Touch calf to hamstring. |
| | | | Extension: 15 degrees |
| | | | Straighten out knee as much as possible. |
| | | | Internal rotation: 10 degrees |
| | | | Twist lower leg toward midline. |

*(continued)*

**Table 11.2** *(continued)*

| Area of Focus | Normal Range. Yes (Y) No (N) | Strength 0–5* | Normal Range Guidelines |
|---|---|---|---|
| 8. Left knee | | | |
| 9. Right hip | | | Flexion: 110–130 degrees |
| | | | Flex knee and bring thigh close to abdomen. |
| | | | Extension: 30 degrees |
| | | | Move thigh backward without moving the pelvis. |
| | | | Abduction: 45–50 degrees |
| | | | Swing thigh away from midline. |
| | | | Adduction: 20–30 degrees |
| | | | Bring thigh toward and across midline. |
| | | | Internal rotation: 40 degrees |
| | | | Flex knee and swing lower leg away from midline. |
| | | | External rotation: 45 degrees |
| | | | Flex knee and swing lower leg toward midline. |
| 10. Left hip | | | |
| 9. Right thumb | | | Adduction/Abduction Contact/45 |
| | | | Interphalangeal hyperextension/Flexion 15H/80 |
| | | | Basal joint palmar adduction/Abduction contact/45 |
| | | | Metacarpophalangeal Hyperextension/Flexion 10/55 |
| 10. Left finger | | | |
| 9. Right finger | | | DIP joints extension/Flexion 0/80 |
| | | | PIP joints extension/Flexion 0/100 |
| | | | MCP joints hyperextension/Flexion (0–45H)/90 |

\* Muscle strength is often rated on a scale of 0/5 to 5/5 as follows:
0/5: no contraction
1/5: muscle flicker, but no movement
2/5: movement possible, but not against gravity (test the joint in its horizontal plane)
3/5: movement possible against gravity, but not against resistance by the examiner
4/5: movement possible against some resistance by the examiner
5/5: normal strength

# Component IV: Making It Happen

A restorative care champion, a nurse on the unit or from quality assurance or administration who has self-identified or was asked to oversee the process, will ideally need to maintain the ongoing encouragement of the nurses and other members of the health care team with regard to engaging patients in restorative care activities. Specifically, this will include monitoring to assure that patient goals are reevaluated and updated, that restorative care activities are documented, and that appropriate systemwide environment changes have occurred as recommended if at all possible. The following

# 11.3   Assessment of Capability for Basic Function Evaluation

Basic Activities of Daily Living

1. Feeding: Ability to independently bring hand to mouth.
2. Dress Upper Extremities: Strength 4 or 5 in upper extremities
3. Dress Lower Extremities: Strength 4 or 5 in upper extremities
4. Don Brace: Strength 4 or 5 in upper extremities
5. Grooming: Unilateral range of motion to at least 90 degrees in shoulder and at least 50% of range in fingers of same arm.
6. Wash: Unilateral range of motion to at least 90 degrees in shoulder and at least 50% of range in fingers of same arm.
7. Perineum: Unilateral range of motion to full elbow extension and at least 50% of range in fingers of same arm.
8. Transfer Chair: Bilateral plantar and dorsiflexion with strength 3/5 or greater and 50% or greater knee and hip extension and strength 3/5 or greater.
9. Transfer Toilet: Bilateral plantar and dorsiflexion with strength 3/5 or greater and 50% or greater knee and hip extension and strength 3/5 or greater.
10. Transfer: Tub/shower: Bilateral plantar and dorsiflexion with strength 3/5 or greater and 50% or greater knee and hip extension and strength 3/5 or greater.
11. Walk 50 Yards: Bilateral plantar and dorsiflexion with strength 3/5 or greater and 50% or greater knee and hip extension and strength 3/5 or greater.
12. Wheel/Chair 50 Yards: Unilateral range of motion to at full elbow extension and at least 50% of range in fingers of same arm.

# Exhibit 11.2

## Risk Factors For Vitamin D Deficiency Checklist

Assessment for Risk of Vitamin D Deficiency:

| Risk Factor | Yes | No |
|---|---|---|
| No vitamin D supplementation | | |
| Little sun exposure | | |
| Crohn's or celiac disease | | |
| Liver of kidney disease | | |
| Dark-colored skin | | |
| Taking any of the following medications: | | |
|   Anticonvulsants (e.g, Dilantin, Phenobarbitol) | | |
|   Cholestyramine | | |
|   Antituberculin medications | | |
|   Chronic alcohol intake | | |
|   Hypoparathyroidism | | |

Score: If ANY risk factor is identified resident is considered high risk; discuss with RCC and Primary Health Care provider.

activities can be used to maintain the motivation of staff to engage in restorative care with patients: (a) positive reinforcement for doing and documenting restorative care activities; (b) meeting in groups or informally with the staff, patients, and/or families to address positive experiences or unpleasant feelings and experiences they have associated with implementing restorative care activities (e.g., frustration, discouragement, lack of support from other staff for nursing and, for patients, pain, fear of falling); (c) ongoing education to strengthen the staff, patients' and families' beliefs about the benefits of participating in functional and PA when in the acute care setting; and (d) helping the staff integrate restorative care activities into routine care (e.g., pushing up in bed versus pulling and repositioning patient, using a commode chair or walking to the bathroom versus using a bedpan).

Implementing a restorative care philosophy into the management of Mrs. Conner during her acute care stay may have helped to prevent some of the subsequent complications postoperatively and to optimize her functional recovery. Restorative care interventions might have included setting goals immediately on her arrival to the unit that established a plan in which she would transfer to void using the bedside commode and would sit up for a set period of time, and bathe and dress with appropriate set up. Exploring with Mrs. Conner her reasons for refusing to transfer to the commode or engaging in functional activities and then eliminating, or at least addressing these concerns and negotiating participation, can be particularly helpful. Pain seemed to be her primary reason for not wanting to get up, with pain management complicated by delirium likely associated with medications. Ice over the incisional area may have helped alleviate some discomfort. Additional concerns such as fear of falling or hurting the hip likewise should be explored with her and addressed. Sometimes just acknowledging these feelings and concerns can help the patient work through them. While eliminating the unpleasant sensations and concerns associated with physical activity post hip replacement, the nurses could focus on the reasons and rational for her to get up and strengthen her belief in the importance of doing so as part of her recovery. Many older adults believe that bed rest is the best way to recover and thus have limited belief in the benefits of engaging so early in the postoperative period in any type of activity. Further reinforcement of what Mrs. Conner did do in therapy and having her continue to perform those activities on the unit is critical. Patients tend to think that it is only with the therapists that they have to, or need to, walk, transfer, or bathe. This might have taken negotiation and bargaining so that she transferred to the commode during daytime hours but could use the bedpan at night.

Identification of a reward with Mrs. Conner may also have been a useful intervention. Getting back to one's home is generally a good source of motivation and a persistent reminder of what she would need to do independently to get back would have been helpful.

The family needed some education about the critical importance of encouraging their mother to engage in daily activities and maintain and regain function. The clear establishment of expectations at the time of admission and development of a goal sheet might have provided this family with the critical care activities they could help their mother with instead of doing everything for her.

Bowel and bladder training and activity provide opportunities to engage patients in transfers and ambulation. Intermittent catheterizations following attempts to sit up and void on a commode could have been initiated prior to reinsertion of the indwelling

Foley catheter. Moreover, from a practical perspective, not having the Foley catheter would have facilitated any transfer and ambulation activities.

Restorative care interventions with Mrs. Conner should not increase nursing time. Motivational discussions can occur during routine nursing activities such as wound care, intermittent catheterizations, medication administration, or when facilitating transfer for therapy or additional work up (e.g., X-ray). Moreover, although nursing, with input from therapies as appropriate, may establish Mrs. Conner's restorative care goals, nursing assistants (or other members of the health care team such as family members or transport staff) as available may implement much of this type of care with appropriate guidance and support to do so.

# Summary

Function of hospitalized older adults is a critical aspect of long-term recovery that is often sacrificed at the expense of a focus on medical management of the acute problem. Many factors influence function, including sociodemographic characteristics, preexisting disability, cognitive status, comorbid conditions, physical status such as low body mass index, elevated erythrocyte sedimentation rate, polypharmacotherapy, as well as the psychosocial state of the patient, particularly his or her motivation and resilience, and the type of care provided. Specifically, nursing care that focuses on completing functional tasks for the individual who has the underlying capability to perform these tasks with verbal cues, minimal assistance, or independently, can result in a decline in the underlying skills needed to engage in the activity and further decline. Conversely, a restorative philosophy of care that focuses on optimizing the function and PA of all patients at the level at which he or she is capable can prevent subsequent decline. Nurses who provide care from a restorative care perspective have an opportunity to decrease the length of stay for these patients by decreasing their risk of associated adverse events such as falls, pressure ulcers, and infections. The Res-Care-AC Intervention provides a practical way in which to implement such a philosophy of care and can be integrated into any acute care unit.

# References

Ackermann, A. D., Kenny, G., & Walker, C. (2007). Simulator programs for new nurses' orientation: A retention strategy. *Journal of Nursing Staff Development, 23*(3), 136–139.

Bandura, A. (1997). *Self-efficacy: The exercise of control.* New York: W.H. Freeman.

Beck, C., Heacock, P., Mercer, S., Walls, R. C., Rapp, C. G., & Vogelpohl, T. S. (1995). Dressing behavior in nursing home residents. *Nursing Research, 46*(3), 126–132.

Bonn, K. (1999). Resuming restorative care. *Nursing Homes, 6*, 72.

Bono, J. E., & Judge, T. A. (2003). Core self evaluations: A review of the trait and its role in job satisfaction and job performance. *European Journal of Personality, 17*, S5–S18.

Bootsma van der Wiel, A., Gussekloo, J., DeCraen, A., Van Exel, E., Knook, D., Lagaay, A., et al. (2001). Disability in the oldest old: "Can do" or "do do"? *Journal of the American Geriatrics Society, 49*, 909–914.

Borson, D., Scanlan, J. M., Chen, P., & Ganguli, M. (2003). The Mini-Cog as a screen for dementia. Validation in a population-based sample. *Journal of the American Geriatrics Society, 51*, 1451–1454.

Bowcutt, M., Rosenkoetter, M. M., Chernecky, C. C., Wall, J., Wynn, D., & Serrano, C. (2008). Implementation of an intravenous medication infusion pump system: Implications for nursing. *Journal of Nursing Management, 16*(2), 188–197.

Boyd, C. M., Zue, Q. L., Guralnik, J. M., & Fried, L. P. (2005). Hospitalization and development of dependence in activities of daily living in a cohort of disabled older women: The women's Health and Aging Study. *Journal of Gerontology Series A: Biological Sciences Medicine and Science, 60*(4), 888–893.

Brown, C. J., Friedkin, R. J., & Inouye, S. K. (2004). Prevalence and outcomes of low mobility in hospitalized older patients. *Journal of the American Geriatrics Society, 52*(8), 1263–1270.

Brown, C. J., Peel, C., Bamman, M. M., & Allman, R. M. (2006). Exercise program implementation proves not feasible during acute care hospitalization. *Journal of Rehabilitation Research and Development, 43*(7), 939–946.

Campbell, P. M. E., & Allain, T. J. (2006). Muscle strength and vitamin D in older people. *Gerontology, 52*, 335–338.

Casado, B. L., Resnick, B., Zimmerman, S., Nahm, E. S., Orwig, D., Macmillan, K. R., et al. (2009). Social support for exercise by experts in older women post hip fracture. *Journal of Women and Aging, 21*(1), 48–62.

Castle, N. G. (1998). The use of physical restraints in nursing homes: Pre- and post-Nursing Home Reform Act. *Journal of Health and Social Policy, 9*(3), 71–89.

Chang, C. C., Wykle, M. L., & Madigan, E. A. (2006). The effect of a feeding skills training program for NAs who feed dementia patients in Taiwanese nursing homes. *Geriatric Nursing, 27*(4), 229–237.

Chaves, P. H., Ashar, B., Guralnik, J. M., & Fried, L. P. (2002). Look at the relationship between hemoglobin concentration and prevalent mobility difficulty in older women: Should the criteria currently used to define anemia in older people be reevaluated? *Journal of the American Geriatrics Society, 50*, 1257–1264.

Covinsky, K. E., Palmer, R. M., Fortinsky, R. H., Counsell, S. R., Stewart, A. L., Kresevic, D., et al. (2003). Loss of independence in activities of daily living in older adults hospitalized with medical illnesses: Increased vulnerability with age. *Journal of the American Geriatrics Society, 51*(4), 451–458.

Davis, K., Schoen, C., Guterman, S., Shih, T., Schoenbaum, S. C., & Weinbaum, I. (2007). *Slowing the growth of U.S. health care expenditures: What are the options?* Available at: http://www.commonwealthfund.org/Content/Publications/Fund-Reports/2007/Jan/Slowing-the-Growth-of-U-S—Health-Care-Expenditures—What-Are-the-Options.aspx

DeFrances, C. J., & Podgornik, M. N. (2006). 2004 National Hospital Discharge Survey. *Advanced Data*, pp. 1–19.

de Morton, N. A., Keating, J. L., & Jeffs, K. (2007). Exercise for acutely hospitalized older medical patients. *Cochrane Database System Review, 1*(CD005955).

Dhesi, J. K., Bearne, L. M., Moniz, C., Hurley, M. V., Jackson, S. H., Swift, C. G., et al. (2002). Neuromuscular and psychomotor function in elderly subjects who fall and the relationship with vitamin D status. *Journal of Bone and Mineral Research 17*, 891–897.

Dunlop, D., Semanik, P., Song, J., Manheim, L. M., Shih, V., & Chang, R. W. (2005). Risk factors for functional decline in older adults with arthritis. *Arthritis Rheumatology, 52*(4), 1274–1282.

Ershler, W. B., Sheng, S., McKelvey, J., Artz, A. S., Denduluri, N., Tecson, J., et al. (2005). Serum erythropoietin and aging: A longitudinal analysis. *Journal of the American Geriatrics Society, 53*, 1360–1365.

Felten, B., & Hall, J. (2001). Conceptualizing resilience in women older than 85: Overcoming adversity from illness of loss. *Journal of Gerontological Nursing, 27*(1), 46–54.

Ferrucci, L., Penninx, B. W., Leveille, S. G., Corti, M. C., Pahor, M., Wallace, R., et al. (2000). Characteristics of nondisabled older persons who perform poorly in objective tests of lower extremity function. *Journal of the American Geriatrics Society, 48*(9), 1102–1110.

Field, C. (2004, February). The 'gift' of restorative nursing: Focusing on restorative care benefits both residents and staff at Cove's Edge Comprehensive Care Center. *Nursing Homes.* Available at: http://findarticles.com/p/articles/mi_m3830/is_2_53/ai_n6094126/? tag=content;col1

Fisher, E., Brownson, C. A., O'Toole, M. L., Shetty, G., Anwuri, V. V., & Glasgow, R. E. (2005). Ecological approaches to self-management: the case of diabetes. *American Journal of Public Health, 95*(9), 1523–1535.

Fleishell, A., & Resnick, B. (1999). *Stayin alive: Developing and implementing a restorative care nursing program.* Laurel, MD: Gerontological Nursing Ventures.

Fletcher, P., & Hirdes, J. (2004). Restriction in activity associated with fear of falling among community-based seniors using home care services. *Age & Ageing, 33*(3), 273–279.

Fortinsky, R., Bohannon, R. W., Litt, M. D., Tennen, H., Maljanian, R., Fifield, J., et al. (2002). Rehabilitation therapy self-efficacy and functional recovery after hip fracture. *International Journal of Rehabilitation Research, 25*(3), 241–246.

Franen, E., Lemkens, N., Van Laer, L., & Van Camp, G. (2003). Age related hearing impairment (ARHI): Environmental risk factors and genetic prospects. *Experimental Gerontology, 38,* 353–359.

Galik, E., & Resnick, B. (2007). Moving beyond behavior. *Topics in Geriatric Rehabilitation, 11*(2), 7–13.

Galik, E., Resnick, B., & Pretzer-Aboff, I. (2008). Pilot testing of the restorative care intervention for the cognitively impaired. *Journal of the American Medical Directors Association., 9*(7), 516–522.

Garg, A. X., Papaioannou, A., Ferko, N., Campbell, G., Clarke, J., & Ray, J. G. (2004). Estimating the prevalence of renal insufficiency in seniors requiring long-term care. *Kidney International, 65,* 649–653.

Gates, D., Fitzwater, E., & Succop, P. (2005). Reducing assaults against nursing home caregivers. *Nursing Research, 54*(2), 119–127.

Gill, T. M., Allore, H., & Guo, Z. (2004). The deleterious effects of bedrest among community-living older persons. *Journal of Gerontology–Series A–Biological Sciences and Medical Sciences, 59*(7), 755–761.

Gill, T. M., Robinson, J. T., Williams, C. S., & Tinetti, M. E. (1999). Mismatches between the home environment and physical capabilities among community-living older persons. *Journal of the American Geriatrics Society, 47*(1), 88–92.

Gitlin, L. N., Mann, W., Tomit, M., & Marcus, S. M. (2001). Factors associated with home environmental problems among community-living older people. *Disability Rehabilitation, 23*(17), 777–787.

Gitlin, L. N., Winter, L., Dennis, M. P., Corcoran, M., Schinfeld, S., & Hauck, W. W. (2006). A randomized trial of a multi-component home intervention to reduce functional difficulties in older adults. *Journal of the American Geriatrics Society, 54*(5), 800–816.

Glantz, M., & Johnson, J. (1999). *Resilience and development positive life adaptations.* New York: Kluwer Academic Press.

Haffenreffer, D., & Gold, M. F. (1991). The rewards of restorative care. *Provider, 12,* 15–21.

Handoll, H., Parker, M., & Sherrington, C. (2004). Mobilization strategies after hip fracture surgery in adults. *Cochrane Database Systems Review, 1*:CD001704.

Handoll, H. H., Sherrington, C., & Parker, M. J. (2004). Mobilization strategies after hip fracture surgery in adults. *Cochrane Database Systems Review, 18*(4), CD001704.

Hicks, G., Simonsick, E. M., Harris, T. B., Newman, A. B., Weiner, D. K., Nevitt, M. A., et al. (2005). Trunk muscle composition as a predictor of reduced functional capacity in the health, aging and body composition study: The moderating role of back pain. *Journal of Gerontology A: Biological Sciences Medicine and Science, 60*(11), 1420–1424.

Hirsch, C. H., Sommers, L., Olsen, A., Mullen, L., & Winograd, C. H. (1990). The natural history of functional morbidity in hospitalized older patients. *Journal of the American Geriatrics Society, 38*(12), 1296–1303.

Holy Cross Hospital Geriatric Emergency Room. (2009). Available at: http://www.holycrosshealth.-org/svc_emergency_seniorcenter.htm

Houston, D. J., & Richardson, L. E., Jr. (2006). Safety belt use and the switch to primary enforcement, 1991–2003. *American Journal of Public Health, 96*(11), 1949–1954.

Houston, D. K., Cesar, M., Ferrucci, L., Cherubini, A., Maggio, D., Bartali, B., et al. (2007). Association between vitamin D status and physical performance: The InCHIANTI Study. *Journal of Gerontology: Medical Sciences, 62A*(4), 440–446.

Irvine, A. B., Bourgeois, M., Bilow, M., & Seeley, J. R. (2007). Internet training for nurse aides to prevent resident aggression. *Journal of the American Medical Directors Association, 8*(8), 519–526.

Isal, M., Montorio, I., Marquez, M., & Losada, A. (2005). Caregivers' expectations and care receivers' competence: Lawton's ecological model of adaptation and aging revisited. *Archives of Gerontology and Geriatrics, 41,* 129–140.

Israel Ministry of Foreign Affairs. (2008)*Public health in Israel.* Retrieved from http://www.jewishvirtu-allibrary.org/jsource/Health/public.html

Iwarsson, S. (2005). A long-term perspective on person-environment fit and ADL dependence among older Swedish adults. *Gerontologist, 45*(3), 327–336.

Iwarsson, S., & Slaug, B. (2001a). *The Housing Enabler.* Lund: Studentlitreratur, Lund.

Iwarsson, S., & Slaug, B. (2001b). *Housing Enabler is an instrument for assessments of accessibility in housing.* Retrieved August 2009, from http://www.enabler.nu/

Johnson, C. S. J., Myers, A. M., Jones, G. R., Fitzgerald, C., Lazowski, D. A., Stolee, P., et al. (2004). Evaluation of the restorative care education and training program for nursing homes. *Canadian Journal on Aging, 24*(2), 115–126.

Kadner, K. (1989). Resilience: Responding to adversity. *Journal of Psychosocial Nursing, 27,* 20–25.

Kolanowski, A., Buettner, L., & Moeller, J. (2006). Treatment fidelity plan for an activity intervention designed for persons with dementia. *American Journal of Alzheimer's Disease and Other Dementias, 21,* 326–332.

Landefeld, C. S. (2003). Improving health care for older persons. *Annals of Internal Medicine, 139*, 421–424.

Lyketsos, C. G., Steele, C., Galik, E., Rosenblatt, A., Steinberg, M., Warren, A., et al. (1999). Physical aggression in dementia patients and its relationship to depression. *American Journal of Psychiatry, 156*(1), 66–71.

Margiotta, A., Bianchetti, A., Ranieri, P., & Trabucchi, M. (2006). Clinical characteristics and risk factors of delirium in demented and not demented elderly medical inpatients. *Nutritional Health Aging, 10*(6), 535–539.

Marrelli, T. M. (2003). Restorative care and home care: New implications for aide and nurse? *Geriatric Nursing, 24*(2), 128–129.

McCusker, J., Kakuma, R., & Abrahamowicz, M. (2002). Predictors of functional decline in hospitalized elderly patients: A systematic review. *Journal of Gerontology Series A: Biological Sciences Medicine and Science, 57*(2), M569–M577.

Morley, J., Haren, M. T., Kim, M. J., Kevorkian, R., & Perry, H. M. III. (2005). Testosterone, aging and quality of life. *Journal of Endocrinology Investment, 28*(3 Suppl.), 76–80.

Mudge, A., Laracy, S., Richter, K., & Denaro, C. (2006). Controlled trial of multidisciplinary care teams for acutely ill medical inpatients: Enhanced multidisciplinary care. *Internal Medicine Journal, 36*(9), 558–563.

Nagi, S. (1976). An epidemiology of disability among adults in the United States. *Milbank Memorial Fund Quality Health Society, 54*, 439–467.

Nair, K. (2005). Aging muscle. *American Journal of Clinical Nutrition 81*(5), 953–963.

Nigg, C., Maddock, J., Yamauchi, J., Pressler, V., Wood, B., & Jackson, S. (2005). The healthy Hawaii initiative: A social ecological approach promoting healthy communities. *American Journal of Health Promotion, 19*(4), 310–313.

Parkes, J., & Shepperd, S. (2004). Discharge planning from hospital to home. *Cochrane Database of Systematic Reviews, 1*(1), CD 000313.

Penninx, B., Pahor, M., Cesari, M., Corsi, A. M., Woodman, R. C., Bandinelli, S., et al. (2004). Anemia is associated with disability and decreased physical performance and muscle strength in the elderly. *Journal of the American Geriatrics Society, 52*(5), 719–724.

Pomeroy, S., & Resnick, B. (2007). Person-environment fit (PE-Fit) and functioning among older adults in a long term care setting. *The Gerontologist, 47*(1), 305.

Pretzer-Aboff, I., Galik, E., & Resnick, B. (2009). Caring for the individual with Parkinson's disease: The experience of caregivers and individuals with Parkinson's disease. *Journal of Rehabilitation Nursing, 34*(2), 55–63, 83.

Remsburg, R., Armacost, K., Radu, C., & Bennet, R. (1999). Two models of restorative nursing care in the nursing home: Designated versus integrated restorative nursing assistants. *Geriatric Nursing, 20*, 321–326.

Resnick, B. (1999). Motivation and the older adult: Can a leopard change its spots? *Journal of Advanced Nursing, 29*, 792–799.

Resnick, B. (2002). Geriatric rehabilitation: The influence of efficacy beliefs and motivation. *Rehabilitation Nursing, 27*(4), 152–159.

Resnick, B., Allen, P., & Ruane, K. (2002). Testing the Effectiveness of a Restorative Care Program. *Long-term Care Interface, 3*(11), 25–30.

Resnick, B., Gruber-Baldini, A. L., Galik, E., Pretzer-Aboff, I., Russ, K., Hebel, J. R., et al. (2009). Changing the philosophy of care in long term care: Testing of the Res-Care Intervention. *The Gerontologist, 49*(2), 175–184.

Resnick, B., Magaziner, J., Orwig, D., Yu-Yahiro, J., Hawkes, W., Shardell, M., et al. (2007). Testing the effectiveness of the Exercise Plus Program in older women post hip fracture. *Annals of Behavioral Medicine, 34*(1), 67–76.

Resnick, B., Pretzer-Aboff, I., Galik, E., Russ, K., Cayo, J., Simpson, M., et al. (2008). Barriers and benefits to implementing a restorative care intervention in nursing homes. *Journal of the American Medical Directors Association, 9*(2), 102–108.

Resnick, B., & Simpson, M. (2003). Restorative care nursing activities: Pilot testing self efficacy and outcome expectation measures. *Geriatric Nursing, 24*(2), 83–87.

Resnick, B., Simpson, M., Bercovitz, A., Galik, E., Gruber-Baldini, A., & Zimmerman, S. (2006). Pilot testing of the restorative care program: Impact on residents. *Journal of Gerontological Nursing, 2*, 11–14.

Resnick, B., Simpson, M., Galik, E., Bercovitz, A., Gruber-Baldini, A., & Zimmerman, S. (2006). Making a difference: Nursing assistants' perspectives of restorative care nursing. *Rehabilitation Nursing, 31*(2), 78–86.

Rigney, T. S. (2006). Delirium in the hospitalized elder and recommendations for practice. *Geriatric Nursing, 27*(3), 151–157.

Robinson-Smith, G., Johnston, M. V., & Allen, J. (2000). Self-care, self-efficacy, quality of life, and depression after stroke. *Archives of Physical Medicine and Rehabilitation, 81*(4), 460–464.

Robinson, B., Artz, A. S., Culleton, B., Critchlow, C., Sciarra, A., & Audhya, P. (2007). Prevalence of anemia in the nursing home: Contribution of chronic kidney disease. *Journal of the American Geriatrics Society, 55,* 1566–1570.

Rodiek, S. (2006). Resident perceptions of physical environment features that influence outdoor usage at assisted living facilities. *Journal of Housing for the Elderly, 19*(3–4), 95–107.

Rogers, J. C., Holm, M. B., Burgio, L. D., Granieri, E., Hsu, C., Hardin, J. M., et al. (1999). Improving morning care routines of nursing home residents with dementia. *Journal of the American Geriatrics Society, 47,* 1049–1057.

Sager, M. A., Rugberg, M. A., & Jalaluddin, M. (1996). Hospital admission risk profile (HARP): Identifying older patients at risk for functional decline following acute medical illness and hospitalization. *Journal of the American Geriatrics Society, 44*(2), 251–257.

Sallis, J. (2003). New thinking on older adults' physical activity. *Journal of Preventive Medicine, 25*(3Sii), 110–112.

Sallis, J., & Glanz, K. (2006). The role of built environments in physical activity, eating, and obesity in childhood. *Future Child, 16*(1), 89–108.

Sandman, P. O., Norberg, A., Adolfsson, R., Axelsson, K., & Hedly, V. (1985). Morning care of patients with Alzheimer-type dementia: A theoretical model based on direct observations. *Journal of Advanced Nursing, 11,* 369–378.

Schalk, B., Visser, M., Penninx, B. W., Baadenhuijsen, H., Bouter, L. M., & Deeg, D. J. (2005). Change in serum albumin and subsequent decline in functional status in older persons. *Aging Clinics and Experimental Research 17*(4), 297–305.

Shanti, C., Johnson, J., Meyers, A. M., Jones, G. R., Fitzgerald, C., & Lazowski, D. A. (2005). Evaluation of the restorative care education and training program for nursing homes. *Canadian Journal of Aging, 24*(2), 115–126.

Singh, A., Chin A Paw, M. J., Bosscher, R. J., & van Mechelen, W. (2006). Cross-sectional relationship between physical fitness components and functional performance in older persons living in long-term care facilities. *Biomedical Central Geriatrics, 6,* 4–6.

Stuck, A. E., Siu, A. L., Wieland, G. D., Adams, J., & Rubenstein, L. Z. (1993). Comprehensive geriatric assessment: A meta analysis of controlled trials. *Lancet, 342,* 1032–1036.

Tabari-Khomeiran, R., Kiger, A., Parsa-Yekta, Z., & Ahmadi, F. (2007). Competence development among nurses: the process of constant interaction. *Journal of Continuing Education in Nursing, 38*(5), 211–218.

Tinetti, M. E., Baker, D., Gallo, W. T., Nanda, A., Charpentier, P., & O'Leary, J. (2002). Evaluation of restorative care vs usual care for older adults receiving an acute episode of home care. *Journal of the American Medical Association, 287*(16), 2098–2105.

Tsauo, J., Leu, W., Chen, Y., & Yang, R. (2005). Effects on function and quality of life of postoperative home-based physical therapy for patients with hip fracture. *Archives of Physical Medicine and Rehabilitation, 86*(10), 1953–1957.

Uhrenfeldt, L., & Hall, E. O. (2007). Clinical wisdom among proficient nurses. *Nursing Ethics, 14*(3), 387–398.

van Wijk, I., Algra, A., van de Port, I. G., Bevaart, B., & Lindeman, E. (2006). Change in mobility activity in the second year after stroke in a rehabilitation population: Who is at risk for decline? *Archives of Physical Medicine and Rehabilitation, 87*(1), 45–50.

Volpato, S., Onder, G., Cavalieri, M., Guerra, G., Sioulis, F., & Maraldi, C. (2007). Characteristics of nondisabled older patients developing new disability associated with medical illnesses and hospitalization. *Journal of General Internal Medicine, 22*(5), 668–674.

Wagner, L. M., Capezuti, E., Brush, B., Boltz, M., Renz, S., & Talerico, K. A. (2007). Description of an advanced practice nursing consultative model to reduce restrictive siderail use in nursing homes. *Research in Nursing & Health, 30,* 131–140.

Wagnild, G. (2003). Resilience and successful aging. Comparison among low and high income older adults. *Journal of Gerontological Nursing, 29*(12), 42–49.

Wakefield, B. J. (2002). Behaviors and outcomes of acute confusion in hospitalized patients. *Applied Nursing Research, 15*(4), 209–216.

Wakefield, B. J., & Holman, J. E. (2007). Functional trajectories associated with hospitalization in older adults. *Western Journal of Nursing Research, 29*(2), 161–177.

Wardh, I., Hallberg, L., Berggren, U., Andersson, L., & Sorensen, S. (2003). Oral health education for nursing personnel; experiences among specially trained oral care aides: One-year follow-up interviews with oral care aides at a nursing facility. Scandinavian Journal of Caring Sciences, 17(3), 250–256.

Winograd, C. H., Lidenberger, E. C., Chavez, C. M., Muauricio, M. P., Shi, H., & Bloch, D. A. (1997). Identifying hospitalized older patients at varying risk for physical performance decline: A new approach. Journal of the American Geriatrics Society, 45(5), 604–609.

Wolfe, S., Nordstrom, C., & Williams, K. (1998). The effect of enhancing self-efficacy prior to job training. Journal of Social Behavior and Personality, 13, 633–651.

# Part III

# Foundations for Clinical Care of Critically Ill Older Adults

# Physiology of Aging: Impact on Critical Illness and Treatment

## 12

Alexandra J. Brock
Rita A. Jablonski

## Introduction

There are many theories of aging that focus on various aspects of the person. Theories and frameworks related to aging arise from many specialties, including sociology, psychology, biology, and spirituality. The simplest definition of aging is the sum of changes that occur with the passage of time (Fletcher, 2007). In physiological terms, normal aging involves the steady erosion of organ system reserve and homeostatic controls, "this erosion is evident only during periods of maximal exertion and stress," (Williams, 2008, p. 13). The more precise term for aging is "senescence," which refers to the usual changes in physiological processes affecting all of the organ systems with different onset, rates, and magnitudes that result in a decline in reserve ending in death (Timiras, 2007). Intrinsic and extrinsic variables that stress bodies affect how one ages and at what rate there is a functional decline of reserve.

As people age, usual physiologic changes occur. These changes have variability among individuals. The impact of these changes inherently begins to reduce the physiologic reserve of the body systems. Unlike younger bodies that have larger reserves from which to draw on and recover, aging bodies have less reserve. Repeated stressors on an aging body result in difficult and prolonged recovery, and, eventually, an inability to recover.

The interplay of genetics, environment, and life choices results in a heterogeneous elderly population with many different levels of vulnerabilities that affect the aging process as well as responses to critical illnesses. Recovery is dependent on each person's inherent physiologic reserve. The magnitude of these aging variations among individuals challenges the health care team in critical care. Early assessment, prevention, and intervention are needed to decrease potential complications and further physical and functional decline in the elderly patient. This requires vigilance; "vigilance by nurses is a central component of nursing care of the older persons who are hospitalized" (Moore & Duffy, 2007, p. 313). In addition to vigilance, critical thinking and a core understanding of usual physiology of aging versus pathologic disease processes establishes an environment in which knowledge and experience are combined. Correctly identifying and treating the vague and sometimes atypical signs and symptoms demonstrated in older adults is paramount in preventing new problems and correcting current deviations in health when caring for older adults in the critical care environment (Rutschmann et al., 2005; Timiras, 2007; Wolf, Foley, & Howard, 2007).

Although older adults represent approximately 50% of the patient population in critical care (Carson, 2003), there is limited research in critical care that focuses on this population exclusively (Fulmer, Flaherty, Bottrell, Fletcher, & Mezey, 2000; Nagappan & Parkin, 2003; Richmond & Jacoby, 2007). As noted previously, the older adult population is quite heterogeneous. The purpose of this chapter is to examine usual changes in physiology that accompany aging by organ system in older adults, and their impact on critical illness; early assessment and clinical recommendations also are discussed.

# The Pulmonary System

## Changes With Aging

Pulmonary age-related changes are a result of several factors and include frequently observed modifications in the musculoskeletal structure such as kyphosis and vertebral collapse secondary to osteoporosis (Timiras, 2007). Changes in the airways discussed below are thought to be the result of cumulative exposure to environmental stressors such as allergies, pollution, or smoking. Many of the changes in the pulmonary system seen in older adults are not appreciable at rest or without stress. During physical activity, however, there is a decrease in oxygen uptake that leads to a decrease in activity tolerance. The older adult then becomes less able to tolerate acute hypoxia or hypercapnia (Peterson, Pack, Silage, & Fisherman, 1981; Timiras).

Changes that lead to a decrease in oxygen uptake include a decline in strength of the respiratory muscles, resulting in muscles that become more prone to fatigue during the increased work of breathing. Calcification of the costal cartilages causes a decrease in chest wall compliance and there is a decrease in elasticity of the lungs when the elastic tissue is replaced with fibrous tissue over time. As the elasticity of the lungs decreases, expiration becomes more difficult and air trapping occurs in the alveoli. There is a concurrent decrease in the number of alveoli as the remaining alveoli increase in size with a resultant decrease in gas exchange. This decline in alveoli creates ventilation–perfusion (V/Q) mismatch resulting in a lower V/Q of the lungs. Lower V/Q and hypoxemia occur together. Multiple small alveoli have greater

## 12.1   The Pulmonary System

| Changes With Aging | Significance to Critical Illness |
|---|---|
| ■ Decrease in respiratory muscle mass and strength | ■ Decreased ability to inhale and exhale<br>■ Increased use of accessory muscles |
| ■ Increase in chest wall stiffness | ■ Increased energy expenditure to breathe<br>■ Increased anterior–posterior diameter |
| ■ Increase in air trapping | |
| ■ Decrease in elasticity of lung tissue | |
| ■ Increase in cross-linked collagen | ■ Lung tissue stiffens<br>■ Increase in residual capacity |
| ■ Decrease in number of alveoli | ■ Decrease in vital capacity |
| ■ Increase in size of alveoli | ■ Decreased FVC |
| ■ Decrease in gas exchange | ■ Increased dead air space<br>■ Decreased V/Q |
| ■ Decrease in mucociliary clearance | ■ Increasing A-a gradient |
| | ■ Decrease in arterial $O_2$ level |
| ■ Decreased cough and gag mechanism (due to changes in musculature and skeletal structure) | ■ Decrease in diffusion of $CO_2$<br>■ Less able to tolerate acute hypoxia and hypercapnia<br>■ Decreased oxygen uptake during stress creating a decreased tolerance to stress<br>■ Mucus is not easily mobilized from lungs<br>■ Increased risk aspiration and infection<br>■ Increased risk of atelectisis<br>■ Obstructed, distant, or displaced heart and lung sounds<br>■ Decreased reserve |

Synthesized from Fletcher (2007), Miller (2009), Timirus (2007), Urden et al. (2006).

surface area for oxygen exchange between the air and the capillaries. When alveoli expand, there is a loss of surface area for ventilation. This results in more deoxygenated blood returning to the left heart and an increasing A-a gradient (alveolar to arterial oxygen pressure difference $PA_{02} - PAO_2$) (Ellstrom, 2006). At rest, these changes do not impede oxygenation sufficiently to cause hypoxemia; during periods of stress or increased activity, the lack of alveolar surface area results in hypoxic conditions. Additionally, lung cilia decrease in both number and activity, resulting in reduced mucociliary clearance. A weakened or impaired cough mechanism, combined with poor ciliary motility, increases the probability of infection in the lungs (see Table 12.1).

### Assessment, Impact on Critical Illness, and Clinical Recommendations

Pulmonary physiology and pathophysiology in the elderly can have a fundamental impact on the older patient in the critical care environment. During a physical assessment, noted changes may include skeletal postural changes that impair chest expansion and an increase in chest anteroposterior diameter caused by air trapping in the alveoli. Pulmonary function tests will show approximately 5–10% per decade increase in residual capacity, a decrease in vital capacity (VC), and a reduction in forced expiratory volume (FEV) (Miller, 2009). Furthermore, maximum inspiratory and expiratory pressure will decrease. Laboratory values will also reflect the effects of physical changes. Arterial oxygen partial pressure ($PaO_2$) will decline slightly but both arterial carbon dioxide partial pressure ($CaO_2$) and hydrogen ion concentration (pH) will remain normal. Higher oxygen delivery ($FiO_2$) may be necessary to meet increased demand. Elderly patients will be more prone to retain secretions because of decreased cough and gag reflexes; they will also be more susceptible to aspiration, infection, pneumonia, and atelectasis influencing length of stay in the hospital and critical care unit (Marik & Kaplan, 2003; Sevransky & Haponik, 2003).

Respiratory status in the critically ill older patient can be central to recovery. During critical illnesses, respiratory reserve is stressed and oxygen demands are increased by many factors, including acute illness, wound healing, blood and fluid loss, and surgery. Additionally, if the older adult either is inactive because of functional limitations or enforced bed rest, the inactivity combined with respiratory changes seen in older adults results in complications such as increased mechanical ventilatory weaning time, or even an inability to wean (Sevransky & Haponik, 2003). To minimize potential complications, nutritional status, pulmonary toileting, chest physiotherapy, oral care, and early mobility require attention. In fact, early mobilization in the ventilated patient is not only possible and safe but also necessary (Bailey et al., 2007; Morris, 2007; Morris & Herridge, 2007; Nelson et al., 2004; Stiller, 2007; Timmerman, 2007). To improve respiratory outcomes in the older adult in the acute care setting, close observation of the respiratory status and relevant laboratory values, with a lower threshold of suspicion as compared to younger adults, is necessary to intervene and protect declining reserve (Sevransky & Haponik).

## Impact on Elderly: Respiratory Problems Common in Critical Care

■ Intubation and Weaning

■ Chronic ventilatory dependence disproportionately affects the elderly (Cox et al., 2007; Kleinhenz & Lewis, 2000).

■ Age does not necessarily impact duration of mechanical ventilation, weaning, or mortality. Mechanical ventilation outcomes are affected by baseline functional status, comorbidities, acute renal failure, multiorgan failure, shock, and a ratio of $PaO_2$ / $FIO_2$ greater than 150* (Esteban et al., 2004; Kleinhenz & Lewis 2000; Kollef, 1993). *Normal is 300–400; less than 300 is representative of acute lung injury (ALI) or acute respiratory distress syndrome (ARDS). This number can show a reduction in oxygenating efficiencies that may be hidden by increases in $FiO_2$ and normal range $PaO_2$ (Matuschak, 2008).

■ Baseline of rapid and shallow breathing as compared to younger adults can slow weaning because critical care nurses attribute the rapid and shallow breathing to respiratory failure. Older adults may breathe slightly faster and shallower than their younger counterparts because of less respiratory reserve. These breathing patterns do not automatically preclude weaning and weaning can continue under closer observation (Sprung, Gajic, & Warner, 2006).

■ Older adults are less likely to recognize the sensation of dyspnea, delaying recognition of respiratory problems until the problems progress to later stages (Torres & Moayedi, 2007).

■ Decreased response to hypoxia and hypercapnia can mask impending failure until critical values are reached (Peterson et al., 1981).

■ Use of arterial blood gases in the elderly may have a greater utility in recognition of changes in older adults when making decisions regarding weaning or impending respiratory failure (Siner & Pisani, 2007).

■ Acute Lung Injury and Acute Respiratory Distress Syndrome

■ Incidence of both increases with age (Manzano et al., 2005; Rubenfeld et al., 2005).

■ Recovery from acute phase of ARDS is equal to younger patients but older adults have an increasingly difficult time recovering from multiorgan failure, remaining extubated and transferring out of the intensive care unit (ICU); as a result older adults have lower survival rates (Ely et al., 2002; Siner & Pisani, 2007).

■ Interventions focused on preventing nonpulmonary complications improve outcomes for elderly patients with ARDS (Eachempati, Hydo, Shou, & Barie, 2005).

■ Rib Fractures/Trauma

■ Older adults have twice the mortality and morbidly of younger patients with the same injury (Bulger, Arneson, Mock, & Jurkovich, 2000).

■ When treating the pain from rib fractures or trauma, epidural analgesia is preferred over intravenous or oral narcotics in elderly patients (Bulger et al., 2000; Wisner, 1990).

■ Early and aggressive respiratory care in older adults is of paramount importance to avoid pulmonary complications and intubation, which are associated with higher mortality in this population (Chelluri et al., 2004).

■ Pneumonia/ventilator-associated pneumonia and higher rates of silent aspiration are noted in elderly patients with decreased cough reflexes and dysphagia (Kikuchi et al., 1994; Marik & Kaplan, 2003).

■ Increased thorax muscle weakness contributes to decreased cough and gag reflexes, increasing the risk for aspiration and associated pneumonia (Timiras, 2007).

# Cardiovascular System

## Changes With Aging

Usual changes that occur with the cardiovascular system have considerable variation in older adults and are often the culmination of genetics, environment, comorbid illnesses, and life choices (Timiras, 2007). Apparent decreases in cardiac reserve may not be appreciable in the daily activity of an older adult "but when that same person experiences physiologic stress such as blood loss, hypoxia, sepsis, or volume depletion, the lack of reserve becomes apparent through cardiac dysfunction" (Marik, 2006, p. S177).

Over time, central arterial structures become thick walled and dilated, with a decrease in elasticity and an increase in peripheral vascular resistance; these changes result in decreased peripheral pulses. Along with these atherosclerotic and vascular changes, there is a modest left-ventricular hypertrophy that may be appreciated on a chest radiograph and may be a clinically normal finding (Lakatta, 2000). Sclerosis and concomitant thickening of heart valves contribute to stenosis or incompetent valves, which impair cardiac blood flow. Collagen and lipid deposits increase in the cardiac muscle as people age (Lakatta, 2002); although the total effect of this is unclear, it may contribute to increase ventricular stiffness and hypertension (Levine & Craven, 2005). Structural and functional changes in the atria may also contribute to the increased prevalence of atrial fibrillation observed in older adults (Timiras, 2007). Changes or decreases in pacemaker cells in the sinoatrial (SA) and atrioventricular (AV) nodes, as well as Bundle of His and bundle branches may contribute to irregular heart rate, increase in myocardial irritability, and decreased heart rate response to stress. Changes may also be attributed to a diminished response to adrenergic stimulation in the heart (Rooke, 2000). Although the resting heart rate remains consistent over time, heart rate variability decreases with age, reflecting changes in the parasympathetic and sympathetic nervous system. These adrenergic changes thus result in the reduction in heart rate variability that predisposes older adults to postural hypotension and increased risks for falls (Timiras) (see Table 12.2).

## Assessment, Impact on Critical Illness, and Clinical Recommendations

Changes in the heart and ventricles result in an increased dependence on adequate filling pressure. As the heart ages it is less responsive to central nervous system (CNS) triggers caused by decreased blood pressure. Adequate fluid volumes are necessary to maintain cardiac output; however, this can become a balancing act to avoid creating conditions of fluid overload in the elderly. Periods of hypervolemia that result when the heart is compromised or stressed can then cause systolic failure resulting in decreased organ perfusion and hypoxemia (Rosenthal & Kavic, 2004).

Decreases in heart rate or minimal increases in heart rate may be an unrecognized response to stress. Using heart rate as an indicator of fever, sepsis, hypovolemia, hypervolemia, and pain may be unreliable in older adults. Prolonged periods of elevated heart rate may be associated with cardiac complications resulting from increased myocardial oxygen demand, decreased cardiac reserve, and functional changes. Extra care should be taken to maintain fluid balance. Ideally, the central venous pressures (CVP) should remain between 8–10 mmHg, pulmonary artery occlusion pressures between 14–18 mmHg, (Rosenthal & Kavic, 2004) and the heart rate under 95 beats per minute during a critical illness (Sander, Welters, Foex, & Sear, 2005). Careful consideration should be given to either invasive or noninvasive hemodynamic monitoring to ensure that optimal fluid status is maintained in the older critical care patient (C. V. R. Brown, Shoemaker, Wo, Chan, & Demetriades, 2005). Atypical and nonspecific signs and symptom presentation in the elderly, especially in the critical

## 12.2   The Cardiovascular System

| Changes With Aging | Significance to Critical Illness |
|---|---|
| ▪ Changes in heart valve—fibrous, thickening, and increased rigidity<br>▪ Decreased pacemaker cells in the SA and AV nodes<br>▪ Increase in myocardial collagen and lipids<br>▪ Arterial stiffening<br>▪ Decreased baroreceptor mechanism<br>▪ Changes to the parasympathetic and sympathetic systems result in changes in adrenergic response | ▪ S3—possible CHF<br>▪ S4—possible hypertensive CV disease, CAD, aortic stenosis, severe anemia<br>▪ Increased peripheral vascular resistance<br>▪ Impaired left ventricular filling with some left ventricular hypertrophy and prolonged contraction and relaxation of ventricle<br>▪ Decreased SV<br>▪ Increased aortic volume and systolic blood pressure<br>▪ Decreased maximal CO<br>▪ Increased dependence on filling pressure; increasing risk of fluid overload<br>▪ Maintenance of CO is achieved by increasing preload and SV instead of HR<br>▪ Decrease in maximal HR<br>▪ Increased myocardial irritability<br>▪ EKG changes<br>▪ Decreased coronary artery blood flow<br>▪ Decreased oxygen use<br>▪ Decrease in inotropic and chronotropic response<br>▪ Increased postural blood pressure changes<br>▪ Decrease in adaptability to stress with increased HR<br>▪ Atypical or silent MI<br>▪ Decreased reserve |

Synthesized from Fletcher (2007), Miller (2009), Timirus (2007), Urden et al. (2006).

care environment, may make it difficult to identify patients who are further compromised until it is too late (Flaherty & Zwicker, 2005).

Deviations from the standard S1, S2 heart sounds assessment can be an indicator of cardiac pathological changes. S3 may indicate congestive heart failure, and S4 can be associated with hypertensive cardiovascular disease and coronary artery disease, aortic stenosis, and severe anemia. A summation gallop of S3 and S4 indicate severe myocardial disease and tachycardia. Both of these extra heart sounds together are NOT an expected finding in usual aging in the absence of other pathological findings (Lakatta, 2002).

## Impact on Elderly: Cardiovascular Problems Common in Critical Care

▪ Tachycardia and bradycardia

▪ Decline in intrinsic and maximal heart rate; and an increase in recovery time to return to resting heart rate after times of stress (Lakatta & Levy, 2003; Levine & Craven, 2005; Rooke, 2000).

- ■ Prolonged increases in heart rate are associated with an increase in cardiac complications (Sander et al., 2005).

- ■ Maintenance of cardiac output in the elderly is achieved by increasing preload and stroke volume unlike younger patients. In younger patients, cardiac output is achieved by increasing the heart rate via beta-adrenergic stimulation (Levine & Craven, 2005; Rooke, 2000).

- ■ Tachyarrhythmias are less tolerated in the older patient because of decreased ventricular compliance resulting in pulmonary edema (Marik, 2006).

■ Myocardial infarction (MI)

- ■ MI may be missed because older adults are less likely to complain of chest pain but are more likely to complain of vague symptoms such as fatigue and nausea (Gregoratos, 2001).

- ■ Shortness of breath is the most common symptom of MI in the elderly (Flaherty & Zwicker, 2005), which may be masked by an endotracheally intubated and mechanically ventilated patient.

# Neurological System

## Changes With Aging

Like the pulmonary and the cardiovascular system, changes in the neurological system reflect the influence of genetics, environment, and life choices. Computerized axial tomography (CAT) scans have uncovered visible decreases in both the size and volume of the brain in older adults (Esiri, 2007). To compensate for reduced brain volume, the ventricle system and cerebral spinal fluid system create a slightly larger subarachnoid space (Esiri). There is also a reduction in neurons, neurotransmitters, dendrites, glial cells, and support cells; however, there is controversy over the meaning of the extent of these decreases and losses (Arking, 2006; Esiri). There are changes in synapses and slowing of nerve conduction velocity and increased neuronal vulnerability with age. There exists additional debate as to whether changes in neurons should be considered a usual pathologic process (Esiri). Other changes include a progressive increase of iron in regions of the brain that are affected by Alzheimer's and Parkinson's disease. The increase in iron may lead to oxidative stress in brain aging (Floyd & Hensley, 2002; Zecca, Youdim, Riederer, Conner, & Crichton, 2004).

The implications of the aforementioned changes in the neurological system can be observed in an overall decrease in muscular strength, a decline in deep tendon reflexes, and slowed motor skills in the majority of older adults (Timiras, 2007). These motor changes, combined with changes in vision, hearing, and balance from the vestibular apparatus can create challenges in balance and coordination. Cognitive-associated changes in the nervous system do not necessarily affect overall intelligence. Reasoning often improves, but the slowing in the processing powers, however, prolongs the time needed to form thoughts and quickly generate words (Albert, Killiany, Birren, & Schaie, 2001; Backman, Small, Wahlin, Birren, & Schaie, 2001; Ketcham,

## 12.3 The Neurological System

| Changes With Aging | Significance to Critical Illness |
|---|---|
| ■ Decrease in brain weight and volume<br>■ Decrease in neuron size, controversy exists over the extent of neuron loss<br>■ Decrease in dendrites and synapses<br>■ Increases in iron<br>■ Increased vulnerability of neurons with age<br>■ Decreased cerebral blood flow (CBF) and impaired auto regulation of perfusion<br>■ Increase in senile plaque in extracellular space of cerebral cortex | ■ Subdural hematomas even possible with minor trauma<br>■ Slowed reaction time<br>■ Slowed speed of cognition in processing and retrieval<br>■ Decrease in attention and memory<br>■ Decline in fluid intelligence<br>■ Decline in ability to quickly generate words<br>■ Increases in iron may lead to oxidative stress<br>■ Decreases tactile senses<br>■ Decrease in muscle strength<br>■ Decline in deep tendon Achilles reflexes<br>■ Slowed motor skills<br>■ Challenges in balance and coordination<br>■ Increased risk of falls<br>■ Altered pain response<br>■ Changes in sleep wake cycles<br>■ Decline or change in vision and hearing<br>■ Increased vulnerability to delirium |

Synthesized from Fletcher (2007), Miller (2009),Timirus (2007), Urden et al. (2006).

Stelmach, Birren, & Schaie, 2001). Changes in cognition and memory can be a usual finding but these changes do not occur homogeneously in the elderly population. Many changes will not be noticed until a person is in a situation of stress and illness that may spotlight minor deficits in motor and cognition otherwise unnoticed in a person's day-to-day activity. Other changes that are considered usual with aging are increased changes in sleep patterns (see chapter 17, this volume), increased risk of delirium (see chapter 26, this volume), and the development of neurodegenerative diseases such as Parkinson's and Alzheimer's dementia (Timiras). Changes in the hypothalamus can affect the neuroendocrine system (Arking, 2006); these changes are addressed in the endocrine section of the chapter. See Table 12.3 for an overview of neurological changes in the older adult.

### Assessment, Impact on Critical Illness, and Clinical Recommendations

Clinical assessment and recommendations for the neurological system focus on the accuracy of diagnosis. The implications for a wrong diagnosis of dementia or the assumption that immobility, changes in level of consciousness, agitation, or any other neurologically based assessment are caused by "usual" aging or are a normative finding can be detrimental and can negatively affect the overall outcome of the hospitalization. In the critical care setting determining what is a usual finding and a baseline assessment can be challenging. Complete history taking and family interviews are important tools in determining what is usual and what constitutes an abnormality for an older patient. With many hospital admissions and critical care admissions in which the patient is not able or is not a reliable source of information, finding resources can be difficult and time consuming, but the impact of accurate diagnosis, treatment plan, outcomes, cost, and ease of care can be enormous.

Assessment findings may include declines in visual acuity and depth perception. Pupillary changes may not necessarily be a neurological finding (Timiras, 2007) and an understanding of the patient history and medications are important when interpreting assessment findings. Difficulty with balance, postural control, and proprioception will have an impact on fall risk and mobility. Sense of touch and vibratory sensation also may be decreased (Timiras), which could have an impact on assessment findings or the patient's ability to move his/her hand away from a negative stimuli while confined to bed in the ICU.

Delirium, an acute neurological change in the elderly, is a reversible finding that may be attributed to nonneurological events (Inouye, 2006). Delirium resulting in alterations in level of consciousness and motor functioning can result from many factors, including changes in electrolytes, infection, medications, pain, surgery, use of indwelling bladder catheters, and use of restraints (Inouye). Delirium can also be caused by emotional stress and lack of sleep. Careful consideration should be taken in the ICU to provide patients with a method to communicate while concomitantly providing additional time for responses. Older adult patients also require access to clean eyeglasses and functioning hearing aids. Frequent orientation to time and place with clocks and visual cues is beneficial as well. Although the need to assess and care for older adults in the ICU is a 24-hour responsibility, nurses working on the evening and night shift can prevent delirium from lack of sleep by clustering their activities to allow for extended periods of rest (see chapters 17 and 26, this volume), and monitoring the older adult as unobtrusively as possible during late evening and night hours to promote quality sleep.

## Impact on Elderly: Neurologic Issues Common in Critical Care

- Delirium

    - Delirium can be superimposed on dementia, making it harder to diagnosis (Fick, Agostini & Inouye, 2002).

    - Delirium is associated with higher mortality, longer hospitalization, and increased costs (Thomason et al., 2005).

    - Rarely caused by a single factor, delirium is usually multifactorial (Morandi, Jackson, & Ely, 2009).

    - Primary prevention is the best treatment strategy for delirium (Milisen, Braes, Fick, & Foreman, 2005)

    - Patients aged 65 and older are at higher risks for delirium (Inouye, 2006).

    - Risk for delirium increases after surgery (Balas et al., 2007).

- Pain

    - Perception and reporting of pain by older adults is complicated by cultural, generational ideology, and personality factors (see chapter 18, this volume).

> Combined with mechanical ventilation and impaired communication, these factors can contribute to underreporting of pain and undertreatment of pain (Happ, Tuite, Dobbin, DiVirgilio-Thomas, & Kitutu, 2004; Horgas & Elliott, 2004).

■ Increased heart rate and blood pressure, along with other sympathetic responses to pain, is not generally a good indicator of pain in the older adult as compared to younger adults because of many factors, including medications and changes in the neurological, neuroendocrine, and cardio-vascular systems.

■ Control of pain can be complicated by the need to prevent under- and oversedation, which along with pain can cause delirium and adverse outcomes.

■ There is evidence to suggest that the cognitively impaired older adult is treated for pain less often then the cognitively intact older adult (Horgas & Elliott, 2004).

■ Nonverbal symptoms of pain can manifest similarly to delirium and be a contributing factor to delirium (Bjoro & Herr, 2008).

# Renal System

## Changes With Aging

Aging-related changes in the renal system initially have minimal impact on renal function until chronic or acute illnesses place additional burdens that exceed renal reserve (Silva, 2005). Renal changes in older adults are thought to reflect the cardiovascular changes observed in older adults, such as increased blood pressure and reduced cardiac functioning, rather than any sole intrinsic change (Fliser et al., 1997). Some of the renal changes observed in older adults include reduction in overall kidney mass, decline in renal blood flow, gradual loss of nephrons secondary to less renal blood flow, diminished glomerular filtration rate (GFR), declining creatinine clearance, and increased blood urea nitrogen (BUN) concentration. These summative changes result in a decrease in the ability to conserve or excrete sodium and potassium, dilute and concentrate urine, and excrete hydrogen ions. In addition to these changes, there is a concurrent decline in renal response to the sympathetic nervous system, the renin–angiotensin–aldosterone system, plus a decreased sensitivity to antidiuretic hormone (ADH) in the renal tubules, resulting in an altered response to hypervolemia and hypovolemia (Silva; Taffett, 2006; Timiras, 2007).

The genitourinary changes that may have an impact on critical illness for both men and women surround the bladder and its ability to empty (see chapter 22, this volume). There is a decrease in muscular tone of the bladder that can result in incomplete bladder empting, and decreased sensation of urge to urinate until the bladder is full. These changes may contribute to urinary incontinence as well as increased postvoid residuals. In men, prostatic hypertrophy can lead to urinary frequency and difficulty (Silva, 2005; Taffett, 2006; Timiras, 2007) (see Table 12.4).

## 12.4  The Renal System

| Changes With Aging | Significance to Critical Illness |
|---|---|
| ■ Some renal changes reflect cardiovascular changes<br>■ Decreased sympathetic response<br>■ Decreased renal blood flow<br>■ Decreased renal mass<br>■ Decrease in functioning nephrons<br>■ Decrease in glomerular filtration rate (GRF)<br>■ Decrease in bladder and urinary tract muscle tone and elasticity<br>■ Decreased renin and aldosterone<br>■ Decreased response to ADH<br>■ Male—benign prostatic hypertrophy | ■ Decreased ability to maintain homeostasis<br>■ Decreased ability to conserve and excrete sodium<br>■ Decreased / impaired secretion of hydrogen ions—once patient is acidotic it may take longer to compensate, remaining in an uncompensated state longer<br>■ Decreased ability to dilute and concentrate urine<br>■ Decreased ability to respond to hypovolemia and hypervolemia<br>■ Decreased clearance of some drugs<br>■ Decreased bladder capacity<br>■ Increased urinary retention or post void residuals<br>■ May not have a sensation to urinate until bladder is completely full<br>■ Increased vulnerability to urinary incontinence<br>■ Increase nocturia<br>■ Increased risk of infections<br>■ Increased vulnerability to nephrotoxins<br>■ Increase vulnerability to renal failure<br>■ Decreased reserve |

Synthesized from Fletcher (2007), Miller (2009),Timirus (2007), Urden et al. (2006).

## Assessment, Impact on Critical Illness, and Clinical Recommendations

Nurses may not be able to visually note changes in kidney function, but rather recognize the impact of these changes in the overall homeostasis of the body. Care decisions pertinent to changes in renal function and specific to the critical care environment include replacement therapy to restore electrolyte balances, acid–base fluctuation, and fluid balances. In other words, the diminished or slower ability to balance electrolytes (in particular sodium and potassium) can predispose to electrolyte increases that affect blood pressure and create fluid shifts. As older adults lose the ability to concentrate urine, they are particularly sensitive to volume depletion and dehydration, which raise blood osmolarity. Hypovolemia and low blood pressure can further contribute to low kidney perfusion, contributing to an already diminished GFR, which further impairs function, creating renal failure (Cheung, Ponnusamy, & Anderton, 2008).

Additionally, the older patient is more likely to suffer from acute renal failure and acidosis, with a decreased ability to eliminate ammonia and acid load in response to stressors such as shock and sepsis (Silva, 2005). In a state of acidosis, it becomes difficult for the already compromised senescent kidneys to regulate pH, predisposing the older patient to acidosis. Furthermore, the decrease in nephrons and the overloading of the existing nephrons with solute decreases renal clearance of drugs, which can lead to a buildup of toxins and adverse drug events (Timiras, 2007).

The use of indwelling bladder catheters interacts with the aforementioned anatomical changes and diminished immune function to create an enhanced risk for bladder infections (Richards, 2003; Suchinski, Piano, Rosenberg, & Zerwic, 1999). Indwelling catheters also restrict mobility in an older adult, which places the elder at risk for delirium, functional decline, and falls. Given these risks, it is necessary to explore alternatives for measuring fluid balance, such as the use of a bedside commode with a urine measurement "hat"; however, this may be difficult in the ICU setting. If a urinary catheter is completely necessary, it should be removed at the earliest opportunity. However, incontinence is never a "usual or common" event but an indication of some other underlying problem such as incomplete bladder emptying. In this instance, straight catheterization may be necessary after voiding to avoid large post-void residuals. With urinary incontinence, meticulous skin care is important to avoid skin breakdown.

## Impact on Elderly: Renal Issues Common in Critical Care

- Acute renal failure (ARF)

  - Senescent renal changes that increase the risk of ARF include decreases in number of glomeruli and capillaries and subsequent decline in GRF, changes in autoregulatory vascular response, renal tubular frailty, and salt and water wasting secondary to reduced tubular reabsorption capability (Cheung, Ponnusamy, & Anderton, 2008; Musso, Liakopoulos, Ioannidis, Eleftheriadis, & Stefanidis, 2006).

  - Because of the predisposition to decreased kidney reserve, prevention is the best treatment.

  - Risk factors are similar to other age groups and include hypovolemic shock, septic shock, cardiovascular events, nephrotoxic agents: antibiotics, nonsteriodal antiinflamatory agents, chemotherapeutics, and contrast dyes. Prenal causes are more common in the elderly then renal causes (Timiras, 2007).

  - Mortality from ARF is high and consequently could benefit from therapy but underlying kidney reserve at admission does affect outcomes (Akposs, et al., 2000; Haas, Spargo, Wit & Meehan, 2000; Van Den Noortgate et al., 2003).

- Electrolyte imbalance

  - Electrolyte imbalances must be carefully monitored and treated. When replacing fluid and electrolytes, baseline kidney function must be considered when assessing for risks of kidney failure (Akposso et al., 2000; Haas et al., 2000; Van Den Noortgate et al., 2003).

  - Changes in renin–angiotensin—aldosterone system can lead to hyponatremia or hypernatremia. (Luckey & Parsa, 2003).

- Hypervolemia and hypovolemia

  - Changes in cardiac and renal functionality and reserve in the elderly result in vulnerability to changes in electrolytes and fluid shifts.

  - Dehydration and hypovolemia can cause worsening function of heart and kidneys.

■ Overhydration from excess fluids can lead to systolic failure and poor organ perfusion. Changes in the kidney with aging decrease the ability to eliminate large fluid volume loads (Rosenthal & Kavic, 2004).

■ Elderly patients have a prolonged period of edema after fluid resuscitation in sepsis as compared to younger patients and this contributes to a poorer outcome from critical illness (Cheng, Plank, & Hill, 1998).

■ Persistent positive fluid balances are associated with increased ventilator days in the elderly (Epstein & Peerless, 2006).

# Endocrine, Hematological, and Immunological Systems

## Changes With Aging

Changes in the endocrine system are not necessarily normal but commonly occur in older adults; there is a high prevalence of endocrine disorders such as diabetes and thyroid disease in the elderly (Timiras, 2007). Many older adults are unable to maintain glucose homeostasis, initially this is a result of insulin resistance, which later is caused by insulin deficiency (Timiras). Overall, there is a decrease in sensitivity to insulin, with a decreased ability to quickly respond to high blood sugar levels and slow return to normal. A critical illness event may accentuate these changes. Type II diabetes is not necessarily a part of usual aging but is associated with increased body fat and obesity, which are also risk factors for many other diseases observed in older adults. Sedentary older adults who become overweight are predisposed to diabetes and atheroslcerosis, both of which, although not a usual part of aging, may accelerate the aging process.

As adults age, thymic mass decreases, whereas thymic nodules increase. These nodules may remain benign in the majority of cases (Timiras, 2007). Triodythyrine (T3) and thyroxine (T4) are slightly decreased but remain within normal range, and thyroid-stimulating hormone (TSH) levels elevate. The changes in thyroid hormones may have a slight affect on decreasing the metabolic rate, decreasing calorigenisis, and decreasing cholesterol metabolism (Timiras). Thermoregulatory responses to either heat or cold are impaired in the elderly because of reductions in hypothalamic and neuroendocrine functions. As a result of this impaired response, older patients in the ICU may have a harder time adjusting to temperature changes and oftentimes have a slightly lower core temperature because of the cool environment and use of intravenous fluids. The immune system changes (see chapter 16, this volume) associated with aging increase infection risks. There is a decrease in T-cell function and a decrease in B-cell production in the bone marrow. These changes can create weaker or delayed hypersensitivity reactions and impaired cell-mediated immune responses. There is an increased incidence of reactivations of latent infections such as tuberculosis and herpes. Increases in circulating IgA (immunoglobulin A) and decreases in circulating IgG (immunoglobulin G) results in susceptibility to infections (Taffett, 2006; Timiras). In addition to these changes, other extrinsic factors seen in older adults that stress the immune system include decreased mobility, environmental exposure to pathogens, medications that lower white blood cell counts (e.g., rheumatoid medications), comorbid conditions such as diabetes, and malnutrition (Mick & Ackerman,

## 12.5 The Endocrine, Hematological, and Immune Systems

| Changes With Aging | Significance to Critical Illness |
|---|---|
| ■ Decreased sensitivity to insulin<br>■ Decrease in thymic mass<br>■ T3 and T4 slightly decreased<br>■ Reduction in hypothalamus and neuroendocrine function<br>■ Decrease in T-cells function<br>■ Decrease in B-cell production<br>■ Increase in circulating IgA<br>■ Decrease in circulating IgG<br>■ Slowing erythrocyte replacement this may be a result of iron levels<br>■ Increased platelet adhesiveness | ■ Decreased response to blood sugar levels slow return to normal. Accentuated during critical illness<br>■ Small affect on decreasing metabolic rate, calorigenisis, cholesterol metabolism<br>■ Thermoregulatory response is impaired affecting response in older patients to adjust to decreases and increases in temp<br>■ Weaker or delayed hypersensitivity reaction<br>■ Impaired cell mediated immune response<br>■ Increase vulnerability to infection<br>■ Atypical or benign signs and symptoms with infection<br>■ Vulnerability to late recognition of infection |

Synthesized from Fletcher (2007), Miller (2009),Timirus (2007), Urden et al. (2006).

2004; Winkelman, 2007). When factors common to aging are combined with elements of a critical illness and its treatment, such as invasive procedures, indwelling lines and catheters, the resulting interactions potentiate risks for nosocomial infections. The thermoregulatory changes, environmental influences on core body temperature, and the diminished ability of the aging immune system to manifest a febrile response to infection contributes to late findings and delayed diagnosis of infection, sepsis, and other immune disorders. Atypical presentations of illness and infection in the elderly can thus result in a late recognition by nurses. Delayed recognition of infection results in delayed treatment, which underscores the need for prevention as a primary goal in the care of the older patient (Timiras).

There are minimal changes in the hematological system, with most changes indicating a pathological process or an iron deficiency. Decreases in hemoglobin are often the result of falling iron levels in the elderly. There is a slowing in erythrocyte replacement, but this may be caused by a decrease in iron intake or absorption (Timiras, 2007). Changes in platelets are also an indication of other issues and are not necessarily specific to changes with aging. There may be an increase in platelet adhesiveness, but evidence concerning hypercoagulability is inconclusive (McCance, 2006). Other factors that may contribute to hypercoagulability of the older adult include dehydration, fluid shifts, immobility, blood stasis, atrial dysrhythmias, and surgery. Table 12.5 indicates the changes that occur with aging in the endocrine, hematological, and immunological systems.

## Impact on Elderly: Issues Common in Critical Care

■ Changes in blood sugar

■ Older adults may require higher doses of insulin than younger adults (Timiras, 2007).

- There is an increased vulnerability to hyperglycemia and resulting dehydration with atypical or subtle signs and symptoms (Gaglia, Wyckoff, & Abrahamson, 2004).

- Delirium, medications, sympathetic changes with aging, other symptoms from critical illness and sensory deficits in the elderly my mask classic signs and symptoms of hypoglycemia (such as tachycardia, palpitations, diaphoresis, tremors, arousal anxiety) (Humbert, Gallagher, Gabby, & Dellasega, 2008).

- Infection and sepsis

  - These are one of the leading causes of death in the critically ill older adult, with risk increasing with age and poorer outcomes (Girard & Ely, 2007; Martin, Mannino, & Moss, 2006).

  - Fever, increased heart rate, and obvious immediate changes in leukocytes may not be an early indicator of infection in the elderly who may have more subtle or atypical signs and symptoms, leading to a late diagnosis and compromised reserve (Fletcher, 2007; Girard & Ely, 2007).

  - Possible indictor of systemic infection can include changes in mental status or delirium, weakness and decreased functional status, anorexia, falls, normothermia or hypothermia, and unexplained hypoglycemia or hyperglycemia (Mick & Ackerman, 2004).

  - Changes in other systems, respiratory, cardiac, renal, neurological, muscular/skeletal, and skin, all can contribute to increased risk of infection when the older patient is further compromised.

# Gastrointestinal System

## Changes With Aging

As with all systems, changes in the gastrointestinal (GI) system have significant heterogeneity among older adults. It is more common today for older adults to have some or all of their own teeth. In the early 1980s, 54% of persons aged 65 or greater had some natural teeth; by 2002, the percentage increased to 70% (The National Institute of Dental and Craniofacial Research, 2002). Dentate older adults are especially vulnerable to caries around previous restorations, such as fillings and crowns (Shay & Ship). Caries can occur when the root surfaces are exposed as a result of periodontal disease in older adults (Shay & Ship, 1995). Older adults may form plaque more quickly than their younger counterparts when oral care is not routinely performed; this may be caused by gingival recession, which exposes more tooth to the oral environment and is also to the result of reduced salivary flow (Shay & Ship). Tooth loss may cause shifting of remaining teeth to the point where occlusal surfaces no longer articulate, interfering with chewing and swallowing functions.

Nearly one third of all older adults experience xerostomia, or dry mouth, because of hyposalivation (Gupta, Epstein, & Sroussi, 2006). Xerostomia causes mouth discomfort, interferes with chewing and swallowing, and supports plaque formation (Gupta et al.). Furthermore, saliva has antibacterial properties; diminished saliva production results in increased bacteria in the mouth. Anticholinergics, antihypertensives, antidepressants, diuretics, anxiolytics, and antihistamines diminish salivary production and alter the ability of the oral environment to fight the effects of pathogens (Ettinger; Shay & Ship). Many medications commonly prescribed for elderly patients, especially calcium channel blockers and antiseizure medications, result in gingival overgrowth, which further predisposes the older adult to caries and periodontal disease (Ettinger, 1996; Shay & Ship, 1995). Oral care is of great importance in critically ill patients in part because of the effect of the various medications that are administered; however the importance of oral care is even greater for those who are orally intubated (Fitch, Munro, Glass, & Pellegrini, 1999; Grap, Munro, Ashtiani, & Bryant, 2003). If older adults do not receive frequent mouth care in the ICU, they are at higher risk for ventilator-associated pneumonia (Berry, Davidson, Masters, & Rolls, 2007).

Other significant changes that occur include a thinning of the gastric mucosa, delayed gastric empting and decreased motility, changes in secretion of gastric enzymes, and decreases in absorption capabilities (Timiras, 2007). Dysphagia can occur as a result of poor dentition and inability to completely masticate food, or can be caused by xerostomia, and from diminished peristaltic contractions in the esophagus (Timiras). In addition, there are changes in the liver size and blood flow, which affect pharmacodynamics and pharmacokenetics; thus, many drugs will reach therapeutic levels at much lower doses (Timiras). Pancreatic changes surround endocrine changes and insulin. Overall GI function is preserved in the elderly and common problems of constipation, gastritis, malnutrition, and other frequent complaints by the elderly are not a function of age alone but may be a combination of other factors, including changes in diet, activity, dentition, medications, body composition, dehydration and other comorbid conditions (Rosenthal & Kavic, 2004; Timiras) (see Table 12.6).

## Assessment, Impact on Critical Illness, and Clinical Recommendations

Assessment findings in the critically ill elderly can be atypical or diffuse and nonspecific, meaning that abdominal pain can be less severe and/or underreported. The elderly may have pathologic processes long before symptoms are appreciable, making them vulnerable to complications (Sanson & O'Keefe, 1996). Fever and other expected assessment findings may be absent when assessing for peritonitis. Dysphagia can lead to aspiration; interventions should focus on prevention, for example, the head of the bed should be elevated to more than 30 degrees to prevent reflux of stomach content caused by a relaxed lower esophageal sphincter. Frequent suctioning of oral secretions will prevent aspiration (Aragon & Sole, 2006; Timirus, 2007). Meticulous mouth care with a soft toothbrush and not a sponge (e.g., toothette) will reduce chances of pneumonia (Sarin, Balasubramaniam, Corcoran, Laudenbach, & Stoopler, 2008). Changes in gastric enzymes and thinning of the mucosal wall combined with the stress of critical illness can increases susceptibility to injury and acute GI bleeding, which in turn diminishes reserve and raises morbidity and mortality of older adults in the ICU (Timiras).

GI complications such as constipation, ileus, and diarrhea are common in ICU patients regardless of age, but the compounding factors of age-related changes in the older adult require prevention, vigilance, and early intervention to avoid additional complications. Evaluation of medications, their appropriateness, and therapeutic levels as affected by both the GI and the renal system can prevent adverse outcomes. Use

## 12.6   The Gastrointestinal System

| Changes With Aging | Significance to Critical Illness |
|---|---|
| ■ Decreased salivary production | ■ Xerostomia |
| ■ Decreased peristaltic contraction in esophagus | ■ Increased mouth bacteria |
| | ■ Mouth more susceptible to injury especially from tubes |
| | ■ Higher risk of ventilator-associated pneumonia |
| ■ Thinning of gastric mucosa | ■ Increased risk of aspiration |
| | ■ Increased dysphagia |
| ■ Decreased motility | ■ Changes in pharmacodynamics and pharmacokinetics—increased potential for adverse medication effects |
| ■ Delayed gastric empting | ■ Increased risk of constipation |
| | ■ Increased risk of gastrointestinal reflux disease (GERD) |
| ■ Changes in secretion of gastric enzymes | ■ Delayed nutrition and vitamin absorption |
| ■ Decreased absorption | ■ Vulnerable to malnutrition |
| ■ Decreased calcium absorption | |
| ■ Decreased or slowed iron absorption | |
| ■ Decrease in size of liver due to changes in flow | |

Synthesized from Fletcher (2007), Miller (2009),Timirus (2007), Urden et al. (2006).

of the Beers criteria (see chapter 13, this text) when making pharmaceutical decisions can help avoid adverse outcomes and elevated costs to care (Bonk, Krown, Matuszewski, & Oinonen, 2006; Fick et al., 2003; Moore & Blount, 2002).

### Impact on Elderly: GI Issues Common in Critical Care

■ Ulcers and GI bleeding

■ Clinical factors that predict mortality from GI bleed in older adults, include hemodynamic instability, hematemesis, hematochezia, failure for blood to clear with gastric lavage, age older then 60, coagulopathy, the presence of a serious comorbidity, and hospitalization (Tariq & Mekhjian, 2007).

■ Cardiovascular, pulmonary, and renal insufficiency can all contribute to difficulties in treating and modifications in management of GI bleeding in the elderly (Wilson, 2006).

■ Medications, particularly NSAIDS (nonsteroidal antiinflammatory drugs), can contribute to an increased risk of ulcers and GI bleeding in the elderly (Wilson, 2006).

- Pain from ulcers may present as chest pain; it is important to identify the correct underlying pathology with any chest pain (Wilson, 2006).

- Nutrition

  - Older adults may already be nutritionally compromised before coming to the critical care environment (Lipschitz, 2006).

  - Protein-calorie malnutrition is common in the elderly during hospitalization and can lead to complications in skin integrity, fluid shifts, delayed healing, increased infections and contributes to morbidity and mortality (Lipschitz, 2006; Nagappan & Parkin, 2003; Rosenthal & Kavic, 2004).

  - Critical care nurses need to advocate for patients in the ICU to prevent delayed nutrition (Reid & Allard-Gould, 2004).

# Musculoskeletal and Integumentary System

## Changes With Aging

Changes in the collagen and connective tissue of the joints from both wear and tear and pathologic processes impair flexibility and movement of the joints. There is compression of the spine because of a decrease in vertebral discs resulting in a loss of height ranging from 1.5 to 3 inches (Oliver & Hill, 2005). With aging, bones decrease in mass for both men and women because of decreased circulating hormones. Bone is dependent on calcium and is affected by changes in circulating levels of calcium. Endogenous calcium is primarily absorbed by the gastrointestinal system; if inadequate levels are consumed or absorbed, calcium blood levels are kept constant by removing it from the bones. The endocrine system and kidneys affect calcium and phosphorus serum levels, which also affect bone mass by contributing to slower remodeling of bones (Timiras, 2007). Bones become more brittle and heal slower after fractures (Inzerillo, Iqbal, Troen, Meier, & Zaidi, 2006; Timiras & Navazio, 2007).

There is a decrease in muscle mass as a result of a loss in muscle fibers called sarcopenia (Timiras & Navazio, 2007). At the same time, there is an infiltrate of fatty tissue into the muscle bundles. The loss of muscle also results in a decrease in metabolic rate of the body, which is directly related to muscle loss. The decrease in muscle mass is related to changes with aging in the nervous system and changes in the skeletal structure. Overall changes with aging in the musculoskeletal system have many variables, some of which are the result of the individual's lifestyle choices prior to illness and some of which are influenced by the health care team's decisions once in the hospital. Muscle breakdown and disuse syndromes can occur quickly independent of age, compounding critical illnesses and resulting in longer lengths of stay (DeJonghe, Bsatuji-Garin, Sharshar, Outin, & Brochard, 2004; Griffiths, Voss, & Allison, 1996; Hirsch, Sommers, Olsen, Mullen, & Winograd,1990; Hopkins, Spuhler, & Thomsen, 2007; Morris & Herridge, 2007; Winkleman, 2007).

Although bones and muscle benefit from increased and continued weight bearing, activity joints will exhibit breakdown. The pain that comes from this wear and tear can contribute to a loss of, or an avoidance of, increased activity. This loss of mobility can affect other systems, in particular the cardiovascular and pulmonary systems. In

## 12.7   The Musculoskeletal System

| Changes With Aging | Significance to Critical Illness |
|---|---|
| ■ Decreased muscle mass<br>■ Increase in fatty tissue<br>■ Slower muscular response to nervous system signals<br>■ Degenerative joint changes<br>■ Decreased/ slowed bone remodeling | ■ Decreased muscle strength<br>■ Impaired shivering<br>■ Decreased exercise tolerance manifesting in endurance, cardio and pulmonary function<br>■ Increased risk of falls<br>■ Increased brittleness of bones<br>■ Increased risk of fracture<br>■ Decrease in height<br>■ Increased joint pain<br>■ Limitations in movement<br>■ Decreased metabolism<br>■ Vulnerable to decreased circulating calcium<br>■ Vulnerable to decreased function<br>■ Vulnerable to malnutrition<br>■ Decreased reserve and endurance |

Adapted from Fletcher (2007), Miller (2009),Timirus (2007), Urden et al. (2006).

turn, the changes in cardiovascular and pulmonary systems may reduce mobility. These feedback loops can result in a decrease in overall function and reserve over time. Table 12.7 lists changes seen with aging in the musculoskeletal system.

Changes in the integumentary system are a result of a loss of subcutaneous fat and elastic and connective tissue. These changes are evident in the wrinkles and sagging tissues observed in older adults. The extent of these changes are determined by other variables such as weight, nutrition, and ultraviolet damage (Timiras, 2007). The dermis loses vasculature supply, which creates the appearance of transparency to the skin (Timiras). Eccrine and sebaceous glands also decline, resulting in less sweating, reducing the body's ability to cool itself and produce less oil, contributing to drier skin (Timiras) (see Table 12.8).

### Assessment, Impact on Critical Illness, and Clinical Recommendations

Changes in the musculoskeletal system and the integumentary system can present unique challenges to ICU nurses caring for older adults. First, it is important to assess initial functional status on admission to both maintain that functional status and to identify any new disability. There are many barriers to mobility that can decondition older adults: intravenous tubes, monitoring wires, an unstable illness trajectory, fatigue, delirium, pain, fear of falling, and prescribed bed rest (C. J. Brown, Williams, Woodby, Davis, & Allman, 2007). Although critical care nurses are in a unique position to help older adults maintain their functional status, other members of the health care team can be helpful. For example, physical therapists can be instrumental in helping to integrate specific exercises into the routine care of older adults as well as to provide devices that prevent functional decline and improve mobility.

## 12.8 The Integumentary System

| Changes With Aging | Significance to Critical Illness |
|---|---|
| ■ Decreased rate of epidermal and dermal cell replacement—epidermis and dermis become thinner | ■ Decreased rate of wound healing |
| | ■ Increased vulnerability to skin breakdown |
| | ■ Dry skin |
| ■ Loss and loosening of subcutaneous fat, collagen, and connective tissue | ■ Inability to cool by sweating |
| | ■ Wrinkled, loose, and thin skin is vulnerable to tearing |
| ■ Decrease in and changes to the vascular supply of the skin | ■ Decreased subcutaneous tissue increases vulnerability to ecchymotic damage |
| ■ Shrinking eccrine glands | ■ Changes in cardiovasculature can affect skin causing arterial ulcers, venous ulcers, diabetic foot ulcers. |
| ■ Stretching of sebaceous glands but decrease in secretion of oil | |

Synthesized from Fletcher (2007), Miller (2009), Timirus (2007), Urden et al. (2006).

Skin care is also important. The standard of care per nearly every nursing textbook is to change positions every 2 hours. Older adults, however, may require more frequent changes in positioning because of diminished capillary blood flow that is compromised by external pressure (Timiras, 2007). Care must be taken to move older adults in a manner that reduces shearing, which contributes to skin breakdown (Timiras). Older adults should be lifted, and not slid, when being repositioned.

## Impact on Elderly: Musculoskeletal and Integumentary Issues Common in Critical Care

■ Skin breakdown and wound healing

■ As compared to younger patients, many older patients are more vulnerable because of delayed wound healing, pressure ulcers, intravenous infiltration, and diminished skin turgor; in addition, thermoregulation is impaired (Stotts & Wu, 2007; Urden et al., 2005).

■ Comorbidities, acute illnesses, and chronic illnesses place the elderly at et al., greater risk for impaired wound healing. The prevention of ulcers can facilitate hospital recovery (Shannon & Lehman, 1996; Stotts & Wu, 2007; Thomas, 2006).

■ Complication in the ICU; edema, infection, malnutrition, cardiovascular, pulmonary, neurological, and musculoskeletal changes can increase risk of wounds and compromise wound healing in all patients. The older patient is at a higher risk as a result of integumentary changes with aging (Shannon & Lehman, 1996; Thomas, 2006).

■ Small wounds and skin tears can present a gateway for larger wounds and infection (Thomas, 2006).

■ Functional decline

   ■ Hospitalized older patients are predisposed to functional decline (Kleinpell, 2007; Kleinpell, Fletcher, & Jennings, 2008).

   ■ Early assessment and intervention of function can be a challenge during an acute illness.

   ■ The ICU environment can contribute to functional decline because of immobilization and sedation. Both increase the incidence of delirium (Inouye, 2006; St. Pierre, 1998; Thomsen, Snow, Rodriguez, & Hopkins, 2008).

## Summary

Older adults are a heterogeneous population, which means that usual changes related to aging follow an overall pattern but may manifest differently in each individual. This chapter described usual changes in physiology that accompany aging that may affect the way older adults respond to critical illness and its treatment. Older adults may present with critical illnesses in unique ways partly as a result of limited physiological reserves. Limited reserves may cause a domino effect, in which compromises in one system result in negative outcomes in another system. Often, symptoms are diffuse and vague and may be undetected unless nurses are proactively caring for these elderly patients. Knowledgeable vigilance on the part of critical care nurses can address health care problems before additional systems are compromised, resulting in better patient outcomes.

## References

Albert, M. S., Killiany, R. J., Birren, J. E., & Schaie, K. W. (2001). Age-related cognitive changes and brain-behavior relationships. In: *Handbook of the psychology of aging* (Vol. 5, pp. 161–185). San Diego: Academic Press.

Akposs, K., Hertig, A., Couprie, R., Flahaut, A., Alberti, C., Karras, G. A., et al. (2000). Acute renal failure in patients over 80 years old: 25 years experience. *Intensive Care Medicine, 26,* 400–406.

Aragon, D., & Sole, M. L. (2006). Implementing best practice strategies to prevent infection in the ICU. *Critical Care Nursing Clinics of North America, 18,* 441–452.

Arking, R. (2006). *The biology of aging* (3rd ed.). New York: Oxford University Press.

Backman, L., Small, B. J., Wahlin, A., Birren, J. E., & Schaie, K. W. (2001). Aging and memory. In *Handbook of the psychology of aging* (Vol. 5, pp. 349–376). San Diego: Academic Press.

Bailey, P., Thomsen, G. E., Spuhler, V. J., Blair, R., Jewkes, J., Bezdjian, L., et al. (2007). Early activity is feasible and safe in respiratory failure patients. *Critical Care Medicine, 35,* 139–145.

Balas, N. E., Deutschman, C. S., Sullivan-Marx, E. M., Strumpf, N. E., Alston, R. P., & Richmond, T. S. (2007). Delirium in older patients in surgical intensive care. *Journal of Nursing Scholarship, 39,* 147–154.

Berry, A. M., Davidson, P. M., Masters, J., & Rolls, K. (2007). Systematic literature review of oral hygiene practices for intensive care patients receiving mechanical ventilation. *American Journal of Critical Care, 16*(6), 552–563.

Bjoro, K., & Herr, K. (2008). Assessment of pain in nonverbal or cognitively impaired older adults. *Clinics in Geriatric Medicine, 24,* 237–262.

Bonk, M. E., Krown, H., Matuszewski, K., & Oinonen, M. (2006). Potentially inappropriate medications in hospitalized senior patients. *American Journal of Health System Pharmacists, 63,* 1161–1165.

Brown, C. J., Williams, B. R., Woodby, L. L., Davis, L. L., & Allman, R. M. (2007). Barriers to mobility during hospitalization from the perspective of older patients and their nurses and physicians. *Journal of Hospital Medicine, 2,* 305–313.

Brown, C. V. R, Shoemaker, W. C., Wo, C. C. J., Chan, L., & Demetriades, D. (2005). Is noninvasive hemodynamic monitoring appropriate for the elderly critically injured patient? *Journal of Trauma Injury, Infection, and Critical Care, 58,* 102–107.

Bulger, E. M., Arneson, M. A., Mock, C. N., & Jurkovich, G. J. (2000). Rib fractures in the elderly. *Journal of Trauma, 48,* 1040–1046.

Carson, S. S. (2003). The epidemiology of critical illness in elderly. *Critical Care Clinics, 19,* 605–617.

Chelluri, L., Im, K. A., Belle, S. H., Schulz, R., Rotondi, A. J., Donahoe, M. P., et al. (2004). Long-term mortality and quality of life after prolonged mechanical ventilations. *Critical Care Medicine, 32,* 61–69.

Cheng, A. T., Plank, L. D., & Hill, G. L. (1998). Prolonged overexpansion of extracellular water in elderly patients with sepsis. *Archives of Surgery, 133,* 745–751.

Cheung, C. M., Ponnusamy, A., & Anderton, J. G. (2008). Management of acute renal failure in the elderly patient. *Drugs & Aging, 25,* 455–476.

Cox, C. E., Carson, S. S., Lindquist, J. H., Olsen, M. K., Govert, J. A., & Chelluri, L. (2007). Differences in one year health outcomes and resource utilization by definition of prolonged mechanical ventilation: Prospective cohort study. *Critical Care, 1.*doi:10.1186/cc5667

De Jonghe, B., Bastuji-Garin, S., Sharshar, T., Outin, H., & Brochard, L. (2004). Does ICU-acquired paresis lengthen weaning from mechanical ventilation? *Intensive Critical Care Medicine, 30,* 1117–1121.

Eachempati, S. R., Hydo, L. J., Shou, J., & Barie, P. S. (2005). Outcomes of acute respiratory distress syndrome in elderly patients. *Journal of Trauma, 63,* 344–350.

Ellstrom, K. (2006). The pulmonary system. In J. G. Alspach (Ed.), *Core curriculum for critical care nursing* (6th ed., pp. 45–183). St. Louis: Saunders.

Ely, E. W., Wheeler, A. P., Thompson, B. T., Ancukiewicz, M., Steinberg, K. P., & Bernard, G. R. (2002). Recovery rate and prognosis in older persons who develop acute lung injury and acute respiratory distress syndrome. *Annuals of Internal Medicine, 136,* 25–36.

Epstein, C. D., & Peerless, J. (2006). Weaning readiness and fluid balance in older critically ill surgical patients. *American Journal of Critical Care, 15,* 54–64.

Esiri, M. M. (2007). Aging and the brain. *Journal of Pathology, 211,* 181–187.

Esteban, A., Anzueto, A., Frutos-Vivar, F., Alia, I., Ely, E. W., Brochard, L., et al. (2004). Outcomes of older patients receiving mechanical ventilation. *Intensive Care Medicine, 30(4),* 639–646.

Ettinger, R. L. (1996). Review: Xerostomia: A symptom which acts like a disease. *Age & Ageing, 25,* 409–412.

Fick, D. M., Agostini, J. V., & Inouye, S. K. (2002). Delirium superimposed on dementia: A systematic review. *Journal of the American Geriatrics Society, 50,* 1723–1732.

Fick, D. M., Cooper, J. W., Wade, W. E., Waller, J. L., Maclean, R., & Beers, M. H. (2003). Updating the beers criteria for potentially inappropriate medication use in older adults. *Archives of Internal Medicine, 163,* 2716–2724.

Fitch, J. A., Munro, C. L., Glass, C. A., & Pellegrini, J. M. (1999). Oral care in the adults intensive care unit. *American Journal of Critical Care, 8,* 314–318.

Flaherty, E., & Zwicker, D. (2005). *Atypical presentation.* Retrieved January 4, 2009, from Hartford Institute for Geriatric Nursing Web site: http://www.consultgerirn.org/topics/atypical_presentation/want_to _know_more

Fletcher, K. (2007). Optimizing reserve in hospitalized elderly. *Critical Care Nursing Clinics of North America, 19,* 285–302.

Fliser, D., Franek, E., Joest, M., Block, S., Mutschler, E., & Ritz, E. (1997). Renal function in the elderly: Impact of hypertension and cardiac function. *Kidney International, 51,* 1196–1204.

Floyd, R. A., & Hensley, K. (2002). Oxidative stress in brain aging: Implications for therapeutics of neurodegenerative disease. *Neurobiology of Aging, 23,* 795–807.

Fulmer, T., Flaherty, E., Bottrell, M. M., Fletcher, K., & Mezey, M. (2000). Acute and critical nursing care. In T. Yoshikawa & D. Norman (Eds.), *Acute emergencies and critical care of the elderly* (pp. 49–65). New York: Marcel Dekker.

Gaglia, M. J., Wyckoff, J., & Abrahamson, M. J. (2004). Acute hyperglycemic crisis in the elderly. *Medical Clinics of North America, 88,* 1063–1084.

Girard, T. D., & Ely, E. W. (2007). Bacteremia and sepsis in the older adult. *Clinics in Geriatric Medicine, 23,* 633–647.

Grap, M. J., Munro, C. L., Ashtiani, B., & Bryant, S. (2003). Oral care interventions in critical care: Frequency and documentation. *American Journal of Critical Care, 12(2),* 113–118.

Gregoratos, G. (2001). Clinical manifestations of acute myocardial infarction in older patients. *American Journal of Geriatric Cardiology, 10(6),* 345–347.

Griffiths, R. D., Voss, A. C., & Allison, S. (1996). Muscle mass, survival and the elderly ICU patient. *Nutrition, 12*(6), 456–458.

Gupta, A., Epstein, J. B., & Sroussi, H. (2006). Hyposalivation in the elderly patients. *Journal of the Canadian Dental Association, 72*(9), 841–846.

Haas, M., Spargo, B. H., Wit, E. J. C., & Meehan, S. (2000). Etiologies and outcomes of acute renal insufficiency in older adults: A renal biopsy study of 259 cases. *American Journal of Kidney Disease, 35*, 433–447.

Happ, M. B., Tuite, P., Dobbin, K., DiVirgilio-Thomas, D., Kitutu, J., (2004). Communication ability, methods, and content among nonspeaking nonsurviving patients treated with mechanical ventilation in the intensive care unit. *American Journal of Critical Care, 13*(3), 210–220.

Hirsch, C. H., Sommers, L., Olsen, A., Mullen, L., & Winograd, C. H. (1990). The natural history of functional morbidity in hospitalized older patients. *Journal of the American Geriatrics Society, 38(12)* 1296–1303.

Hopkins, R. O., Spuhler, V. J., & Thomsen, G. E. (2007). Transforming ICU culture to facility early mobility. *Critical Care Clinics, 23,* 81–96.

Horgas, A. L., & Elliott, A. F. (2004). Pain assessment and management in persons with dementia. *Nursing Clinics of North America, 39,* 593–606.

Humbert, J., Gallagher, K., Gabby, R., & Dellasega, C. (2008). Intensive insulin therapy in the critically ill geriatric patient. *Critical Care Nurse Quarterly, 31,* 14–18.

Inouye, S. I. (2006). Delirium in older persons. *New England Journal of Medicine, 354,* 1157–1165.

Inzerillo, A., Iqbal, J., Troen, B., Meier, D. E., & Zaidi, M. (2006). Skeletal fragility in the elderly. In C. K., Cassel, R. M., Leipzig, H. J., Cohen, E. B., Larson, & D. E. Meier (Eds.), *Geriatric medicine an evidenced-based approach* (4th ed., pp. 621–650). New York: Springer Publishing Company.

Ketcham, C. J., Stelmach, G. E., Birren, J. E., & Schaie, K. W. (2001). Age-related declines in motor control. In *Handbook of the psychology of aging* (vol. 5, pp. 313–348). San Diego: Academic Press.

Kikuchi, R., Watabe, N., Konno, T., Mishina, N., Sekizawa, K., & Sasaki, H. (1994). High incidence of silent aspiration in elderly patients with community acquired pneumonia. *American Journal of Respiratory Critical Care Medicine, 150,* 251–253.

Kleinhenz, M. E., & Lewis, C. Y. (2000). Chronic ventilator dependence in elderly patients. *Clinics in Geriatric Medicine, 16*(4), 735–756.

Kleinpell, R. (2007). Supporting independence in hospitalized elders in acute care. *Critical Care Nursing Clinics of North America, 19,* 247–252.

Kleinpell, R. M., Fletcher, K., & Jennings, B. M. (2008). *Reducing functional decline in hospitalized elderly.* Retrieved January 15, 2009, from Agency for Healthcare Research and Quality Web site: http://www.ahrq.gov/qual/nurseshdbk

Kollef, M. H. (1993). Do age and gender influence outcomes from mechanical ventilation. *Heart & Lung, 22,* 442–449.

Lakatta, E. G. (2000). Cardiovascular health in aging. *Clinics in Geriatric Medicine, 16*(3), 1–10

Lakatta, E. G. (2002). Age-associated cardiovascular changes in health: Impact on cardiovascular disease in older adults. *Heart Failure Reviews, 7,* 29–49.

Lakatta, E. G., & Levy, D. (2003). Arterial and cardiac aging: Major shareholders in cardiovascular disease enterprises. Part II: The aging heart in health: Links to heart disease. *Circulation, 2003*(107), 346–354.

Levine, B. S., & Craven, R. F. (2005). Physiology adaptations with aging. In S. L. Woods, E. S. Froelicher, S. U. Motzer, & E. J. Bridges (Eds.), *Cardiac nursing* (5th ed., pp. 220–226). Philadelphia: Lippincott, Willams & Wilkins.

Lipschitz, D. A. (2006). Nutrition. In C. Cassel, R. Leipzig, H. Cohen, E. Larson, & D. Meier (Eds.), *Geriatric medicine an evidenced-based approach* (4th ed., pp. 1009–1021). New York: Springer Publishing Company.

Luckey, A. E., & Parsa, C. J. (2003). Fluid and electrolytes in the aged. *Archives of Surgery, 138,* 1055–1060.

Manzano, F., Yuste, E., Colmenero, M., Aranda, A., Garcia-Horcajadas, A., Rivera, R., et al. (2005). Incidence of acute respiratory distress syndrome and its relation to age. *Journal of Critical Care, 20,* 274–280.

Marik, P. E. (2006). Management of the critically ill geriatric patient. *Critical Care Medicine, 34*(9 Suppl.), S176–182.

Marik, P. E., & Kaplan, D. (2003). Aspiration pneumonia and dysphagia in the elderly. *Chest, 124,* 328–336.

Matuschak, G. M. (2008). Acute respiratory failure and acute lung injury ARDS. In P. G. Schmitz & K. J. Martin (Eds.). *Internal medicine; Just the facts* (pp. 654–661). New York: McGraw–Hill.

McCance, K. L. (2006). Structure and function of the hematologic system. In K. L. McCance & S. E. Huether (Eds.), *Pathophysiology the biologic basis for Disease in adults and children* (5th ed., pp. 893–926). Philadelphia: Elsevier Mosby.

Mick, D. J., & Ackerman, M. H. (2004). Critical care nursing for the older adult: Pathophysiological and functional considerations. *Nursing Clinics of North America, 39,* 473–493.

Milisen, K., Braes, T., Fick, D. M., & Foreman, M. D. (2005). Cognitive assessment and differentiating the 3 Ds (dementia, depression, delirium). *Nursing Clinics of North America, 41,* 1–22.

Miller, C. A. (2009). *Nursing for wellness in older adults* (5th ed.). Philadelphia: Lippincott, Williams & Wilkins.

Moore, L. A., & Blount, K. A. (2002). Medications and the elderly in the critical care setting. *Critical Care Nursing Clinics of North America, 14,* 111–119.

Moore, S. M., & Duffy, S. (2007). Maintaining vigilance to promote best outcomes for hospitalized elders. *Critical Care Clinics of North America, 19,* 313–319.

Morandi, A., Jackson, J. C., & Ely, E. W. (2009). Delirium in the intensive care unit. *International Review of Psychiatry, 21*(1), 43–58.

Morris, P. E. (2007). Moving our critically ill patients: Mobility barriers and benefits. *Critical Care Clinics, 23,* 1–20.

Morris, P. E., & Herridge, M. S. (2007). Early intensive care unit mobility: Future directions. *Critical Care Clinics, 23,* 97–110.

Musso, C. G., Liakopoulos, V., Ioannidis, I., Eleftheriadis, T., & Stefanidis, I. (2006). Acute renal failure in the elderly: Particular characteristics. *International Urology Nephrology, 38,* 787–793.

Nagappan, R., & Parkin, G. (2003). Geriatric critical care. *Critical care clinics, 19,* 253–270.

The National Institute of Dental and Craniofacial Research. (2002). *A plan to eliminate craniofacial, oral, and dental health disparities.* Bethesda, MD: Author.

Nelson, A., Powell-Cope, G., Gavin-Dreschnack, D., Quigley, P., Bulat, T., Baptiste, A. S., et al. (2004). Technology to promote safe mobility in the elderly. *Nursing Clinics of North America.* doi:10.1016/j.cnur.2004.05.001

Oliver, S., & Hill, J. (2005). Arthritis in the older person. *Nursing Older People, 17*(4), 25–28.

Peterson, D. D., Pack, A. I., Silage, D. A., & Fisherman, A. P. (1981). Effects of aging on ventilatory and occlusion pressure response to hypoxia and hypercapnia. *American Review of Respiratory Disease, 124,* 387–391.

Reid, M. B., & Allard-Gould, P. (2004). Malnutrition and the critically ill elderly patient. *Critical Care Nursing Clinics of North America, 16,* 531–536.

Richards, C. L. (2003). Urinary tract infections in the frail elderly: Issues for diagnosis treatment and prevention. *International Urology and Nephrology, 36,* 457–463.

Richmond, T., & Jacoby, S. F. (2007). Cultivating responsive system for the care of acutely and critically ill older adult. *Critical Care Nursing Clinics of North America, 19,* 263–268.

Rooke, G. A. (2000). Autonomic and cardiovascular function in the geriatric patient. *Anesthesiology Clinics of North America, 18,* 31–46.

Rosenthal, R. A., & Kavic, S. M. (2004). Assessment and management of the geriatric patient. *Critical Care Medicine, 32,* S92–105.

Rubenfield, G. D., Caldwell, E., Peabody, E., Weaver, J., Martin, D. P., Neff, M., et al. (2005). Incidence and outcomes of acute lung injury. *New England Journal of Medicine, 353,* 1685–1693.

Rutschmann, O., Chevalley, T., Zumwald, C., Luthy, C., Vermeulen, B., & Sarasin, F. (2005). Pitfalls in the emergency department triage of frail elderly patients without specific complaints. *Swiss Medicine Weekly, 135,* 145–150.

Sander, O., Welters, I. D., Foex, P., & Sear, J. W. (2005). Impact of prolonged elevated heart rate on the incidence of major cardiac events in critically ill patients with high risk of cardiac complications. *Critical Care Medicine, 33,* 81–88.

Sanson, T. G., & O'Keefe, K. P. (1996). Evaluation of abdominal pain in the elderly. *Emergency Medicine Clinics of North America, 14,* 615–627.

Sarin, J., Balasubramaniam, R., Corcoran, A. M., Laudenbach, J. M., & Stoopler, E. T. (2008). Reducing the risk of aspiration pneumonia among elderly patients in long-term care facilities through oral health interventions. *Journal of the American Medical Directors Association, 9*(2), 128–135.

Sevransky, J. E., & Haponik, E. F. (2003). Respiratory failure in elderly patients. *Clinics in Geriatric Medicine, 19,* 205–224.

Shannon, M. L., & Lehman, C. A. (1996). Protecting the skin of the elderly patient in the intensive care unit. *Critical Care Nursing Clinics of North America, 8*(1) 17–28.

Shay, K., & Ship, J. A. (1995). The importance of oral health in the older patient. *Journal of the American Geriatrics Society, 43*(12), 1414–1422.

Silva, F. G. (2005). The aging kidney: A review part I. *International Urology and Nephrology, 37,* 185–205.

Siner, J. M., & Pisani, M. A. (2007). Mechanical ventilation and acute respiratory distress syndrome in older patients. *Clinics in Chest Medicine, 28,* 783–791.

Sprung, J., Gajic, O., & Warner, D. O. (2006). Review article: Age related alterations in respiratory function anesthetic considerations. *Canadian Journal of Anesthesia, 53*(12) 1244–1257.

St. Pierre, J. (1998). Functional decline in hospitalized elders: Preventive nursing measures. *AACN Clinical Issues, 9*(1), 109–118.

Stiller, K. (2007). Safety issues that should be considered when mobilizing critically ill patients. *Critical Care Clinics, 23,* 35–53.

Stotts, N. A., & Wu, H. S. (2007). Hospital recovery is facilitated by prevention of pressure ulcers in older adults. *Critical Care Nursing Clinics of North America, 19,* 269–275.

Suchinski, G. A., Piano, M. R., Rosenberg, N., & Zerwic, J. J. (1999). Treating urinary tract infections in the elderly. *Dimensions in Critical Care Nursing, 18,* 21–27.

Taffett, G. E. (2006). Physiology of aging. In C. Cassel, R. Leipzig, H. Cohen, E. Larson, & D. Meier (Eds.), *Geriatric medicine an evidenced-based approach* (4th ed., pp. 27–35). New York: Springer Publishing Company.

Tariq, S. H., & Mekhjian, G. (2007). Gastrointestinal bleeding in older adults. *Clinics in Geriatric Medicine, 23,* 769–784.

Thomas, D. R. (2006). Management of chronic wounds. In C. K. Cassel, R. M. Leipzig, H. J. Cohen, E. B. Larson, & D. E. Meier (Eds.), *Geriatric medicine an evidenced-based approach* (4th ed., pp. 967–977). New York: Springer Publishing Company.

Thomason, J., Wu, W., Shintani, A., Peterson, J. F., Pun, B. T., Jackson, J. C., & Ely, E. W. (2005). Intensive care unit delirium is an independent predictor of longer hospital stay: A prospective analysis of 261 non-ventilated patients. *Critical Care, 9,* R375–R381.

Thomsen, G. E., Snow, G. L., Rodriguez, L., & Hopkins, R. O. (2008). Patients with respiratory failure increase ambulation after transfer to an intensive care unit where early activity is priority. *Critical Care Medicine, 36*(4), 1119–1124.

Timiras, P. S. (2007). *Physiological basis of aging and geriatrics* (4th ed.). New York: Informa.

Timiras, P. S., & Navazio, F. M. (2007). The skeleton, joints, and skeletal and cardiac muscles. In P. S Timiras (Ed.), *Physiological basis of aging and geriatrics* (4th ed., pp. 329–344). New York: Informa.

Timmerman, R. A. (2007). A mobility protocol for the critically ill adult. *Dimensions in Critical Care Nursing, 26,* 175–179.

Torres, M., & Moayedi, S. (2007). Evaluation of the acutely dyspneic delderly patient. *Clinics in Geriatric Medicine, 23,* 307–325.

Urden, L. D., Stacy, K. M., & Lough, M. E. (2006). Gerontological alterations and management. In L. D. Urden, K. M . Stacy, & M. E. Lough (Eds.), *Thelan's critical care nursing* (5th ed., pp. 227–248). St Louis: Mosby Elsevier.

Van Den Noortgate, N., Mouton, V., Lamot, C., Van Nooton, G., Dhondt, A., Vanholder, R., et al. (2003). Outcome in post-cardiac surgery population with acute renal failure requiring dialysis: Does age make a difference? *Nephrology Dialysis Transplantation, 18,* 732–736.

Williams, M. E. (2008). *Geriatric physical diagnosis: A guide to observation and assessment.* Jefferson, NC: McFarland.

Wilson, J. A. P (2006). Gastroenterologic disorders. In C. K. Cassel, R. M Leipzig, H. J. Cohen, E. B. Larson, & D. E. Meier (Eds.), *Geriatric medicine an evidenced-based approach* (4th ed., pp. 835–849). New York: Springer Publishing Company.

Winkelman, C. (2007). Inactivity and inflammation in the critically ill patient. *Critical Care Clinics, 23,* 21–34.

Wisner, D. (1990). A stepwise logistic regression analysis of factors affecting morbidity and mortality after thoracic trauma: Effect of epidural analgesia. *Journal of Trauma, 30,* 799–805.

Wolf, L., Foley, A. L., & Howard, P. K. (2007). How normal are normal vital signs? Effective triage of the older patient. *Journal of Emergency Nursing, 33,* 587–589.

Zecca, L., Youdim, M. B., Riederer, P., Connor, J. R., & Crichton, R. R. (2004). Iron, brain aging and neurodegenerative disorders. *Nature Reviews—Neuroscience, 5,* 863–873.

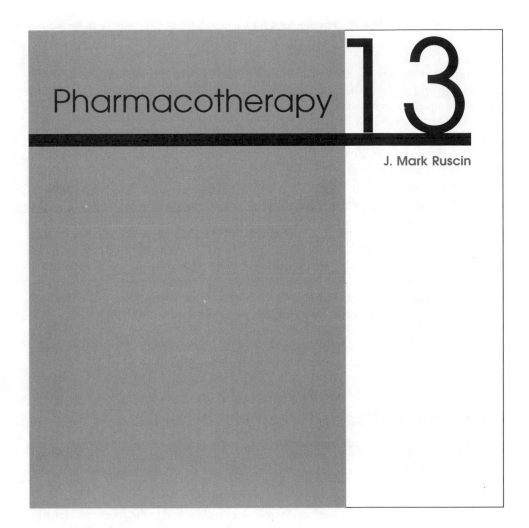

# Pharmacotherapy 13

J. Mark Ruscin

## Introduction

Medication-related morbidity and mortality continues to be a significant challenge among older adults, contributing to thousands of deaths each year and costing the U.S. health care system billions of dollars (Bootman, Harrison, & Cox, 1997; Hanlon et al., 1997; Johnson & Bootman, 1995; Perry, 1999). Adverse drug events (ADEs) in the acute care setting occur frequently, particularly among older patients, and have been shown to increase the risk of morbid and fatal events, as well as increase the costs of care (Bates et al., 1997; Clasen, Pestotnik, Evans, Lloyd, & Burke, 1997; Lazarou, Pomeranz, & Corey, 1998). Morbidity and mortality related to medication use can result from any of a number of possible problems, including adherence issues; drug–drug interactions; drug–disease interactions; drug dosing; medication misuse by patients; and even transcription, prescribing, or dispensing errors (Goulding, 2004). Medications are the most common intervention used to prevent or treat medical problems. Because older adults more commonly have multiple medical problems relative to younger populations, they generally use more medications. Although medications can cure or palliate disease and enhance health-related quality of life, medications can also be detrimental to quality of life and can cause adverse effects, including functional impairment and decline. The risk of adverse drug events is frequently associated with advanced age; however, studies have demonstrated that medication problems are more strongly associated with an increasing number of medications being used, rather than the age of the patient (Gurwitz et al., 2003; Hanlon et al., 2006; Hanlon, Schmader, & Gray, 2000). Relatively little information is available regarding the optimal use of most medications in older patients, particularly in patients greater than 85 years of age. Usual medication doses are often extrapolated from younger and healthier adult populations, which may not be appropriate for older more frail patients.

There is a progressive decline in many organ systems with advancing age that may impact pharmacotherapy. Age- and disease-related changes leading to a decline in functional reserve capacity can affect the ability of a patient to respond to physiological challenges or stresses. The decline in functional reserve and the response to pharmacotherapeutic interventions can be most challenging during times of acute illness. Medication-related problems associated with pharmacokinetic changes, polypharmacy, and inappropriate prescribing are common issues in all settings of care. A fundamental understanding of pharmacokinetic and pharmacodynamic changes in aging and of principles of appropriate medication prescribing can be critical to minimizing adverse events and drug-related functional decline in older adults.

## Pharmacokinetics and Pharmacodynamics

### Case Study 1

B.L. is a 73-year-old African American female who is admitted to the medical intensive care unit following presentation to the emergency department with new-onset symptoms consistent with stroke. B.L. was found to be in atrial fibrillation at the time of admission and was started on digoxin, metoprolol and intravenous heparin infusion. Her symptoms were consistent with a large left hemispheric ischemic stroke, confirmed by MRI (magnetic resonance imaging) testing. Two hours after the heparin was started, B.L. deteriorated neurologically, and she has a repeat MRI that demonstrates an intracerebral hemorrhage, and the heparin is stopped. The physician writes orders to start the patient on phenytoin to reduce the risk of seizures associated with the bleed.

Many age-related and disease-related physiologic changes can affect drug pharmacokinetics and pharmacodynamics. *Pharmacokinetics* relates to how medications are handled by the body, including absorption, distribution, metabolism, and elimination. *Pharmacodynamics* refers to the physiologic effect of the drug on the body, such as decreasing blood pressure or alleviating pain. Although the changes in these parameters related to aging and disease are common, they are also quite variable and difficult to predict in individual patients.

# Absorption

Physiologic changes associated with aging and disease can alter the absorption of drugs that are administered orally. Changes commonly observed include an increase in gastric pH caused by a decrease in gastric acid production, decreases in gastrointestinal blood flow, and slowed gastric emptying and gastrointestinal transit (Cusack, 2004). Despite these age-related changes, there are relatively few medications that are affected by aging and disease to a clinically significant degree and most medications that are absorbed by passive diffusion are affected little by aging and disease (Iber, Murphy, & Connor, 1994). For many medications, the rate of absorption may change, but the overall extent is not affected to a clinically significant degree. However, the changes may be clinically relevant for certain medications. Some medications require the acidic environment of the stomach to assist with appropriate absorption, including ketoconazole and calcium carbonate. Also, a decrease in gastric acid and an increase in gastric pH can cause inappropriate release of enteric-coated dosage forms, such as some aspirin and erythromycin products. Slowed or delayed gastric emptying can alter pharmacokinetics, depending on the absorption site of the drug. For example, acetaminophen is largely absorbed in the small intestine. Slowed gastric emptying can interrupt the presentation of acetaminophen to the site of absorption, leading to lower peak concentrations of the drug and a reduction and delay in the analgesic effect. Medical problems, such as diabetic gastroparesis can have a similar effect. Some medications undergo first-pass metabolism, either in the gut wall or the liver, before reaching the systemic circulation. Aging is associated with a decrease in first-pass metabolism, which may lead to increased concentrations of certain drugs, such as morphine or propranolol (Iber et al.).

# Distribution

Once a drug is absorbed and enters the systemic circulation, it is then distributed throughout the body. Characteristics of the drug (lipid/water solubility) and of the patient (body composition, blood flow, plasma protein levels) can alter how a drug is distributed. Generally with age, total body water decreases and body fat increases (Cusack, 2004). As a result, the distribution of water-soluble drugs (gentamicin, digoxin) decreases and the distribution of fat (lipid)-soluble drugs (diazepam) increases, leading to differences in drug concentrations when compared to younger populations. Distribution can also be affected by changes with protein binding of drugs. It is important to note that only the free portion of a drug exerts a pharmacologic effect, not the protein-bound portion. With advancing age, serum albumin concentrations tend to decline, particularly in patients with nutrition problems (Grandison & Boudinot, 2000). For drugs that are highly bound to albumin, such as phenytoin, free (nonprotein bound) concentrations of the drug may be increased, leading to an exaggerated pharmacologic effect or drug toxicity. Alpha-1 acid glycoprotein is another plasma protein that can bind medications and can be increased in patients with acute illnesses such as trauma, cancer, or inflammatory disorders. As a result, the free fraction of medications that bind to alpha-1 acid glycoprotein can be reduced (lidocaine, propranolol, quinidine) (Grandison & Boudinot).

## Metabolism

The major site of drug metabolism is the liver. Although aging is thought to affect some aspects of metabolism, others aspects are left relatively unaffected by aging. The metabolic reactions that occur in the liver are generally divided into two types: phase I (oxidative) and phase II (conjugative). Phase I reactions have been shown to be reduced with aging and may affect the metabolism of drugs via this route (diazepam, flurazepam, theophylline), leading to a decline in drug clearance and prolonged pharmacologic activity (Herrlinger & Klotz, 2001; Sotaniemi, Arranto, Pelkonen, & Pasanen, 1997). Medications metabolized by phase II reactions do not appear to be substantially affected by aging (lorazepam, temazepam) and may be preferred in older patients, if feasible. Blood flow to the liver can also affect metabolism, with metabolism decreasing with decreased blood flow to the liver, as may be seen in heart failure. Other factors that can affect drug metabolism include smoking, genetics, gender, diet, and drug interactions, particularly those involving the cytochrome P450 enzyme system (Herrlinger & Klotz).

## Elimination

Of the drugs that are not metabolized in the liver, most are eliminated by the kidneys. Even some drugs that are metabolized in the liver have metabolites that are eliminated by the kidneys. Some common medications that are eliminated by renal excretion include: gentamicin, digoxin, lithium, vancomycin, many of the cephalosporins, allopurinol, and atenolol. Meperidine, morphine, and propxyphene are examples of medications that are metabolized in the liver, but have metabolites that are eliminated by the kidneys. The calculated creatinine clearance is a commonly used tool to estimate glomerular filtration and to dose medications for patients (Cockroft & Gault, 1976; Levey et al., 1999). Glomerular filtration is thought to decline fairly consistently with age, however, current methods used to estimate glomerular filtration by calculating the creatinine clearance do have limitations. The Cockcroft and Gault equation is one of the most commonly used equations, and most recommendations for medication dose adjustments are based on this equation (Cockroft & Gault). However, many labs report estimations of glomerular filtration and renal function by reporting the Modified Diet in Renal Disease equation for patients who have had their serum creatinine tested (Levey et al.). Many older patients have a serum creatinine that looks normal, however, factors such as inactivity and reduced lean muscle tissue can make the serum creatinine look quite low, and overestimate the patients renal function when used to estimate the creatinine clearance in standard equations (Muhlberg & Platt, 1999).

## Pharmacodynamics

Pharmacodynamic changes associated with aging are not as well defined as pharmacokinetic changes. There is evidence of altered drug response with some medications that appear to make older adults more sensitive to the pharmacologic effects. Older adults have greater analgesic response to opioids, greater central nervous system response to benzodiazepines, and greater response to warfarin and heparin compared to younger populations (Greenblatt et al., 1991; Gurwitz, Avorn, Ross-Degnan, Choodnovskiy, & Ansell, 1992; Herrlinger & Klotz, 2001). Increased pharmacodynamic sensitivity can only be clearly determined when pharmacokinetic parameters are simultaneously evaluated. If pharmacokinetic parameters are similar between older patients and younger patients, yet an exaggerated response is observed in older patients, then increased sensitivity may explain the difference. This change may be the result of changes in receptor affinity, receptor numbers, or postreceptor response (Herrlinger & Klotz, 2001). Similarly, it is suggested that older patients may be less sensitive to other classes of medications, including beta-blockers and beta agonists.

## Case Study 1

How might changes in pharmacokinetics and pharmacodynamics associated with aging alter the response to medications with B.L.?

Several factors may alter B.L.'s response to the medications she is taking. Digoxin, commonly used for atrial fibrillation and heart failure, primarily distributes into body water and lean tissue. With age, total body water generally declines, decreasing the volume of distribution of digoxin and increasing serum concentrations of the drug. Additionally, digoxin is primarily eliminated by glomerular filtration in the kidneys, and with reduced renal function, the total clearance of digoxin is reduced, the half-life is prolonged, and serum concentrations can increase over time, increasing the risk for digoxin toxicity. Studies have also demonstrated that older patients may be more sensitive to the effects of anticoagulants, such as warfarin and heparin, putting B.L. at increased risk of bleeding. Whether this was the sole cause of the intracerebral bleeding incident in B.L. is difficult to say. Evaluation of the aPTT (activated partial thromboplastin time) at the time that the bleeding was identified may be able to tell us whether she was being overtreated with heparin. Frequent evaluation of the aPTT is important to prevent bleeding complications with heparin therapy in older patients. The initiation of phenytoin for the prevention of seizures would also require monitoring because of pharmacokinetic changes associated with aging. Phenytoin is highly protein bound, approximately 90%, with only 10% of the drug free to exert the pharmacologic effect. In patients with decreased albumin, the free fraction can be increased and can cause toxicity, such as nystagmus and ataxia. Dilantin toxicity can also increase the risk of falls caused by ataxia. For patients with low serum albumin, free phenytoin concentrations can be obtained to more accurately evaluate serum concentrations.

# Inappropriate Medication

Inappropriate medication prescribing in older adults has received a significant amount of attention in the medical literature (Aparasu & Mort, 2000; Fick et al., 2003; Garcia, 2006; Goulding, 2004; Zhan et al., 2001). The primary reason is that inappropriate medication prescribing is considered a common cause of ADEs in all types of patient care settings (Chang et al., 2005; Cooper, 1999; Field et al., 2004; Gurwitz et al., 2003;

## 13.1 Selected Potentially Inappropriate Medications for Older Patients From the Beer's Criteria List (Not All-Inclusive)

| | |
|---|---|
| Amiodarone (Cordarone) | Amitriptyline (Elavil) |
| Barbiturates | Belladonna alkaloids (Donnatal) |
| Carisoprodol (Soma) | Chlordiazepoxide (Librium) |
| Chlorpropamide (Diabenese) | Cimetidine (Tagamet) |
| Clonidine (Catapres) | Clorazepate (Tranxene) |
| Cylcobenzaprine (Flexeril) | Dessicated thyroid |
| Diazepam (Valium) | Dicyclomine (Bentyl) |
| Diphenhydramine (Benadryl) | Doxazosin (Cardura) |
| Doxepin (Sinequan) | Ergot mesyloids (Hydergine) |
| Fluoxetine (Prozac) | Flurazepam (Dalmane) |
| Guanedrel (Hylorel) | Hydroxyzine (Vistaril, Atarax) |
| Indomethacin (Indocin) | Ketoralac (Toradol) |
| Meperidine (Demerol) | Meprobamate (Miltown, Equanil) |
| Methocarbamol (Robaxin) | Methyldopa (Aldomet) |
| Nifedipine (Procardia) | Nitrofurantoin (Macrodantin) |
| Oxazepam (Serax) | Oxybutynin (Ditropan) |
| Pentazocine (Talwin) | Piroxicam (Feldene) |
| Propantheline (Probanthine) | Propoxyphene (Darvon, Darvocet) |
| Thioridazine (Mellaril) | Triazolam (Halcion) |

Hajjar et al., 2005; Hanlon et al., 1997; Lindley, Tully, Paramsothy, & Tallis, 1992). Criteria for evaluating medication appropriateness have been developed and evaluated. One method, commonly known as the Beer's Criteria, is a list of specific medications that are considered potentially inappropriate for older adults (Fick et al., 2003). Table 13.1 lists some of the medications included among the Beer's Criteria. Medications included within the Beer's list are generally considered ineffective or to have potential risks that exceed the potential benefits. Therefore, the likelihood of older patients experiencing ADEs from these medications is quite high. Most clinicians would agree that the medications included in this list are suboptimal choices for the majority of older patients, however, several studies have shown that use of these medications has continued and remains fairly constant, with 20 to 25% of older patients continuing to use medications found on the list (Hajjar et al., 2005; Zhan et al., 2001).

Acutely ill older patients may be more susceptible to the adverse effects of medications during times of reduced physiologic reserves, and therefore may be at greater risk for experiencing ADEs related to the use of potentially inappropriate medications. However, a recently published Italian study showed that potentially inappropriate drug use (defined as use of Beer's Criteria medications) in hospitalized older patients was not significantly associated with ADEs, length of stay, or in-hospital mortality (Onder et al., 2005). Another study published in the United States found that nearly one third of hospitalized elderly patients were prescribed a medication from the Beer's Criteria list (Page & Ruscin, 2006). One in 10 adverse drug events was related to the use of a Beer's Criteria medication, but no significant relationship was found between the use of Beer's medications and length of stay, risk of ADEs, or in-hospital mortality. Limiting the definition of inappropriate medication to the Beer's Criteria minimizes the possibility that other (nonlisted) medications can be potentially inappropriate in certain patients and may significantly underestimate the problem (Goulding, 2004; Ruscin & Page). For example, in the case study of B.L., the use of phenytoin would not be considered inappropriate based on the Beer's Criteria. However, if the drug was not dosed properly based on B.L.'s serum albumin, the risk for an ADE related to phenytoin toxicity would be high. The results of these previous studies in acute care settings demonstrate that interventions to reduce the risk of medication-related morbidity and mortality in older adults need to be broader than that which can be achieved with use of the Beer's Criteria alone.

## Drug Interactions

In the situation of multiple drug use, drug–drug interactions can be quite common. Whether or not a drug–drug interaction is clinically significant can be difficult to determine in some situations. Drug–drug interactions can occur through multiple mechanisms, but generally are considered either pharmacokinetic or pharmacodynamic interactions (Herrlinger & Klotz, 2001; Sotaniemi et al., 1997) Drug absorption can be altered when one drug influences the absorption of another drug. For example, the bile acid binding resin cholestyramine can bind and decrease the absorption of many medications if the medications are administered in close proximity to one another. The absorption of warfarin, thyroid hormones, digoxin, valproic acid, and many other orally administered medications can be reduced if administered with cholestyramine. To prevent problems, medications should be given either 1 hour before or 4 to 6 hours after the administration of cholestyramine. Drug distribution can be altered if two drugs are given that are both highly protein bound. For example, if a patient is taking a stable dosage regimen of warfarin, and a new medication is started that is also highly protein bound, the second drug may displace warfarin from protein binding sites, increasing the amount of free warfarin as well as increasing the antithromotic effect and the potential risk of bleeding. Frequent monitoring of the antithrombotic effect of warfarin would be warranted in this situation. There are numerous drug–drug interactions that can occur involving drug metabolism in the liver. Drugs metabolized by the cytrochrome P450 enzyme system in the liver are commonly involved (Herrlinger & Klotz). When two drugs are metabolized by the same enzyme there may be competition for the enzymes that changes the metabolism of one or both of the medications. Also, some of the enzymes can be inhibited by medications or induced by other medications. For example, warfarin is metabolized by cytochrome P450 enzymes 2C9 and 3A4. Medications that influence either of these enzymes can interact with warfarin. Fluconazole can inhibit the metabolism of warfarin by P450-3A4 and increase the anticoagulant effect of warfarin. Amiodarone, metronidazole, and sulfamethoxazole can inhibit the metabolism of warfarin by P450-2C9 and increase the anticoagulant effect of warfarin. On the other hand, phenytoin can induce the metabolism of warfarin by P450-2C9 and reduce the anticoagulant effect of warfarin. Pharmacodynamic drug interactions can occur when two medications are used that either have antagonistic effects or have similar receptor effects. Beta-agonists, like albuterol, are frequently used in patients who have pulmonary disease to improve airflow to the lungs. However, nonselective beta blockers, such as propranolol, can have the opposite effect, reducing airflow to the lungs in patients with pulmonary disease. In this instance, selective beta-blockers, such as metoprolol, are preferred.

There are numerous computerized programs available to help search for possible drug interactions. These programs can be difficult to use clinically because the programs often do not give useful information to describe how likely the interactions are to occur and how clinically relevant the interaction may be. Involving pharmacists in the assessment of potential drug interactions can be useful in helping to make clinically sound decisions about the risk and potential severity of drug–drug interactions.

## Principles of Drug Use in the Elderly

Several approaches can be used successfully to help minimize the risk of a negative impact of medications in older patients. The use of standard adult doses may not be appropriate in all patients, and starting with lower doses in more frail patients may be appropriate. Trying to achieve this can sometimes be difficult when the commercial availability of smaller dosage forms is lacking. This is generally more problematic with oral dosage forms than with parenteral dosage forms. The frequent use of drug levels or concentrations may help avoid problems with drug overdoses and toxicity (Greenblatt, Sellers, & Koch-Weser, 1982). It is important to consider any new symptoms as though they are a possible drug side effect. Drug cascades and polypharmacy can be a negative consequence when additional medications are added to treat the side effects of other medications. Minimizing the use of medications should be a high-priority goal when at all possible. However, it is just as important to avoid situations in which medications are withheld from older patients when treatment may be beneficial.

## Summary

Physiologic changes associated with aging and disease have the potential to alter how medications are handled within the body and thereby affect the patient's response to treatment. Understanding how these changes may affect drug therapy can help prevent negative outcomes associated with drug therapy. Some medications should be avoided all together because the risk of use generally outweighs the potential benefits. Close monitoring of therapy, particularly in older patients who are acutely ill, can significantly reduce the risk of adverse events and medication-related morbidity and mortality.

## References

Aparasu, R. R., & Mort, J. R. (2000). Inappropriate prescribing for the elderly: Beers criteria-based review. *Annals of Pharmacotherapeutics, 34*, 338–346.

Bates, D. W., Spell, N., Cullen, D. J., Burdick, E., Laird, N., Petersen, L. A., et al. (1997). The costs of adverse drug events in hospitalized patients. Adverse Drug Events Prevention Study Group. *Journal of the American Medical Association, 277*, 307–311.

Bootman, J. L., Harrison, D. L., & Cox, E. (1997). The health care cost of drug-related morbidity and mortality in nursing facilities. *Archives of Internal Medicine, 157*, 2089–2096.

Chang, C. M., Liu, P. Y., Yang, Y. H., Yang, Y. C., Wu, C. F., & Lu, F. H. (2005). Use of the Beers criteria to predict adverse drug reactions among first-visit elderly outpatients. *Pharmacotherapy, 25*, 831–838.

Clasen, D. C., Pestotnik, S. L., Evans, R. S., Lloyd, J. F., & Burke, J. P. (1997). Adverse drug events in hospitalized patients: Excess length of stay, extra costs, and attributable mortality. *Journal of the American Medical Association, 277*, 301–306.

Cockroft, D. W., & Gault, M H. (1976). Prediction of creatinine clearance from serum creatinine. *Nephron, 16*, 31–41.

Cooper, J. W. (1999). Adverse drug reaction-related hospitalizations of nursing facility patients: A 4-year study. *Southern Medical Journal, 92*, 485–490.

Cusack, B. J. (2004). Pharmacokinetics in older persons. *American Journal of Geriatric Pharmacotherapy, 2*, 274–302.

Fick, D. M., Cooper, J. W., Wade, W. E., Waller, J. L., Maclean, J. R., & Beers, M. H. (2003). Updating the Beers criteria for potentially inappropriate medication use in older adults: Results of a US consensus panel of experts. *Archives of Internal Medicine, 163*, 2716–2724.

Field, T. S., Gurwitz, J. H., Harrold, L. R., Rothschild, J., DeBellis, K. R., Seger, A. C., et al.(2004). Risk factors for adverse drug events among older adults in the ambulatory setting. *Journal of the American Geriatrics Society, 52*, 1349–1354.

Garcia, R. M. (2006). Five ways you can reduce inappropriate prescribing in the elderly: A systematic review. *Journal of Family Practice, 55*, 305–312.

Goulding, M. R. (2004). Inappropriate medication prescribing for elderly ambulatory care patients. *Archives of Internal Medicine, 164*, 305–312.

Grandison, M. K., & Boudinot, F. D. (2000). Age-related changes in protein binding of drugs: Implications for therapy. *Clinical Pharmacokinetics, 38*, 271–290.

Greenblatt, D. J., Harmatz, J. S., Shapiro, L., Englhardt, N., Gouthro, T. A., & Shader, R. I. (1991). Sensitivity to triazolam in the elderly. *New England Journal of Medicine, 324*, 1691–1698.

Greenblatt, D. J., Sellers, E. M., & Koch-Weser, J. (1982). Importance of protein-binding for the interpretation of serum or plasma drug concentrations. *Journal of Clinical Pharmacology, 22*, 259–263.

Gurwitz, J. H., Avorn, J., Ross-Degnan, D., Choodnovskiy, I., & Ansell, J. (1992). Aging and the anticoagulant response to warfarin. *Annals of Internal Medicine, 116*, 901–904.

Gurwitz, J. H., Field, T. S., Harrold, L. R., Rothschild, J., Debellis, K., Seger, A. C., et al. (2003). Incidence and preventability of adverse drug events among older persons in the ambulatory setting. *Journal of the American Medical Association, 289*, 1107–1116.

Hajjar, E. R., Hanlon, J. T., Sloane, R. J., Lindblad, C. I., Pieper, C. F., Ruby, C. M., et al. (2005). Unnecessary drug use in frail older people at hospital discharge. *Journal of the American Geriatrics Society, 53*, 1518–1523.

Hanlon, J. T., Pieper, C. F., Hajjar, E. R., Sloane, R. J., Lindblad, C. I., Ruby, C. M., et al. (2006). Incidence and predictors of all and preventable adverse drug reactions in frail elderly post hospital stay. *Journals of Gerontology: Medical Sciences, 61A*, 511–115.

Hanlon, J. T., Schmader, K., & Gray, S. L. (2000). Adverse drug reactions. In J. C. Delafuente & R. B. Stewart (Eds.), *Therapeutics in the elderly* (3rd ed., pp. 289–314). Cincinnati, OH: Harvey Whitney.

Hanlon, J. T., Schmader, K. E., Koronkowski, M. J., Weinberger, M., Landsman, P. B., Samsa, G. P., et al. (1997). Adverse drug events in high risk older outpatients. *Journal of the American Geriatrics Society, 45*, 945–948.

Herrlinger, C., & Klotz, U. (2001). Drug metabolism and drug interactions in the elderly. *Best Practices: Research in Clinical Gastroenterology, 15*, 897–918.

Iber, F. L., Murphy, P. A., & Connor, E. S. (1994). Age-related changes in the gastrointestinal system: Effects on drug therapy. *Drugs & Aging, 5*, 34–48.

Johnson, J. A., & Bootman, J. L. (1995). Drug-related morbidity and mortality. A cost-of-illness model. *Archives of Internal Medicine, 155*, 1949–1956.

Lazarou, J., Pomeranz, B. H., & Corey, P. N. (1998). Incidence of adverse drug reactions in hospitalized patients: A meta-analysis of prospective studies. *Journal of the American Medical Association, 279*, 1200–1205.

Levey, A. S., Bosch, J. P., Lewis, J. B., Greene, T., Rogers, N., & Roth, D. for Modification of Diet in Renal Disease Study Group. (1999). A more accurate method to estimate glomerular filtration rate from serum creatinine: A new prediction equation. *Annals of Internal Medicine, 130*, 461–470.

Lindley, C. M., Tully, M. P., Paramsothy, V., & Tallis, R. C. (1992). Inappropriate medication is a major cause of adverse drug reactions in elderly patients. *Age & Ageing, 21*, 294–300.

Muhlberg, W., & Platt, D. (1999). Age-dependent changes of the kidneys: Pharmacological implications. *Gerontology, 45*, 243–253.

Onder, G., Landi, F., Liperoti, R., Fialova, D., Gambassi, G., & Bernabei, R. (2005). Impact of inappropriate drug use among hospitalized older adults. *European Journal of Clinical Pharmacology, 61*, 453–459.

Page, R. L., & Ruscin, J. M. (2006). The risk of adverse drug events and hospital-related morbidity and mortality among older adults with potentially inappropriate medication use. *American Journal of Geriatric Pharmacotherapeutics, 4,* 297–305.

Perry, D. P. (1999). When medicine hurts instead of helps. *Consultant Pharmacist, 14,* 1326–1330.

Ruscin, J. M., & Page, R. L. II. (2002). Inappropriate prescribing for elderly patients. *Journal of the American Medical Association, 287,* 1264–1265.

Sotaniemi, E. A., Arranto, A. J., Pelkonen, O., & Pasanen, M. (1997). Age and cytochrome P450-linked drug metabolism in humans. *Clinical Pharmacology and Therapeutics, 61,* 331–339.

Zhan, C., Sangl, J., Bierman, A. S., Miller, M. R., Friedman, B., Wickizer, S. W., & Meyer, G. S. (2001). Potentially inappropriate medication use in the community-dwelling elderly: Findings from the 1996 Medical Expenditure Panel Survey. *Journal of the American Medical Association, 286,* 2823–2829.

# Nutrition and Hydration

# 14

Kathryn A. Wilt
Donna M. Fick

In this age of epidemic obesity and the ever ubiquitous plastic bottle of water, it's hard to imagine that malnutrition and dehydration would be a practical concern. Yet in the intensive care unit, a high percentage of malnourished and dehydrated persons continue to present, complicating treatments and hindering patient outcomes. Complications from trauma, elective surgeries, and sepsis can compound patient presentation and hinder nutritional and hydration interventions. The critical care nurse must identify patients at risk, understand the effects of malnutrition and dehydration in the older adult, and implement nursing interventions to improve patient outcomes both during hospitalization and postdischarge. This chapter highlights the etiology of these conditions, describes appropriate geriatric assessment tools for nutrition and hydration, and discusses evidence-based nursing interventions to improve outcomes.

Problems with nutrition and hydration are common in older adults. Prevalence estimates of nutritional deficiency and dehydration in these patients range from 40 to 70% with little improvement in these percentages over the last 30 years. Over 60% of patients experience deterioration of their nutritional status during their hospital stay (Barr, Hecht, Flavin, Khorana, & Gould, 2004). Older persons are at higher risk for dehydration and electrolyte imbalances, with elders aged 85 to 99 being six times more likely to be hospitalized for dehydration than those aged 65 to 69. As our nation's older adults enjoy increased longevity (by the year 2030, persons over 65 will double in number in the United States, growing from 35 million to 71.5 million [Federal Interagency Forum on Aging-Related Statistics, 2008]), those at risk for nutritional and hydrational deficiencies will continue to increase. Although these statistics are alarming in themselves, many health care practitioners do not recognize malnutrition as a risk factor and fail to establish early interventions for these patients (Adams, Bowie, Simmance, Murray, & Crowe, 2008).

## Risk Factors With the Older Adult Patient and Associated Outcomes From Poor Nutrition/Hydration Status

Why have older adults continued to be at such high risk for poor nutrition and hydration deficiencies? Both systemic and individual risk factors can be identified. From the systematic viewpoint, the lack of nutritional training of health care providers, a failure to regard malnutrition as important, scarcity of clinical nutritionists, and lack of hospital policy are indicated (Pironi, Paganelli, Merli, & Miglioni, 2000). From the older adult's vantage point, the answer is multifactorial in nature, as shown in Figure 14.1. Chronic disease, prevalent in 75% of older persons over age 65, leads to compromised nutrient intake and absorption (Reid & Allard-Gould, 2004). Social isolation, economic hardship, and polypharmacy are also major contributors to compromised intake. Once in the intensive care unit (ICU), their consumption may be restricted by prolonged NPO (nothing by mouth) status, lack of attention to oral care, changes in mental status including delirium, and use of restraints. Malnutrition is also compounded by health care practitioners minimizing nutritional concerns in lieu of other more acute health issues, resulting in therapy delays (Bachrach-Lindström, Jensen, Lunkin, & Christensson et al., 2007; Barr et al., 2004; Ennis, Saffel-Shrier, & Verson, 2001). A lack of understanding of the normal age-related changes that occur in the older adult, which impact thirst, taste, hunger, and digestive function, may affect nursing diagnoses and interventions. Absence of a hospital nutritional protocol also delays nutrition and hydration interventions (Bachrach-Lindström et al.). Finally, from the nursing research perspective, few high-quality investigations document the relationship between interventions and associated outcomes in the older adult.

Both malnutrition and dehydration result in a cascade of negative physiologic effects as well as long-term negative outcomes. Catabolic depletion of muscle protein results in higher rates of infection, decreased rates of wound healing, and increased length of hospital stays. Poorly managed nutrition results in more days of mechanical ventilation, higher incidence of delirium (Culp & Cacchione, 2008) increasing medical complications and associated health care costs (Barr et al., 2004; Braunschweig, Gomez, & Sheean, 2000). Hospital length of stays and mortality rates are three times higher in patients with moderate to severe malnutrition (Barr et al.).

## Aging Changes and Common Geriatric Problems

The older adult undergoes normal physiologic changes that can impact his/her nutritional and hydration status. Decreases in lean muscle mass, total body water, and metabolic rate, along with accompanying increases in body fat are typical in the older

# 14.1

**Hospitalization and physiologic responses leading to malnutrition.**

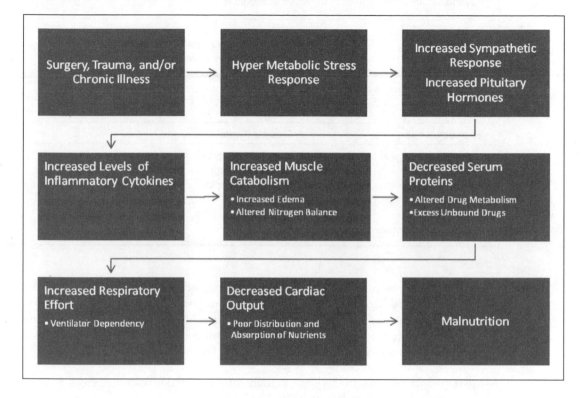

adult. This latter factor and the high prevalence of obesity in the older adult hinder identification of nutritional issues. Older adults lose taste/thirst sensation and visual acuity, and may lose hand/eye coordination, resulting in less desire and/or ability to feed themselves. Increased frequency of urination or nocturia may lead older adults to drink less fluids causing dehydration leading to constipation, whereas many medications may alter taste/thirst, cause decreased gastrointestinal motility, and decreased nutrient absorption. Although cognitive decline is not a normal change in aging adults, benign forgetfulness results in neglect to eat and drink at regular intervals, particularly for those living alone. A summary of physiologic changes in the older adult is shown in Table 14.1.

## Defining Malnutrition and Dehydration

Malnutrition refers to a series of complex interactions in the body that result in reduced (or excessive) nutrient intake leading to an alteration in body composition or serum

## 14.1 Risk Factors Leading to Poor Nutrition and Hydration in Critical Care

| Psychosocial | Physiological |
|---|---|
| ■ Depression | ■ Dysphagia |
| ■ Grief | ■ Disabilities and loss of self-care capacity |
| ■ Living alone | ■ Polypharmacy & medication interactions |
| ■ Lower health literacy | ■ Edentulism or lack of/poorly fitting dentures |
| ■ Overconsumption of alcohol | ■ Dry mouth or taste bud atrophy |

| Socioeconomic | Chronic Illness |
|---|---|
| ■ Fixed incomes and high cost of food | ■ Inability to prepare or ingest food |
| ■ Lack of dietary variety | ■ Decreased appetite |
| ■ Lack of health care provider knowledge | ■ Poor oral health |
| ■ Lack of early interventions | |

chemistry. It can be caused by diminished (or excessive) intake, malabsorption of nutrients, impaired digestion, excessive losses from vomiting and diarrhea, or from increased nutrient use during hypercatabolic states like trauma and fever. In the older adult, malnutrition and dehydration are influenced by chronic diseases that compromise food intake and nutrient absorption. Other relevant terms include:

*food insufficiency*: an inadequate amount of food intake resulting from lack of resources (Briefel & Wotecki, 1992);

*protein energy malnutrition*: the presence of clinical and laboratory signs such as body wasting, low body mass index (BMI), low albumin and prealbumin levels caused by insufficient protein/calorie consumption (DiMaria-Ghalili & Guenter, 2008).

Dehydration is usually a term associated with water deficiency—a rare condition as most people have access to water. In most cases of clinical dehydration, hypernatremia (serum sodium greater than 145 mEq/L) is also seen, resulting from depletion in total body water content resulting from pathological fluid loss, diminished water intake, or a combination of these factors. In the older adult, renal efficiency decreases with age because of tubular dysfunction or the inability to concentrate the urine. Comatose or paralyzed older patients will also exhibit insensible water losses through the skin and lungs with minimal formation of urine. Inadequate hydration causes numerous negative biological effects in the older adult, ranging from fatigue, headache, muscle weakness and spasms, renal dysfunction and gastric disorders, and blood pressure anomalies that contribute to the dizziness, which can lead to falls (Mukand, Cai, Zielinski, Danish, & Berman, 2003).

Dehydration may be exacerbated in the older adult by excessive consumption of caffeinated beverages or alcoholic beverages and their effects on antidiuretic hormones.

Concerns with incontinence and nocturia, as well as the use of anticholinergic medications may contribute to dehydration. Each of these factors should be considered by the critical care nurse when assessing oral intake.

## Assessing the Older Adult for Nutritional and Hydration Deficiencies

Assessment of the critically ill patient for nutritional and hydration deficiencies is an ongoing process throughout hospitalization. The Joint Commission now mandates that a systematic nutritional assessment be completed at patient admission (Joint Commission, 2008). Ideally, an initial risk screening by the nurse is completed, followed by a detailed assessment if warranted. A comprehensive data review by an interdisciplinary team should then identify patient-specific needs and goals, and establish how patient progress will be monitored. Components of a complete assessment are shown in the bulleted points that follow; the ICU nurse may need to be creative to elicit this information in critically ill adults. The nurse should consider the following prior to conducting the initial screening:

- Is the patient verbal? A reliable historian? Or is a caretaker/guardian available for consultation? Special considerations may need to be provided for the person with dementia.
- Are physiologic measures distorted because of an emergent condition or medications (e.g., fluid retention masking weight loss; burn victims with fluid and electrolyte shifts)?
- Will this patient be NPO for more than 3 days because of tests/surgeries?
- Has the patient had a temperature of >100.4° F for more than 3 days inducing an accelerated catabolic state?
- Are pain, agitation, and/or delirium present, which are known to elevate nutrition requirements?
- Is the patient in a shock state, hypothermic, or will she/he be routinely sedated which will decrease energy needs?

Of particular importance in the initial phase of patient assessment is the use of an interdisciplinary team to provide a comprehensive evaluation of the patient. Ideally this team includes the patient (and knowledgeable family member), physician or gastrointestinal specialist, pharmacist, hospital dietician, occupational therapist (for feeding and swallowing concerns) and speech pathologist if dysphagia is suspected. Creating a timetable for periodic follow-up assessments (including postdischarge evaluation) is critical for continued patient improvement.

### Which Nutritional Assessment Tool to Use?

Many nutritional screening/assessment tools exist for the nurse professional with Green and Watson (2005) identifying 71 of them in their systematic review; 21 of these are designated to be used with an older population. Green and Watson caution that many of these instruments have not been subjected to validity and/or reliability testing, and that sensitivity/specificity of the tools have not been investigated.

Typically a screening tool is a short instrument that can quickly identify an at-risk adult, the results of which would lead to use of further assessments or measurements. The Mini Nutritional Assessment (MNA) incorporates both of these elements and remains one of the most frequently used and highly validated clinical tools for use with older adults (DiMaria-Ghalili & Guenter, 2008; Feldblum et al., 2007). It consists of two sections: the first six screening questions comprise the MNA-SF (for Short Form)—an initial patient screening that takes less than 5 minutes to administer. The MNA does not use any laboratory measures to establish nutritional status. If this tool indicates a risk for malnutrition, the 12-question assessment section of the MNA is completed and referrals for nutritional consulting should be initiated. See LINKS section at the end of this chapter for additional MNA resources.

Other geriatric-specific nutrition assessments exist but validity in the critical care setting has not been established. They include the Nutrition Screening Initiative: DETERMINE Your Nutritional Health—a 10-item checklist Developed by American Academy of Family Physicians, in partnership with the American Dietetic Association and the National Council on Aging (see LINKS at end of chapter). This tool also does not use laboratory values and relies heavily on the patient as an accurate historian. The Geriatric Nutritional Risk Index (Bouillanne et al., 2005) is a modified version of the Nutritional Risk Index (Buzby et al., 1988) that combines two nutritional indicators (albumin and weight loss). However, limited validity data is available for this index.

## Anthropometric Measures

Simple anthropometric measurements (height, weight, weight history, BMI) can provide baseline information on nutritional status of the critical care patient, but should be used with caution. Unintentional weight loss of 10 pounds in the last 6 months, or loss of 5 pounds in the previous month is commonly considered a red flag to the clinician. However, weight measures are less indicative of nutritional status in the critically ill patient because of fluid retention. Typically anthropometric measures are more useful for establishing long-term malnutrition versus acute deficiencies (Harrington, 2004) but normative BMI data for the older adult is lacking and may be inappropriate for nutritional screening in this population (Bonnefoy, Jauffret, Kostka, & Jusot, 2002). Obtaining a reliable height for the older adult is difficult if she/ he cannot stand erect. Consider obtaining a demi-span length—measured as the distance from the middle of the sternal notch to the tip of the middle finger—or knee height measurement, which does not vary with advancing age (see Chumlea, Roche, & Steinbaugh, 1985; and LINKS for a knee-height calculator).

## Laboratory Indicators

Laboratory indicators of nutritional and hydration status should be routinely reviewed by the critical care nurse (see Table 14.2). No single laboratory test is indicative of malnutrition or dehydration, as many of the indicators are affected by disease states, stress levels, immune and hydration status (Green & Watson, 2005; Vivanti, Harvey, Ash, & Battistutta, 2008). The most common nutrition indicators include serum prealbumin, serum albumin, transferrin, and total lymphocyte count. Abnormal hematological measures may not correlate with low (at-risk) nutritional screening scores, however (Alves de Rezende, Cunha, Junior, & Penha-Silva, 2005; Feldblum et al., 2007). Albuminemia is considered to be an indicator of long-term protein deficiency and has been

## 14.2 Common Laboratory Markers for Nutrition and Hydration

| Indicator | Normal Value | Comment |
|---|---|---|
| Nutrition Markers | | |
| Serum albumin | 3.4–5.4 g/dL | Low levels of albumin may also result from ascites, burns, glomerulonephritis, liver disease, malabsorption diseases (e.g., Crohn's disease), and nephrotic syndrome. |
| Prealbumin | 15–35 mg/dl | Generally considered a more sensitive indicator of protein malnutrition than albumin because of its shorter half life. Level may be elevated in dialysis patients or those prescribed steroids. |
| Transferrin | >200 mg/dl | A serum protein that binds and transfers iron, it is increased with iron-deficiency anemia. A predictor of protein depletion. Decreased with chronic illness and liver disease. |
| Total lymphocyte count | >1500 mm$^3$ | Affected by many disease processes. |
| Hydration Markers | | |
| BUN/creatinine ratio | < 20 | Values greater than 25 indicate dehydration. |
| Serum osmolality | 280–300 mmol/kg | A measure of protein, BUN, sodium, potassium, and glucose in the serum. |
| Serum sodium | <150 mEq/L | |
| Urine-specific gravity | 1.005–1.030 | Elevated values (>1.030) indicate dehydration with urine becoming progressively more concentrated in color. |
| Urine volume | >1200cc/day or 50cc/hour | |

shown to be associated with skeletal muscle mass and protein intake. Serial prealbumin levels are considered a more sensitive indicator of nutrition and should be assessed routinely along with urine urea nitrogen to estimate nitrogen balance using a 24-hour urine collection (L. Bernstein et al., 1995). Hydration indicators can include urine color, urine-specific gravity, blood urea nitrogen (BUN) and creatinine, as well as osmolarity measures. A normal-appearing BUN and creatinine in older patients can underestimate the degree of renal problems.

## Oral Health Care Assessment

Assessment of patient oral health can provide clues to the causes of poor nutrition and hydration. Missing teeth or dentures, dental caries, inadequate salivation, mouth

## 14.3   Common Medications Used in the Older Adult Patient and Effects on Digestion

| Effect | Drugs |
|---|---|
| Causes dry mouth | Anticholinergics, antidepressants, antihypertensives, and bronchodilators |
| Increases appetite | Alcohol, antihistamines, corticosteroids, dronabinol, insulin, megestrol, acetate, mirtazapine, sulfonylureas, thyroid hormone |
| Decreases appetite | Antibiotics, bulk agents (methylcellulose, guar gum), cyclophosphamide, digoxin, glucagon, indomethacin, morphine, fluoxetine |
| Increases plasma glucose level | Octreotide, opioids, phenothiazines, phenytoin, probenecid, thiazide diuretics, corticosteroids, warfarin |
| Decreases plasma glucose level | ACE inhibitors, aspirin, barbiturates, alpha-blockers, insulin, monoamine oxidase inhibitors (MAOIs), oral antihyperglycemic drugs, phenacetin, phenylbutazone, sulfonamides |
| Increases plasma lipid level | Adrenal corticosteroids, chlorpromazine, ethanol, growth hormone, oral contraceptives (estrogen–progestin type), thiouracil, vitamin D |
| Decreases plasma lipid level | Aspirin and $p$-aminosalicylic acid, l-asparaginase, chlortetracycline, colchicine, dextrans, glucagon, niacin, phenindione, statins, sulfinpyrazone, trifluperidol |
| Decreases protein metabolism | Chloramphenicol, tetracycline |

lesions, and periodontal diseases can hinder both the functional and social aspects of eating and drinking. The Kayser-Jones Brief Oral Health Status Examination (BOHSE) is a simple 10-item tool developed for nursing-home residents that the critical care nurse can use to evaluate mouth and dentition conditions that may impact eating and drinking (Kayser-Jones, Bird, Paul, Long, & Schell, 1995). This tool is available on the Internet from The Hartford Institute for Geriatric Nursing as listed in the LINKS section at the end of this chapter.

## Polypharmacy and Drug Interactions

Older adults represent only 12% of the population but consume approximately 30% of prescription medications (Williams, 2002). Prescribed medications can significantly affect appetite, nutrient motility, gastrointestinal distress, energy level, and mental outlook, leading to decreased water and nutrient intake. Digoxin use in the older adult is considered one of the most problematic drugs because of its narrow therapeutic range (Ennis et al., 2001). Table 14.3 lists the effects of common drugs on nutrition. The Food and Drug Administration and National Institute for Health also publish nutrient–drug interaction guidelines (See LINKS). The health care team should be alert for possible food/drug interactions and teach the patient means to minimize medication effects postdischarge.

# Interventions

Interventions to improve the nutrition and hydration status of the critically ill adult begin during admission and continue postdischarge. Involvement of the entire health care team *and* the patient with his or her family/caregiver provides a solid foundation for success. The critical care nurse may be involved in the following specific interventions with the older adult patient:

- Improve the mealtime experience in the ICU
- Increase fluid intake
- Use of oral supplements
- Use of parenteral nutrition or total parenteral nutrition (TPN)
- Provide oral care

## Determining Energy Requirements

The general approach to the nutritional care of the critically ill patient involves delivery of a balanced diet, including carbohydrate, fat, protein, and essential nutrients. Specialists agree that critically ill patients have better outcomes when they are fed early—ideally within 24 to 48 hours of admission, although the literature is conflicting in this area (Cresci, 2005). Protein requirements for a patient will vary depending on the severity of the illness, but in general, most patients require 0.8 to 1.5 grams of protein per kilogram mass weight per day. Those patients with severe stress levels, traumatic crushing injuries, GI (gastrointestinal) bleeds, or those undergoing hemodialysis may require more than 2 grams per kilogram per day. End-stage liver disease patients' protein needs may be lessened because of their inability to metabolize higher protein levels. The Harris–Benedict equation (Harris & Benedict, 1919) can be used to predict resting-energy expenditure requirements and modified for use with differing patient conditions (Parrish & Falls-McCray, 2003). There are English and metric versions of the Harris–Benedict equation that can be accessed at: http://www.bmi-calculator.net/bmrcalculator/bmr-formula.phb (accessed December 4, 2008).

## Improving the Mealtime Experience in the Critical Care Unit

Along with the biological aspects associated with food, eating and drinking have complex social and psychological implications that remain relevant even in a critical care setting. Establishing an atmosphere conducive to these elements may be difficult in an ICU, but some interventions can be readily accomplished as shown in the text box that follows.

---

### Improving Mealtime in the Critical Care Unit

- Reposition patient prior to setting his or her meal tray in place.
- Reduce portion sizes to accommodate reduced appetites.
- Reduce distractions during mealtime, including well-meaning visitors who may interrupt a patient's focus on the meal.

---

*(continued)*

**Improving Mealtime in the Critical Care Unit** *(continued)*

- Remove or eliminate noxious odors, including used urinals, bedpans, over-flowing trash receptacles, soiled laundry, and so on.
- Provide ample space on the patient's bedside table for a meal tray, utensils, and napkins and ensure they are within the patient's reach.
- Provide a towel or napkin across the patient's chest so that unexpected drips or food spillage don't distract the patient.
- Ensure that the patient is in a safe and comfortable position for eating prior to the meal.

Another hindrance to patient nutrition may be that persons bearing responsibility for patient nutrition and hydration assistance are not defined within the institution (Dickinson, Welch, & Ager, 2007). Helping patients with eating and hydration is delegated to ancillary staff members, perhaps reinforcing the mistaken notion that mealtime care is unskilled and unimportant. Particularly for high-risk patients, clarification of staff responsibilities and necessary resources should be addressed at patient admission. Patient mealtimes can also be a hectic period for nursing staff, who often must yield to physician visits, scheduled diagnostic tests, and staffing changeovers. On a personal level, oversight of patient mealtime may conflict with the nurse taking a much-needed break. Making the mealtime experience a priority in a critical care setting will continue to be an ongoing challenge.

Can nurse attitudes affect the delivery of hydration and nutrition care for the critical care patient? Research has shown that a high percentage (47%) of nursing staff displayed lack of knowledge toward proper nutritional care, and either neutral or negative attitudes toward the importance of nutritional nursing care (Bachrach-Lindström et al., 2007; Kowanko, Simon & Wood, 1999). Of further concern is that nurse aides and assistants who provide a majority of the hands-on assistance to patients have the greatest negative attitude toward these tasks (Bachrach-Lindström et al.)

## Increasing Fluid Intake

Most fluid intake in the ICU occurs during mealtime and medication administration. Although scientific research has not established specific guidelines for fluid intake for the older adult, researchers and the Institute of Medicine's Food and Nutrition Board recommend 1 milliliter (ml) of water for each kilocalorie expended or 30 ml/kg body weight per day with a minimum intake of 1500 ml daily based on medical status (Chernoff, 1999; Juan, Basiotis, & the USDA Center for Nutrtiton Policy, 2002). The following list offers specific interventions to improve the hydration status of older adults in the ICU:

- Teach the patient that his/her thirst sensation decreases with age.
- Determine if psychological barriers exist to increased fluid intake (incontinence worries, fear of nocturia).
- Determine the patient's preferred beverage and accommodate where possible.
- Calculate a daily fluid goal with the client.
- Provide fluids to the patient consistently during the day.

■ Accommodate at-risk individuals' (those with impaired swallowing or who require thickened liquids) needs.

Most critical care patients are dependent on the nurse or assistant for fluid access. Encourage nursing support staff to vigilantly monitor the patient's beverage cup and to ask if the patient needs refreshment. Providing soaked toothettes for older adults who are cognitively impaired is also suggested as an alternate means to deliver fluids: chewing or sucking on the wet toothette provides oral stimulation and increases salivation, which can lead to enhanced swallowing capability.

## Use of Oral Supplements

Some evidence exists that use of liquid oral supplements (e.g., Ensure™, Jevity™, Nepro™, Pulmocare™, among others) increases weight of older adult patients (Joanna Briggs Institute, 2007), however, the research is not straightforward (Milne, Potter, & Avenell, 2002). Specifically, a review of 49 clinical trials showed little evidence of improvement in clinical outcomes with oral supplements, including reduction in length of hospital stay. If they are used, researchers advise that they be served at room temperature, ascertain that the patient can open the package, use them when administering medications, and finally, encourage a sip-style of consumption for these beverages.

## Enteral and Parenteral Nutrition

Enteral nutrition has generally been preferred over the parenteral route for physiologic reasons, the availability of nutrient-complete formulations, a lower cost, and the reduced hepatobiliary and metabolic disruptions experienced by the patient. Maintaining bowel function via the enteral route enhances secretion of mucosal immune factors, which can limit possible septic complications (Landzinski, Kiser, Fish, Wischmeyer, & MacLaren, 2008). Total parenteral nutrition (TPN) is associated with higher levels of bacteria translocation, resulting in hospital-acquired pneumonias and other respiratory compromises, as well as increased incidence of infection, gut atrophy, GI bleeding, electrolyte imbalances, and immune system dysfunction (Heyland et al., 2003). TPN is also approximately four times as expensive as enteral formulas and is not nutritionally complete. However, in the presence of gastrointestinal feed intolerance or fluid restrictions, parenteral nutrition remains an important option. Current practice in the critical care setting may now use a combination or concomitant enteral and parenteral feedings.

The type of enteral product chosen can affect patient outcomes and the critical care nurse must evaluate each patient's reaction to the formulation. The American Society for Parenteral and Enteral Nutrition (ASPEN) publishes guidelines for specific supplements to be used with various disease states (available at http://www.nutritioncare.org/wcontent.aspx?id=532 (also see ASPEN 2002a, 2002b, 2007). Specialty immune-boosting formulations have also been developed and are under investigation (Cresci, 2005). ASPEN recommends initiating enteral therapy early (within 36 hours of admission or surgery) as early initiation is associated with lower incidence of infection and reduced length of hospital stay (Marik & Zaloga, 2001). Use of calorically dense dietary formulas is common in the critical care setting, but evidence to support improved patient outcomes is not straightforward (Bryk, Zenati, Forsythe, Peitzman, & Ochoa, 2008). There are also specialty recipes formulated for patients with decreased digestive and absorption capacity.

ICU nurses play a critical role in the successful implementation of both enteral and parenteral feedings. With enteral feeds, routine monitoring of tube placement is critical, with abdominal radiographs remaining the gold standard for checking position. The practice of injecting air into the tube with auscultation verification is not a valid technique to verify tube placement (Fulbrook, Bongers, & Albarran, 2007). Vigilant adherence to aseptic practice and adherence to facility protocol regarding care of long-term vascular access devices used with TPN is mandated to prevent infections. Critical care nurses must monitor the amount of supplement that patients actually receive; patients rarely receive the prescribed amounts of calories and protein (Elpern, Stutz, Peterson, Gurka, & Skipper, 2004; Heyland et al., 2003). The most common reason for the deficit between ordered amount and that delivered is diagnostic testing, but another common reason is to the result of "high" residual volume. Little clinical evidence exists that adequately defines excessive residual volume. Malnourished patients receiving either enteral or parenteral nutrition must be carefully monitored for both hyperglycemic episodes and refeeding syndrome, which results in significant fluid shifts and electrolyte imbalances (Griffiths & Bongers, 2005; Yantis & Velander, 2008). Potassium, magnesium, and phosphorous levels should be routinely tested in these patients. Overfeeding of critically ill patients can cause hyperglycemia, fatty liver, and increase $CO_2$ production. Promotility agents such as metoclopramide may also be initiated to improve tolerance to enteral nutrition in critically ill patients, reduce gastroesophageal reflux, and pulmonary aspiration (Booth, Heyland, & Paterson, 2002; Landzinski et al., 2008). These agents accelerate gastric emptying and increase tolerance to enteral nutrition. See Table 14.4 for a listing of problems associated with enteral nutrition.

## When Should Oral Feedings Be Restarted?

With use of either enteral or parenteral nutrition, the critical care nurse and nutrition specialist must establish an effective transition program to oral feedings (Grossman & Bautista, 2001). Exact answers as to when this should occur have not been scientifically studied. ASPEN recommends that nutritional support be halted when oral intake meets 50 to 75% of requirements, although there is dispute on the exact requirement and the protocol used to achieve it (ASPEN, 2002a; Grossman & Bautista). A transitional feeding program may be preferred to an abrupt stop to nutritional support particularly for patients with renal, hepatic, or pancreatic disorders. Critical care nurses must be alert for changes in electrolyte levels, gastrointestinal symptoms, daily bowel habits, and changes in patient mental status throughout the transitional period.

## Providing Oral Health Care

The critical care nurse should alert the primary health care provider and family if professional dental care is required and document assessment findings from routine oral cavity inspections. Providing oral health care, although normally delegated to a nursing assistant, should be routinely monitored and documented by the nurse. Teeth and/or dentures as well as the tongue should be brushed or swabbed with a toothette after each meal and before bedtime. Swabbing the teeth and gums using a toothette

# 14.4 Complications of Enteral Nutrition

| Complication | Cause | Intervention |
| --- | --- | --- |
| **Feeding tube misplaced** | Tube located in the endobronchial tree or pleural space | Tape tube in place and mark tube at exit point. Measure and record length of tubing extending from nose. Monitor external length of tube every 4 hours. Obtain confirmation X-rays; Do not use auscultation method to check tube placement as it is not reliable. Measure pH of residual fluid. pH of gastric contents ranges from 0–4; pH for patients receiving $H_2$ antagonists is higher (4–6); in lungs, pH normally greater than 6. Observe and document volume and appearance of residual fluid every 4 hours. (Note: There is no scientific consensus on how much residual fluid is considered excessive.) |
| **Aspiration** | Tube improperly placed Nasogastric feeding when nasal jejunal is appropriate Gastric reflux Patient improperly positioned for feeding | Confirm feeding-tube placement. Discuss feeding-tube location with physician. Residual volume high. Lack of gastric motility. Elevate head of bed 30–45 degrees during feeding and for 30 minutes post meals. |
| **Clogged feeding tube** | Inadequate tube maintenance. Medications Thickened Formulas | Flush tube before and after administration of medications. Finely crush medications and administer with sufficient liquid. Unclog feeding tube with carbonated beverage or specific enzymatic dissolving solution. |
| **Feeding intolerance (cramps, nausea, high residual)** | Use of calorically dense dietary formula Infusion rate too high Decreased gastric emptying Obstruction | Assess for nausea, distended abdomen. Assess residual. Confirm tube placement. Confirm bowel integrity. Consult with dietician to reduce formula concentration. Decrease rate of infusion. Consider promotility agents. |
| **Metabolic dehydration** | Insufficient fluids Inappropriate use of hyperosmolar or high-protein formulas. | Provide adequate fluid intake (30/ml/kg/day). Consult with dietician on formula selection. Monitor intake and output. Monitor electrolyte levels. |

(continued)

**Table 14.4** *(continued)*

| Complication | Cause | Intervention |
|---|---|---|
| **Diarrhea** | Gut atrophy Hyperosmolar formulas (> 500 mOsm/kg) Magnesium, potassium, phosphorus supplements Antibiotics Pancreatic Insufficiency Rapid infusion rate, high-fat intake Hypoalbuminemia Fecal Impaction | Consider whether liquid medications (prepared in sorbitol base)—may cause osmotic diarrhea. Dilute medication boluses and assess for medication intolerance. Slow down infusion rate. Consult dietician regarding formula change. Assess liver function. Screen for *C. difficile* or other infections. Consider use of fiber in supplement. |

| Total Parenteral Nutrition Complications | Cause | Intervention |
|---|---|---|
| Risk for infection | Use of large-bore IV; frequent access to line | Use sterile procedure for dressing and line changes. Minimize access to line. Change tubing per facility protocol. |
| Fluid overload and imbalanced electrolytes | Infusion rate too fast/inappropriate for patient | Monitor for hyperglycemia, signs of fluid volume overload (daily weight, central venous pressure). |

saturated with antimicrobial mouthwash (0.2% chlorhexidine gluconate) is also recommended (Gil-Montoya, de Mello, Cardenas, & Lopez, 2006) . Additional oral-hygiene care tips are available from the University of Iowa College of Nursing Evidence-Based Practice Guidelines Website (See LINKS).

# Special Considerations

## Patients Using Mechanical Ventilation

Maintaining diaphragmatic strength in the ventilated patient is a key reason for starting early nutritional support in the ventilated patient (Parrish & Falls-McCray, 2003). Parrish and Falls-McCray suggest that nutrition support be started within 3 days of hospitalization. Loss of lean muscle in the respiratory cavity can lead to diminished inspiratory ability and ineffective cough reflexes. Heightened precautions must be used to prevent aspiration in these at-risk patients receiving enteral nutrition. Critical care nurses must be alert to signs of silent aspiration, changes in lung sounds, and use caution when repositioning these clients. Overfeeding can result in increased $CO_2$ production, which can compromise respiratory homeostasis.

## Persons With Dementia

Weight loss and worsening nutritional status have been associated with severity and progression of persons with Alzheimer's disease (AD) (Holm & Soderhamn, 2003). The unfamiliar environment and disruptive sensory experience of the ICU negatively affects the older adult's ability to maintain adequate nutrient intake. Accordingly, the ICU nurse must insist that resources be allocated at mealtimes to assist these patients. Specific interventions for those assisting persons with dementia include providing smaller portions, frequently offering small sips of liquids, and demonstrating chewing/swallowing practices to these older adults. Patients in the later stages of AD were shown to respond better to frequent prompts to drink versus offering their favorite beverage (Simmons, Alessi, & Schnelle, 2001).

## The Patient With Dysphagia

The impairment of any part of the swallowing process increases the risk of aspiration, and ICU patients with acute stroke are at increased risk. Dysphagia can result from behavioral, sensory, or motor deficits and is prevalent in older adults with neurologic disease and dementia (Easterling & Robbins, 2008). Dysphagia and aspiration are associated with the development of aspiration pneumonia. Online resources at http://www.hartfordign.org/publications/trythis/issue_20.pdf show best practices for assessment and prevention of aspiration among older adults who are being hand-fed or fed by tube. To view an accompanying online video, go to http://links.lww.com/A226.

---

### Tips for Preventing Aspiration in the Hospitalized Older Adult

- Allow the patient to rest for 30 minutes before meals.
- Sit the person upright in a chair or elevate the bed to a 90-degree angle.
- Slightly flex the older adult's head to maintain a "chin-down" position.
- Adjust rate of feeding and portion of food/drink to patient tolerance level. Don't Rush!
- Alternate feeding of solids with liquids.
- Avoid foods that are easily aspirated (corn, peas, rice).
- Frequently assess for unswallowed food (food pocketing) in the mouth.
- Vary placement of food in the mouth.
- Determine whether thicker or thinner food viscosity is better tolerated.
- Use caution regarding sedatives and hypnotics as these agents may impair the swallowing and the cough reflex.

---

## Nutrition/Hydration Protocols in the Critical Care Setting

Availability and adherence to a facility-wide nutrition/hydration algorithm benefits those patients who are malnourished, those older adults with expected prolonged

NPO status, and those identified at risk (Barr et al., 2004; Bozzonetti, Calderone & Romano, 2004; Heyland et al., 2003). Ideally this protocol is an interdisciplinary collaborative effort by nutritional, nursing, and medical professionals and is based on established protocols as supported by the American Society of Parenteral and Enteral Nutrition (ASPEN, 2007) and the American College of Chest Physicians (1997). These protocols, when started within the first 24–48 hours, are associated with multiple positive patient outcomes. By establishing earlier enteral or parenteral feeds, these ICU nutritional protocols may result in less days of mechanical ventilation and reduced risk of death (Barr et al.). Critical care nurses can be instrumental in establishing and monitoring adherence to facility nutrition/hydration protocols and ensuring that positive outcomes are documented and publicized.

## Nutritional Support for Chronic Disease and Specific Illnesses

The American College of Chest Physicians (ACCP, 1997) has developed specific nutritional guidelines for patients with systemic inflammatory response syndrome (SIRS), multiple organ dysfunction syndrome (MODS), renal and liver failure, diabetes mellitus, and other diseases. To help health care professionals meet the challenges of providing specialized nutritional support for older patients with chronic disease, the Nutrition Screening Initiative (NSI) has published: *The Role of Nutrition in Chronic Disease Care* (see Exhibit 14.1). This manual addresses nutritional strategies for adults with cancer, chronic obstructive pulmonary disease, coronary heart disease, dementia, diabetes, failure to thrive, osteoporosis, and hypertension.

## Patient Teaching

Increasing the older adult patient's awareness and motivation to restore or maintain nutritional balance is the primary goal of patient teaching. Health care professionals should establish a nutritional care plan prior to patient discharge (Reid & Allard-Gould, 2004). Be sure that the discharge instructions specifically state the need for nutritional follow-up for at-risk patients. Involving the patient and caregiver in this planning where practical has been shown to reduce nutritional deficiencies (Pedersen, 2005). The ICU nurse and health care team should pay attention to specific patient nutritional needs and identify patients' perceptions about proper nutrition. Teach the patient that a diverse dietary intake of different food, fruit, and vegetable choices is associated with better nutritional status as well as improved cardiovascular status and decreased obesity (M. A. Bernstein et al., 2002).

Identifying community resources for the older adult patient can also ameliorate nutritional deficiencies. The critical care nurse along with the dietician should provide contact information for local Meals on Wheels programs, senior centers, and charitable organizations that sponsor free or reduced meals. The Department of Health and Human Services has developed a search engine for older adults to locate community services in their area at http://www.eldercare.gov/Eldercare/Public/Home.asp. However, health care providers must be cognizant that many older adults may not have access to a computer and will need assistance in getting this information.

# Exhibit 14.1

## LINKS: Nutrition and Hydration Resources on the Web

Mini-Nutritional Assessment (MNA) (in English) can be downloaded from the MNA Web site http://www.mnaolder adult.com/forms/MNA english.pdf.

Mini Nutritional Assessment Homepage (http://www.mna-older_adult.com/) offers a training guide and other resource materials.

A video demonstration of the MNA is available at http://links.lww.com/A221.

DETERMINE your nutritional health (part of the Nutrition Screening Initiative) available at http://www.dphhs.mt.gov/sltdaboutsltc/reports/2007NutritionSurvey.pdf

**Other Assessment Tools**

Estimating Height in Bedridden Patients. Available at http://www.rxkinetics.com/height_estimate.html.

**Drug–Nutrient Interactions**

http://www.cc.nih.gov/ccc/patient_education/drug_nutrient/

Drug–Nutrient Interactions: What you should know: http://www.fda.gov/cder/consumerinfo/druginteractions.htm

**Oral Health Assessment and Resources**

Oral Hydration can be assessed using the Kayser-Jones Brief Oral Health Status Examination (BOHSE) available at http://www.hartfordign.org/publications/trythis/issue18.pdf.

http://www.consultgerirn.org/topics/oral_healthcare_in_aging/

University of Iowa College of Nursing Evidence-Based Practice Guidelines Web site: http://www.nursing,uiowa.edu/products_services/evidence_based.htm

**Assessing and Preventing Aspiration**

The Hartford Institute for Geriatric Nursing, College of Nursing, New York University http://www.hartfordign.org/publications/trythis/issue_20.pdf

**General Nutrition Web Sites**

Gerontological Nutritionists, a Practice Group of the American Dietetic Association, has a resource-filled Web site at: http://www.gndpg.org/

Nutritional information from the Food and Nutrition Information Center (FNIC), National Agricultural Library (NAL), and United States Department of Agriculture (USDA) and Department of Health and Human Services (DHHS) is found at: http://www.nutrition.gov

Nutrition Insights—a publication of the Center for Nutrition Policy and Promotion, affiliated with the U.S. Department of Agriculture—is available at http://www.usda.gov/cnpp

Nutrition Management resources are available from: Nutrition Screening Initiative, PO Box 753, Waldorf, MD 20604-0753 Phone; 202-625-1662 e-mail; NSI@gmmb.com

## Summary

Critical care nurses increasingly bear more responsibility than in the past for total patient care (Guenter, Curtas, Murphy, & Orr, 2003). As the impact of nutritional/ hydration status relative to hospital outcomes becomes more visible to regulatory personnel, it is probable that nutritional status will become another milestone by which hospital care is measured. To this end, the critical care nurse must diligently document and advocate for the older adult's nutritional welfare as strongly as any other impairment.

Research has shown that well-nourished and hydrated older adults are healthier and less susceptible to chronic disease, have stronger immune systems, and may possess improved response to vaccinations (Hara, Tanaka, & Hirota, 2005). However, additional high-quality randomized controlled trials are needed to validate current ICU nursing and dietician practices relative to improving nutrition and hydration care for older adult patients. Specifically, the effectiveness of intravenous nutrition must be rigorously studied (Koretz, 2007a, 2007b), protocols for transitioning from enteral/parenteral to oral feeds is lacking, culturally appropriate nutrition interventions should be developed, and the psychosocial /environmental aspects of patient intake in a busy ICU setting require further investigation. The critical care nurse remains in the forefront in contributing to both the development of appropriate evidence-based nursing practices and serving as the older adult's advocate in obtaining nutrition and hydration support while hospitalized.

## References

Adams, N. E., Bowie, J. J., Simmance, N., Murray, M., & Crowe, T. C. (2008). Recognition by medical and nursing professionals of malnutrition and risk of malnutrition in elderly hospitalized patients. *Nutrition & Dietetics, 65*, 144–150.

Alves de Rezende, C. H., Cunha, T. M., Junior, V. A., & Penha-Silva, N. (2005). Dependence of mini-nutritional assessment scores with age and some hematological variables in elderly institutionalized patients. *Gerontology, 51*, 316–321.

American College of Chest Physicians. (1997). Applied nutrition in ICU patients: A consensus statement of the American College of Chest Physicians. *Chest, 111*(3), 769–778.

American Society for Parenteral and Enteral Nutrition (ASPEN). (2002a). Standards for specialized nutrition support: Adult hospitalized patients. *Nutrition in Clinical Practice, 17*(6), 384–391.

American Society for Parenteral and Enteral Nutrition (ASPEN). (2002b). Board of Directors and the Clinical Guidelines Task Force. *Journal of Parenteral and Enteral Nutrition, 26S*, 51SA–52SA.

American Society for Parenteral and Enteral Nutrition (ASPEN). (2007). Statement on parenteral nutrition standardization: *Journal of Parenteral and Enteral Nutrition, 31*(5), 441–449.

Bachrach-Lindström, M., Jensen, S., Lunkin, R., Christensson, L. (2007). Attitudes of nursing staff working with older people towards nutritional nursing care. *Journal of Clinical Nursing, 16*, 2007–2014.

Barr, J., Hecht, M., Flavin, K. E., Khorana, A., Gould, M. K. (2004). Outcomes in critically ill patients before and after the implementation of an evidence-based nutritional management protocol. *Chest, 125*, 1446–1457.

Bernstein, L., Bachman, T., Meguid, M., Ament, M., Baumgartner, T., Kinosian, B., et al. (1995). Measurement of visceral protein status in assessing protein and energy malnutrition: Standard of care. Prealbumin in Nutritional Care Consensus Group. *Nutrition, 11*, 169–171.

Bernstein, M. A., Tucker, K. L., Ryan, N. D., O'Neill, E. F., Clements, K. M., Nelson, M. E., et al. (2002). Higher dietary variety is associated with better nutritional status in frail elderly people. *Journal of the American Dietetic Association, 102*(8), 1096–1104.

Bonnefoy, M., Jauffret, M., Kostka, T., & Jusot, J. F. (2002). Usefulness of calf circumference measurement in assessing the nutritional state of hospitalized elderly people. *Gerontology, 48*, 162–169.

Booth, C. M., Heyland, D. K., & Paterson, W. G. (2002). Gastrointestinal promotility drugs in the critical care setting: A systematic review of the evidence. *Critical Care Medicine, 30*(7), 1429–1435.

Bouillanne, O., Morineau, G., Dupont, C., Coulombel, I., Vincent, J. P., Nicolis, I., et al. (2005). Geriatric Nutritional Risk Index: A new index for evaluating at-risk elderly medical patients. *American Journal of Clinical Nutrition, 82,* 777–783.

Bozzonetti, P., Calderone, K., & Romano, K. (2004). An interdisciplinary consultation team approach to the nutritional needs of patients with dementia. *The Gerontologist, 44* (1), 257.

Braunschweig, C., Gomez, S., & Sheean, P. M. (2000). Impact of declines in nutritional status on outcomes in adult patients hospitalized for more than 7 days. *Journal of the American Dietetic Association, 100*(11), 1316–1322.

Briefel, R. R., & Wotecki, C. E. (1992). Development of the food sufficiency questions for the third National Health and Nutrition Examination Survey. *Journal of Nutrition Education, 24,* 24S–28S.

Bryk, J., Zenati, M., Forsythe, R., Peitzman, & Ochoa, J. B. (2008). Effect of calorically dense enteral nutrition formulas on outcome in critically ill trauma and surgical patients. *Journal of Parenteral and Enteral Nutrition, 32* (1), 6–11.

Buzby, G. P., Knox, L. S., Crosby, L. O., Eisenberg, J. M., Haakenson, C. M., McNeal, G. E., et al.(1988). Study protocol: A randomized clinical trial of total parenteral nutrition in malnourished surgical patients. *American Journal of Clinical Nutrition, 47* (Suppl.), 366–381.

Chernoff, R. (1999). Nutritional support in the elderly. In *Geriatric nutrition: The health professional's handbook* (2nd ed.). Gaithersburg, MD: Aspen Publishers.

Chumlea, W. C., Roche, A. F. &, Steinbaugh, M. L. (1985). Estimating stature from knee height for persons 60 to 90 years of age. *Journal of the American Geriatrics Society, 33*(2), 116–120.

Cresci, G. (2005). Targeting the use of specialized nutritional formulas in surgery and critical care. *Journal of Parenteral and Enteral Nutrition, 29*(1), S92–S95.

Culp, K. R., & Cacchione, P. Z. (2008). Nutritional status and delirium in long-term care elderly individuals. *Applied Nursing Research, 21,* 66–74.

Dickinson, A., Welch, C., & Ager, L. (2007). No longer hunger in hospital: Improving the hospital mealtime experience for older people through action research. *Journal of Clinical Nursing, 17,* 1492–1502.

DiMaria-Ghalili, R. A., & Guenter, P. A. (2008). The Mini Nutritional Assessment. *American Journal of Nursing, 108* (2), 50–59.

Easterling, C., & Robbins, E. (2008). Dementia and dysphagia. *Geriatric Nursing, 29*(4), 275–285.

Elpern, E. H., Stutz, L., Peterson, S., Gurka, D. P., & Skipper, A. (2004). Outcomes associated with enteral tube feedings in a medical intensive care unit. *American Journal of Intensive Care, 13* (3), 221–227.

Ennis, B. W., Saffel-Shrier, S., & Verson, H. (2001). Malnutrition in the elderly: What nurses need to know. *Dimensions of Critical Care Nursing, 20* (6), 28–34.

Federal Interagency Forum on Aging-Related Statistics. (2008). *Older Americans 2008: Key indicators of well-being.* Retrieved July 6, 2008, from http://www.agingstats.gov/agingstatsdotnet/Main_Site/Data/Data_20 08.aspx

Feldblum, I., German, L., Casterl, H., Harman-Boehm, I., Bilenko, N., Eisinger, M., et al. (2007). Characteristics of undernourished older medical patients and the identification of predictors for undernutrition status. *Nutrition Journal, 6* (37). Retrieved May 14, 2008, from http://www.nutritionj,com/content/6/1/37

Fulbrook, P., Bongers, A., & Albarran, J. W. (2007). A European survey of enteral nutrition practices and procedures in adult intensive care units. *Journal of Clinical Nursing, 16,* 2132–2141.

Gil-Montoya, J. A., de Mello, A. F., Cardenas, C., & Lopez, I. (2006) Oral health protocol for the dependent institutionalized elderly. *Geriatric Nursing, 27* (2), 95–101.

Green, S. M., & Watson, R. (2005). Nutritional screening and assessment tools for use by nurses: literature review. *Journal of Advanced Nursing, 50* (1), 69–83.

Griffiths, R. D., & Bongers, T. (2005). Nutrition support for patients in the intensive care unit. *Postgraduate Medical Journal, 81,* 629–636.

Grossman, S., & Bautista, C. (2001). A transitional feeding protocol for critically ill patients. *Dimensions of Critical Care Nursing, 20* (5), 46–51.

Guenter, P. Curtas, S., Murphy, L., & Orr, M., (2003). The impact of nursing practice on the history and effectiveness of total parenteral nutrition. *Journal of Parental and Enteral Nutrition, 28* (1), 54–59.

Hara, M., Tanaka, K., & Hirota, Y. (2005). Immune response to influenza vaccine in healthy adults and the elderly: Association with nutritional status. *Vaccine, 23,* 1457–1463.

Harrington, L. (2004). Nutrition in critically ill adults: Key processes and outcomes. *Critical Care Nursing Clinics of North America, 16*, 459–465.

Harris, J. A., & Benedict, F. G. (1919). *A biometric study of basal metabolism in man.* Washington, DC: Carnegie Institution of Washington.

Heyland, D. K., Schroter-Noppe, D., Drover, J. W., Jain, M., Keefe, L., Rupinder, D., et al. (2003). Nutrition support in the critical care setting: Current practice in Canadian ICUs—Opportunities for improvement? *Journal of Parental and Enteral Nutrition, 27* (1), 74–83.

Holm, B., & Soderhamn, O. (2003). Factors associated with nutritional status in a group of people in an early stage of dementia. *Clinical Nutrition, 22*(4), 385–389.

Hudgens, B. S., Lagnkamp-Henken, B., Stechmiller, J. K., Herrlinger-Garcia, K. A., & Nieves, C. (2004). Malnutrition as indicated by Mini-Nutrition Assessment is associated with impaired immune function in elderly nursing home residents with pressure ulcers. *Journal of Parenteral and Enteral Nutrition, 28*(1), S20.

Joanna Briggs Institute. (2007). Effectiveness of interventions for under nourished older inpatients in the hospital setting. *Australian Nursing Journal, 15* (5), 28–31.

The Joint Commission. (2008). *Provision of care, treatment, and services, item B17.* Retrieved July 3, 2008, from http://www.jointcommission.org/NR/rdonlyres/D315C586-0D2B-4DB4-A9E4-FFC7681A55CC/0/LTC2008PCChapter.pdf

Juan, W. Y., Basiotis, P. P., and the USDA Center for Nutrition Policy and Promotion Aging Interest Group. (2002, September). *Nutrition insights: More than one in three older Americans may not drink enough water.* Retrieved June 20, 2008, from http://www.cnpp.usda.gov

Kayser-Jones, J., Bird, W. F., Paul, S. M., Long, L., & Schell, E. S. (1995). An instrument to assess the oral health status of nursing home residents. *The Gerontologist, 35* (6), 814–824.

Koretz, R. L. (2007a). Do data support nutrition support? Part I: Intravenous nutrition. *Journal of the American Dietetic Association, 107*(6), 988–996.

Koretz, R. L. (2007b). Do data support nutrition support? Part II: Enteral artificial nutrition. *Journal of the American Dietetic Association, 107*(8), 1374–1380.

Kowanko, I., Simon, S., & Wood, J. (1999). Nutritional care of the patient: Nurses' knowledge and attitudes in an acute care setting. *Journal of Clinical Nursing, 8*, 217–224.

Landzinski, J., Kiser, T. H., Fish, D., Wischmeyer, P. E., & MacLaren, R. (2008). Gastric motility function in critically ill patients tolerant vs. intolerant to gastric nutrition. *Journal of Parenteral and Enteral Nutrition, 32*(1), 45–50.

Marik, P. E., & Zaloga, G. P. (2001). Early enteral nutrition in acutely ill patients: A systematic review. *Critical Care Medicine, 29* (12), 2264–2270.

Milne, A. C., Potter, J., & Avenell, A. (2002). Protein and energy supplementation in elderly people at risk from malnutrition. *Cochrane Database of Systematic Reviews, 3*, Art. No.: CD003288. doi: 10.1002/14651858.CD003288.pub2

Mukand, J. A., Cai, C., Zielinski, A., Danish, M., & Berman, J. (2003). The effects of dehydration on rehabilitation outcomes of elderly orthopedic patients. *Archives of Physical Medicine and Rehabilitation, 84* (1), 58–61.

Parrish, C. R., & Falls-McCray, S. (2003). Nutrition support for the mechanically ventilated patient. *Critical Care Nurse, 23*(1), 77–80.

Pedersen, P. U. (2005). Nutritional care: The effectiveness of actively involving older patients. *Journal of Clinical Nursing, 14*, 247–255.

Pironi, L., Paganelli, F., Merli, C., & Miglioni, M. (2000). Timely nutrition screen for hospital patients. *Clinical Nutrition, 19* (3), 209–210.

Reid, M. B., & Allard-Gould, P. (2004). Malnutrition and the critically ill elderly patient. *Critical Care Nursing Clinics of North America, 16*, 531–536.

Simmons, S. F., Alessi, C., & Schnelle, J. F. (2001). An intervention to increase fluid intake in nursing home residents: Prompting and preference compliance. *Journal of the American Geriatrics Society, 49*, 926–933.

Vivanti, A., Harvey, K., Ash, S., & Battistutta, D. (2008). Clinical assessment of dehydration in older people admitted to the hospital: What are the strongest indicators? *Archives of Gerontology & Geriatrics, 47*, 340–355.

Williams, C. M. (2002). Using medications appropriately in older adults. *American Family Physician, 66* (10), 1919–1924.

Yantis, M. A., & Velander, R. (2008). How to recognize and respond to refeeding syndrome. *Nursing 2008, 38*(5), 35–39.

# Physical Restraints in Critical Care: Practice Issues and Future Directions

# 15

Lorraine C. Mion
Cheryl M. Bradas

## Introduction

*Physical restraint* is defined as any manual method, physical or mechanical device, material, or equipment that immobilizes or reduces the ability of the patient to move his or her arms, legs, body or head freely (§482.13(e)1, *Federal Register*, 2006). It is not the device per se, but the intent of use that determines whether a device qualifies as a physical restraint. Examples include, but are not limited to, limb restraints, hand mitts or splints, elbow immobilizers, and full side rails. Nurses and other health care professionals use physical restraints to protect the patient or others. However, the use of physical restraints for the involuntary immobilization of the patient may not only be an infringement of the patient's rights, but can result in patient harm, including soft-tissue injury, fractures, delirium, and even death (Bower, McCullough, & Timmons, 2003; D. Evans, Wood, & Lambert, 2003; Miles, 1993). Because of the growing body of literature and case reports of adverse events with the use of physical restraints, accrediting and regulatory agencies have limited their use, first in long-term-care settings, then in the acute care settings. Despite these regulations, the use of physical restraints for the management of patients in acute nonpsychiatric settings, especially critical care, remains a controversial and challenging practice. This chapter focuses on the issues of physical restraint in critical care settings with recommendations for changing practice.

# Legal Issues

## Regulations and Accrediting Standards

The first set of regulations pertaining to physical restraints in hospitals occurred in 1992. At that time, the U.S. Food and Drug Administration (FDA) issued a Medical Alert on the potential hazards of restraint devices (USFDA, 1992). Any harm that arises from the use of a restraining device, which now includes bed side rails, must be reported to the FDA. The Joint Commission established standards related to the use of physical restraints in the mid-1990s; over the ensuing years these have become increasingly prescriptive as well as more difficult for acute care settings to meet (Joint Commission, 2009).

In 1999, the Health Care Finance Administration, now Centers for Medicare and Medicaid Services (CMS), established an interim rule for hospitals' Conditions of Participation that regulated the use of physical restraints in all settings that accepted Medicare or Medicaid participants. In December 2006, CMS made a final rule on the Patients' Rights Conditions of Participation (*Federal Register*, 2006; 42 CFR Part 482). These conditions establish the *minimum* protection of patients' rights and safety that may be superseded by state regulations or accrediting agencies, but can never be less. In brief, use of physical restraint is an intervention of last resort, only used when less restrictive mechanisms have been determined to be ineffective, the use of restraint must be in accordance with a written modification to the patient's plan of care, used in accordance with the order of a physician or licensed independent practitioner, must never be written as a PRN, that is, an as needed order, each order must be renewed every 24 hours for violent or self-destructive behavior, each order for restraint use for nonviolent reasons must be renewed according to hospital policy, and restraint must be discontinued at the earliest possible time.

## Risks of Liability

One factor in clinicians' reluctance to forgo the use of physical restraints is the fear of liability in cases of injury or death when restraints were not used. Unfortunately, case law has been mixed on use of physical restraints in hospitals. In a review of cases filed against hospitals that alleged wrongdoing for using or not using physical restraints, Kapp (1994, 1999) reported that hospitals have been found liable for both. Although hospitals have a clear duty to protect patients from harm, they do not have a duty to restrain patients (Kapp, 1999). As the practice in hospitals becomes one of reduced restraint use because of changing legal and accrediting standards, it will become easier for hospitals to justify nonuse of restraints in instances of patient injury in cases in which nonrestraint interventions were clearly demonstrated (Kapp, 1999). However, it will also become harder for a hospital to justify its use of restraints in instances of patient harm (Kapp, 1999).

## Professional Standards of Care

Professional organizations establish evidence-based guidelines that become the standard for usual and customary practice. These standards are then used in legal cases as an appropriate standard of care for care processes and practices. A number of professional organizations have established guidelines for the use of physical restraints, including the Society for Critical Care (Macciolli et al., 2003). As early as 1994, a set of voluntary standards on physical restraints were developed for hospital nurses by the Nurses Improving Care of the Hospitalized Elderly Project, sponsored by the John A. Hartford Foundation (Mion et al., 1994). Professional guidelines, in combination with the Joint Commission and CMS requirements, are used to establish hospital-based policies and procedures and quality-of-perfomance activities.

Several organizations and coalitions have made efforts to standardize performance measures and to quantify the impact of care on the quality of patient outcomes. Perhaps the most significant organization is the National Quality Forum (NQF, 2004). By law, federal agencies, such as CMS, must defer to the NQF consensus standards when establishing policy; which includes 15 nurse-sensitive indicators. One of these indicators is the use of physical restraints. Besides CMS, the Joint Commission has adopted the NQF nurse-sensitive indicators. Last, as part of the condition for participation as a Magnet facility, hospitals must examine use of physical restraint in relation to nursing skill mix and hours.

In summary, physical restraint as a routine intervention is prohibited by CMS and the Joint Commission, is refuted by professional organizations, and considered a lack of quality in nursing care.

## Prevalence and Rationale of Staff

### Extent of Use

The use of physical restraints in hospitals was first examined in the 1980s, but studies were limited to non-ICU adult units. The overall prevalence of physical restraint use on general units ranged from 6 to 13% with higher rates (18 to 22%) among elderly patients (Mion, Minnick, Palmer, Kapp, & Lamb, 1996). More recent studies demonstrate much higher rates of use in intensive care unit (ICU) settings (Minnick, Mion, Leipzig, Lamb, & Palmer 1998; Mion et al., 2001; Minnick, Mion, Johnson, Catrambone, & Leipzig, 2007). Several important practice patterns have emerged from these studies.

First, physical restraint use varies by the type of ICU. Pediatric ICUs have consistently shown the lowest rates of use with an overall rate of 50.6 restraint days/1000 patient-days (Minnick et al., 1998; Minnick, Mion, et al., 2007). Highest rate of use occurs in neuroscience ICUs (267.9/1000 patient-days) followed by surgical ICUs (219.9/1000 patient-days) (Minnick et al; Minnick, Mion, et al., 2007; Mion et al., 2001).

Second, rates vary substantially among similar ICUs (Minnick, Mion, et al., 2007; Mion et al., 2001). For example, among 41 general ICUs, rates varied from 9 to 351/ 1000 patient-days, more than a 10-fold difference (Minnick, Mion, et al.). This variation among similar ICUs across hospitals could not be explained by differences in nursing staffing ratio or nursing skill mix; the ICUs were remarkably similar in these staffing measures (Minnick, Fogg, Mion, Catrambone, & Johnson, 2007). We also examined whether the type of hospital (academic or nonacademic), geographic region of the country, size of the hospital, or type of hospital (nonprofit, profit, governmental) had any association with use of physical restraint. There were no associations found among these variables.

There also appears to be a cultural difference. Physical restraints in ICUs have been reported absent in England and Norway (Martin & Mathisen, 2005; Nirmalan, Dark, Nightingale, & Harris, 2004). On the other hand, a small study in one Korean ICU of 51 patients reported that 46% of their patients had bilateral wrist restraints applied at some point during their ICU stay (Choi & Song, 2003).

In summary, physical restraint use is common in ICUs. But the practice varies widely by type of ICU and within types of ICUs. Clearly, there are patient populations associated with clinicians' decisions to use physical restraint, but more important, there are major practice differences *even when controlling for patient population.*

## Rationale for Use

In the 1980s, hospital nurses cited fall prevention as the primary reason for restraint use (56 to 77%) (Mion et al., 1996). Although fall risk is still a concern, today's hospital nurses cite prevention of patient therapy disruption as the primary reason for restraint use (reported for 75% of restraint-days) (Minnick et al., 1998; Minnick, Mion, et al., 2007). Most nurses cited patient care issues for the rationale to use physical restraint. However, a small proportion (1–2%) of nurses have cited insufficient staffing as the reason for restraining patients (D. Evans & Fitzgerald, 2002; Minnick et al., 1998; Minnick, Mion et al., 2007).

Researchers have examined the perceptions of caregiving staff as well as their attitudes and beliefs regarding physical restraint. Clinicians rarely questioned the use of physical restraints in the 1980s, instead assuming that this widespread practice was necessary as well as appropriate (Frengley, 1996). Early studies on attitudes toward restraints, mostly conducted at single sites with small sample sizes, found that 75 to 82% of nursing staff were "comfortable" using restraints and up to 78% believed that restraints prevented injury (Houston & Lach, 1990; Scherer, 1991). In the late 1990s, well after the Joint Commisssion had begun more restrictive standards, a study of 799 nurses and physicians at three teaching hospitals found that 46% felt a patient suffered loss of dignity when placed in restraints, 17% felt guilty using restraints, and 16% felt embarrassment when family entered the room of a restrained patients (Lamb, Minnick, Mion, Palmer, & Leipzig, 1999). Despite the negative reactions, most of these respondents believed that the benefits of restraints outweighed the risks.

Now that we have had more than 5 years of federal regulations restricting their use, to what extent have attitudes or knowledge changed among acute care personnel? Given the variation in knowledge, attitudes, and huge variation in actual use of restraint, it appears that the decision to use physical restraint continues to be one based on individual judgment and beliefs rather than on scientifically validated protocols.

## Ethical Issues in the Use of Physical Restraint

The use of physical restraints has been examined from an ethical perspective in multiple settings, including critical care (Nirmalan et al., 2004; Reigle, 1996; Slomka,

Agich, Stagno, & Smith, 1998). The primary ethical dilemma is the tension between the clinician's value of beneficence or protection versus the patient's autonomy. Physical restraint is applied against a patient's wishes; thus the practice compromises the individual's dignity and demonstrates a diminished respect for the person. The virtue of beneficence is that good will result from the action; at the very least no harm should arise from the use of physical restraint. Although the lack of beneficial results from the use of physical restraints has been well documented in many health care settings, we do not know the risk-to-benefit ratio of use or nonuse of physical restraint in patients who are critically ill (Maccioli et al., 2003).

One must also consider the socioculture and political contexts of restraint use. For example, in the United Kingdom, physical restraint use is low to nonexistent. This is likely the result of the legal mandate prohibiting its use since the 1800s. U.S. clinicians tend to frame their assessments of older adults in terms of risk aversion, for example, to prevent falls or to prevent functional decline (Kaufman, 1994). This risk aversion shapes much of our approach to older patients. If the primary focus is on the likelihood of harm, one is less likely to see self-esteem or dignity as the more important value to guide clinical decisions (Slomka et al., 1998). Interestingly, Slomka and associates point out the contradictory nature of the frequent use of physical restraint in the United States, that is, a society that places a high value on autonomy yet is so willing to violate that autonomy in the interest of perceived patient benefit.

Ethics not only focus on the individual patient, but on society. We must acknowledge the realities of reduced resources and escalating health care costs (Minnick, Mion, et al., 2007; Slomka et al., 1998). Any protocols or methods to reduce or eliminate restraints must be weighed against costs. This is a time of a shortage of registered nurses coupled with sicker patients and more complex technology (Johnson, Billingsley, & Costa, 2006). If the restraint-alternative protocols strain the existing resources, then clinicians and administrators alike will be reluctant to adopt these measures (Slomka et al.). On the other hand, if alternatives to physical restraints in critical care settings can be shown to contribute to quality outcomes (e.g., patient safety, patient dignity/satisfaction) *and* are within existing cost-containment efforts, then there is an increased likelihood of successfully implemeting and maintaining practice guidelines.

## Administrative Responsibilities

Changing established practices and philosphies of care requires much effort and can take years. Education and training are important, but certainly not sufficient in changing practice behavior. Probably the single most important factor to shift practices to restraint-free care is the commitment by administrators and key clinical leaders (Amato, Salter & Mion, 2006; Mion et al., 2001). The huge variation seen in the rates of restraint use among 40 hospitals that cannot be explained by size of hospital, type of hospital, or geographic location supports this observation. Administrators, including nurse managers, set the tone for the unit. Care providers have to feel supported during any transition period. Reducing health care providers' reliance on physical restraint in managing confused or agitated patients, especially in the critical care units, is a major shift that leaves many staff uneasy. Administrators can set a goal for a restraint-free environment and then put in place actions that enhance the achievement of the goal. For example, use of physical restraint could be viewed as a sentinel event requiring a full analysis. The findings from the case would then be used to help direct care for other patients. These analyses are also useful for uncovering system or organizational issues that can be barriers or facilitators to change.

## Critical Care Settings

The use of physical restraint in acute care hospitals occurs predominantly in the intensive care units . Nurses use physical restraints to maintain life-sustaining therapies or life-maintaining therapies. Unfortunately, strategies that have been used with such great success in long-term-care settings, rehabilitation settings, and general hospital units are not as successful in critical care environments (Mion et al., 2001). The severity of illness of patients; the intensity and delivery of care; the pace of activity; and the consequences of interruptions, delays, or disruptions of therapeutic devices differ significantly between non-ICUs and ICUs. The fear or concern of delirious patients dislodging chest tubes requiring return to the (operating room) OR, disturbing external ventricular drains with subsequent brain damage, pulling out central lines with the possibility of hemorrhage, or self-extubation from mechanical ventilation is one that heavily influences critical care nurses' decisions to use physical restraints.

Part of the difficulty in changing practice is the lack of information regarding the extent of therapy disruption in these units or the resulting immediate and subsequent harm to patients (Mion et al., 2007). There have been many studies, primarily single site, that have specifically examined self-extubation from mechanical ventilation. The rates range greatly from 0.3 to 14.3%, with higher rates in medical ICUs (Mion, 1996; Mion et al.). Reintubation after self-extubation also varies considerably, from 11 to 76%. It is important to note that 33 to 91% of those who self-extubated *did so while physically restrained*. What other therapy, for example, antihypertensive medication, would be tolerated with such a high failure rate?

We examined the prevalence of patient-initiated device removal, the patient contexts, patient risk-adjusted factors and consequences among 49 ICUs in 39 hospitals (Mion et al., 2007). Data were collected on 49,470 patient-days. Patients removed 1,623 devices on 1,097 occasions for an overall rate of 22.1 episodes/1000 patient-days. Wide variation in rates were noted: from none to 102.1 episodes/1000 patient-days. Events occurred fairly evenly between days and nights. Forty-four percent of the patients were in physical restraint at the time of the episode. In 250 (23%) events, patients sustained some level of harm, mostly minor in nature. In 10 (< 1%) episodes, patients incurred major harm. Yet, no deaths occurred.

We looked at the frequency of reinserting the device. Depending on the type of device, the reinsertion rates varied. If devices were easily applied or reinserted, such as oxygen masks or peripheral intravenous lines, then the reinsertion rates were high. On the other hand, devices that are more complex and difficult to insert (such as endotracheal tubes or surgical drains) were much less likely to be reinserted. Some have conjectured in the self-extubation literature the reason for nonuniversal reinsertion is because the devices are left in place too long. This could contribute to prolonged use of physical restraint, which in turn, contributes to agitation and delirium (Inouye & Charpentier, 1996). Additional hospital resources (e.g., X-rays, laboratory tests) were used in slighly more than half the episodes. This has important cost implications for the hospital; Fraser and colleagues (Fraser, Riker, Prato, & Wilkins, 2001) commented that in one ICU, the costs of patient removal of devices reached $250,000 annually.

Among these 49 ICUs, we found that the staffing levels and staff mix were remarkably similar; hence, there was no association between staffing ratios and therapy disruptions. Two of three studies that examined whether nurse staffing levels were associated with self-extubation reported no association (Boulain, 1998; Chevron et al., 1998; Marcin et al., 2005). The relationship between physical restraint rates and self-extubation rates is also unclear, with studies reporting positive, negative, or no association (Carrion et al., 2000; Frezza, Carleton, & Valenziano, 2000; Kapadia, Bajan, & Raje, 2000; Mion et al., 2001; Tominaga, Rudzwick, Scannell, & Waxman, 1995).

Finally, the pattern of sedation and analgesia in these units was unclear. Almost one third of the patients had received *no* analgesia or sedation in the 24 hours prior to the episode. In an earlier cohort study, we examined medical intensive care unit (MICU) patient outcomes after implementing sedation and analgesia guidelines and found that those cared for with the guidelines had less self-extubations and use of physical restraints as compared to those who were provided care outside the guidelines (Bair et al., 2001). It would seem that if we examined appropriate strategies for sedation and analgesia in critically ill patients, it may well result in improved clinical outcomes while providing care in a more humane fashion.

Attention to the environment of the ICU is important because environment affects vulnerable persons more strongly. Indeed, there is an inverse relationship of the individual's level of vulnerability with environmental insults on subsequent delirium development among hospitalized older adults (Inouye & Charpentier, 1996). Environmental features such as noise, light, and unit design have been shown to be associated with agitation, anxiety, and disorientation of ICU patients (Williams, 1988).

Care providers' lack of communication with ICU patients results in distress, anxiety, and confusion (Fontaine, 1994). There are a number of suggestions, most largely untested, that make sense in relieving the ICU patient's distress, anxiety, and agitation: attention to the physical environment, use of communication techniques with seemingly noncommunicative patients, encouragement of collaborative practice among ICU disciplines, and nonpharmacologic approaches (Maccioli et al., 2003). If we use strategies to prevent delirium as well as to manage delirium when it does develop and provide adequate pain control, there is the very likely outcome that the patient will be less agitated, obviating the need to use physical restraint.

# Alternatives to Physical Restraints

This book has provided the reader with a number of protocols addressing care issues such as delirium, sleep, nutrition, medications, and function. The reader is encouraged to review these protocols closely. Implementing best practices aimed at these areas will in itself reduce the use of physical restraints. A brief overview of an approach found successful in reducing restraints in various health care settings follows.

## Restraint Reduction Program

Because physical restraints are affected by patient-specific factors, clinician-specific factors, environmental factors, and administrative/organizational factors, one must take an interdisciplinary, multicomponent approach to their use. A unit-based planning committee for the project could consist of staff nurses, a unit manager, advanced practice nurse, therapist(s), and physician leader (Amato et al., 2006; Mion et al., 2001). Baseline information is gathered on (a) extent of use on the unit, (b) type(s) of restraints commonly employed, (c) rationale for use, and (d) types of patients (e.g., all ventilated). Depending on the ease of data gathering, the duration of use (number of days) could also be collected for each patient (Amato et al.; Mion et al., 2001). The planning committee uses this information to set goals to be achieved. For example, if the overall prevalence of use is 400 days/1,000 patient-days (i.e., 40%), then the initial goal could be a reduction of 10%. Alternatively, a given ICU could set duration of use as its goal. For instance, at one surgical intensive care unit, all patients were transferred to the unit with bilateral restraints in place. Thus, instead of prevalence, the planning committee focused on reducing duration of use from an average of 5 days to 3 days (40% reduction) (Mion et al., 2001).

Successful programs have been shown to have four components: administrative support, education, consultation, and feedback (Amato et al., 2006; D. Evans, Wood, & Lambert, 2002; L. K. Evans et al., 1997; Mion et al., 2001). Adminstrative support involves not only nursing leadership but physicians, therapists, and pharmacy. (Note: These may be the same individuals who are on the planning committee.) We have found that a staff nurse who is an informal leader of the unit, acting as a "restraint reduction champion," should be part of the administrative support group. Someone with the authority to make purchasing decisions should also be included in this group. If other ancillary support departments are affected by the plan, such as central supply or information systems, then a management representative from these departments should be included. At regularly scheduled meetings these key leaders are provided updates on progress, barriers to implementation, and discussions on facilitating adoption of practices among the unit staff.

Education is necessary, but not sufficient as the only measure (Vance, 2003). Formal and informal sessions for all levels of nursing staff focus on restraint and seclusion policy; hospital's philosophy regarding patient rights and restraints; overview of physical restraints and adverse consequences; and content specific to delirium, agitation, and falls. Content for these conditions needs to draw on best evidence for implementing nonrestraint approaches to assessment, prevention, and management. Local vendors of companies that sell equipment to replace restraints or serve as less restrictive types of restraints are very willing to meet with nursing personnel and demonstrate the various products. Staff can usually conduct a trial of the products and provide input for the purchasing decision; active participation among staff for these decisions facilitates the adoption of less or nonrestraint alternatives (Amato et al., 2006).

Consultation has been provided in previous projects by advanced practice nurses, physicians, and/or therapists (Amato et al., 2006; L. K. Evans et al., 1997; Mion et al., 2001). Consultation can be done by a single individual or a team. Each unit and hospital will have its own set of available resources to determine the most feasible resource. The consultant(s) round with the nurses at set intervals (e.g., daily, three times a week, weekly). During these rounds, nurses present patients who are in restraints and/or who keep trying to disrupt therapies. The consultant can do a brief, targeted assessment of the patient with the staff nurse. Together, the staff nurse and consultant set mutual goals and plan of care aimed at either avoiding the restraint or getting the restraints off as soon as possible. During subsequent sessions, the consultant and staff nurse review the action plan, evaluate its effectiveness, and adjust as needed.

Feedback is essential. We have found that two levels of feedback are effective (Amato et al., 2006; Mion et al., 2001). First, the individual nurse and adherence to the plan of care is monitored and reviewed during the consultation sessions. Positive feedback is always provided, negative feedback is avoided. Second, at the unit level, posted monthly graphs of the restraint prevalence against the targeted benchmark provides essential information on how well the unit as a whole is reaching its goal. If more than one ICU is doing a restraint reduction program, then side-by-side graphs can be developed to provide some incentive in competing to reach the benchmark (Amato et al., 2006; Mion et al., 2001; Note: the readers are referred to these two studies for example graphs).

## Patient-Specific Strategies

The two major reasons for using physical restraints, to prevent therapy disruption and falls, require targeted approaches. The act of self-terminating therapy among hospitalized, acutely ill older adults is most likely a manifestation of delirium, pain, or agitation and less likely an impulse to enact a desire (i.e., advanced directive). Both falls and delirium are well-known syndromes with significant morbidity and mortality among older adults. Both are complex syndromes with multiple underlying etiologies that require a combination of individual-specific, environmental-specific, and organizational-specific strategies. Inouye and colleagues have demonstrated an approach to preventing delirium in a randomized controlled trial, but the study was done on non-ICUs (Inouye et al., 1999). To what extent these strategies would work in critical care is not known. Given the complexity of falls and delirium, no single intervention will suffice as an alternative to physical restraint. Rather, attention to the environment and organization of the unit combined with patient-specific approaches provides the most successful approach to this issue (Amato et al., 2006; Mion et al., 2001).

## Falls

Although falls do not occur as commonly in ICUs as on general units, they are still a major care issue, especially in light of the current Centers for Medicare and Medicaid Services stance that costs of care for hospital falls is no longer covered. The goal is to minimize the risk or probability of falling without resorting to physical restraint. Using a systematic or standardized approach, the nurse assesses the patient for intrinsic (personal), extrinsic (environment), and situational (activity) factors. The evaluation need not be complex or time consuming and a number of fall-risk assessment guidelines are available. For example, the patient's strength, balance, and mobility can be assessed by simply observing the person's ability to turn him- or herself in bed, to get into a sitting position in the bed, or to transfer in and out of bed or chair. The nurse can quickly note any difficulty with mobility in the bed, ability to stand up independently without using a rocking motion or use of upper extremities, ability to sit down without "plopping" onto the surface of the chair, and for those patients in critical care units such as coronary care who are able to walk, the ability to walk steadily to the bathroom without holding onto objects or the wall. Note whether the person complains of lightheadedness or dizziness; if present, check for orthostatic hypotension and whether the person has sedating medications or aggressive antihypertensive regimens. Extrinsic factors include clothing and footwear. Slippers should be nonskid, bare feet and socks are not recommended. Furniture design, particularly beds at a proper height and chairs with extended arm rests for easier leverage, can facilitate mobility. Although beds that are low to the floor assist with preventing fall injury, they may actually contribute to a fall in persons with weak quadricep. Full side rails raise the issue of whether the side rails help keep a sedated or somnolent person from rolling out of the bed (i.e., protective device) or whether they are used to prevent the person from voluntarily getting out of the bed (i.e., restraint device). Clinical experience has shown that there is a population of patients, even in ICUs, who are capable of trying to get out of bed. These are the ones most at risk for sustaining injuries from side rails. Patients can either be caught between side rails and/or fall from a greater height and sustain a fracture. In these cases, a lowered bed height with a floor mat can be a sound clinical decision in preventing falls from beds (Healey, Oliver, Milne, & Connelly, 2008).

Hospital equipment can also contribute to falls such as legs collapsing on bedside commodes, bedside tables on wheels that move when patients lean on them, or tripping over tubing during transfers. All patients should have beds at appropriate heights for ease of exiting and entering, have call bells within reach, and have clear pathways. Targeted interventions are implemented for any intrinsic or extrinsic factor. Depending on the type of unit, some units may elect to incorporate "universal" interventions that other floors would consider a targeted intervention. For example, a coronary care unit or heart failure unit may elect to assess for orthostatic hypotension in all patients because of the type and amount of medications used for their conditions. For a more comprehensive overview of fall-prevention strategies, the reader is encouraged to use existing protocols through the John A. Hartford Foundation Insitute for Geriatric Nursing.

## Try This Series

The *Try This Series* translates best evidence of tools or assessment approaches for multiple conditions affecting older adults, including falls. Each condition has a 2-page overview of the tool and supporting evidence, Web-based resources, free demonstration videos, and corresponding articles in the *American Journal of Nursing*. The John A. Hartford Foundation Institute for Geriartic Nursing also produces a book of evidence-based geriatric nursing protocols that is updated every 2 to 3 years (see http://www.hartfordign.org./resources/education/tryThis.html). The reader is referred to the most recent edition's chapter on fall prevention (Gray-Miceli, 2008).

## Patient-Initiated Device Disruption

Patients who purposefully attempt to remove their devices do so because of pain, discomfort, agitation, or cognitive impairment (dementia, delirium, or delirium superimposed on dementia). Patients may "accidentally" remove devices because of restlessness or agitated movement. Addressing the underlying cause(s) of the behavior will assist in implementing targeted interventions. In many cases, nurses will identify "confusion" as the underlying cause. The nurse must differentiate whether the "confusion" is caused by dementia, delirium, or delirium superimposed on dementia (Tullman, Mion, Fletcher, & Foreman, 2008). This is because the strategies one uses aren't necessarily the same for each condition. A systematic approach to determine the cause of the cognitive disturbance and/or behavior is necessary for treatment and the reader is referred to chapter 26 in this book. An excellent Web site demonstrating assessment of delirium in ICU patients can be found at http://www.icudelirium.org.

Family members are the best resource to determine the older adult's baseline cognition and behavior and efforts to obtain this information must be made as early as possible. Targeted interventions will vary by the underlying causes and include institution of an alchol-withdrawal protocol for management of alcohol/drug dependency, pain management strategies for those with pain, pharmacologic and nonpharmacologic measures to manage anxiety, pharmacologic and nonpharmacologic measures to manage discomfort (e.g., lighting, warmth, noise).

In addition to treating the underlying causes of the delirium or agitation, strategies to protect the device from self-termination can be implemented. First, determine whether the device is absolutely necessary. Even in the critical care environment, major therapy devices are not necessarily reinserted once a patient pulls it out (Mion et al., 2007). This raises the question of how long should these devices be kept in place? CMS continues to identify and expand the "never" hospital-acquired conditions or events that result in no payment to the hospitals. A number of these involve noscomial infections from devices or catheters, such as ventilator-associated pneumonia and catheter-associated nosocomial infection. Thus, always question whether the device is absolutely necessary or whether a less noxious device or approach may be used instead. For example, if a nasogastric tube is used for nutrition, request the assessment of other disciplines, such as speech or occupational therapists, to determine whether oral feeding could be introduced. If long-term enteral feeding is required, a fuller interdisciplinary team plan with the patient and family is warranted given the known deleterious effects of tube feedings with certain conditions. Second, use anchoring or camouflaging techniques to secure the device against the patient's attempts to dislodge the device and/or to "hide" the device from the patient. For instance, nasogastric tubes cannot be hidden or disguised. The tube, however, can be taped so it doesn't interrupt the person's visual field or pull on the nares as an obvious irritant. Abdominal binders can be used to cover abdominal tubes. Commercial products are available to secure various tubes, including nasogastric tubes, endotracheal tubes, intravenous lines, and indwelling bladder catheters. Although none of these devices is likely to prevent a determined person from pulling out a device, they do provide anchoring and stability of the device that are probably more secure than taping methods.

## Summary

The pattern and rationale for physical restraint use has changed over the past 2 decades. Focusing on assessment and prevention of delirium and falls will minimize their use. Further work is needed in the ICU settings for best strategies to identify delirium, prevent delirium, and manage hyperactive delirium that would include nonpharmacologic as well as pharmacologic approaches. To avoid the use of physical restraints, practical and cost-effective strategies need to be devised and tested. This would best be done in an interdisciplinary patient-centered fashion. Many ICUs have already achieved very low rates of physical restraint; sharing best practices or quality improvement projects at professional meetings and in publications would facilitate adoption of safe and quality practices that would eliminate the need for restraints.

## Case Study

# Preventing Falls

Mrs. M., an 87-year-old widow living independently in a nearby senior citizens apartment complex, was admitted to the general 10-bed ICU of the local community hospital. She is admitted in respiratory distress with community-acquired pneumonia. She has a history of mild cognitive impairment, hypertension, heart failure, coronary artery disease, previous myocardial infarction 3 years ago, and bilateral hip replacements for osteoarthritis over 10 years previously. Oxygen mask at 40%, respiratory treatments, intravenous antibiotics, and aggressive management of fluid overload are begun.

When Mrs. M. needed to urinate, she told the nurse she was strong enough to walk to the bathroom. During the attempt to stand up from the bed, it was obvious that Mrs. M. was too weak to ambulate. The nurse got a bedside commode and instructed Mrs. M. to call her before trying to get in or out of the bed herself. The patient agreed to call. The nurse checked back a few minutes later and found Mrs. M. attempting to get up unassisted. The nurse was able to catch Mrs M. and lower her gently and without any harm to the floor in an assisted fall. After getting Mrs. M. situated in bed, Mrs. M. was easily oriented and assured the nurse she would call if she needed help. The nurse left the room, returning 10 minutes later to find Mrs. M. with her oxygen mask off and attempting to climb out of the foot of the bed. Mrs. M. was clearly short of breath, disoriented to place and to time, telling the nurse she had to go home to get her children off the school bus. At that time, the nurse applied a waist restraint and requested a consultation from the acute care geriatric clinical nurse specialist (GCNS).

The GCNS completed a Confusion Assessment Method (CAM) and determined that Mrs. M. met the criteria for delirium: acute fluctuating changes in cognition, inability to focus, and disorganized thinking. A medication review was conducted with the pharmacist to screen for potentially psychoactive medications contributing to the delirium; none were noted. Mrs. M. was moved closer to the main nurses' station to allow more frequent contact and surveillance by staff. Because her glasses and hearing aids were not brought to the hospital with her, her daughter was called and asked to bring them to the hospital. Until then, Mrs. M. was given a pair of reading glasses and a pocket listenator. A toileting regime was established so Mrs. M. would not try to climb out of bed to get to the bathroom. Because Mrs. M. was weak and had difficulty standing, a low-height bed was ordered. The low bed was to be kept in the lowest position with a bedside floor mat at all times that care was not being provided. This would decrease the likelihood of sustaining any injury if Mrs. M. was to roll out of the bed. A skin sleeve was placed over her IV site and an activity board was given to her to allow for diversion. The waist restraint was removed. Mrs. M. did not sustain any falls during her ICU stay. By time of discharge from the ICU to the general unit, Mrs. M.'s delirium had cleared and she was consistent in requesting assistance from the nurses when needing to use the bathroom.

## Case Study

### Preventing Patient-Initiated Device Disruption

Mr. T. is a 67-year-old married man who was admitted to the surgical ICU after undergoing an emergency splenectomy, and open reduction of a right hip fracture from a motor vehicle collision. He also sustained a lumbar vertebral fracture, three rib fractures, and a pneumothorax. He was noted to have vomited at the scene and aspiration was suspected. Lab work drawn in the emergency department revealed blood alcohol twice the legal limit. No family could be located to provide a medical history. He comes to the SICU with an oral endotracheal tube and mechanical ventilation, an arterial line, nasogastric tube to low suction, chest tube, two peripheral IV lines, and an indwelling bladder catheter. He is somnolent and difficult to arouse on ICU admission. On postoperative day 1 he was responsive to questioning and followed level 1–2 commands. On postoperative day 2 he started experiencing some restlessness. The surgical resident ordered the alcohol-withdrawal protocol as a precaution. Despite the alcohol-withdrawal protocol, Mr. T.'s restlessness increased. He attempted to sit up and dislodged the NG tube and chest tube in the process. The SICU nurse placed him in bilateral wrist restraints. Mr. T. became agitated, thrashing his legs about in bed and fighting against the restraints. The surgical clinical nurse specialist (CNS) was called to provide consultation.

The CNS reviewed Mr. T.'s medications and noted that the surgical resident had decreased the fentanyl drip on the previous day. Discussions with the attending physician and other members of the team (pharmacist, respiratory therapist, nutritionist) centered on viability of discontinuing some of the devices. The NG tube was removed. A trial weaning proved successful and Mr. T. was extubated and nasal cannula applied. At that point, he could be heard to be groaning and seen to be grimacing. His fentanyl drip was discontinued and he was started on morphine for pain management. The social worker was able to contact the family and the adult children agreed to take turns staying at Mr. T.'s bedside until his agitation subsided. On questioning the adult children it was learned that Mr. T. rarely drank alcohol and that the night of the collision he was at a friend's retirement party. The benzodiazepine drip from the alcohol-withdrawal protocol was stopped. Over the next few hours, Mr. T.'s agitation subsided and the wrist restraints were removed. No further attempts were made to dislodge the devices.

## References

Amato, S., Salter, J. P., & Mion, L. C. (2006). Physical restraint reduction in the acute rehabilitation setting: A quality improvement study. *Rehabilitation Nursing, 31*(6), 235–241.

Bair, N., Bobek, M. B., Hoffman-Hogg, L., Mion, L. C., Slomka, J., & Arroliga, A. (2000). Introduction of sedation guidelines in an intensive care unit: Physician and nurse adherence. *Critical Care Medicine, 28*, 707–713.

Boulain, T. (1998). Unplanned extubations in the adult intensive care unit: A prospective multicenter study. *American Journal of Respiratory and Critical Care Medicine, 157*(4), 1131–1137.

Bower, F., McCullough, C., & Timmons, M. (2003). A synthesis of what we know about the use of physical restraints in psychiatric and acute care settings: 2003 update. *Online Journal of Knowledge Synthesis in Nursing, 10*(1), document number 1.

Carrion, M. I., Ayuso, D., Marcos, M., Paz Robles, M., de la Cal, M. A., Alia, I., et al. (2000). Accidental removal of endotracheal and nasogastric tubes and intravascular catheters. *Critical Care Medicine, 28*(1), 63–66.

Chevron, V., Menard, J. F., Richard, J-C., Girault, C., Leroy, J., & Bonmarchand, G. (1998). Unplanned extubation: Risk factors of development and predictive criteria for reintubation. *Critical Care Medicine, 26*(6), 1049–1053.

Choi E., & Song, M. (2003). Physical restraint use in a Korean ICU. *Journal of Clinical Nursing, 12*, 651–659.

Evans, D., & Fitzgerald, M. (2002). Reasons for physically restraining patients and residents: A systematic review and content analysis. *International Journal of Nursing Studies, 39*, 735–743.

Evans, D., Wood, J., & Lambert, L. (2002). A review of physical restraint minimization in the acute and residential care settings. *Journal of Advanced Nursing, 40*(6), 616–625.

Evans, D., Wood, J., & Lambert, L. (2003). Patient injury and physical restraint devices: A systematic review. *Journal of Advanced Nursing, 41*(3), 274–282.

Evans, L. K., Strumpf, N. E., Allen-Taylor, S. L., Capezuti, E., Maislin, G., & Jacobsen, B. (1997). A clinical trial to reduce restraints in nursing homes. *Journal of the American Geriatrics Society, 45*, 675–681.

*Federal Register.* (2006, December 8). Part IV. Department of Health and Human Services. Centers for Medicare and Medicaid Services. 42 CFR Part 482 Medicare and Medicaid programs; hospital conditions of participation: Patients' rights; final rule. (pp. 71377–71428). Available at http://www.access.gpo.gov/su_docs/aces/fr-cont.html

Fontaine, D.K. (1994). Nonpharmacologic management of patient distress during mechanical ventilation. *Critical Care Clinics, 10*, 695–708.

Fraser, G. L., Riker, R .R., Prato, B. S., & Wilkins, M. L. (2001). The frequency and cost of patient-initiated device removal in the ICU. *Pharmacotherapy, 21*(1), 1–6.

Frengley, J. D. (1996). The use of physical restraints and the absence of kindness. *Journal of the American Geriatrics Society, 44*, 1125–1127.

Frezza, E. E., Carleton, G. L., Valenziano, C. P. (2000). A quality improvement and risk management initiative for surgical ICU patients: A study of the effects of physical restraints and sedation on the incidence of self-extubation. *American Journal of Medical Quality, 15*(5), 221–225.

Gray-Miceli, D. (2008). Preventing falls in acute care. In E. Capezuti, D. Zwicker, M. Mezey, & T. Fulmer (Eds.), *Evidence-based geriatric nursing protocols for best practice* (pp. 161–198). New York: Springer Publishing Company.

Healey, F., Oliver, D., Milne, A., & Connelly, J. B. (2008). The effect of bedrails on falls and injury: A systematic review of clinical studies. *Age and Ageing, 37*, 368–378.

Houston, K., & Lach, H. (1990). Restraints: How do you score? *Geriatric Nursing, 4*, 231–232.

Inouye, S. K., Bogardus, S. T., Charpentier, P. A., Leo-Summers, L., Acampora, D., Holford, T. R., et al. (1999). A multicomponent intervention to prevent delirium in hospitalized older adults. *New England Journal of Medicine, 340*, 669–676.

Inouye, S. K., & Charpentier, P. A. (1996). Precipitating factors for delirium in hospitalized elderly persons: Predictive model and interrelationship with baseline vulnerability. *Journal of the American Medical Association, 340*(9), 669–676.

Johnson, J. E., Billingsley, M. C., & Costa, L. L. (2006). Xtreme nursing and the nursing shortage. *Nursing Outlook, 54*(4), 294–299.

The Joint Commission. (2009). *Standards: Hospital deeming application.* March 2009 update. www.jointcommission.org/Standards/

Kapadia, F. N., Bajan, K. B., Raje, K. V. (2000). Airway accidents in intubated intensive care unit patients: An epidemiologic study. *Critical Care Medicine, 28*(3), 659–664.

Kapp, M. B. (1994). Physical restraints in hospitals: Risk management's reduction role. *Journal of Healthcare Risk Management, 14*(1), 3–8.

Kapp, M. B. (1999). Physical restraint use in acute care hospitals: Legal liability issues. *Elder's Advisor, 1*(1), 1–10.

Kaufman, S. R. (1994). Old age, disease, and the discourse of risk: Geriatric assessment in U.S. health care. *Medical Anthropology Quarterly, 8*(4), 430–447.

Lamb, K., Minnick, A., Mion, L. C., Palmer R., & Leipzig, R. (1999). Help the health care team release its hold on restraint. *Nursing Management, 30*(12), 19–24.

Maccioli, G. A., Dorman, T., Brown, B. R., Mazuski, J. E., McLean, B. A., Kuszaj, J .M., et al. (2003). Clinical practice guidelines for the maintenance of patient physical safety in the intensive care unit: Use of restraining therapies—American College of Critical Care Medicine Task Force 2001–2002. *Critical Care Medicine, 31*(11), 2665–2676.

Marcin, J. P., Rutan, E., Rapetti, P. M., Brown, J. P., Rahnamayi, R., & Pretzlaff, R. K. (2005). Nurse staffing and unplanned extubation in the pediatric intensive care unit. *Pediatric Critical Care Medicine, 6*(3), 254–257.

Martin, B., & Mathisen, L. (2005). Use of physical restraint in adult critical care: A bicultural study. *American Journal of Critical Care, 14*(2), 133–142.

Miles, S. H. (1993). Restraints and sudden death. *Journal of the American Geriatrics Society, 41*, 1013.

Minnick, A. F., Fogg, L., Mion, L. C., Catrambone, C., & Johnson, M. E. (2007). Resource clusters and variation in physical restraint use. *Journal of Nursing Scholarship, 39*(4), 363–370.

Minnick, A. F., Mion, L. C., Johnson, M. E., Catrambone, C., & Leipzig, R. (2007). Prevalence and variation of physical restraint use in US acute care settings. *Journal of Nursing Scholarship, 39*(1), 30–37.

Minnick, A. F., Mion, L. C., Leipzig, R., Lamb, K., & Palmer, R. M. (1998). Prevalence and patterns of physical restraint use in the acute care setting. *Journal of Nursing Administration, 28*(11), 19–24.

Mion, L. C. (1996). Establishing alternatives to physical restraint in the acute care setting: A conceptual framework to assist nurses' decision making. *AACN Clinical Issues, 7*(4), 592–602.

Mion, L. C., Fogel, J., Sandhu, S., Palmer, R. M., Minnick, A. F., Cranston, T., et al. (2001). Outcomes following physical restraint reduction programs in two acute care hospitals. *Joint Commission Journal on Quality Improvement, 27*(11), 605–618.

Mion, L. C., Minnick, A. F., Leipzig, R., Catrambone, C., & Johnson, M. E. (2007). Patient-initiated device removal in intensive care units: A national prevalence study. *Critical Care Medicine, 35*(12), 2714–2720.

Mion, L. C., Minnick, A., Palmer R., Kapp, M. B., & Lamb, K. (1996). Physical restraint use in the hospital setting: Unresolved issues and directions for research. *Milbank Quarterly, 74*(3), 411–433.

Mion, L. C., Strumpf, N., with the NICHE Faculty. (1994). Use of physical restraints in the hospital setting: Implications for the nurse. *Geriataric Nursing, 15*(3), 127–131.

National Quality Forum. (2004). *Nursing care quality at NQF.* Retrieved September 19, 2009, from http://216.122.138.39/nursing

Nirmalan, M., Dark, P. M., Nightingale, P., & Harris, J. (2004). Physical and pharmacological restraint of critically ill patients: Clinical facts and ethical considerations. *British Journal of Anaesthesia, 92*(6), 789–792.

Reigle, J. (1996). The ethics of physical restraints in critical care. *AACN Clinical Issues, 7*(4), 585–591.

Scherer, Y. K. (1991). The nursing dilemma of restraints *Journal of Gerontological Nursing, 17*(2), 14–17, 32–34.

Slomka, J., Agich, G. J., Stagno, S., & Smith, M. L. (1998). Physical restraint elimination in the acute care setting: Ethical considerations. *Healthcare Ethics Committee Forum, 10*(3–4), 244–262.

Tominaga, G. T., Rudzwick, H., Scannell, G., & Waxman, K. (1995). Decreasing unplanned extubations in the surgical intensive care unit. *American Journal of Surgery, 170*(6), 586–589.

Tullmann, D. F., Mion, L. C., Fletcher, K., & Foreman, M.D. (2008). Delirium: Prevention, early recognition, and treatment. In E. Capezuti, D. Zwicker, M. Mezey, & T. Fulmer (Eds.), *Evidence-based geriatric nursing protocols for best practice* (pp. 111–126). New York: Springer Publishing Company.

U.S. Food and Drug Administration. (1992). *FDA safety alert: Potential hazards with restraint devices.* Rockville, MD: Author.

Vance, D. (2003). Effect of a treatment interference protocol on clinical decision making for restraint use in the intensive care unit. *AACN Clinical Issues, 14*(1), 82–91.

Williams, M. A. (1988). The physical environment and patient care. *Annual Review of Nursing, 6*, 356–362.

# Infection, Sepsis, and Immune Function

# 16

Matthew R. Sorenson

## Introduction

Aging has traditionally been associated with increased disease mortality and morbidity. As individuals age, causes of death begin to reflect changes in immune function. Although cancer is consistently one of the leading causes of death for all age groups, its mortality rate rises with age. Septicemia consistently becomes one of the 10 leading causes of death for females and males over age 55, and in those over 65 years of age, influenza and pneumonia enter as the top 10 leading causes of death and remain there along with chronic lower respiratory diseases (Kung, Hoyert, Xu, & Murphy, 2008). Several theories have been postulated to explain this increased risk, ranging from the cumulative effects of wear and tear on the body to the accumulation of free radicals (Weinert & Timiras, 2003). Regardless of the theoretical perspective, there are changes in the immune system associated with aging, changes that interact with other medical conditions and risk factors to result in the development of infection or disease. These changes have been referred to as *immunosenescence*.

*Senescence* is a term used to describe the process of aging, in particular age-related physiologic changes. Taking a lead from that word, immunosenescence has become a term used specifically to refer to age-related changes in immune function. As individuals age, there are changes in select aspects of the immune system that put the elderly at greater risk for the development of infection, cancer, and autoimmune disease. These changes are not necessarily universal, with some research indicating that a person who routinely exercises and practices good nutritional habits may be able to avoid immunosenescence for quite some time, whereas an individual with other medical conditions may experience declines in immune function. There is also evidence that, although usually considered negative, immunosenescence can lead to some positive outcomes such as a decrease in the possibility of tissue rejection through the presence of a less potent immune system (Bradley, 2002).

Immunosenescence is probably best viewed then as a predisposing condition that is not sufficient in and of itself to result in disease or physical decline. Select changes in immune function have been associated more strongly with the presence of chronic disease, rather than with chronological age (Castle, Uyemura, Rafi, Akande, & Makinodan, 2005), indicating that age-related immune changes alone are insufficient to result in adverse consequences. Immune function in the elderly is best viewed as part of a larger multifactorial disease model (Castle, Uyemura, Fulop, & Makinodan, 2007), which also includes genetic variables, lifestyle, place of residence, preexisting conditions, previous viral or chemical exposure, medications, diet, and the presence of physical or psychological stress. In the frail or critically ill elder, there may even be certain immunologic markers that identify the presence of risk ahead of time (DelaRosa et al., 2006).

This chapter identifies age-related changes in immune function and briefly reviews the relevance of these changes and elements of the immune system. In doing so, the chapter builds on concepts expressed in chapter 10 on the chronically critically ill, and uses concepts from other chapters on pressure ulcers, wound healing, and nutrition. Attention is paid to the interaction between comorbid conditions and immunity. Areas significant to the assessment and evaluation of immune function in the elderly are highlighted, and the chapter concludes with nursing interventions.

## Immunosenescence as Contributory Risk

The pathogenic processes associated with several chronic illnesses result in effects on the immune system; effects that may place the individual at risk for the development of infection or other disease. These illnesses interact with other variables such as place of residence, exposure to viral and other disease-causing factors throughout the life span, nutritional habits, and existent treatments. Exhibit 16.1 provides a brief overview of elder health risk factors associated with the development of infection and sepsis.

The care environment, either hospital, private home or nursing care facility, can expose the elder to a variety of infectious agents, many of which may be resistant to antibiotics. Placement in a homeless shelter or crowded environment can also put the elder at risk for developing tuberculosis, pneumonia, influenza, and several skin diseases. This could also lead to colonization with several potential organisms, some of which may await immunosuppression or comprise of the immune system to fully develop into an infection (Htwe, Mushtaq, Robinson, Rosher, & Khardori, 2007).

The factors associated with the development of infection risk are those that place the individual more at risk for exposure to pathogens, and include others that represent frailty, whereas factors associated with sepsis reflect an individual who already has

# Exhibit 16.1

## Risk Factors Associated With Infection and Septic Shock in the Elderly

### Increased Risk of Infection

**Cognitive Changes**
- Delirium
- Dementia

**Dysphagia**

**Aspiration**

**Immunosenescence**
- Reduced antigen response
- Reduced vaccine responsiveness

**Sensory Deficits**
- Neuropathy
- Dysthesia

**Immobility**

**Loss of Skin Integrity**
- Burns
- Pressure ulcers
- Surgical incisions

**Invasive Devices**
- Indwelling urinary catheters
- Central lines
- Implanted devices

**Pharmaceuticals**
- Steroids
- Immunosuppressive medication

### Increased Risk of Septic Shock

**Concomitant Medical Disease**

**Diminished Cardiovascular Function**
- Circulatory deficits
- Peripheral vascular disease
- Peripheral occlusive disease

**Malnutrition**

**Endocrine Disorder**
- Diabetes mellitus
- Thyroid disorders
- Cushing's disease

**Chronic Inflammation**
- Chronic inflammatory disease
- Prolonged production of cytokines in response to systemic infection

Adapted from Opal, S. M., Girard, T. D., & Ely, E. W. (2005). The immunopathogenesis of sepsis in elderly patients. *Clinics in Infectious Disease, 41*(Suppl. 7), S504–S512.

a degree of health impairment resulting from the presence of chronic or acute disease or injury.

The presence of invasive devices, either feeding tubes, intravenous lines, indwelling catheters, or tracheostomies, provide routes of access for organisms. The presence of implanted devices such as artificial joints could be associated with the development of septic arthritis, or place the individual at risk for the development of infection. The adverse consequences of immobility not only include circulatory issues (deep vein thrombus, pulmonary embolism), but also increase the possibility of pressure sores providing another portal of entry for pathogens. Also associated with immobility are urinary tract infections, pneumonia, and often malnutrition. These factors present a host of challenges to the health status of the elder.

## Comorbidity and Immune Function in the Aged

The immune system is intimately linked with several other physiologic systems, such as the neuroendocrine and central nervous system. A disturbance of immunologic function can have consequence for the regulation of other bodily processes and vice versa. As aging aspects of the immune system interact with aging aspects of other biological systems, their response mechanisms may weaken. As a result, nursing must consider the presence of other illness and comorbidity that the individual elder may be experiencing.

The pathogenic disease process may result in an inflammatory immune cascade that places the elder at risk for the development of autoimmune conditions or result in a suppression of immune function, placing the elder at risk for infection and the development of cancer. Such inflammatory processes are seen with heart disease (pericarditis, myocarditis), inflammatory bowel disease, hyperglycemia, and several other chronic conditions. Immune system suppression is associated with acquired immunodeficiencies, aplastic anemia, as well as several categories of medications and chemotherapies.

### Diabetes Mellitus

Although a disease may have an inflammatory etiology, or result in chronic inflammation, this by no means provides protection against infection. Diabetes is a condition characterized by ongoing inflammation that also places the individual at significant risk for infection. Diabetes is considered an inflammatory process, and the presence of acute or chronic hyperglycemia reduces the degranulative capacity of neutrophils (the process through which these cells begin destruction of targets), and contributes to the activation of coagulation pathways (Alba-Loureiro et al., 2007). Individuals with type II diabetes in particular appear to be at increased risk for the development of thrombi during periods of hyperglycemia (Stegenga et al., 2008). Hyperglycemia also further activates inflammatory pathways and contributes to an increase in plasma fatty acids (Blondet & Beilman, 2007).

Diabetes also has well-known effects on wound healing and contributes to the development of neuropathy, further placing the elder at risk for pressure ulcer. The presence of obesity itself is associated with a chronic inflammatory response (Wellen & Hotamisligil, 2005) as well as with the development of type II diabetes. These findings highlight the importance of glycemic control in a critically ill population. Insulin has antiinflammatory effects and has been shown to reverse several of the immunologic effects of hyperglycemia (Blondet & Beilman, 2007).

## Cardiovascular and Circulatory Conditions

Circulatory problems such as peripheral vascular disease in conjunction with immobility can contribute to the development of cellulitis (Adedipe & Lowenstein, 2006); a bacterial infection that becomes common in the elderly. Immobility, regardless of cause, interacts with circulatory deficits, loss of sensation, and poor nutrition, which contribute to the development of pressure ulcers. Pressure or stasis ulcers are likely to display more than one organism, and are the second leading cause of bacteremia in the elderly behind urinary tract infections. Such wounds are often difficult to treat because of the presence of multiple microorganisms and can lead to osteomyelitis or become septic (Htwe et al., 2007). In turn, bed rest, which is often implemented in intensive care settings, can be associated with muscle wasting and further circulatory deconditioning. It has also been speculated that bed rest and immobility have effects on immune function that contribute to muscle wasting through the release of proinflammatory cytokines. Hypoxic episodes and fatigue may also be associated with the activation of inflammatory pathways (Winkelman, 2007). Although it is not possible to prevent the patient from all potential forms of harm, it is important to keep in mind the underlying disease process responsible for hospitalization and its potential effects on immune function.

Acute coronary syndrome has also been thought to be related to inflammatory processes, with several studies demonstrating a relationship (Werba et al., 2008). Infection itself may also result in increased lipid levels, providing a mechanism through which infection could contribute to the worsening of atherosclerosis (Khovidhunkit, Memon, Feingold, & Grunfeld, 2000).

## Cerebrovascular Accident (Brain Attack or Stroke)

Immunosenescence-related changes in the production of proinflammatory proteins may be associated with stroke risk (Singh et al., 2008). The production of immune proteins normally occurs in a balanced system. As an individual ages, that balance could be disrupted, leading to a production of immune proteins that can contribute to vessel instability within the brain. There also appears to be a relationship between the development of infection and the development of ischemic stroke. Infections can induce inflammatory changes within local tissue that appear to contribute to atherosclerotic plaques. Both bacterial and viral infections appear associated with the development of stroke up to 30 days postinfection, with the highest risk occurring within 7 days of infection. This risk appears to develop through the release of inflammatory mediators such as C-reactive protein and cytokines, which in turn influence coagulation (Emsley & Hopkins, 2008). This relationship demonstrates the need to carefully monitor the critically ill elder who has recently experienced an infectious process. Coagulation studies should be carefully evaluated.

## Rheumatoid Arthritis

Atherosclerosis and rheumatoid arthritis (RA) appear to share several common pathways. Each condition is considered an inflammatory condition and there appear to be intimate ties between the two. Heart disease is one of the leading causes of death in individuals with rheumatoid arthritis, and the presence of RA itself is considered a risk factor of cardiovascular disease (Szekanecz et al., 2007). Markers of RA-related inflammation appear to provide an independent contribution to endothelial cell dysfunction (Dessein, Joffe, & Singh, 2005). The elder with RA needs careful cardiovascular evaluation, with attention paid to the potential for the development of acute coronary syndrome.

### Viral Exposure

The presence of a previous viral etiology can place the elder adult at risk for the development of reactivation and new infection. There is a profile of immunologic changes in the older adult that appear characteristic of previous viral exposure. This immune-risk phenotype is associated with a greater risk of mortality and morbidity. This phenotype, or profile, is associated with a decreased responsiveness to new infections and a correspondent likelihood of viral reactivation. The presence of a viral infection provides a continuing stimulation of the immune system that is believed to be associated with the development of atherosclerosis, cognitive deficits, and the development of cancer in association with aging (Sansoni et al., 2008). A classic example is the reactivation of herpes zoster, which affects a significant proportion of the aging population.

*Herpes Zoster.* The likelihood of varicella-zoster virus reactivation is significantly increased in the elderly and appears associated with a decrease in cell-mediated immunity. Out of the approximately 1 million cases of herpes zoster in the United States each year, the majority of cases occur in individuals 50 years of age or older. Half of all elders are expected to experience herpes zoster by age 85 (Weinberg, 2007). Pain and paresthesia are experienced in the affected dermatome as many as 4 weeks prior to the development of the classic rash presentation (Weinberg, 2007). This pain may be easily mistaken as having a cardiac or abdominal etiology, which leads to treatment delays (Adedipe & Lowenstein, 2006). Although 50% of all patients develop thoracic lesions, 10 to 15% may develop lesions along the trigeminal nerve, which may result in permanent visual loss associated with nerve damage (Weinberg). The elder individual treated in a critical care situation is under physiologic and psychologic stress. This stress can contribute to the reactivation of varicella, as could the use of immunosuppressant medications. Nursing personnel need to evaluate carefully for the reactivation of this viral etiology in the critical care setting.

## Key Points

The inflammatory processes associated with chronic diseases can have adverse effects on symptoms and other conditions. When evaluating the chronically ill elder, the nurse must keep in mind the potential for infection to contribute to the development of thrombic events such as stroke.

## Overview of the Immune System Changes Associated With Age

There are two major aspects of the immune system involved in defending the host: innate (natural or nonspecific) and adaptive (acquired, specific). The innate immune

## 16.1 Immune Cell Changes in Immunosenescence

| Cell Population | Number of Cells | Functional Capability of Cells | Relevance |
|---|---|---|---|
| B Cells | Increased | Decreased | Decline in amount and functional ability. Increase in number of self-recognizing antibodies. |
| Macrophages | No change | Decreased | Decrease in ability to clear organisms. |
| Natural Killer | Increased | Decreased | Decreased viral defense, but increase in number may compensate. |
| Neutrophils | No change | Decreased | Decreased efficacy in responding to microorganisms. Cells die quickly, are effective for a shorter period of time. |
| T cells | | | |
| Naïve | Decreased | Reduced ability to clonally expand. | Diminished immune response to new antigens. |
| Memory | Increased | Decreased | Appear more sensitive to programmed cell death (apoptosis). |

system is generally considered the first line of defense as it reacts first to the presence of pathogens, often serving to signal aspects of the adaptive immune system. The innate immune system could then be viewed as providing a means of controlling an infection until the adaptive immune system becomes fully functional in 4 to 7 days. This period of time is required for the proliferation and development of sufficient numbers of effector immune cells.

The innate immune system is comprised of physical barriers that prevent easy passage of foreign pathogens and a set of phagocytic cells. The adaptive immune system is concerned with cell-mediated and humoral immunity. The innate and the adaptive immune systems are interdependent, with a significant degree of interaction and interreliance between them, particularly on the part of T cells. There are also specialized forms of lymphoid tissue in the lungs (bronchial-associated lymphoid tissue), mucosa (mucosal-associated lymphoid tissue), and the gastrointestinal tract (gut-associated lymphoid tissues) that serve as defenses against a large number of pathogens with large numbers of phagocytic cells that help present antigens to the immune system.

The innate immune system in general appears to lose effectiveness during immunosenescence, whereas the adaptive immune system undergoes more pronounced changes in select cell populations. Changes in the innate immune system include increased permeability of physical barriers and a loss of effectiveness. In terms of adaptive immunity, there is a general loss of naïve T cells and decrease in the functionality of immunoglobulin. These changes not only place the elder at greater risk for exposure to infectious agents, they also decrease the organism's ability to defend against such agents. These changes are reviewed in Table 16.1.

## The Innate Immune System

The innate immune system is so named as it is present at birth and does not require exposure to antigens to be effective against pathogens. The first elements of the innate immune system are physical barriers, such as the skin, that protect the organism from infection. These barriers are comprised of epithelial cells that bar and defend against most pathogens. For example, mucosal epithelial cells produce mucus, hindering the ability of pathogens to bind to the epithelial wall and traffic through; the cilia of the respiratory tract can aid in clearing organisms. The pH environment and flora of the gastrointestinal tract provide defenses; peristaltic motion aids in ensuring continual clearance of food and any pathogens it contains. Epithelial cells also produce enzymes and proteins that aid in phagocytosis of bacteria and inhibit microbial growth (Janeway, 2005). However, with aging and illness come changes to these physiologic defenses that can place the individual at greater risk for pathogenic invasion.

The loss of skin tissue in the elderly can serve to compromise the skin barrier, lessening its effectiveness in preventing the entry of foreign organisms. Dehydration in elder individuals concomitant with poor nutrition has adverse consequences for skin turgor and, in combination with immobility from a host of chronic conditions, can contribute to the development of pressure ulcers providing access for pathogenic organisms. Changes in the ability of cilia to clear the respiratory tract, along with decreased compliance and weakening of chest musculature can contribute to the development of pneumonia and other respiratory diseases even without considering exposure to smoking. With age comes slowing of peristalsis and delayed gastric emptying, along with changes in gastric-wall permeability, which may increase an individual's exposure to pathogens found in food or liquids. These innate protective barriers are then affected by aging and a complete assessment of the patient is required to fully evaluate for the presence of age-related changes that place the individual at risk. However, these barriers are not the only aspects of the immune system influenced by aging, the cells of the innate immune system are also affected. These are granulocytes (neutrophils, eosinophils, basophils) and natural killer cells that provide the second line of immunologic defense once a pathogen passes physical barriers.

## Neutrophils and the Shift

Neutrophils are granulocytes present in peripheral circulation and are the first immune cells to respond to the site of an infection. Once at the site of infection, the half-life of neutrophils is extended, allowing neutrophils to have a prolonged period of phagocytosis at the site of infection. These cells then engulf bacteria or other targets through phagocytosis and release enzymatic mediators that destroy the target. Among these mediators is superoxide, which is influenced by certain hormones. Neutrophils are an important player in the innate immune response, one that is sensitive to age.

In critical care settings, *a shift to the left* is a term used to describe the appearance of increased numbers of neutrophils and immature precursor cells in circulation. The presentation of an infectious organism will stimulate the release of neutrophils into the circulation. Mature neutrophils are accompanied by immature neutrophils often known as "bands" because of their appearance under a microscope.

In the elderly, there appears to be little decrease in the number of neutrophils. The effectiveness of neutrophils, however, decreases with age. Neutrophils in elder populations do not destroy bacterial targets as effectively, and also appear to die prematurely. Although neutrophil life is prolonged at the site of an infection in younger populations,, this does not appear to occur in ill elders (Crighton & Puppione, 2006). Therefore, a shift to the left may be present, demonstrating an increase in cell numbers, but the functional capacity of these cells is diminished. Thus, the presence of a left shift in an ill elderly patient should be considered a potential sign of bacterial infection whether or not there is fever (Bentley et al., 2001).

Neutrophil function is possibly influenced by hormonal release in response to physical or psychological stress (Butcher et al., 2005). In individuals over 65 years of age, there appears to be a gradual reduction of dehydroepiandrosterone (DHEA), a hormone that antagonizes cortisol. Cortisol is a glucocorticoid associated with the stress response. In elder individuals the physical stress associated with surgery has been shown to result in elevated levels of cortisol that appear to suppress the generation of superoxide on the part of neutrophils (Butcher et al.). Physical or psychological stress in the elderly may then further suppress immune function.

## Cell Markers

Toll (or Toll-like) receptors are present on antigen presenting cells and are considered part of the innate immune system. These receptors provide a means of recognizing pathogens without requiring prior experience with the pathogen. These receptors also stimulate the production of immune proteins known as cytokines, which signal other aspects of the immune system. In elderly adults, this signaling capacity of Toll receptors appears diminished. This loss or lessening of function may impair immunologic activation and lead to a less potent vaccine response (van Duin & Shaw, 2007). This may result in a need to repeat vaccinations for the vaccine to be effective in elder populations.

## The Complement System

The complement system involves a series of proteins released into the circulation that enhance the ability of phagocytic cells to locate targets and aids in the process of phagocytosis. The complement system also aids in the development of immunologic memory and facilitates antibody response. Although aging appears to have little overall effect on the activity of the complement system, this system is intimately linked with coagulation pathways that are in turn influenced by inflammatory processes.

## Natural Killer Cells

Natural killer or NK cells are lymphocytes with antiviral and antitumor effects. These cells mature predominately in the thymus and to some degree in the liver. As the thymus atrophies with age, the importance of the liver as a site of maturation becomes more important. In relationship to aging, the number of these cells seems to increase while their overall effectiveness appears diminished. It has been speculated that the increased number of these cells created in association with aging makes up for their reduced effectiveness. Yet, even with increased numbers, there is an overall reduction in the cytotoxic capacity of NK cells and a decrease in their ability to release important proteins known as cytokines. This can lead to a functional decrease in the ability to fight infection and precancerous cells (Mocchegiani & Malavolta, 2004). In an older individual with liver disease or an endocrine disorder the maturation of NK cells would be further reduced. Nutritional concerns will also influence NK cell counts. Zinc and vitamin E levels appear to influence both the number and functional capability of

NK cells (DelaRosa et al., 2006) highlighting a recurrent theme in terms of immune function in the elderly. The existence of dysphagia, anorexia, or poor nutrition often has significant consequences on immune function.

## Key Point

Nutritional deficits are associated with cognitive deficits and immune suppression in older adults. The nutrition and hydration status of the critically ill elder should be closely monitored. Prealbumin and retinol binding protein levels are markers of protein depletion and should also be monitored in the critically ill older adult.

## Adaptive Immunity

In terms of the cells of the innate immune system, there seems to be some decrease in the functional capacity of neutrophils, with unclear findings as to their affects on other aspects of the innate system. The findings in terms of adaptive immunity indicate a general decrease in cell immunity through effects on cell signaling, T cell subsets, and overall functionality of immunoglobulin. Overall, there is a decease in both cell-mediated and humoral immunity. Concomitant with these changes is an overall increase in autoimmune responses, with the potential for the development of immune-mediated neuropathies (Pletz, Duda, Kappos, & Steck, 2003).

## Cell Markers and Signaling

Signal transduction is the process by which messages are relayed from the cell membrane into the cell interior and nucleus. This process involves enzymes and signals elements of the immune system and is involved in genetic regulation. One particular molecule involved in signal transduction is CD28, which stimulates cytotoxic T cells and aids in the development of T and B cells. In older adults, this marker appears to be either missing or less responsive to regulatory influences (Thewissen et al., 2007). Cells lacking this marker have been found to be associated with the development of rheumatoid arthritis (Michel et al., 2007). Cells that lack CD28 do not respond to the presence of an antigen that would normally trigger T cells responses. Diet offers a possible explanation for this lack of response. A major electrolyte in the signaling pathway is calcium. In elder populations that may be malnourished or have osteoporosis, it is possible that signaling pathways may be disrupted. Chronic viral infection has also been proposed as an explanatory factor, such exposure gradually shifts the production of immune proteins known as cytokines toward an antiinflammatory type response (Castle et al., 2007). Either consideration highlights the importance of recognizing the value of history taking and assessment in evaluating immune function in the elderly.

## T Cells

Several factors contribute to immunosenescence in relation to T cells. With aging, atrophy or involution of the thymus interacts with diminished T cell responsiveness to result in a loss of select T cell classes. This loss of T cell classes results in significant effects on the production and secretion of immune proteins known as cytokines. There is also a reduction in the number of T cells that aid in regulation of viral epitopes and survey the system for the presence of potential tumors.

T cells are divided into three general groups: helper, cytotoxic, and memory cells. Helper T cells tend to display a protein marker identified as cluster of differentiation (CD) marker four, thus are referred to as CD4 helper cells. Cytotoxic cells display CD8 and are referred to as CD8+ cells, and are present in naïve, effector, and memory groups. Naïve T cytotoxic cells are mature cells prepared to respond to antigens. The presence of a large number of naïve cells is considered helpful in an organism adjusting to new challenges such as infection. Memory T cells have encountered antigens (often through prior infection or vaccination) and are prepared to respond in the face of a re-exposure. This results in a stronger and more pronounced immune response when the infectious organism is re-encountered. Although the number of memory cells in the elderly remains high, there is a reduction in the number of naive T cells. This is related to atrophy of the thymus, where T cells mature. This atrophy leads to a gradual reduction in the production and release of naive T cells over time, leading to a decline in their numbers (Pawelec et al., 2002).

The large number of memory cells may be associated with previous viral exposure and may even result in a diminished response to vaccination (Xie & McElhaney, 2007). Previous experience with cytomegalovirus or other viral epitopes could be associated with several of the immune changes that are considered hallmarks of immunosenescence (Pawelec et al., 2005). Therefore, physical history and lifestyle are important elements to consider when trying to identify whether an elder individual is at risk for immune-related disease (Pawelec et al.). In turn, decreased responsiveness on the part of T cells may contribute to the reactivation or viral epitopes such as varicella or other chronic viral infections (Effros, 2003a, 2003b; Schmader, 2007).

Helper T cells are involved in the development of cell-mediated and humoral immunity. In cell-mediated immunity T cells release proteins that attract other cells such as macrophages to the site of infection to aid in the process of phagocytosis. In humoral immunity, T cells interact with B cells to stimulate the production of antibodies. With aging, comes a loss of cell-mediated immunity with gradual declines in the functionality of most T cell subclasses. There is also an increase in the number of available B cells that appear to target the organism itself. There is then a decrease in the responsiveness of T cells to stimulation concomitant with a reduction in the number of certain types of T cells that aid in the response to novel pathogens.

## B Cells

Once T cells aid B cells in recognizing an antigen, B cells proliferate in lymphoid tissue and develop into plasma cells. These plasma cells, or activated B cells, then produce antibodies that are released into the circulatory system. There is also a subgroup of B cells, memory B cells, which can provide the organism a stronger and more immediate response on re-encountering an antigen. Reductions in the functional capability of T cells, especially T helper cells, will ultimately affect B cell function. Several of the changes in T cell subsets associated with immunosenescence reduce the ability of T cells to interact effectively with B cells. This results in a restriction in the quantity and quality of immunoglobulin produced by B cells (Prelog, 2006).

In the elderly, there also appear to be larger numbers of memory B cells that are producing self-antigens which target the individual's own tissue. The presence of these cells is believed to be associated with increased risk for autoimmune conditions in association with aging. As the production of immune proteins shifts with aging toward an increase in the production of proteins (cytokines) associated with an antibody-mediated response, the elder is placed at even more risk for the development of autoimmune conditions (Prelog, 2006).

## Cytokines

Cytokines are soluble proteins that serve as signaling mechanisms for the immune system. These proteins possess both proinflammatory and anti-inflammatory properties, often with one cytokine serving to balance the other. Those cytokines associated with inflammatory processes and pronounced T cell-mediated immune responses are referred to as Th1 cytokines. These cytokines are viewed as being produced by type one T helper cells. Cytokines associated with antibody production and the suppression of inflammatory responses are referred to as Th2 cytokines. These Th2 cytokines are believed to be produced by a group of T lymphocytes known as type two T helper cells. These proteins are important and necessary parts of an effective immune response. Aging, medications, and the presence of chronic disease can all serve to alter the production of these proteins, potentially affecting not only immune function, but also increasing the development of inflammatory disease associated with aging (Castle, 2000).

## The Immunologic Risk Profile

The study of differences between immune function in healthy older adults and those considered frail has generated findings that have identified certain parameters that could be considered an immunologic risk profile. This immunologic risk phenotype is associated with a reduction in immune function that contributes to morbidity and mortality. The risk profile consists of the functionality of several cell types. Reduced functional capacity in terms of natural killer cells along with reduced functionality on the part of antibodies is considered to be associated with illness and frailty in elders (DelaRosa et al., 2006). Certain comorbidities, malnutrition, autoimmune disorders, or recurrent infection seem to trigger an increase in the production of Th2 or anti-inflammatory cytokines. In the elderly, there are then decreased numbers of T helper cells and an increase in the number of suppressing (CD8) cells. This could lead to a situation in which an elder cannot generate an adequate antibody response in response to vaccination (Castle et al., 2007). Although implementation of a risk profile of this kind is difficult in the clinical setting, it does help demonstrate the tie between chronic disease and immune function. The changing balance of immune cells in an elder could lead to a process of immunologic suppression of immune response, increasing vulnerability to infectious disease.

## Review of Immune Changes in the Ill Elderly

Immunologic changes in the elderly appear to be associated more with the presence of comorbid disease than with aging itself. Phagocytic cells display a reduction in their ability to clear microorganisms and there is a decrease in the release of superoxide by neutrophils. NK cell count appears to increase, but the overall effectiveness of these cells is diminished. The ability of T cells to engage B cells is reduced, resulting in a decrease in the production of antibodies and a loss of effectiveness. There is an increased production of proinflammatory cytokines leading to a process of inflammation, which through a complex series of events, is ultimately associated with a suppression of T cell response. Overall there is a reduced responsiveness to vaccine and a slowed adaptive immune risk that may place the critically ill elder at risk for the development of infection and sepsis.

## Key Points

In the elderly, the number of cells may not change greatly, but their functional capacity is diminished. The elder patient may require more than one vaccination for an adequate amount of antibody to be produced. The critically ill elder may be more vulnerable to new infectious organisms because of decreased capacity of the immune system.

# Assessment and Evaluation of the Elderly

In the face of the immune changes experienced by the critically ill elder, the ability to assess for the appearance of infection becomes paramount. There are several issues associated with aging that influence assessment findings and the potential meaning of those findings. The elder may view the presenting symptom as a symptom of aging rather than a new indicator of disease. The presence of chronic disease (e.g., diabetes, chronic obstructive pulmonary disease) may mask the presentation of symptoms or make it difficult to determine the source. Infection may also present subtlely and without some of the classic cardinal signs in the older adult. The intent of this section is to explore issues related to fever, infection, and sepsis along with reviewing areas that should be included as part of the nursing assessment.

## Fever

An increased body temperature or fever is an inflammatory response that can occur from tissue injury or other trauma to the body. This trauma stimulates release of cytokines, which act on select regions of the brain to elicit a pyrogenic response. The increased body temperature stimulates the growth of several classes of immune cells and can actually suppress the growth of several microorganisms. The development of pathogenic fever begins with presentation of a pathogen to macrophages, which then release cytokines into the circulation. These cytokines stimulate the release of prostaglandin from the brain, which results in the autonomic responses typically associated with fever (Moltz, 1993).

In the elderly, these responses are often found to be blunted or absent, possibly because of a lower baseline temperature or through a decrease in the release of prostaglandin within the central nervous system in response to pyrogen. In certain elders, there may be an inability to release adequate amounts of prostaglandin resulting in a lack of fever (Grahn, Norman, & Yoshikawa, 1987). It has been estimated that 20 to 30% of all elderly patients will either not exhibit fever or its presentation will be minimized (Norman & Yoshikawa, 1996). Pharmacologic therapies may also result in a fever of unknown origin in elders (Norman, Wong, & Yoshikawa, 2007).

In light of these findings, three alternative definitions of fever in the elderly have been provided.

1. The presence of a persistent temperature (oral or tympanic) of 37.2° C (99° F) or greater has been offered as a criterion for fever in the elderly.
2. Should the need to determine a core temperature exist, either because of inaccessibility of the oral route as in a patient with a tracheostomy, a persistent rectal temperature of 37.5° C (99.5° F) or greater would also meet criteria.
3. An increase of 1.3° C (2.4° F) or more over baseline temperature, regardless of the route of measurement, could also represent fever (Norman, 2000).

Using these parameters provides a method of evaluating elders who have either a blunted pyrogenic response or lower baseline temperature.

## Bacteremia

Bacteria can often be found within the bloodstream or in other bodily fluids such as urine. However, the presence of bacteria in the circulation does not always elicit a physiologic response from the organism. In fact, asymptomatic bacteremia is a common finding among the elderly. What distinguishes bacteremia from sepsis is the presence of an immunologic-mediated inflammatory response known as systemic inflammatory response syndrome (SIRS). This inflammatory cascade involves the release of several proinflammatory cytokines (interleukin-1, tumor necrosis factor-alpha) that serve to activate leukocytes and promote the adhesion of leukocytes to the endothelial cell wall, leading to endothelial damage. This damage leads to the activation of clotting mechanisms that contribute to the development of micro thrombi and clotting complexes that impair capillary blood flow, which ultimately further enhance hypoxia.

Unfortunately, SIRS is not unique to infectious disease. It can be associated with trauma, burns, or endocrine pathologies (Gullo, Bianco, & Berlot, 2006), although the response is generally initiated and supported by exposure to infectious agents, either gram-negative or gram-positive bacteria, viral epitopes, or yeasts (Gullo et al.).

## Sepsis

Sepsis may be underdiagnosed in the elderly (Girard, Opal, & Ely, 2005) and should be considered as part of an inflammatory response continuum. In the absence of a clear etiologic infection, this process may be referred to as SIRS. When an infection results in SIRS, sepsis exists. Infection is ultimately an inflammatory response elicited by physiologic trauma or exposure to pyrogenic substances and should be considered part of a larger continuum along which lies sepsis, severe sepsis, septic shock, and organ failure. *Sepsis*, characterized by the presence of tachycardia accompanied by leukocytosis or leukopenia and increased $PaCO_2$ or tachypnea. *Severe sepsis* is defined as a state of organ dysfunction brought about through either infection or hypoperfusion. Further along the continuum is *septic shock*, defined as a state of hypotension that is not reversible through fluid administration. This state of hypotension develops as a result of organ dysfunction associated either with infection or hypoperfusion.

## 16.2   Sepsis-Related Definitions and Criteria

| Term | Definition or Criteria |
| --- | --- |
| Infection | An inflammatory response generated in response to pathogen exposure. |
| Systemic Inflammatory Response Syndrome | A systemic inflammatory response to a variety of stimuli manifested by two or more of the following: |
| | 1. Fever (greater than 38° C |
| | 2. Heart rate in excess of 90 beat per minute. |
| | 3. Respiratory rate greater than 20 per minute, or a $PaCO_2$ less than 32 mmHg. |
| | 4. White blood cell count of less than 4,000 or greater than 12,000 |
| | 5. Greater than 10% of white blood cells are immature (bands). |
| Severe Sepsis | Acute organ dysfunction that is secondary to infection. |
| Septic Shock | Acute organ dysfunction secondary to infection that is accompanied by hypotension not reversible by fluid administration. |
| Sepsis-Induced Hypotension | Systolic blood pressure that is less than 90 mmHg<br>*or*<br>A mean arterial pressure less than 70 mmHg<br>*or*<br>a decrease in SBP of 40 mmHg or two standard deviations below age-appropriate norms. |
| Sepsis-Induced Tissue Hypoperfusion | The presence of septic shock, elevated serum lactate or oliguria |

Adapted from Bone et al. (1992). Definitions for sepsis and organ failure and guidelines for the use of innovative therapies in sepsis: The ACCP/SCCM consensus conference. The American College of Chest Physicians/Society of Critical Care Medicine, *Chest 101*(6), 1644–1655.
Dellinger, R. P., et al. (2008). Surviving sepsis campaign: International guidelines for management of severe sepsis and septic shock: 2008. *Critical Care Medicine, 36*(1), 296–327.

Untreated this can progress to multiple organ dysfunction syndrome (MODS; Dellinger et al., 2004, 2008). Septic shock could then result in disseminated intravascular coagulation or organ failure (heart, liver, or kidney). Recently it was found that the onset of sepsis-related organ dysfunction and functional status are associated with 1-year mortality in the elderly (Regazzoni et al., 2008). Table 16.2 provides common sepsis-related definitions and criteria.

The diagnostic criteria for sepsis are reflective of an inflammatory response to infection and are purposively broad. The association between organ dysfunction and sepsis led to the inclusion of such parameters as changes in mental status, oliguria, hypoxemia, and altered liver function. These criteria are perhaps better thought of as a list of potential signs associated with sepsis, for none are considered to be truly specific for sepsis alone (Levy et al., 2003). Exhibits 16.2 and 16.3 provide a list of potential signs for SIRS. Of note is that many of these findings may be commonplace in elderly populations, especially those with comorbidity. In an older patient, one might expect some alteration in kidney or liver function, along with some confusion

# Exhibit 16.2

## Sepsis Diagnostic Criteria

**General**

   Fever or hypothermia

   Tachypnea

   Significant edema or positive fluid balance (>20 mL/kg over 24 hr)

**Inflammatory variables**

   Leukocytosis (WBC count >12,000 l)

   Leukopenia (WBC <4000 l)

   A normal WBC with >10% immature forms

   Plasma C-reactive protein >2 SD above the normal value

**Hemodynamic variables**

   Arterial hypotension

   Cardiac index >3.5 L/min/m$^2$

**Organ dysfunction variables**

   Acute oliguria

   Creatinine increase (>0.5 mg/dL)

   Coagulation abnormalities (INR >1.5 or PTT >60 sec)

   Ileus

   Thrombocytopenia

**Tissue perfusion variables**

   Hyperlactatemia (>1 mmol/L)

   Decreased capillary refill or mottling

Adapted from Levy, M. M., et al., (2003). 2001 SCCM/ESICM/ACCP/ATS/SIS International Sepsis Definitions Conference. *Critical Care Medicine, 31*(4), 1250–1256.

on a normative basis. It is then imperative to closely observe the elderly patient for changes from baseline levels that may indicate the development of sepsis.

## Septic Shock and the Elderly

Elderly patients are at significant risk for the development of septic shock. This is in part a result of the presence of chronic disease, significant comorbidity, and the use of invasive devices for monitoring and providing airway or circulatory access. A significant number of ill elderly also reside in care facilities that place them at risk for acquisition of antibiotic-resistant organisms. Treatment of sepsis in this population requires early identification and aggressive management.

In terms of establishing a diagnosis, blood or sputum cultures should be obtained. Samples should be obtained from two or more sites, and a sample should be obtained from each vascular access device that has been in place longer than 48 hours. The administration of intravenous fluids should be initiated immediately in hypotensive patients, and it has been argued that broad spectrum antibiotic therapy be started within 1 hour of sepsis recognition (Girard et al., 2005).

Intravenous treatment of hypotension or elevated serum lactate should be initiated immediately with a central venous pressure goal of 8 to12 mmHg, 12 to 15 mmHg in ventilated patients. Elevated serum lactate levels indicate the presence of metabolic acidosis. Other goals are a mean arterial pressure of 65 mmHg and urine output of .5 ml/kg/hr. Central venous oxygen saturation should be at least 70%. If this goal is not achieved further fluid administration may be considered along with the possibility of an infusion of packed red blood cells. The nurse should also anticipate starting a dobutamine continuous drip (Dellinger et al., 2008).

## Common Infections and Sites

Beyond the location of invasive lines, there are several potential sites for infection in elder individuals. Some are less apparent than others. Aspiration in the elderly is significantly associated with respiratory infection (Kikawada, Iwamoto, & Takasaki, 2005). Influenza and pneumonia are frequent in the elderly and often present in an atypical manner. In terms of influenza, headache and fatigue may be the only presenting signs, whereas an increase in respiratory rate with a diminishing $PaO_2$ often is the initial presentation of pneumonia in the elderly (Meyer, 2004). Indeed, sepsis in the elderly has been found to be more likely respiratory or genitourinary in nature than sepsis in younger patient populations (Martin, Mannino, Eaton, & Moss, 2003).

Abdominal disease has a greater prevalence in elder populations. Diverticulitis is common and often reoccurs. The incidence of choledocholithiasis (gallstones in the common bile duct) and cholelithiasis (stones in the gallbladder) is higher in the elderly; elderly patients with these conditions often experience a more complicated course and are at increased sepsis risk. The incidence of sepsis in patients with cholelithiasis has been found to be 80%, and 73% of these septic patients develop multiple organ dysfunction (Stewart, Grifiss, Jarvis, & Way, 2008).

The presence of cerebrovascular events or other brain injury may be associated with dysphagia and impulsivity contributing to the risk of aspiration. It is then important to monitor patients for the presence of cognitive deficits as well as dysphagia. Hospitalization is more frequently associated with the development of urinary tract infections. Exhibit 16.3, which is derived from several sources, identifies frequent infectious agents in relationship to location. Another consideration is that immunosenescence results in a decreased ability to defend against viral epitopes. As indicated previously, one of the most common viral etiologies associated with aging is reactivation of varicella.

## Assessment

The following are signs the critical care nurse should look for when assessing the critically ill elder for signs of possible infection:

# Exhibit 16.3

## Common Infective Organisms in the Elderly

**Biliary and Gastrointestinal**
  *Clostridium difficile*
  *Enterobacter*
  *Enterococcus*
  *Escherichia coli*
  *Helicobacter pylori*
  *Klebsiella*

**Central Nervous System**
  *Cryptococcus neoformans*
  *Herpes simplex virus*
  *Listeria monocytogenes*
  *Neisseria meningitidis*
  *Streptococcus pneumoniae*

**Respiratory**
  *Bordetella pertussis*
  *Chlamydiae pneumoniae*
  *Haemophilus influenzae*
  *Influenza A and B*
  *Mycobacterium tuberculosis*
  *Parainfluenza*
  *Respiratory Syncytial Virus*
  *Staphylococcus aureus*
  *Streptococcus pneumoniae*

**Skin**
  *Cytomegalovirus*
  *Staphylococcus aureus*
  *Streptococcus pyogenes*
  *Varicella-zoster virus*

**Urinary**
  *Coagulase-negative staphylococci*
  *Escherichia coli*
  *Kiebsiella pneumoniae*
  *Proteus mirabilis*
  *Pseudomonas aeruginosa*
  *Staphylococcus aureus*

**Wounds**
  *Bacteroides fragilis*
  *Proteus mirabilis*
  *Staphylococcus aureus*

*Note:* Information is provided in alphabetical order and not in order of incidence.

**1. Mental Status**: Changes in cognitive status are considered one of the first and potentially most relevant indications of infection in the elderly. Any change in functional status could be indicative of infection, such as increasing or new-onset confusion, loss of balance, or irritability (Norman, 2000). In the critical care setting, neurologic function checks may help determine the presence of mental status change and the Folstein Mini-Mental Examination (Tombaugh & McIntyre, 1992) is performed as an evaluative measure in many settings. The presence of dementia or delirium may influence decision making and make communication with the patient more difficult. Evaluating symptoms may be more difficult in the elder with aphasia or other communicative deficits.

The older patient with dementia or delirium may also present with anxiety or confusion. This can place the ventilated patient at increased risk for aspiration or contamination of invasive lines. Consultation with the treatment team for a sedative may be necessary. Avoiding restraints is preferred as it places the patient at increased risk for complications associated with immobility (see chapter 26).

**2. Vital Signs**: Although little change in vital signs may be associated with the development of infection, an increase in respiratory rate may be indicative of pneumonia, particularly if the rate increases above 25 breaths/minute. As vital signs are evaluated, the nurse should keep in mind the possibility of dehydration in the elder. If dehydration is suspected, an orthostatic blood pressure should be performed as appropriate. A rapid, bounding pulse may be indicative of developing sepsis, along with a decreasing blood pressure. Sepsis is also characterized by increasing $PaCO_2$ levels or tachypnea. Heart and lung sounds should also be performed. The presence of crackles in the lungs could indicate pneumonia, whereas new-onset heart murmur could indicate valvular damage from endocarditis. The detection of pericardial rubs could indicate tuberculosis or pericarditis. Heart sounds should be auscultated in all positions.

**3. Nutrition and Hydration**: A decrease in oral intake can also be associated with infection. A dehydrated elder is at increased risk for changes in mental status and other complications that contribute to disease risk. In addition to an evaluation of skin turgor, the elder should be evaluated for dry mucous membranes along with tongue furrows or dryness. Aside from the considerations related to dehydration are separate issues related to vitamin and electrolyte intake.

Nutritional status can have relevance not only for the onset of mental confusion and cognitive deficits as in the case of Vitamin B (folate, $B_6$, $B_{12}$) deficiency, but can also contribute to overall immune function. Adequate intake of the B vitamins and antioxidants such as Vitamin C and E, are viewed as essential for promotion of a strong proinflammatory defensive response and influence the functional capacity of several immune cell classes. Administration of nutritional supplements is capable of reversing a trend toward anti-inflammatory antibody-mediated responses in the elderly (Langkamp-Henken et al., 2006). Zinc has been shown to reverse the loss of function in natural killer cells associated with aging and has been found to reduce the incidence and duration of pneumonia in older individuals (Meydani et al., 2007). Additionally, the contribution of nutrition to tissue wasting and wound healing should not be overlooked as pressure and stasis ulcers are a common route to infection.

**4. Oral and Dental Condition:** The presence of dental infections is associated with the development of endocarditis, and a dry mouth can quickly develop candidiasis. The teeth can harbor organisms that may play a role in the development of aspiration pneumonia (Htwe et al., 2007).

**5. Cough and Dysphasia**: Cough may be the only initial indicator of pneumonia or other lower respiratory tract disease. Decreased cough reflex and dysphagia can contribute to aspiration pneumonia, a leading cause of respiratory infections in the elderly. It is also important to recall, however, that the presence of cough may indicate GERD (gastroesophageal reflux disease), cardiovascular complications, or the use of an ACE (angiotensin-converting enzyme) inhibitor or other medication. It is then important to consider a previous history of dysphasia or the possibility of transient ischemic attack or other neurologic disease.

**6. Changes in Bladder or Bowel Function**: New-onset incontinence, dysuria, hematuria, or frequency may be the first signs of a developing urinary tract infection. Infections of the urinary tract are common in healthy elders and are even more frequent in those with comorbid disease. In elders living in residential care facilities, bacteremia can occur in up to 55% of females and 31% of males. Often these infections involve more than one infectious organism, particularly in those with indwelling urinary catheters. In the elder with limited range of motion or impaired motor function, obtaining a clean catch urine specimen may prove difficult (Adedipe & Lowenstein, 2006). Obtaining a catherized specimen should be considered either through the use of a sterile intermittent catherization or after changing the indwelling urinary catheter apparatus. The use of a freshly applied external catheter may be sufficient for a male patient, although attention needs to be paid to cleansing the site prior to application to avoid sample contamination.

In older patients with bacteriuria and no other symptoms, treatment is often discouraged. The side effects that may be experienced from antibiotics can have adverse health consequences for the elder and the development of resistant organisms is a real concern. In the individual with symptoms, a urine analysis and culture should be obtained. In the severely ill elder, treatment may be started at the time a specimen is obtained, and continued for at least 14 days in those with an indwelling urinary catheter (Htwe et al., 2007).

Because of changes in the gastrointestinal tract associated with aging, the elder may be exposed to pathogenic diarrhea. Diarrhea is potentially associated with fluid loss and dehydration in the elderly, particularly loss combined with already reduced intake. The use of antibiotics is associated with the development of *Clostridium difficile*, which leads to colitis. If the patient is experiencing watery diarrhea or abdominal pain and has been recently treated with an antibiotic course, *Clostridium difficile* should be suspected. Diverticulitis is also common in the elderly and results in abdominal pain, nausea, and anorexia.

**7. Social History**: The use of injectable medications could expose the elder to hepatitis and human immunodeficiency virus. The presence of indigestible agents used to dilute an illicit injectable drug could accumulate in the lungs and contribute to the development of pneumonia or pleural effusion. Smoking history has a significant effect on lung function and in time may contribute to the development of respiratory infection. Chronic smokers are particularly at risk for the development of sinusitis.

## Nursing Care Recommendations

The following are a list of related nursing interventions to use for the patient with infection.

- In the septic patient, monitor heart rate, blood pressure, and respiratory rate every 5 minutes until stable. The development of infection may contribute to the development of thrombic and coagulation abnormalities. Monitor clotting times and assess for the presence of petechiae.
- Monitor cardiac rhythm and electrolyte status, particularly in individuals thought to be malnourished. Inflammatory changes may contribute to the development of cardiovascular dysfunction.
- Strict intake and output records should be kept particularly for those with a comorbid head injury who may develop syndrome of inappropriate antidiuretic hormone (SIADH).
- Oral care and examination of denture fit is important for both patients with and without tracheostomy. This will help reduce the possibility of aspiration.
- Examine dressings over central lines and assess other ports of entry for invasive lines such as indwelling urinary catheters. Note any drainage, redness, swelling, or tenderness. If the invasive line is removed and infection suspected, ensure that catheter is preserved and the insertion tip is sent for culture.
- Report any clots or sediment noted in indwelling urinary catheter line.
- Turn patient when possible and examine skin areas for evidence of pressure ulcer formation. Note any redness, tenderness, skin sloughing, or coolness.
- In the presence of surgical wounds or traumatic skin injury, examine the site at least once during the shift for signs and symptoms of infection.

## Alleviating Immunosenescence

Many of the preceding interventions target complications of immunosenescence. Unfortunately, many of the cellular changes associated with immunosenescence reflect a lifetime of exposure and lifestyle. Engaging in a pattern of vigorous exercise and proper eating habits can help stave off immunosenescence, but these activities need to have been engaged in for a period of several years. A moderate level of physical activity on a regular basis over the span of several years appears to improve immune function in the older adult population (Senchina & Kohut, 2007). However, in the critical care setting, one is unlikely to encounter an older adult who is able to participate in such activity. In the face of chronic disease in a potentially frail elder, there are certain interventions that may be able to decrease patient vulnerability but not eliminate it:

1. It is critical to ensure adequate levels of nutrition and hydration. Although doing so may not fully ameliorate immunosenescence, it can reverse some deficits and leave the elder better armed to fight infection. Caloric restriction may have a benefit in conjunction with appropriate nutrition, although this area requires greater study (Bengmark, 2006).
2. Standard precautions need to be maintained with vigilance. Preventing the development of an infection in the first place is perhaps the best intervention for a critically ill elder facing immunosenescence.
3. Although the critically ill elder cannot engage in the levels of physical activity necessary to combat immunosenescence, nursing can assist in the performance of active and passive range–of–motion exercises. This will help reduce the incidence of contracture and reduce muscle atrophy and wasting. As well, proper positioning and turning of the patient are important considerations in reducing the formation of pressure ulcers and compression neuropathies.

4. Ultimately, monitoring the elder for the development of complications and minimizing the development of infections and pressure sores are the most effective nursing interventions currently available. Most preventive health measures need to be implemented years in advance to help avoid the development of chronic illness states and prevent age-associated immune change. Unfortunately at present there is no means of rapidly reversing immunosenescence.

## Preventive Measures

An annual influenza vaccination is suggested for all elders and should be considered while the elder is still hospitalized. A newer recommendation is for the administration of Zoster vaccine to all adults over the age 60. This vaccination can be administered to those with a previous history of zoster outbreak and as yet there are no recommendations for repeat administration. Pneumococcal vaccine should be given to all adults 65 years of age or over and a readministration given to those elders whose immune system may be comprised either because of viral infections or medications (as in the case of transplant patients) (Zimmerman, Middleton, Burns, Clover, & Kimmel, 2007).

Routine screening for tuberculosis and tetanus infection is encouraged for those elders living in multiple-person dwellings. Dental care should be provided on a regular basis along with a regular physical. Podiatric care should be provided annually or more frequently in individuals with diabetes or other forms of neuropathy.

Instruction of the elder or care providers in infection control measures is important. Hand washing remains one of the most effective measures to prevent transmission of microorganisms and should be taught to those family members assisting with in-home care. Considering the prevalence of in home dialysis, antibiotic therapy, blood transfusions, and other advanced procedures, ensuring that the family members and the elder individual are aware of infection-control measures is imperative.

## Case Study

The patient is a 75-year-old male admitted 2 days earlier with a diagnosis of acute coronary syndrome. He has a number of chronic conditions: Type II diabetes mellitus, hypertension, and rheumatoid arthritis. His prior medical history includes chickenpox and rubella.

The patient presented to the emergency room with a complaint of chest pain worsening on exertion with shortness of breath. Pain was accompanied by recurrent headaches with a bi-temporal throbbing sensation occurring two to three times over last 2 weeks. Headaches primarily occurred while he engaged in physical activity.

His vital signs were as follows: temperature = 99.4° Fahrenheit (otic), pulse 68 (3+), respirations 22. Initial blood pressures: 140/110 (right arm), 152/108 (left arm). Height 74 inches (187.9 cm), weight 294 lbs (133.6 kg).

The patient was alert and oriented in all spheres. He was able to follow all instructions and initiate conversation. He makes and maintains eye contact. Speech is intact and clear. No slurring or dysarthria are evident.

No increase in diameter of chest was noted on inspection. Respirations not labored, no use of accessory muscles. No pursing of lips or clubbing of extremities noted. No diaphoresis noted. Lungs clear in all fields.

His cardiovascular assessment indicated an apical pulse loud on auscultation, RRR. No deviation in rate between apical and radial pulse. Radial pulses 3+.

His laboratory results indicated a white blood cell count of 14,000 µl, neutrophils 75%, lymphocytes 20%, monocytes 3%, eosinophils 1%, and basophils 1%. Absolute neutrophil count (ANC): 1,064. C-reactive protein: 3.4 *mg/L*.

## The Immunologic Relevance of Prior Medical History

The etiology of rheumatoid arthritis (RA) includes the systemic production of proinflammatory cytokines. This process of systemic inflammation appears to contribute to more rapid progression of atherosclerosis and is considered a risk for cardiovascular disease. Obesity and diabetes also have inflammatory influences predisposing this patient to the development of heart disease along with increasing risk of infection. The presence of these conditions in combination most likely have contributed to the cardiovascular dysfunction this patient is currently experiencing. These conditions can also complicate the posttreatment course. The immunological effects of the prior medical history then require consideration in relationship to present health status.

Exposure to varicella in childhood also places this patient at risk of viral reactivation in the advent of treatment with antibiotics or immunosuppressant medication. It is also possible that age-related changes in immune function could also result in suppression of select elements of the immune system allowing for varicella reactivation. Nurses need to be aware of the significant frequency in which varicella reactivation occurs in the elder population and remain attentive to symptom presentation.

### Management of Present Course

The presence of an elevated c-reactive protein is generally more indicative of a bacterial or fungal infection than of a viral etiology. The presence of an elevated blood count could indicate the start of an infectious process, or leukocytosis. The patient should then be evaluated for any other signs and symptoms of infection, along with the implementation of tight glucose monitoring and control. Carefully evaluate for the development of thrombic events, maintaining an awareness of the potential for stroke or the potential worsening of cardiovascular status. Provide education to the patient and family for postdischarge management of heart disease, with education to address the possible use of statins and immunosuppressant medications. The management of RA and other inflammatory conditions often involves the use of medications that suppress or modulate elements of immune function. These medications place the elder at increased risk for viral reactivation and exposure to new infections.

## Summary

The immune changes associated with aging place older individuals at increased risk for the development of infections, cancer, and autoimmune conditions. Evaluating this population requires awareness of the age-related changes and of presenting symp-tomatology. Nursing needs to exert vigilance in the evaluation of the elder and ensure prompt follow up.

# References

Adedipe, A., & Lowenstein, R. (2006). Infectious emergencies in the elderly. *Emergency Medicine Clinics of North America, 24*(2), 433–448.

Alba-Loureiro, T. C., Munhoz, C. D., Martins, J. O., Cerchiaro, G. A., Scavone, C., Curi, R., et al. (2007). Neutrophil function and metabolism in individuals with diabetes mellitus. *Brazilian Journal of Medical and Biological Research, 40*(8), 1037–1044.

Bengmark, S. (2006). Impact of nutrition on ageing and disease. *Current Opinion in Clinical Nutrition and Metabolic Care, 9*(1), 2–7.

Bentley, D. W., Bradley, S., High, K., Schoenbaum, S., Taler, G., & Yoshikawa, T. T. (2001). Practice guideline for evaluation of fever and infection in long-term care facilities. *Journal of the American Geriatrics Society, 49*(2), 210–222.

Blondet, J. J., & Beilman, G. J. (2007). Glycemic control and prevention of perioperative infection. *Current Opinion in Critical Care, 13*(4), 421–427.

Bone, R. C., Balk, A., Cerra, F. B., Dellinger, R. P., Fein, A. M., Knaus, W. A., et al. (1992). Definitions for sepsis and organ failure guidelines for the use of innovative therapies in sepsis: The ACCP/ SCCM consensus conference the American College of Chest Physicians Society of Critical Care Medicine. *Chest, 101* 1644–1655.

Bradley, B. A. (2002). Rejection and recipient age. *Transplant Immunology, 10*(2–3), 125–132.

Butcher, S. K., Killampalli, V., Lascelles, D., Wang, K., Alpar, E. K., & Lord, J. M. (2005). Raised cortisol: DHEAS ratios in the elderly after injury: potential impact upon neutrophil function and immunity. *Aging Cell, 4*(6), 319–324.

Castle, S. C. (2000). Clinical relevance of age-related immune dysfunction. *Clinical Infectious Diseases, 31*(2), 578–585.

Castle, S. C., Uyemura, K., Fulop, T., & Makinodan, T. (2007). Host resistance and immune responses in advanced age. *Clinics in Geriatric Medicine, 23*(3), 463–479, v.

Castle, S. C., Uyemura, K., Rafi, A., Akande, O., & Makinodan, T. (2005). Comorbidity is a better predictor of impaired immunity than chronological age in older adults. *Journal of the American Geriatrics Society, 53*(9), 1565–1569.

Crighton, M. H., & Puppione, A. A. (2006). Geriatric neutrophils: Implications for older adults. *Seminars in Oncology Nursing, 22*(1), 3–9.

DelaRosa, O., Pawelec, G., Peralbo, E., Wikby, A., Mariani, E., Mocchegiani, E., et al. (2006). Immunological biomarkers of ageing in man: Changes in both innate and adaptive immunity are associated with health and longevity. *Biogerontology, 7*(5–6), 471–481.

Dellinger, R. P., Carlet, J. M., Masur, H., Gerlach, H., Calandra, T., Cohen, J., et al. (2004). Surviving Sepsis Campaign guidelines for management of severe sepsis and septic shock. *Critical Care Medicine, 32*(3), 858–873.

Dellinger, R. P., Levy, M. M., Carlet, J. M., Bion, J., Parker, M. M., Jaeschke, R., et al. (2008). Surviving Sepsis Campaign: International guidelines for management of severe sepsis and septic shock: 2008. *Critical Care Medicine, 36*(1), 296–327.

Dessein, P. H., Joffe, B. I., & Singh, S. (2005). Biomarkers of endothelial dysfunction, cardiovascular risk factors and atherosclerosis in rheumatoid arthritis. *Arthritis Research & Therapy, 7*(3), R634–643.

Effros, R. B. (2003a). Genetic alterations in the ageing immune system: Impact on infection and cancer. *Mechanisms of Ageing and Development, 124*(1), 71–77.

Effros, R. B. (2003b). Problems and solutions to the development of vaccines in the elderly. *Immunology and Allergy Clinics of North America, 23*(1), 41–55.

Emsley, H. C., & Hopkins, S. J. (2008). Acute ischaemic stroke and infection: Recent and emerging concepts. *Lancet Neurology, 7*(4), 341–353.

Girard, T. D., Opal, S. M., & Ely, E. W. (2005). Insights into severe sepsis in older patients: From epidemiology to evidence-based management. *Clinical Infectious Diseases, 40*(5), 719–727.

Grahn, D., Norman, D. C., & Yoshikawa, T. T. (1987). Fever and aging: Central nervous system prostaglandin E2 in response to endotoxin. *Experimental Gerontology, 22*(4), 249–255.

Gullo, A., Bianco, N., & Berlot, G. (2006). Management of severe sepsis and septic shock: Challenges and recommendations. *Critical Care Clinics, 22*(3), 489–501.

Htwe, T. H., Mushtaq, A., Robinson, S. B., Rosher, R. B., & Khardori, N. (2007). Infection in the elderly. *Infectious Disease Clinics of North America, 21*(3), 711–743.

Janeway, C. (2005). *Immunobiology: The immune system in health and disease* (6th ed.). New York: Garland Science.

Khovidhunkit, W., Memon, R. A., Feingold, K. R., & Grunfeld, C. (2000). Infection and inflammation-induced proatherogenic changes of lipoproteins. *Journal of Infectious Disease, 181* (Suppl. 3), S462–472.

Kikawada, M., Iwamoto, T., & Takasaki, M. (2005). Aspiration and infection in the elderly: Epidemiology, diagnosis and management. *Drugs & Aging, 22*(2), 115–130.

Kung, H., Hoyert, D. L., Xu, J., & Murphy, S. L. (2008). *National Vital Statistics Reports: Deaths: Final Data for 2005*. Washington, DC: NCHS.

Langkamp-Henken, B., Wood, S. M., Herlinger-Garcia, K. A., Thomas, D. J., Stechmiller, J. K., Bender, B. S., et al. (2006). Nutritional formula improved immune profiles of seniors living in nursing homes. *Journal of the American Geriatrics Society, 54*(12), 1861–1870.

Levy, M. M., Fink, M. P., Marshall, J. C., Abraham, E., Angus, D., Cook, D., et al. (2003). 2001 SCCM/ESICM/ACCP/ATS/SIS International Sepsis Definitions Conference. *Critical Care Medicine, 31*(4), 1250–1256.

Martin, G. S., Mannino, D. M., Eaton, S., & Moss, M. (2003). The epidemiology of sepsis in the United States from 1979 through 2000. *New England Journal of Medicine, 348*(16), 1546–1554.

Meydani, S. N., Barnett, J. B., Dallal, G. E., Fine, B. C., Jacques, P. F., Leka, L. S., et al. (2007). Serum zinc and pneumonia in nursing home elderly. *American Journal of Clinical Nutrition, 86*(4), 1167–1173.

Meyer, K. C. (2004). Lung infections and aging. *Ageing Research Reviews, 3*, 55–67.

Michel, J. J., Turesson, C., Lemster, B., Atkins, S. R., Iclozan, C., Bongartz, T., et al. (2007). CD56-expressing T cells that have features of senescence are expanded in rheumatoid arthritis. *Arthritis and Rheumatism, 56*(1), 43–57.

Mocchegiani, E., & Malavolta, M. (2004). NK and NKT cell functions in immunosenescence. *Aging Cell, 3*(4), 177–184.

Moltz, H. (1993). Fever: Causes and consequences. *Neuroscience and Biobehavioral Reviews, 17*(3), 237–269.

Norman, D. C. (2000). Fever in the elderly. *Clinical Infectious Diseases, 31*(1), 148–151.

Norman, D. C., Wong, M. B., & Yoshikawa, T. T. (2007). Fever of unknown origin in older persons. *Infectious Disease Clinics of North America, 21*(4), 937–945.

Norman, D. C., & Yoshikawa, T. T. (1996). Fever in the elderly. *Infectious Disease Clinics of North America, 10*(1), 93–99.

Opal, S. M., Girard, T. D., & Ely, E. W. (2005). The immunopathogenesis of sepsis in elderly patients. *Clinics in Infectious Disease, 41* (Suppl. 7), S504–5512.

Pawelec, G., Akbar, A., Caruso, C., Solana, R., Grubeck-Loebenstein, B., & Wikby, A. (2005). Human immunosenescence: Is it infectious? *Immunological Reviews, 205*, 257–268.

Pawelec, G., Barnett, Y., Forsey, R., Frasca, D., Globerson, A., McLeod, J., et al. (2002). T cells and aging, January 2002 update. *Frontiers in Bioscience, 7*, d1056–1183.

Pletz, M. W., Duda, P. W., Kappos, L., & Steck, A. J. (2003). Immune-mediated neuropathies: Etiology and pathogenic relationship to aging processes. *Journal of Neuroimmunology, 137*(1–2), 1-11.

Prelog, M. (2006). Aging of the immune system: A risk factor for autoimmunity? *Autoimmunity Reviews, 5*(2), 136–139.

Regazzoni, C. J., Zamora, R. J., Petrucci, E., Pisarevsky, A. A., Saad, A. K., Mollein, D. D., et al. (2008). Hospital and 1-year outcomes of septic syndromes in older people: a cohort study.*Journals of Gerontology. Series A, Biological Sciences and Medical Sciences, 63*(2), 210–212.

Sansoni, P., Vescovini, R., Fagnoni, F., Biasini, C., Zanni, F., Zanlari, L., et al. (2008). The immune system in extreme longevity. *Experimental Gerontology, 43*(2), 61–65.

Schmader, K. (2007). Herpes zoster and postherpetic neuralgia in older adults. *Clinics in Geriatric Medicine, 23*(3), 615–632.

Senchina, D. S., & Kohut, M. L. (2007). Immunological outcomes of exercise in older adults. *Clinical Interventions in Aging, 2*(1), 3–16.

Singh, A. K., Singh, V., Pal Singh, M., Shrivastava, P., Singh, N., Gambhir, I. S., et al. (2008). Effect of immunosenescence on the induction of cardiovascular disease pathogenesis: Role of peripheral blood mononuclear cells. *Immunopharmacology & Immunotoxicology, 30*(2), 411–423.

Stegenga, M. E., van der Crabben, S. N., Blumer, R. M., Levi, M., Meijers, J. C., Serlie, M. J., et al. (2008). Hyperglycemia enhances coagulation and reduces neutrophil degranulation, whereas hyperinsulinemia inhibits fibrinolysis during human endotoxemia. *Blood, 112*(1), 82–89.

Stewart, L., Grifiss, J. M., Jarvis, G. A., & Way, L. W. (2008). Elderly patients have more severe biliary infections: Influence of complement-killing and induction of TNFalpha production. *Surgery, 143*(1), 103–112.

Szekanecz, Z., Kerekes, G., Der, H., Sandor, Z., Szabo, Z., Vegvari, A., et al. (2007). Accelerated atherosclerosis in rheumatoid arthritis. *Annals of the New York Academy of Sciences, 1108,* 349–358.

Thewissen, M., Somers, V., Hellings, N., Fraussen, J., Damoiseaux, J., & Stinissen, P. (2007). CD4+CD28 null T cells in autoimmune disease: Pathogenic features and decreased susceptibility to immuno-regulation. *Journal of Immunology, 179*(10), 6514–6523.

Tombaugh, T. N., & McIntyre, N. J. (1992). The Mini-Mental State Examination: A comprehensive review. *Journal of the American Geriatrics Society, 40*(9), 922–935.

van Duin, D., & Shaw, A. C. (2007). Toll-like receptors in older adults. *Journal of the American Geriatrics Society, 55*(9), 1438–1444.

Weinberg, J. M. (2007). Herpes zoster: epidemiology, natural history, and common complications. *Journal of the American Academy of Dermatology, 57*(6 Suppl.), S130–135.

Weinert, B. T., & Timiras, P. S. (2003). Invited review: Theories of aging. *Journal of Applied Physiology, 95*(4), 1706–1716.

Wellen, K. E., & Hotamisligil, G. S. (2005). Inflammation, stress, and diabetes. *Journal of Clinical Investigation, 115*(5), 1111–1119.

Werba, J. P., Veglia, F., Amato, M., Baldassarre, D., Massironi, P., Meroni, P. L., et al. (2008). Patients with a history of stable or unstable coronary heart disease have different acute phase responses to an inflammatory stimulus. *Atherosclerosis, 196*(2), 835–840.

Winkelman, C. (2007). Inactivity and inflammation in the critically ill patient. *Critical Care Clinics, 23*(1), 21–34.

Xie, D., & McElhaney, J. E. (2007). Lower GrB+ CD62Lhigh CD8 TCM effector lymphocyte response to influenza virus in older adults is associated with increased CD28null CD8 T lymphocytes. *Mechanisms of Ageing and Development, 128*(5–6), 392–400.

Zimmerman, R. K., Middleton, D. B., Burns, I. T., Clover, R. D., & Kimmel, S. R. (2007). Routine vaccines across the life span, 2007. *Journal of Family Practice, 56*(2 Suppl. Vaccines), S1–S73.

# Understanding and Managing Sleep Disorders in Older Adult Patients in the Intensive Care Unit

# 17

Elisabeth Marie
Nirav Patel
Nalaka S. Gooneratne

## Case Study

A 67-year-old man with alcoholic cirrhosis, complicated by hepatocellular carcinoma and hepatic hydrothorax (pleural effusion caused by advanced liver disease), and a history of narcotic drug abuse was admitted to the intensive care unit (ICU) with acutely progressive dyspnea. The dyspnea was attributed to worsening hepatic hydrothorax based on a chest X-ray and therapeutic thoracentesis (sampling of pleural effusion with a needle inserted into pleural space). The course of the patient's hospital stay was dominated by his tenuous respiratory status as evidenced by dyspnea with minimal exertion, a requirement for supplemental oxygen at rest, and markedly abnormal chest X-rays.

The patient underwent frequent medical tests and procedures, including multiple thoracenteses, paracenteses (sampling of fluid in the abdominal cavity), arterial blood gases, and a transjugular intrahepatic portosystemic shunt (TIPS) procedure. He initially demonstrated extreme respiratory insufficiency requiring 100% oxygen supplementation as a result of massive right hepatic hydrothorax, which was also having a compressive effect on his right heart, manifesting as cardiac tamponade physiology. After the TIPS procedure the patient's hydrothorax reaccumulated but at a much lower rate and his respiratory condition, though not normal, stabilized.

A recurrent complaint of this gentleman's stay was his inability to sleep well in the ICU. A variety of reasons were expressed during the course of his stay. Initially, his breathing was so laborious that he could not get comfortable due to a "suffocating feeling." Emerging anxiety and ruminations about death compounded his difficulty to initiate sleep. As his respiratory condition stabilized, he began to experience diffuse body pain and required regular doses of intravenous narcotic (hydromorphone). The pain was described as 8 on a scale of 1 to 10 and was particularly intense in the lumbar region of his back. This pain was cited on numerous occasions to be an impediment to sleep attainment.

It was clear that sleep was being adversely affected by the patient's illness. In addition, it was stated that frequent interruptions by hospital environment or staff were also sources of sleep disturbance. Specific examples included nursing staff patient-centered duties, audible monitor alarms, and ambient light in the unit.

The medications he was being administered were also challenging his ability to sleep. For example, high doses of furosemide prescribed to treat his hydrothorax led to a frequent need to micturate during the night. Lactulose, administered to avoid hepatic encephalopathy, required the patient to exit the bed and sit on the adjacent commode every 2 to 3 hours. The patient developed anxiety concerning the possibility that he may defecate in the bed, further perpetuating his sleep problems.

The patient was hospitalized for several weeks, distancing him from friends. As he considered the possibility of death, he began to share his feelings of lost opportunity with family who visited infrequently. It was readily apparent that in addition to severe medical illness, he was carrying a heavy burden of psychosocial stress. The patient's general outlook on life became increasingly negative and he indicated that he felt depressed.

---

This case history illustrates the challenges of being an acutely ill patient with particular attention to disturbances in sleep. Several sources of sleep disturbance are exemplified, including medical illness, pain, psychosocial stress, isolation, medical technology, hospital environment, and health care providers. The illustrated sources of sleep disturbance are broad, and hence approaches to addressing them involve a multidisciplinary and multimodality strategy.

Treatment of the sleep difficulties of this patient focused on the following:

1. Treatment of the underlying medical disorder (hepatic hydrothorax)
2. Treatment of pain with appropriate analgesia
3. Emotional support by the nursing staff and support staff
4. Anxiolysis with lorazepam (treatment options limited because of liver disease)

5. Reduced frequency of unnecessary vitals checks
6. Discontinuation of telemetry monitoring to reduce discomfort, noise, and anxiety.

# Introduction

## Our Biological Clock: Circadian Rhythms and Physiological Changes During Sleep

The interplay of various physiological systems keeps our bodies on a roughly 24-hour sleep–wake cycle. These systems promote wakefulness specifically during daylight and sleep at night. In addition, a number of hormones can influence, or are influenced by, the biological clock. Melatonin, produced by the pineal gland of the brain, is one element of this circadian regulatory process and its production peaks at night. Bright light, however, can suppress the nocturnal melatonin surge and thereby impair sleep. Levels of thyroid-stimulating hormone peak during sleep onset and decrease throughout the night. Growth hormone and prolactin secretion increase with sleep onset. Gamma aminobutyric acid (GABA) is released after sleep onset and inhibits excitatory activity promoting wakefulness. After declining throughout the day, adrenocorticotropic hormone and cortisol reach their lowest level around midnight, increasing again in the early morning. Body temperature, saliva flow, and swallowing all decrease during sleep.

## Stages of Sleep

Sleep is a dynamic state, with variation in both electrophysical output and autonomic nervous system behavior. Distinct electrophysiological characteristics, captured by electroencephalographic (EEG) monitoring, form the basis of the division of the sleep cycle into four distinct stages: stage 1, stage 2, stage 3, and rapid-eye-movement sleep (REM sleep) (Iber, Ancoli-Israel, Chesson, & Quan, 2007). Stages 1 to 3 are together referred to as nonrapid-eye-movement sleep, or NREM sleep.

Stage 1 is a light sleep, from which one can be easily awakened. As muscle activity slows, one may experience sudden muscle contractions. There is also a decrease in minute ventilation (Henke, Dempsey, Kowitz, & Skatrud, 1990). The respiratory rate remains stable in most cases, however. In stage 2, EEG waves slow, but with bursts of rapid waves called *sleep spindles*. Stage 2 is also characterized by *k-complexes*, which are high voltage waves. Stage 3 is also known as slow-wave sleep, or SWS, because of the low-frequency EEG waves characteristic of the stage. There is a lack of eye movement or other muscle activity as well. Stage 3 is the deepest sleep stage, when awakening is most difficult and is often accompanied by grogginess and/or confusion. In the past, SWS was further separated into two separate stages (3 and 4), but those two stages have been combined in the newer classification system (Iber et al., 2007).

REM sleep is characterized not only by episodic rapid eye movement but also by loss of muscle tone. During REM sleep, minute ventilation decreases further as our breathing becomes shallower, rapid, and irregular, accompanied by an increase in blood pressure and heart rate (Collop, Salas, Delayo, & Gamaldo, 2008). It is upon awakening from REM sleep that people most vividly remember their dreams.

A single cycle through the sleep stages takes between 70 and 120 minutes, with the first cycle usually being the shortest. Thus, a normal individual sleeping 8 hours will complete between four and six sleep cycles. SWS (Stage N3) is postulated to be the most restorative sleep stage. For example, growth hormone secretion is elevated during SWS, and body metabolism is reduced (Akerstedt & Nilsson, 2003). REM also is potentially necessary for the restorative impact of sleep on cognition and memory formation. This is indicated in part by the finding that the time one spends in the various sleep cycles changes in response to sleep deprivation. After an extended period of wakefulness, a patient will enter SWS more quickly–thus spending less time in stages 1 and 2–and will spend an extended time in SWS and REM sleep (Collop et al., 2008). The phenomenon of increased time spent in SWS and REM sleep after a period of total or partial sleep deprivation is known as SWS rebound and REM sleep rebound, respectively. In some cases REM rebound is associated with nightmares.

Sleep is interrupted by *arousals* and *awakenings*. An awakening is a sudden change into full wakefulness, whereas arousals are an abrupt shift into a lighter stage of sleep, represented by an accompanying change in the EEG frequency for at least 3 seconds. Both arousals and awakenings contribute to *sleep fragmentation*. Repeated arousals and awakenings decrease the amount of time spent specifically in SWS and REM sleep.

## Physiologic Role of Sleep

On average, about one third of a typical day is spent in the sleep state. It is a phylogenetic phenomenon common to all mammals, and has been proposed to occur even in insects and worms. The amount of time that a given species spends in the sleep state can vary considerably, however. Considering the amount of time spent in the sleep state and the variability across species, a key question here relates to the specific role of sleep. One theory is that sleep is necessary for growth and repair functions. Evidence to support this comes from the observation that growth hormone levels peak during the sleep phase. Animal studies, for example, have shown that wound healing is decreased in the event of sleep deprivation (Gumustekin et al., 2004). Others have suggested a primary role of sleep in energy metabolism and regulation (Laposky, Bass, Kohsaka, & Turek, 2008). Research in sleep deprivation in animal models has shown that chronic sleep deprivation is associated with weight loss despite hyperphagia, and hypothermia with subsequent death (Rechtschaffen & Bergmann, 1995). In addition, there are reductions in growth hormone levels; prolactin; leptins; and an increase in insulin resistance. Chronic low-grade inflammation may also result from sleep deprivation (Akerstedt & Nilsson, 2003). These are discussed in more detail in the section on "Consequences of Inadequate Sleep." For these reasons, sleep is postulated to play a central role in growth, tissue restoration, and energy metabolism.

## Sleep Changes in Older Adults

Physiological changes that occur as one ages make it more likely for an elderly person entering the ICU to have sleep difficulties than someone in the general population.

Older adults tend to have less slow-wave sleep (Ohayon, Carskadon, Guilleminault, & Vitiello, 2004). They also experience an increase in nocturnal awakenings and an increase in the amount of time it takes to fall back asleep after an awakening, leading to a decreased sleep efficiency (Ohayon et al.). Interestingly, sleep latency (i.e., the amount of time it takes to initially fall asleep) tends to remain fairly stable (Ohayon et al.). There is also a decrease in melatonin production and a general decline in the regulation of the circadian rhythm (Cajochen, Munch, Knoblauch, Blatter, & Wirz-Justice, 2006). Older adults are particularly at risk for a circadian rhythm disorder (CRD) of the advanced phase type, in which the person experiences early-morning awakenings and increased daytime napping. Conversely, they may also have a delayed sleep phase as well, in which they go to bed late and wake late, in part because of a less structured schedule associated with retirement (Youngstedt, Kripke, Elliott, & Klauber, 2001). Elderly individuals who are visually impaired are especially prone to nighttime sleep disturbances (Asplund, 2000) because external light levels help to set the internal circadian clock. An awareness of patients' preexisting sleep disorders on the part of the clinical care team is important, as these conditions may influence care.

# Common Sleep Disturbances

## Insomnia

Insomnia is generally defined as difficulty in falling or staying asleep that is associated with daytime impairments resulting from sleepiness or fatigue. Insomnia symptoms occur in approximately 15 to 30% of older adults (Ohayon, 2002). Insomnia is often secondary to illness, pain and discomfort, medication, or another sleep disorder, such as sleep apnea or restless leg syndrome (see below). Though as we age we are susceptible to primary disturbances in sleep, other medications, medical conditions, and sleep disorders also contribute to insomnia in the elderly. A list of medications associated with insomnia is found in Exhibit 17.1. In general, poor sleep quality in the ICU may fall under the *International Classification of Sleep Disorders-2* (American Academy of Sleep Medicine, 2005, p. 31) diagnoses of "physiologic (organic) insomnia, unspecified," which applies to cases in which a medical disorder or physiological state is suspected to be causing the insomnia, or "nonorganic insomnia, NOS (not otherwise specified)" for situations in which sleep-disruptive or psychological factors are potentially contributing to the insomnia, but the diagnosis is not certain. More specific insomnia diagnoses are available, but because of the multifactorial nature of sleep disruption in the ICU, these more specific diagnoses are difficult to firmly establish.

## Sleep Apnea

Sleep apnea is a condition in which the individual repeatedly stops breathing during sleep. An observer may notice that the patient initially snores loudly, then suddenly stops snoring and has a cessation of airflow despite evidence of continued chest and abdominal wall movements lasting for 10 seconds or longer, followed by a sudden gasping or choking as he/she resumes breathing again. Obstructive sleep apnea (OSA) occurs when the cessation of breathing results from the collapsing of the upper airway by the soft-tissue structures, such as the tongue, which then obstructs the airway.

## Exhibit 17.1

| Selected List of Medications That Impair Sleep | |
|---|---|
| **Category** | **Examples** |
| Antihypertensive medications | Alpha-blockers, beta-blockers, methyldopa, reserpine |
| Central nervous system stimulants | Amphetamines, dextroamphetamine, methylphenidate, modafinil |
| Hormones | Corticosteroids, thyroid hormone replacement therapy |
| Respiratory medications | Albuterol, theophylline |
| Decongestants | Phenylephrine, pseudoephedrine |

In patients who are intubated, obstructive sleep apnea does not occur because the endotracheal tube bypasses the areas that are associated with upper airway collapse. A tracheostomy also bypasses this area and essentially cures obstructive sleep apnea. Central sleep apnea is caused by a failure in the brain's respiratory center (located in the medulla) to signal the muscles involved to breathe. Some patients have mixed sleep apnea, with both obstructive and central apnea events occurring. Regardless of the cause of the apnea, the intermittent and repetitive deprivation of oxygen throughout the course of the night puts a strain on the heart and other bodily organs. Consequently, sleep apnea puts an individual at greater risk for cardiac disease, stroke, and high blood pressure (Yaggi et al., 2005). In response to a prolonged apnea event, the brain signals the individual to wake up to start breathing again. Thus, sleep apnea often involves frequent arousals, which the individual may or not be aware of, but which result in fragmented sleep. Thus, the quality of sleep of individuals with untreated sleep apnea is often poor, as reflected in the existence of daytime fatigue and impaired daytime functioning. Older adults are especially at risk for sleep apnea, with prevalence rates approaching 20 to 25% when defining sleep apnea as the occurrence of abnormal breathing events 15 or more times per hour (Young et al., 2002).

Another sleep disorder seen in the ICU that often coexists with OSA is obesity-hypoventilation syndrome (OHS). The main factor that differentiates OHS from sleep apnea is that patients with OHS also have daytime hypercapnia. This is caused by a reduced ventilatory drive, thus leading to daytime hypercapnia. It is important to note that most obese patient's do not manifext reduced ventilatory drive.

## Restless Leg Syndrome and Periodic Leg Movement Disorder

Restless leg syndrome (RLS) is a neurological disorder characterized by unpleasant sensations in the legs, accompanied by an urge to move the legs. On moving or flexing the legs, the uncomfortable feeling disappears, only to return when the legs are still again. Though more rare, the sensation may also occur in the feet, arms, or hands. The sensation is usually at its worst when in an otherwise relaxed state, such as when one is lying down and trying to fall asleep, and can cause insomnia (see previous section for more information on insomnia). Though RLS can develop at any age, it is more common in older adults (Allen & Earley, 2001; Hening, Allen, Tenzer, & Winkelman, 2007). People with iron deficiency, anemia, kidney failure, pregnancy, diabetes, Parkinson's disease, and peripheral neuropathy are more prone to developing RLS. In cases resulting from iron deficiency, treatment of the iron deficiency can often improve the RLS symptoms, thus checking iron levels is an important part of the evaluation (Allen & Earley; Lopes et al., 2005). In about 85% of people, RLS is accompanied by periodic limb movement disorder (PLMD; Allen & Earley), defined by involuntary limb jerking or twitching during sleep that may last throughout the night. It is distinguished from RLS in that the movements occur while the person is asleep, and are completely involuntary. The movements can lead to frequent arousals, leading to daytime sleepiness and dysfunction. Periodic leg movement disorder (PLMD) can also present without RLS.

# Consequence of Inadequate Sleep

Sleep is essential for the healthiest of people. Inadequate sleep has been linked to impairment of numerous physiological systems. The extensive body of research on the effects of sleep deprivation, and more generally, poor sleep, has largely concentrated on healthy individuals, but the undeniable conclusion is that inadequate sleep is linked to the impairment of numerous biological and physiological systems. For the critically ill patient, this can lead to an increased burden on both the patient and the health care system in the form of increased length of hospital stay. Long term, there is a growing body of evidence indicating that poor sleep in the ICU can affect patient mortality both during the hospital stay and after discharge (Salas & Gamaldo, 2008).

## Cognitive and Behavioral Functioning

Inadequate sleep can have a severe impact on daytime function. Daytime fatigue or sleepiness, short-term memory loss, poor concentration, increased reaction time, and irritability are just some of the consequences of insufficient or disrupted sleep. These effects have been observed after just one night of sleep deprivation in healthy individuals (Thomas et al., 2000). Individuals who have undergone extended sleep deprivation react to negative events in an exacerbated fashion, whereas their responses to positive events are muted (Zohar, Tzischinsky, Epstein, & Lavie, 2005). There is an increase in self-reported negative feelings, such as depression, frustration, anxiety, and anger (Orton & Gruzelier, 1989). This may be caused by sleep deprivation-related abnormalities in the prefrontal cortex, a region of the brain involved in regulating emotions and behaviors (Salas & Gamaldo, 2008).

## Immune, Metabolic, and Endocrine System Functioning

Research indicates that sleep deprivation can alter immune system function. Modest sleep loss, such as a reduction from 8 to 6 hours over a week-long period, in healthy males was associated with increased serum proinflammatory cytokines such as IL-6 and TNF-alpha (Vgontzas et al., 2004). Both IL-6 and TNF-alpha are markers of systemic inflammation that have been linked with the development of cardiovascular disease, insulin resistance, and osteoporosis (Vgontzas, Bixler, Papanicolaou, & Chrousos, 2000). The association of elevated IL-6 with reduced pain tolerance may explain the increased sensitivity to pain (*hyperalgesia*) frequently reported after sleep deprivation (Salas & Gamaldo, 2008). Short-term partial sleep loss has also been shown to lead to an increase in high-sensitivity C-reactive protein, which has been correlated with higher cardiovascular morbidity (Meier-Ewert et al., 2004). Even a single night of partial sleep deprivation has been linked to a decrease in natural killer cell number and activity in healthy subjects (Irwin et al., 1996).

Sleep deprivation also causes changes in energy metabolism. During sleep deprivation, patients often experience hyperphagia, or a desire to increase their food intake (Laposky et al., 2008). This increased desire to eat may be mediated by abnormal leptin levels (Spiegel et al., 2004). In addition, insulin and glucose metabolism are adversely affected. Patients demonstrate increased insulin resistance and poor glycemic control when subjected to sleep deprivation, for example (Spiegel, Knutson, Leproult, Tasali, & Van Cauter, 2005).

Despite these findings, there is a lack of data on a connection between short-term sleep deprivation and acute clinical implications in the ICU setting. This could be caused, in part, by the difficulty of conducting clinical research in the ICU. It is possible that poor sleep could both leave one more susceptible to illness onset and impair one's ability to recover from illness and injury. One study of vaccination responses found that healthy subjects had a weakened response to immunization when the vaccination was received after sleep deprivation (Spiegel, Sheridan, & Van Cauter, 2002). However, whether sleep loss in the ICU impairs the immune system's capability to recover from critical illness is a question that needs further investigation.

## Cardiovascular System Functioning

Frequent arousals from sleep are linked to increased blood pressure and catecholamine release (Loredo, Ziegler, Ancoli-Israel, Clausen, & Dimsdale, 1999; Tochikubo, Ikeda, Miyajima, & Ishii, 1996). The elevated sympathetic nervous system activity seen with sleep deprivation (Zhong et al.) leads to an increased risk of heart attack (Liu, Tanaka, & Fukuoka Heart Study Group, 2002). Sleep deprivation also leads to a decreased sensitivity of the baroreflex, which regulates blood pressure (Zhong et al.). The increased amount of REM sleep that follows a period of sleep deprivation, fragmentation, or REM sleep suppression (a side effect of many medications; see the text that follows) is also problematic for the critically ill because of the increased and variable heart rate, blood pressure, and respiration associated with REM sleep.

## Gastrointestinal Injury

Sleep deprivation has been associated with increased risk for peptic ulcer disease. Research in rats has shown that partial sleep deprivation resulted in gastric mucosal damage in 30 to 50% of the rats (Guo, Chau, Cho, & Koo, 2005). This may be the

## Exhibit 17.2

### Characteristics of Sleep in the ICU

Severely fragmented

Noncircadian

Decreased time in SWS and REM sleep

Increased time in stage 1 and stage 2 sleep

Increased arousals and awakenings

Total sleep time over 24 hours may be normal

result of increased gastric acid levels and decreased gastric mucosal blood flow (Guo et al.).

## Sleep Patterns in the ICU

Patients often report problems falling and staying asleep while in the ICU (Freedman, Kotzer, & Schwab, 1999; Novaes, Aronovich, Ferraz, & Knobel, 1997; Rotondi et al., 2002; Southwell & Wistow, 1995). Objective study measurements support subjective patient reports of sleep difficulties. Polysomnography (PSG) studies have shown that patients in the ICU experience decreased sleep time, fragmentation of sleep, and atypical sleep architecture (Aurell & Elmqvist, 1985). Arousals and awakenings have been reported between 22 and 79 times per hour (Gabor, Cooper, & Hanly, 2001; Gabor et al., 2003; Parthasarathy & Tobin, 2002). Many ICU patients spend increased time in stage 1 sleep and a corresponding decreased time in SWS and REM sleep (Aurell & Elmqvist; Cooper et al., 2000), with the percentage of REM sleep ranging from none to 11% of total sleep time (Aurell & Elmqvist; Cooper et al.; Freedman, Gazendam, Levan, Pack, & Schwab, 2001; Parthasarathy & Tobin), a marked contrast to the norm of 20 to 25% of total sleep time. Patients in the ICU are also susceptive to REM rebound after a period of suppressed REM sleep, often occurring after the discontinuation of medication (see Effects of Medications section) or during postoperative recovery (Cooper, Gabor, & Hanly, 2001). The circadian rhythm of sleep is typically lost in the ICU, with much of patients' sleep occurring during the day (Cooper et al., 2001; Sareli & Schwab, 2008) (see Exhibit 17.2).

## Effects of Environment

There are multiple aspects of the ICU environment that do not make it conducive to adequate restful sleep. These factors may exacerbate preexisting sleep disturbances as well as create new ones present for the length of the hospital stay. Because of the changes in sleep–wake regulation previously discussed, older adults are especially likely to enter the ICU with a preexisting sleep disturbance.

## Noise

Alarms, pagers, intercoms, ventilation machines, ringing phones, housekeeping activities, televisions, and conversations are common sources of noise in the ICU environment (Salas & Gamaldo, 2008). The U.S. Environmental Protection Agency (EPA) recommends that hospital noise levels do not exceed 35 dB during the night and 45 dB during the day, yet these levels are often exceeded in ICU settings (Salas & Gamaldo, 2008). Loud noises are particularly troublesome for older adults as they are more sensitive to the awakening effects of sound than younger patients (Bonnet, 1989).

Though most of the research has focused on peak noise level, recent investigations have examined the effect that deviation from the baseline noise level may have in causing arousals and awakenings. In a recent study, the arousal threshold (i.e., the noise level that caused an arousal) of healthy volunteers exposed to ICU noise recordings was diminished when investigators decreased the difference between the baseline and peak noise level by means of white noise (Stanchina, Abu-Hijleh, Chaudhry, Carlisle, & Millman, 2005).

Instinctively, it is easy to consider noise in the ICU as the cause for sleep disruption. Much of the research done in the last quarter of the 20th century that looked at the effect of ICU noise on sleep used healthy subjects exposed to audio recordings of ICU noise overnight (Gabor et al., 2003). However, a polysomnographic study of ICU patients using noise recordings showed that on average 15% of arousals and awakenings were caused by noise (Freedman et al., 2001). Findings from other studies also support a role of ICU-related noise in disrupting patients' sleep, but note that it is not the paramount cause of sleep disturbances in the ICU (Gabor et al., 2001, 2003). This corresponds to subjective patient reporting after a stay in the ICU (Freedman et al., 1999). Still, 15% is a significant percentage of arousals and awakenings and thus noise level is an important consideration in creating the optimal ICU environment. An example of the effects of a loud noise on sleep architecture is provided in Figure 17.1.

## Light

Studies show that light levels in ICU do mimic a day–night rhythm, with peak levels occurring during the day and lower levels at night (Meyer et al., 1994). Light exposure affects the secretion of melatonin, with research indicating that light levels in the 100- to 500-lux range can affect nighttime melatonin secretion (Boivin, Duffy, Kronauer, & Czeisler, 1996). As discussed earlier, many elderly patients already have decreased levels of melatonin production; thus, they are particularly susceptible to suppression of sleep by exposure to light in the evening and nighttime hours. Furthermore, there is evidence that the circadian rhythm of melatonin secretion is often disturbed in mechanically ventilated and critically ill patients. Keeping the light levels low at night is not necessarily a panacea, as at least one study has found that lower light levels in the ICU corresponded with greater variation in light level, another potential source of sleep disruption (Walder, Francioli, Meyer, Lancon, & Romand, 2000). Bursts of light during sleep can cause awakenings or arousals, even if they are below the

# 17.1

**Effects of loud noises on sleep architecture.**

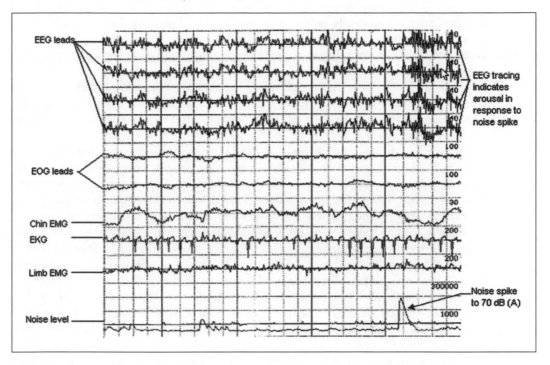

threshold necessary to affect melatonin secretion or other aspects of the human circadian rhythm (Meyer et al.).

## Medical Tests and Care Activities

ICU patients undergo frequent interruption because of medical tests and care activities. One study found an average of almost eight patient-care activities per hour of sleep, with most of these being nursing procedures such as changing dressings, adjusting intravenous drips, and giving medication (Gabor et al., 2003). Another study found the taking of vital signs was the most common intervention during the nighttime hours (excluding vital signs recorded from arterial catheters), followed by assessing intake and output (excluding patients who had urinary catheters), administration of medication, patient assessments, and turning (Tamburri, DiBrienza, Zozula, & Redeker, 2004). Routine baths took place between 2 a.m. and 5 a.m. on 61% of the study nights, and out of 147 study nights, periods of at least 2 hours without interventions occurred only nine times, or 6% of the nights studied (Tamburri et al.). Interestingly, this same study found only one sleep-promoting intervention noted in patient records for the 147 nights studied.

## Mechanical Ventilation and Sleep

About 40% of patients in the ICU are on some form of mechanical ventilation during their stay (Parthasarathy, 2004). Any independent effect of mechanical ventilation on sleep is difficult to parse out from the other sources of sleep disruption in the ICU, such as the ICU environment, medications, and the illness itself, and investigations into this area are relatively recent. It is known that poor sleep can adversely affect the respiratory system by weakening both respiratory muscle function and blunting the ventilatory response to carbon dioxide. Sleep deprivation in a patient with respiratory failure may, therefore, impair recovery and weaning from mechanical ventilation (Meyer et al., 1994). With studies indicating that patients receiving mechanical ventilation have between 20 to 63 arousals and awakenings per hour (Parthasarathy), the impact of mechanical ventilation on sleep merits awareness and attention on the part of both researchers and health care workers.

Research indicates that the mode of ventilation can influence the patient's quality of sleep. Data indicates that fewer central apneas occur with assist-control ventilation than with pressure-support ventilation (Meza, Mendez, Ostrowski, & Younes, 1998; Parthasarathy & Tobin, 2002). For those who did develop central apneas, assist-control ventilation also resulted in fewer arousals and awakenings than pressure-support ventilation, though there was no difference between the two modes in the individuals who did not have central apneas. A resting partial pressure of carbon dioxide ($PCO_2$) close to the apnea threshold has been associated with central apnea events (Parthasarathy & Tobin). For this reason, adding dead space may also improve sleep, as it increases the patient's resting $PCO_2$. In one study, adding dead space decreased the total number of arousals and awakenings in patients who experienced central apneas during pressure-support ventilation from 83 events to 44 events per hour, and sleep efficiency improved from 63 to 81% (Parthasarathy & Tobin).

Dyssynchronous breathing is another potential cause of sleep disturbance in mechanically ventilated patients. During NREM sleep, the range of respiratory frequencies in which a person can entrain is diminished (Weinhouse & Schwab, 2006).

## Effects of Medication on Sleep

It is important to understand that the sedating effects of many of the drugs administered in the ICU, although they calm the patient, reduce pain, and in some cases promote sleep, generally do not mimic naturally induced sleep. The differences between naturally occurring sleep and that occurring under medications commonly prescribed in the ICU will be described in the text that follows.

### Sedatives

Sedative-hypnotics are often administered to older adults in the ICU both for their calming effect on agitated and anxious patients and specifically to promote sleepiness. However, although sedatives increase total sleep time, they do not promote a "normal" circadian sleep cycle (see Exhibit 17.3). The most commonly used sedatives in the ICU are those that act on GABA receptors. Benzodiazepines and propofol, both of which activate inhibitory GABA receptors, decrease sleep latency and increase total

# Exhibit 17.3

## Physiologic Characteristics of Sleep in Comparison to Sedation

| Sleep | Sedation |
| --- | --- |
| **Differences** | |
| Spontaneous | Not spontaneous |
| Circadian | Not circadian |
| Essential function | Nonessential |
| Reversible with external stimuli | Not completely reversible with external stimuli |
| Cyclic progression by EEG | No cyclic progression by EEG |
| **Similarities** | |
| Altered sensorium | |
| Overlapping neurophysiological | |
| pathways | |
| Respiratory depression | |
| Disconjugate eye movements (REM) | |
| Muscle hypotonia | |
| Temperature dysregulation | |

Adapted from Weinhouse et al., (2008).

sleep time. However, they also decrease the amount of time spent in SWS, the most restorative sleep stage, with a corresponding increase in stage 2 sleep (Bourne & Mills, 2004). The spindles of stage 2 sleep under sedation are different than those recorded in nonsedative sleep (Feshchenko, Veselis, & Reinsel, 1997), though the implications of this are unclear.

## Analgesics

### Opioids

Opioids are the principal class of drugs used for pain alleviation in the ICU. In healthy individuals, opioids increase wakefulness and inhibit both SWS and REM sleep (Cronin, Keifer, Baghdoyan, & Lydic, 1995; Dimsdale, Norman, DeJardin, & Wallace, 2007). Nevertheless, if pain or discomfort are the chief causes of poor sleep, there is evidence that the administering of opioids can improve sleep (Caldwell, 2004; Caldwell et al., 2002). However, it is important to be mindful of the fact that sleep under the effects of opioids is unlikely to be of optimal quality, as even with increased sleep time, the time spent in restorative sleep is likely to be diminished. Abrupt discontinuation of opioids can result in REM sleep rebound (Bourne & Mills, 2004). The increased time in REM sleep is often problematic for the elderly in the ICU because of the reduction of accessory muscle function during REM sleep, causing respiratory problems and hypoxemia. Hypoxemia during REM sleep is especially prevalent among those with chronic obstructive pulmonary disease (COPD) and obstructive sleep apnea (Douglas, 1998; Weinhouse, 2008)

## Cardiovascular Drugs

Beta-blockers are administered in the ICU to those who have hypertension, acute coronary syndrome, and acute burn injuries, and as a preventive against dysrhythmias after cardiothoracic surgery (Arbabi et al., 2004; Egan, Basile, Chilton, & Cohen, 2005). The most lipid-soluble drugs (i.e., those with the greatest ability to cross the blood–brain barrier) have the strongest negative impact on sleep, being associated with insomnia and REM suppression, as well as nightmares (McAinsh & Cruickshank, 1990). These include propranolol and pindolol. Atenolol and sotalol as less likely to cause sleep disturbances, because of their lack of lipid solubility. The alpha2-agonist clonidine is REM suppressive; it and methyldopa, another alpha2-agonist, can cause insomnia (Gentili et al., 1996).

Many drugs used to treat hypotension are associated with insomnia and suppression of SW and REM sleep, including norepinephrine/epinephrine and dopamine (Bourne & Mills, 2004).

## Respiratory Drugs

Theophylline, used in the treatment of asthma and COPD, is linked with sleep fragmentation, decreased SW and REM sleep, and poor sleep efficiency (Bailey et al., 1990). Other medications used to treat asthma and COPD, such as albuterol, can also have an alerting effect that reduces sleep efficiency. It can be difficult, however, to separate out the effects of the medication from the effects of the medical condition they are treating. Patients with COPD have decreased total sleep time and REM sleep, they shift between sleep stages more frequently. Hypercapnia has been implicated in the arousals of those with COPD as well (Fleetham et al., 1982).

## Corticosteroids

Corticosteroid medications are used to decrease inflammation; their most prevalent use among the elderly is in the treatment of arthritis and related conditions. They are also used to control some of the symptoms of lupus, and, in an inhaled form, to control asthma. Corticosteriods stimulate the nervous system and thus can cause insomnia. Their use has been linked to an increase in arousals as well as suppression of SWS and REM sleep (Turner & Elson, 1993).

## Gastric Acid Blockers

Patients on mechanical ventilation are often given gastric acid blockers to treat GI bleeding as well as to protect against stress ulcers. H2 receptor antagonists can cause insomnia in some cases (Orr, Duke, Imes, & Mellow, 1994).

## Antidepressants

Tricyclic antidepressants, selective serotonin-reuptake inhibitors (SSRIs), and mono-amine oxidase inhibitors (MAOIs) are all antidepressants commonly prescribed to older adults. Tricyclic antidepressants tend to increase total sleep time, whereas SSRIs and MAOIs are associated with decreased total sleep time, as well as with insomnia and daytime sedation (Armitage, 2000; Gursky & Krahn, 2000). All three classes of antidepressants, however, are associated with decreased time in REM sleep (Armitage; Gursky & Krahn; Staner et al., 1995; von Bardeleben, Steiger, Gerken, & Holsboer, 1989). Tricyclic antidepressants and SSRIs also worsen RLS and PLMD (Weinhouse, 2008).

The effects of antidepressant withdrawal are also prevalent in the ICU. As tricy-clics, SSRIs and MAOIs all suppress REM, sudden stoppage of medication can result in REM sleep rebound (Staner et al., 1995). The increased time spent in REM sleep is problematic for the critically ill elderly because of the accompanying loss of accessory muscle tone and resulting respiratory difficulty. Those with COPD and/or OSA (obstructive sleep apnea) are especially at risk for hypoxemia during REM sleep (Hiestand & Phillips, 2008; Parthasarathy, 2004).

## Anticonvulsants

Anticonvulsants may worsen the sleep disturbances often present in epileptic patients. Dopamine antagonists worsen RLS and PLMD in particular (Weinhouse, 2008).

## Recreational Drugs

Withdrawal from recreational drugs is another potential source of disturbed sleep in the ICU. Both nicotine and alcohol withdrawal disrupt sleep, causing insomnia and a decrease in SWS (Gann et al., 2004; Hughes, Higgins, & Bickel, 1994). Cannabis withdrawal can also cause insomnia, whereas amphetamine and cocaine withdrawal are associated with nightmares and rebound REM sleep (Weinhouse, 2008).

# Improving Sleep in the ICU

## Obstructive Sleep Apnea

The treatment of sleep apnea relies on relieving the upper airway obstruction character-istic of sleep apnea. The most commonly used and effective treatment is external (noninvasive) positive airway pressure ventilation. Two examples of this are continu-ous positive airway pressure ventilation (CPAP), in which case the patient is adminis-tered one set level of external pressure applied either to the nose or mouth via a sealed mask, or bilevel positive airway pressure ventilation (bilevel or BiPAP), in which the patient has different pressures for inhalation and exhalation. When initially starting PAP, the most commonly used initial pressure is a continuous airway pressure of 5-cm $H_2O$, and the PAP is titrated up at 2-cm $H_2O$ every 30 to 60 minutes until the patient's apnea episodes resolve. Patients rarely require more than 20-cm $H_2O$ of airway pressure, and in cases where higher settings are required, bilevel ventilation may be needed to allow for a lower exhalation setting (thus an inhalation pressure may be 22-cm $H_2O$ while an exhalation setting may be 10-cm $H_2O$). Although positive airway pressure therapy (PAP) is effective, patient compliance can be a major challenge, with approximately 30 to 50% of patients having difficulty tolerating PAP.

Several factors have been studied in regard to their possible association with PAP compliance. A history of active cigarette smoking (Russo-Magno, O'Brien, Panciera, & Rounds, 2001) and nocturia (Russo-Magno et al.) are known to reduce PAP compliance. With regard to the patient's sleep apnea, the presence of mild or moderate sleep apnea (Pelletier-Fleury, Rakotonanahary, & Fleury, 2001), and minimal daytime sleepiness symptoms at presentation (Pelletier-Fleury et al.) may lead to reduced compliance. Treatment-related factors include whether the patient had resolution of sleep apnea symptoms with treatment (Russo-Magno et al.) or the need for higher PAP pressures (Pelletier-Fleury et al., 2001). Increasing age has been associated with greater degrees of noncompliance in univariate analysis, but when controlling for other factors, was no longer found to be significant (Pelletier-Fleury et al.). This is possibly to the result of the limited sample size of the studies that have focused on older subjects.

Patients with insomnia may also have particular difficulty adapting to the noninvasive positive pressure ventilation (Barthlen & Lange, 2000; Haynes, 2005; Hoffstein, Viner, Mateika, & Conway, 1992; Roehrs et al., 1985). These patients spend considerable portions of the night awake, and thus have a heightened awareness of the discomfort of the equipment (Krakow et al., 2001). The net result is that it can be very difficult to start noninvasive positive pressure ventilation on patients with significant insomnia complaints (Krakow et al.).

Interventions that can improve compliance include patient education on the importance of PAP therapy, adjustment of mask types (nasal mask, nasal pillow, or face mask) to find one that is associated with increased patient comfort, and addition of a humidifier to the unit to help reduce dryness. Frequent checks to determine whether there are mask leaks are helpful as well. All masks have a blow-off valve that allows exhaled carbon dioxide to leave the system—this usually blows directly away from the patient. However, air that leaks out from the sides of the mask near where it attaches to the face or nose suggests the presence of an air leak that requires adjustment of the mask straps. Some patients find the bilevel setting more comfortable than the continuous positive airway pressure setting because it reduces the work of breathing associated with exhalation. Patients may also find it helpful to get acclimated to PAP therapy while they are awake, such as while watching TV, before trying to use it at night. Lastly, it may be necessary to tolerate subtherapeutic PAP settings to help the patient become acclimated to the unit, thus although a setting of 10-cm $H_2O$ may be ideal, the patient may only be able to tolerate 5-cm $H_2O$ initially and can gradually be worked up to 10-cm $H_2O$ the next night.

## Insomnia

### Environment

Although there is frequently a tendency to think of environmental noise as coming from equipment and other patients, it is worth noting that noise levels can also be increased because of staff vocalizations. Thus one important measure that can reduce the noise level in the ICU is to institute quiet times when the staff is asked to speak softly. In addition, monitors with central stations can be set to alarm only at the central station and not at the bedside to help reduce loud, disruptive noises next to the patient. Providing patients with earplugs is another low-cost way to decrease the noise level they experience (Patel, Chipman, Carlin, & Shade, 2008).

Though it may seem counterintuitive to add noise to the ICU environment, adding white noise may decrease arousals and awakenings caused by noise by decreasing the difference between baseline and peak noise levels (Stanchina et al., 2005). Along the same lines, though it is important to maintain a day–night rhythm for environmental light, drastic changes in light levels during sleep can also cause disturbances. Thus, as nursing and care duties that require a certain level of light may be unavoidable during nighttime hours, striving for the minimum possible baseline light level is not necessarily desirable either, as it will create greater variability in light levels.

## Music Therapy

The use of music to decrease anxiety has been well documented, and though few of these studies evaluate sleep as an outcome measure, there is interest in the use of music therapy to promote sleep in postoperative and critically ill patients (Patel et al., 2008). A study by Zimmerman et al. looked at the effect of music and music videos in improving sleep among postoperative cardiac surgery patients. There was a significant improvement in sleep among those who received the music video intervention compared to the control group, whereas the improvement in sleep among those who received the music (without video component) intervention approached significance (Zimmerman, Nieveen, Barnason, & Schmaderer, 1996). Music that is of low tone, played by string instruments, and with a tempo of approximately 60 beats per minute is considered ideal to promote relaxation (K. Richards, Nagel, Markie, Elwell, & Barone, 2003; White, 1999). Ocean sounds have also been found to improve sleep in postoperative coronary artery bypass graft patients (Williamson, 1992). Proper infection-control is important for headphones and other equipment that may be provided by the ICU.

## Massage

Massage can promote relaxation as measured by physiological indicators such as reductions in heart rate, respiratory rate, muscle tension, and oxygen consumption (K. C. Richards, Gibson, & Overton-McCoy, 2000). A 5- to 10-minute massage can promote sleep (K. C. Richards, 1994), with its effectiveness documented specifically among the critically ill. For example, a study by Richards and colleagues of men with cardiovascular disease in the ICU found an improved sleep efficiency following a 6-minute effleurage back massage (Richards, 1998). The effleurage technique involves stroking in a slow, rhythmic manner, with the palms of the hands providing firm, steady pressure, and maintaining contact with the skin whenever possible.

## Aromatherapy

Aromatherapy is the use of essential oils such as thyme, rosemary, lavender, and jasmine to promote healing and/or improve mood. There is little experimental data on its use in promoting sleep; however, evidence of its ability to reduce anxiety and promote relaxation may mean it may be useful in lessening some of the psychological factors that contribute to poor sleep in the ICU (Brownfield, 1998; K. Richards et al., 2003). Aromatherapy can be incorporated into other sleep-promoting techniques, such as massage, or used during bathing. Though it has not been studied, health care providers should be mindful that aromatherapy may be contraindicated for patients with reactive airway disease and certain allergies.

## Mechanical Ventilation

Sleep quality is improved with assist-control ventilation over pressure-support ventilation (Meza et al., 1998; Parthasarathy & Tobin, 2002). Maintaining the patient's own respiratory efforts and physiologic baseline are important, and appropriate adjustments to the level of ventilator support has been shown to improve both quantity and quality of sleep (Patel et al., 2008). Adding dead space can also decrease arousals and awakenings (Parthasarathy & Tobin). See the section Effect of Mechanical Ventilation for more information.

## Pharmacology

There is a broad range of therapeutic options for the treatment of insomnia in older adults (Dolder, Nelson, & McKinsey, 2007). These agents can be divided into those that act on the GABA receptor and those that act on non-GABA sites. The GABA agents can also be divided into benzodiazepines that act nonselectively on the GABA receptor, or a nonbenzodiazepine category in which the drugs act via the alpha-1 receptor subtype of the GABA unit. We will initially discuss the GABA agents then consider non-GABA agents. All of the GABA agents can lead to weakness and/or gait instability because of their sedative effects, and may lead to excessive sedation, although this effect is less prominent with the nonbenzodiazepine category of GABA agents.

Temazepam is commonly used in the outpatient setting because of its price, long history of use, and effectiveness for treating sleep-maintenance insomnia. However, it tends to have a long half-life (approximately 8 to 15 hours) and thus may lead to next-day sedation effects, especially in patients with impaired drug metabolism/ clearance, such as in the ICU setting. Common starting doses in older adults are 7.5 mg, or half the usual starting dose of 15 mg, up to a maximum dose of 30 mg. Other commonly used nonbenzodiazepine agents include:

1. Zolpidem, a short-acting sedative-hypnotic with a half-life of approximately 2 to 4 hours, with a starting dose of 2.5-5 mg up to a maximum dose of 10 mg. Recently, a continuous-release formulation has been developed that is more effective for patients with frequent nocturnal awakenings and early-morning awakenings.
2. Eszopiclone, which has a half-life of 5 to 7 hours and a starting dose of 1 mg for older adults, up to a maximum dose of 3 mg.
3. Zaleplon, an ultra-short–acting agent with a half-life of 1 hour. This makes it less likely to be associated with next-day sedative effects; however, it is less effective for maintaining sleep throughout the night. It can be used in a middle-of-the-night dosing regimen in which the patient can receive one dose at bedtime and then another dose with a nocturnal awakening (Walsh, Pollak, Scharf, Schweitzer, & Vogel, 2000). The starting dose is 5 mg, up to a maximum dose of 10-20 mg.

# Exhibit 17.4

## List of Nursing Interventions to Improve Sleep

| Category | Examples |
|---|---|
| Reduce environmental noise | Limit alarms to alert at central station only |
| | Institute set periods of quiet time during which staff are asked to speak softly |
| | Consider using white noise/nature sounds to minimize acute ambient sound level changes |
| Adjust light levels | Daytime: Place patient in a room with a window and open blinds during late morning/afternoon hours |
| | Nighttime: Reduce light levels |
| Structure sleep–wake times | Administer night-time medications at consolidated times to minimize patient disruption |
| | Adopt a regular sleep–wake pattern for the patient |
| | Attempt to minimize napping |
| Other | Avoid caffeinated beverages (coffee, tea, chocolates, sodas) after noon |
| | Perform bath in early evening |
| | Massage: Brief massage to help initiate sleep |

In the category of non-GABA agents, there is growing interest in the possibility of therapeutic use of the hormone melatonin as a means of promoting sleep and maintaining the circadian rhythm of ICU patients. A small (24 patients) double-blind placebo-controlled 2008 study found that administering melatonin in the evening led to increased nocturnal sleep efficiency in ICU patients (Bourne, Mills, & Minelli, 2008). Though these results are encouraging, larger clinical trials are necessary to determine whether there is a place for melatonin therapy in the ICU, either in routine clinical care or as an option in certain subgroups of the ICU patient population. Because of the decrease in melatonin production that occurs with aging (see Sleep Changes in Older Adults section), this is of particular interest to the care of the elderly in the ICU.

The selective melatonin receptor agonist is a newer class of hypnotic, approved for use by the FDA in 2005. Rozerem is currently the only formulation approved for use, though others are in development (Ahmed, 2008). Rozerem is known to promote sleep without psychomotor impairment, and lacks the withdrawal symptoms associated with other hypnotics, such as benzodiazepines (Griffiths & Johnson, 2005; Johnson, Suess, & Griffiths, 2006). Rozerem is primarily successful in promoting sleep onset, and does not tend to decrease awakenings. However, its lack of side effects, and the fact that it has not been found to either decrease respiration in patients with moderate to severe COPD (Kryger, Roth, Wang-Weigand, & Zhang, 2008) or to worsen mild to moderate obstructive sleep apnea (Kryger, Wang-Weigand, & Roth, 2007) make rozerem a useful pharmacological option, alone or in conjunction with other medications, for older adults in the ICU. Rozerem is available in one formulation, 8 mg, and higher doses are not associated with added benefit. Patients generally report a less prominent sedative effect with rozerem, and it may not be associated with a subjective improvement in sleep.

Other agents that are frequently used in the outpatient setting include diphenhydramine and antidepressants. Treatment with diphenhydramine in the ICU setting should be discouraged because of the risk of anticholinergic effects, such as urinary retention. There is relatively little data regarding the efficacy and safety of treatment of insomnia with antidepressants, especially in the hospitalized setting, and these agents should generally be avoided as well. Exhibit 17.4 lists nursing interventions that promote sleep in the ICU.

## Summary

Medical illness and health care environments can be particularly obstructive to obtaining adequate and restful sleep. Poor sleep (quality and/or quantity) in the ICU, especially among the elderly, is multifactorial in origin, involving environmental, pharmacological, and medical components. Likewise, the optimal approach to improving sleep among ICU patients must also be comprehensive. An understanding of the various elements contributing to sleep disturbance in the ICU, as well as an appreciation of individual patient medical profiles as they relate to sleep, is crucial in promoting improved sleep in the ICU. As we learn more about the vital role that human sleep plays in the function of body systems the importance of promoting and facilitating sleep continues to grow.

## References

Ahmed, Q. A. (2008). Effects of common medications used for sleep disorders. *Critical Care Clinics, 24*(3), 493–515.

Akerstedt, T., & Nilsson, P. M. (2003). Sleep as restitution: An introduction. *Journal of Internal Medicine, 254*(1), 6–12.

Allen, R. P., & Earley, C. J. (2001). Restless legs syndrome: A review of clinical and pathophysiologic features. *Journal of Clinical Neurophysiology: Official Publication of the American Electroencephalographic Society, 18*(2), 128–147.

American Academy of Sleep Medicine. (2005). *International classification of sleep disorders, 2nd ed.: Diagnostic and coding manual.* Westchester, IL: Author.

Arbabi, S., Ahrns, K. S., Wahl, W. L., Hemmila, M. R., Wang, S. C., Brandt, M. M., et al. (2004). Beta-blocker use is associated with improved outcomes in adult burn patients. *Journal of Trauma, 56*(2), 265–269; discussion 269–271.

Armitage, R. (2000). The effects of antidepressants on sleep in patients with depression. *Canadian Journal of Psychiatry. 45*(9), 803–809.

Asplund, R. (2000). Sleep, health and visual impairment in the elderly. *Archives of Gerontology and Geriatrics, 30*(1), 7–15.

Aurell, J., & Elmqvist, D. (1985). Sleep in the surgical intensive care unit: Continuous polygraphic recording of sleep in nine patients receiving postoperative care. *British Medical Journal (Clinical Research Ed.), 290*(6474), 1029–1032.

Bailey, W. C., Richards, J. M., Jr., Manzella, B. A., Brooks, C. M., Windsor, R. A., & Soong, S. J. (1990). Characteristics and correlates of asthma in a university clinic population. *Chest, 98*(4), 821–828.

Barthlen, G. M., & Lange, D. J. (2000). Unexpectedly severe sleep and respiratory pathology in patients with amyotrophic lateral sclerosis. *European Journal of Neurology : The Official Journal of the European Federation of Neurological Societies, 7*(3), 299–302.

Boivin, D. B., Duffy, J. F., Kronauer, R. E., & Czeisler, C. A. (1996). Dose–response relationships for resetting of human circadian clock by light. *Nature, 379*(6565), 540–542.

Bonnet, M. H. (1989). The effect of sleep fragmentation on sleep and performance in younger and older subjects. *Neurobiology of Aging, 10*(1), 21–25.

Bourne, R. S., & Mills, G. H. (2004). Sleep disruption in critically ill patients—pharmacological considerations. *Anaesthesia, 59*(4), 374–384.

Bourne, R. S., Mills, G. H., & Minelli, C. (2008). Melatonin therapy to improve nocturnal sleep in critically ill patients: Encouraging results from a small randomised controlled trial. *Critical Care (London, England), 12*(2), R52.

Brownfield, A. (1998). Aromatherapy in arthritis: A study. *Nursing Standard (Royal College of Nursing [Great Britain]: 1987], 13*(5), 34–35.

Cajochen, C., Munch, M., Knoblauch, V., Blatter, K., & Wirz-Justice, A. (2006). Age-related changes in the circadian and homeostatic regulation of human sleep. *Chronobiology International, 23*(1-2), 461–474.

Caldwell, J. R. (2004). Avinza - 24-h sustained-release oral morphine therapy. *Expert Opinion on Pharmacotherapy, 5*(2), 469–472.

Caldwell, J. R., Rapoport, R. J., Davis, J. C., Offenberg, H. L., Marker, H. W., Roth, S. H., et al. (2002). Efficacy and safety of a once-daily morphine formulation in chronic, moderate-to-severe osteoarthritis pain: Results from a randomized, placebo-controlled, double-blind trial and an open-label extension trial. *Journal of Pain and Symptom Management, 23*(4), 278–291.

Collop, N. A., Salas, R. E., Delayo, M., & Gamaldo, C. (2008). Normal sleep and circadian processes. *Critical Care Clinics, 24*(3), 449–460, v.

Cooper, A. B., Gabor, J. Y., & Hanly, P. J. (2001). Sleep in the critically ill patient. *Seminars in Respiratory and Critical Care Medicine, 22*(2), 153–164.

Cooper, A. B., Thornley, K. S., Young, G. B., Slutsky, A. S., Stewart, T. E., & Hanly, P. J. (2000). Sleep in critically ill patients requiring mechanical ventilation. *Chest, 117*(3), 809–818.

Cronin, A., Keifer, J. C., Baghdoyan, H. A., & Lydic, R. (1995). Opioid inhibition of rapid eye movement sleep by a specific mu receptor agonist. *British Journal of Anaesthesia, 74*(2), 188–192.

Dimsdale, J. E., Norman, D., DeJardin, D., & Wallace, M. S. (2007). The effect of opioids on sleep architecture. *Journal of Clinical Sleep Medicine: JCSM: Official Publication of the American Academy of Sleep Medicine, 3*(1), 33–36.

Dolder, C., Nelson, M., & McKinsey, J. (2007). Use of non-benzodiazepine hypnotics in the elderly: Are all agents the same? *CNS Drugs, 21*(5), 389–405.

Douglas, N. J. (1998). Sleep in patients with chronic obstructive pulmonary disease. *Clinics in Chest Medicine, 19*(1), 115–125.

Egan, B. M., Basile, J., Chilton, R. J., & Cohen, J. D. (2005). Cardioprotection: The role of beta-blocker therapy. *Journal of Clinical Hypertension (Greenwich, Conn.), 7*(7), 409–416.

Feshchenko, V. A., Veselis, R. A., & Reinsel, R. A. (1997). Comparison of the EEG effects of midazolam, thiopental, and propofol: The role of underlying oscillatory systems. *Neuropsychobiology, 35*(4), 211–220.

Fleetham, J., West, P., Mezon, B., Conway, W., Roth, T., & Kryger, M. (1982). Sleep, arousals, and oxygen desaturation in chronic obstructive pulmonary disease. The effect of oxygen therapy. *American Review of Respiratory Disease, 126*(3), 429–433.

Freedman, N. S., Gazendam, J., Levan, L., Pack, A. I., & Schwab, R. J. (2001). Abnormal sleep/wake cycles and the effect of environmental noise on sleep disruption in the intensive care unit. *American Journal of Respiratory and Critical Care Medicine, 163*(2), 451–457.

Freedman, N. S., Kotzer, N., & Schwab, R. J. (1999). Patient perception of sleep quality and etiology of sleep disruption in the intensive care unit. *American Journal of Respiratory and Critical Care Medicine, 159*(4 Pt 1), 1155–1162.

Gabor, J. Y., Cooper, A. B., Crombach, S. A., Lee, B., Kadikar, N., Bettger, H. E., et al. (2003). Contribution of the intensive care unit environment to sleep disruption in mechanically ventilated patients and healthy subjects. *American Journal of Respiratory and Critical Care Medicine, 167*(5), 708–715.

Gabor, J. Y., Cooper, A. B., & Hanly, P. J. (2001). Sleep disruption in the intensive care unit. *Current Opinion in Critical Care, 7*(1), 21–27.

Gann, H., van Calker, D., Feige, B., Cloot, O., Bruck, R., Berger, M., et al. (2004). Polysomnographic comparison between patients with primary alcohol dependency during subacute withdrawal and patients with a major depression. *European Archives of Psychiatry and Clinical Neuroscience, 254*(4), 263–271.

Gentili, A., Godschalk, M. F., Gheorghiu, D., Nelson, K., Julius, D. A., & Mulligan, T. (1996). Effect of clonidine and yohimbine on sleep in healthy men: A double-blind, randomized, controlled trial. *European Journal of Clinical Pharmacology, 50*(6), 463–465.

Griffiths, R. R., & Johnson, M. W. (2005). Relative abuse liability of hypnotic drugs: A conceptual framework and algorithm for differentiating among compounds. *Journal of Clinical Psychiatry, 66* (Suppl. 9), 31–41.

Gumustekin, K., Seven, B., Karabulut, N., Aktas, O., Gursan, N., Aslan, S., et al. (2004). Effects of sleep deprivation, nicotine, and selenium on wound healing in rats. *International Journal of Neuroscience, 114*(11), 1433–1442.

Guo, J. S., Chau, J. F., Cho, C. H., & Koo, M. W. (2005). Partial sleep deprivation compromises gastric mucosal integrity in rats. *Life Sciences, 77*(2), 220–229.

Gursky, J. T., & Krahn, L. E. (2000). The effects of antidepressants on sleep: A review. *Harvard Review of Psychiatry, 8*(6), 298–306.

Haynes, P. L. (2005). The role of behavioral sleep medicine in the assessment and treatment of sleep disordered breathing. *Clinical Psychology Review, 25*(5), 673–705.

Hening, W., Allen, R. P., Tenzer, P., & Winkelman, J. W. (2007). Restless legs syndrome: Demographics, presentation, and differential diagnosis. *Geriatrics, 62*(9), 26–29.

Henke, K. G., Dempsey, J. A., Kowitz, J. M., & Skatrud, J. B. (1990). Effects of sleep-induced increases in upper airway resistance on ventilation. *Journal of Applied Physiology (Bethesda, MD.: 1985), 69*(2), 617–624.

Hiestand, D., & Phillips, B. (2008). The overlap syndrome: Chronic obstructive pulmonary disease and obstructive sleep apnea. *Critical Care Clinics, 24*(3), 551–63, vii.

Hoffstein, V., Viner, S., Mateika, S., & Conway, J. (1992). Treatment of obstructive sleep apnea with nasal continuous positive airway pressure. Patient compliance, perception of benefits, and side effects. *American Review of Respiratory Disease, 145*(4 Pt 1), 841–845.

Hughes, J. R., Higgins, S. T., & Bickel, W. K. (1994). Nicotine withdrawal versus other drug withdrawal syndromes: Similarities and dissimilarities. *Addiction (Abingdon, England), 89*(11), 1461–1470.

Iber C, Ancoli-Israel, S., Chesson A. L., & Quan S. (2007). *The AASM manual for the scoring of sleep and associated events: Rules, terminology and technical specifications.* Westchester, IL: American Academy of Sleep Medicine.

Irwin, M., McClintick, J., Costlow, C., Fortner, M., White, J., & Gillin, J. C. (1996). Partial night sleep deprivation reduces natural killer and cellular immune responses in humans. *The FASEB Journal: Official Publication of the Federation of American Societies for Experimental Biology, 10*(5), 643–653.

Johnson, M. W., Suess, P. E., & Griffiths, R. R. (2006). Ramelteon: A novel hypnotic lacking abuse liability and sedative adverse effects. *Archives of General Psychiatry, 63*(10), 1149–1157.

Krakow, B., Melendrez, D., Ferreira, E., Clark, J., Warner, T. D., Sisley, B., et al. (2001). Prevalence of insomnia symptoms in patients with sleep-disordered breathing. *Chest, 120*(6), 1923–1929.

Kryger, M., Roth, T., Wang-Weigand, S., & Zhang, J. (2008). The effects of ramelteon on respiration during sleep in subjects with moderate to severe chronic obstructive pulmonary disease. *Sleep & Breathing, 13*(1), 79–84.,

Kryger, M., Wang-Weigand, S., & Roth, T. (2007). Safety of ramelteon in individuals with mild to moderate obstructive sleep apnea. *Sleep & Breathing, 11*(3), 159–164.

Laposky, A. D., Bass, J., Kohsaka, A., & Turek, F. W. (2008). Sleep and circadian rhythms: Key components in the regulation of energy metabolism. *FEBS Letters, 582*(1), 142–151.

Liu, Y., Tanaka, H., & Fukuoka Heart Study Group. (2002). Overtime work, insufficient sleep, and risk of non-fatal acute myocardial infarction in Japanese men. *Occupational and Environmental Medicine, 59*(7), 447–451.

Lopes, L. A., Lins Cde, M., Adeodato, V. G., Quental, D. P., de Bruin, P. F., Montenegro, R. M., Jr., et al. (2005). Restless legs syndrome and quality of sleep in type 2 diabetes. *Diabetes Care, 28*(11), 2633–2636.

Loredo, J. S., Ziegler, M. G., Ancoli-Israel, S., Clausen, J. L., & Dimsdale, J. E. (1999). Relationship of arousals from sleep to sympathetic nervous system activity and BP in obstructive sleep apnea. *Chest, 116*(3), 655–659.

McAinsh, J., & Cruickshank, J. M. (1990). Beta-blockers and central nervous system side effects. *Pharmacology & Therapeutics, 46*(2), 163–197.

Meier-Ewert, H. K., Ridker, P. M., Rifai, N., Regan, M. M., Price, N. J., Dinges, D. F., et al. (2004). Effect of sleep loss on C-reactive protein, an inflammatory marker of cardiovascular risk. *Journal of the American College of Cardiology, 43*(4), 678–683.

Meyer, T. J., Eveloff, S. E., Bauer, M. S., Schwartz, W. A., Hill, N. S., & Millman, R. P. (1994). Adverse environmental conditions in the respiratory and medical ICU settings. *Chest, 105*(4), 1211–1216.

Meza, S., Mendez, M., Ostrowski, M., & Younes, M. (1998). Susceptibility to periodic breathing with assisted ventilation during sleep in normal subjects. *Journal of Applied Physiology, 85*(5), 1929–1940.

Novaes, M. A., Aronovich, A., Ferraz, M. B., & Knobel, E. (1997). Stressors in ICU: Patients' evaluation. *Intensive Care Medicine, 23*(12), 1282–1285.

Ohayon, M. M. (2002). Epidemiology of insomnia: What we know and what we still need to learn. *Sleep Medicine Reviews, 6*(2), 97–111.

Ohayon, M. M., Carskadon, M. A., Guilleminault, C., & Vitiello, M. V. (2004). Meta-analysis of quantitative sleep parameters from childhood to old age in healthy individuals: Developing normative sleep values across the human lifespan. *Sleep, 27*(7), 1255–1273.

Orr, W. C., Duke, J. C., Imes, N. K., & Mellow, M. H. (1994). Comparative effects of H2-receptor antagonists on subjective and objective assessments of sleep. *Alimentary Pharmacology & Therapeutics, 8*(2), 203–207.

Orton, D. I., & Gruzelier, J. H. (1989). Adverse changes in mood and cognitive performance of house officers after night duty. *BMJ (Clinical Research Ed.), 298*(6665), 21–23.

Parthasarathy, S. (2004). Sleep during mechanical ventilation. *Current Opinion in Pulmonary Medicine, 10*(6), 489–494.

Parthasarathy, S., & Tobin, M. J. (2002). Effect of ventilator mode on sleep quality in critically ill patients. *American Journal of Respiratory and Critical Care Medicine, 166*(11), 1423–1429.

Patel, M., Chipman, J., Carlin, B. W., & Shade, D. (2008). Sleep in the intensive care unit setting. *Critical Care Nursing Quarterly, 31*(4), 309–318; quiz 319–320.

Pelletier-Fleury, N., Rakotonanahary, D., & Fleury, B. (2001). The age and other factors in the evaluation of compliance with nasal continuous positive airway pressure for obstructive sleep apnea syndrome. A cox's proportional hazard analysis. *Sleep Medicine, 2*(3), 225–232.

Rechtschaffen, A., & Bergmann, B. M. (1995). Sleep deprivation in the rat by the disk-over-water method. *Behavioural Brain Research, 69*(1–2), 55–63.

Richards, K., Nagel, C., Markie, M., Elwell, J., & Barone, C. (2003). Use of complementary and alternative therapies to promote sleep in critically ill patients. *Critical Care Nursing Clinics of North America, 15*(3), 329–340.

Richards, K. C. (1994). Sleep promotion in the critical care unit. *AACN Clinical Issues in Critical Care Nursing, 5*(2), 152–158.

Richards, K. C. (1998). Effect of a back massage and relaxation intervention on sleep in critically ill patients. *American Journal of Critical Care: An Official Publication, American Association of Critical-Care Nurses, 7*(4), 288–299.

Richards, K. C., Gibson, R., & Overton-McCoy, A. L. (2000). Effects of massage in acute and critical care. *AACN Clinical Issues, 11*(1), 77–96.

Roehrs, T., Conway, W., Wittig, R., Zorick, F., Sicklesteel, J., & Roth, T. (1985). Sleep–wake complaints in patients with sleep-related respiratory disturbances. *American Review of Respiratory Disease, 132*(3), 520–523.

Rotondi, A. J., Chelluri, L., Sirio, C., Mendelsohn, A., Schulz, R., Belle, S., et al. (2002). Patients' recollections of stressful experiences while receiving prolonged mechanical ventilation in an intensive care unit. *Critical Care Medicine, 30*(4), 746–752.

Russo-Magno, P., O'Brien, A., Panciera, T., & Rounds, S. (2001). Compliance with CPAP therapy in older men with obstructive sleep apnea. *Journal of the American Geriatrics Society, 49*(9), 1205–1211.

Salas, R. E., & Gamaldo, C. E. (2008). Adverse effects of sleep deprivation in the ICU. *Critical Care Clinics, 24*(3), 461–476, v–vi.

Sareli, A. E., & Schwab, R. J. (2008). The sleep-friendly ICU. *Critical Care Clinics, 24*(3), 613–626, viii.

Southwell, M., & Wistow, G. (1995). In-patient sleep disturbance: The views of staff and patients. *Nursing Times, 91*(37), 29–31.

Spiegel, K., Knutson, K., Leproult, R., Tasali, E., & Van Cauter, E. (2005). Sleep loss: A novel risk factor for insulin resistance and type 2 diabetes. *Journal of Applied Physiology (Bethesda, MD.: 1985), 99*(5), 2008–2019.

Spiegel, K., Leproult, R., L'hermite-Baleriaux, M., Copinschi, G., Penev, P. D., & Van Cauter, E. (2004). Leptin levels are dependent on sleep duration: Relationships with sympathovagal balance, carbohydrate regulation, cortisol, and thyrotropin. *Journal of Clinical Endocrinology and Metabolism, 89*(11), 5762–5771.

Spiegel, K., Sheridan, J. F., & Van Cauter, E. (2002). Effect of sleep deprivation on response to immunization. *JAMA: The Journal of the American Medical Association, 288*(12), 1471–1472.

Stanchina, M. L., Abu-Hijleh, M., Chaudhry, B. K., Carlisle, C. C., & Millman, R. P. (2005). The influence of white noise on sleep in subjects exposed to ICU noise. *Sleep Medicine, 6*(5), 423–428.

Staner, L., Kerkhofs, M., Detroux, D., Leyman, S., Linkowski, P., & Mendlewicz, J. (1995). Acute, subchronic and withdrawal sleep EEG changes during treatment with paroxetine and amitriptyline: A double-blind randomized trial in major depression. *Sleep, 18*(6), 470–477.

Tamburri, L. M., DiBrienza, R., Zozula, R., & Redeker, N. S. (2004). Nocturnal care interactions with patients in critical care units. *American Journal of Critical Care : An Official Publication, American Association of Critical-Care Nurses, 13*(2), 102–112; quiz 114–115.

Thomas, M., Sing, H., Belenky, G., Holcomb, H., Mayberg, H., Dannals, R., et al. (2000). Neural basis of alertness and cognitive performance impairments during sleepiness. I. effects of 24 h of sleep deprivation on waking human regional brain activity. *Journal of Sleep Research, 9*(4), 335–352.

Tochikubo, O., Ikeda, A., Miyajima, E., & Ishii, M. (1996). Effects of insufficient sleep on blood pressure monitored by a new multibiomedical recorder. *Hypertension, 27*(6), 1318–1324.

Turner, R., & Elson, E. (1993). Sleep disorders. Steroids cause sleep disturbance. *BMJ (Clinical Research Ed.), 306*(6890), 1477–1478.

Vgontzas, A. N., Bixler, E. O., Papanicolaou, D. A., & Chrousos, G. P. (2000). Chronic systemic inflammation in overweight and obese adults. *JAMA : The Journal of the American Medical Association, 283*(17), 2235; author reply 2236.

Vgontzas, A. N., Zoumakis, E., Bixler, E. O., Lin, H. M., Follett, H., Kales, A., et al. (2004). Adverse effects of modest sleep restriction on sleepiness, performance, and inflammatory cytokines. *Journal of Clinical Endocrinology and Metabolism, 89*(5), 2119–2126.

von Bardeleben, U., Steiger, A., Gerken, A., & Holsboer, F. (1989). Effects of fluoxetine upon pharma-coendocrine and sleep-EEG parameters in normal controls. *International Clinical Psychopharmacology, 4* (Suppl. 1), 1–5.

Walder, B., Francioli, D., Meyer, J. J., Lancon, M., & Romand, J. A. (2000). Effects of guidelines implementation in a surgical intensive care unit to control nighttime light and noise levels. *Critical Care Medicine, 28*(7), 2242–2247.

Walsh, J. K., Pollak, C. P., Scharf, M. B., Schweitzer, P. K., & Vogel, G. W. (2000). Lack of residual sedation following middle-of-the-night zaleplon administration in sleep maintenance insomnia. *Clinical Neuropharmacology, 23*(1), 17–21.

Weinhouse, G. L. (2008). Pharmacology I: Effects on sleep of commonly used ICU medications. *Critical Care Clinics, 24*(3), 477–491, vi.

Weinhouse, G. L., & Schwab, R. J. (2006). Sleep in the critically ill patient. *Sleep, 29*(5), 707–716.

White, J. M. (1999). Effects of relaxing music on cardiac autonomic balance and anxiety after acute myocardial infarction. *American Journal of Critical Care: An Official Publication, American Association of Critical-Care Nurses, 8*(4), 220–230.

Williamson, J. W. (1992). The effects of ocean sounds on sleep after coronary artery bypass graft surgery. *American Journal of Critical Care: An Official Publication, American Association of Critical-Care Nurses, 1*(1), 91–97.

Yaggi, H. K., Concato, J., Kernan, W. N., Lichtman, J. H., Brass, L. M., & Mohsenin, V. (2005). Obstructive sleep apnea as a risk factor for stroke and death. *New England Journal of Medicine, 353*(19), 2034–2041.

Young, T., Shahar, E., Nieto, F. J., Redline, S., Newman, A. B., Gottlieb, D. J., et al. (2002). Predictors of sleep-disordered breathing in community-dwelling adults: The sleep heart health study. *Archives of Internal Medicine, 162*(8), 893–900.

Youngstedt, S. D., Kripke, D. F., Elliott, J. A., & Klauber, M. R. (2001). Circadian abnormalities in older adults. *Journal of Pineal Research, 31*(3), 264–272.

Zhong, X., Hilton, H. J., Gates, G. J., Jelic, S., Stern, Y., Bartels, M. N., et al. (2005). Increased sympathetic and decreased parasympathetic cardiovascular modulation in normal humans with acute sleep deprivation. *Journal of Applied Physiology (Bethesda, MD: 1985), 98*(6), 2024–2032.

Zimmerman, L., Nieveen, J., Barnason, S., & Schmaderer, M. (1996). The effects of music interventions on postoperative pain and sleep in coronary artery bypass graft (CABG) patients. *Scholarly Inquiry for Nursing Practice, 10*(2), 153–170; discussion 171–114.

Zohar, D., Tzischinsky, O., Epstein, R., & Lavie, P. (2005). The effects of sleep loss on medical residents' emotional reactions to work events: A cognitive-energy model. *Sleep, 28*(1), 47–54.

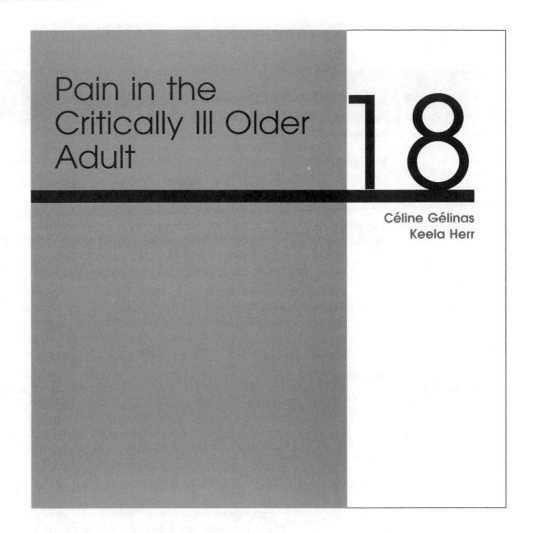

# Pain in the Critically Ill Older Adult

**18**

Céline Gélinas
Keela Herr

## Prevalence and Challenges in Pain Assessment and Management

Dramatic increases in the aged of America and other countries will affect the makeup of patients in all care settings. Adults 65 years and older will compose 20% of the population by the year 2030 (U.S. Census Bureau, 2000), and increases in the older adult critical care population are expected (Groeger et al., 1993). Because older adults currently account for more than 50% of all intensive care unit (ICU) days (Angus, Kelley, Schmitz, White, & Popovich, 2000), critical care nurses must be prepared to provide high-quality care, including excellent pain management.

Use of evidence-based pain management practices appropriate for the older adult is the foundation of effective pain assessment and treatment. Critical care nurses need to be knowledgeable of existing evidence-based guidelines and consensus recommendations in caring for critically ill older persons and patients in pain. Although evidence-based guidelines here are limited, existing resources are readily adapted to the setting and environment of critical care. See Table 18.1 for resources and access information.

## 18.1   Resources for Evidence-Based Pain Management in Older Persons

| Name of Site | Web Address | Summary of Resource |
|---|---|---|
| Agency For Healthcare Research And Quality | www.ahcpr.gov | Lists AHRQ supported clinical practice guidelines, which can be downloaded; links to National Guideline Clearinghouse. |
| American Geriatrics Society | www.american geriatrics.org | AGS provides clinical practice guidelines on problems prevalent in older persons. A guideline on *Persistent Pain in Older Persons* published in 2002 and available via the Web site, as well as resources to use with families. A revision is in progress. |
| American Society For Pain Management Nursing | www.aspmn.org | ASPMN supported a task force to develop recommendations for pain assessment in nonverbal persons. The position statement as well as other resources related to pain practice are available on their Web site. |
| International Association For The Study Of Pain | www.iasp-pain.org | IASP is a nonprofit professional organization dedicated to furthering research on pain and improving the care of patients with pain. The target audience is scientists, physicians, dentists, psychologists, nurses, physical therapists, and other health professionals actively engaged in pain research and those who have special interest in the diagnosis and treatment of pain. |
| PainEDU | www.painedu.org | PainEDU is an educational Web site for clinicians teaching about pain assessment and management. This site is a comprehensive resource and is based on the latest scientific information about pain treatment. This Web site provides a free downloadable manual: *The PainEDU Manual: A Clinical Companion*. |
| National Comprehensive Cancer Network | www.nccn.org | The National Comprehensive Cancer Network is an alliance of 20 of the world's leading cancer centers working together to develop treatment guidelines for most cancers, and dedicated to research that improves the quality, effectiveness, and efficiency of cancer care. NCCN offers a number of programs to give clinicians access to tools and knowledge that can help guide decision making in the management of cancer. |
| Beth Israel Medical Center Department of Pain Medicine & Palliative Care | www.stoppain.edu | Offers a module entitled "Symptom Management at End of Life: Pain Module." This module guides learners through critical assessment, diagnosis, treatment planning, implementation of interventions and outcomes assessment in an interactive problem-based format using learner feedback. |

## Table 18.1 *(continued)*

| Name of Site | Web Address | Summary of Resource |
| --- | --- | --- |
| Medscape | www.medscape.com/nurses | Offers robust and integrated medical information and educational tools. Many online CEU activities, as well as timely clinical information to improve patient care. There is a link to palliative care-specific educational offerings and resources on the homepage side. |
| National Pain Education Council | www.npec.org | Two modules for CME/CEU provide in-depth, evidence-based information related to one aspect in the treatment of chronic pain: assessment, treatment decisions, long-term management strategies, and more. Together, the series presents evidence-based processes portraying current best practices for the management of chronic pain, with the ultimate goals of relieving patients' suffering and improving their health and quality of life. |
| Partners Against Pain | www.partnersagainstpain.com | This Web site includes a Professional Education Center. By clicking on the Healthcare Professionals tab at top, the components of the "Pain Management Kit" are listed with links to downloadable tools or a site where materials can be purchased. This site includes information for patients and caregivers, healthcare professionals, and health systems. *The Medical Education Resource Catalog* lists a variety of formats for accredited and nonaccredited education. |
| American Pain Society | www.ampainsoc.org | The American Pain Society's CME program is designed to assess, plan, implement, and evaluate high-quality professional education. The American Pain Society offers an excellent, comprehensive pain management CME/CEU for 4 hours of credit, free of charge. The APS offers evidence-based guidelines for pain management on topics related to older persons including cancer pain, osteoarthritis, fibromyalgia, low back pain. |
| National Initiative On Pain Control | www.painknowledge.org | This site offers numerous educational venues with the use of innovative, interactive, and practical activities that support the Initiative's goals. NIPC educational activities highlight the magnitude of the problem, providing guidance in pain assessment, and offer proven strategies for pain management, all with the aim of improving patient outcomes. |
| University of Iowa College of Nursing Evidence-Based Guidelines | www.nursing.uiowa.edu | The College of Nursing hosts access to evidence-based guidelines developed to guide practice in caring for older persons. In 2006, *Acute Pain Management in Older Adults—Evidence Based Guideline* was published. Access to this and other guidelines via the Web site. |

## Pain Prevalence

Pain is a major concern of patients and their families experiencing acute health situations but particularly so for those critically ill. Indeed, pain is highly prevalent and a major stressor in patients in the critical care setting. In interviews with patients about their critical care experience, researchers found most patients recall having pain and anxiety over loss of control (Stanik-Hutt, Soeken, Belcher, Fontaine, & Gift, 2001). The intensity of pain is often described as moderate to severe (Desbiens et al., 1996; Gélinas, 2007a; Puntillo et al., 2001; Stanik-Hutt et al., 2001). A large prospective study involving mostly older adults, the SUPPORT study, found that 50% of patients reported pain and 15% of these reported extreme or moderate pain that occurred at least half of the time (SUPPORT Investigators, 1995). Significant levels of pain were associated with chronic obstructive lung disease and heart failure. More importantly, pain is often undermanaged in the critically ill in general, and in older adults specifically. Reports of undermanaged pain in the critically ill are consistently noted (Dracup & Bryan-Brown, 1995; Gélinas, 2007a; Meehan, McRae, Rourke, Eisenring, & Imperial, 1995; Puntillo, 1990; Puntillo & Weiss, 1994; Puntillo, Reitman, et al., 2002; Stein-Parbury & McKinley, 2000; Tittle & McMillan, 1994), with older patients commonly administered less analgesia than those younger than 65 years old (Lay, Puntillo, Miaskowski, & Wallhagen, 1996). Numerous reports in varied care settings document the problem of undertreated pain in older adults, particularly those with cognitive impairment. Cognitively impaired older adults hospitalized with hip fracture received significantly less opioid analgesia than those with less or no impairment (Feldt, Ryden & Miles, 1998: Morrison & Siu, 2000). Moreover, less analgesia is prescribed and administered for cognitively impaired nursing home residents, even when the impaired residents have similar numbers of painful diagnoses as cognitively intact residents (Bernabei et al., 1998; Horgas & Tsai, 1998). Thus, inability to communicate in older adults with dementia is a major barrier to both assessment and treatment and thus affects recognition of pain in the critical care setting, as well. Recognition and effective treatment of pain in older persons in any setting of care is challenging and improvements in use of evidence-based practices are needed.

## Problems Associated With Untreated Pain

Acute pain, often unrelieved, is a major stressor that has both physiologic and psychological consequences that contribute to poor patient outcomes and impaired quality of life. Unmanaged pain has been shown to have serious physiological and psychological consequences (Carr & Goudas, 1999), including increased morbidity and mortality (Dracup & Bryan-Brown, 2000), increased pulmonary complications (Puntillo & Weiss, 1994), increased cardiac work (Pooler-Lunse & Price, 1992), and depression and anxiety (Desbiens et al., 1996). Moreover, older adults who experience poor pain relief have poorer outcomes (Ardery, Herr, Titler, & Hannon, 2003; Brown, Klein, Lewis, Johnston, & Cummings, 2003; Feldt, Ryden, & Miles, 1998, Glasson, Sawyer, Lindley, & Ginsberg, 2002; Morrison, Magaziner, McLaughlin, et al., 2003). Older patients with pain demonstrate greater dependence in activities of daily living (ADLs), increased depression, increased anxiety, and poorer quality of life, reinforcing the significance of pain in older persons (Desbiens et al., 1996). Given the profound impact of ineffectively managed pain, efforts to recognize and manage pain in this population are essential.

## Challenges in Assessment and Treatment

The critical care nurse is faced with many challenges in caring for older persons that affect pain assessment and management. The following discussion addresses selected factors of particular importance when working with this population.

### Aging Changes

Pharmacokinetics and pharmacodynamic alterations in older adults result in changes in response to analgesics (higher circulating plasma levels of drug and longer duration of drug action) and their adverse effects that impact the ability to provide effective pain management (American Geriatrics Society, 2009). Knowledge of these factors can assist the critical care nurse to advocate for appropriate treatment and to monitor carefully for adverse events and response to treatment (See Pharmacological Management Section). Additionally, aging can affect the presentation of illness and related pain. Older persons are much more likely to present atypically with absence of pain in myocardial infarction, peptic ulcer disease, and pneumothorax (Moore & Clinch, 2004). Thus, serious consequence, such as delayed diagnosis, longer hospital stays, and altered outcomes can occur if health care providers are unaware of these unique aging changes. Critical care nurses need to be aware of atypical presentations as part of the pain-assessment process.

### Cognitive Impairment

Frail older adults who suffer from severe dementia and other forms of cognitive impairment who are unable to verbally express their pain are at particularly high risk for poor pain assessment and management (Ardery, Herr, Hannon, et al., 2003; Feldt, Ryden, et al., 1998; Morrison, Magaziner, Gilbert, et al., 2003; Morrison & Siu, 2000). There is no empirical evidence that cognitively impaired older adults experience less pain than cognitively intact individuals (Manfredi et al., 2003; Miller & Talerico, 2002; Morrison & Siu, 2000; Rakel & Herr, 2004), yet recognizing and treating pain in older persons who are cognitively impaired or critically ill is a challenge.

### Delirium

Delirium is a form of transient cognitive impairment and can interfere with the ability to communicate and thus report pain reliably. Delirium is characterized by recent onset of fluctuating awareness and inability to focus attention, change in cognition (e.g., memory deficit, disorientation), or perceptual disturbance, and the presence of an underlying organic illness (American Psychiatric Association, 2000). The incidence of delirium in older adults in the intensive care setting is 62% (McNicholl et al., 2003), making it a significant factor affecting pain assessment. Although older adults with delirium may be able to speak, the content may not be understandable or reliable. Identification of pain in nonverbal older adults and those with delirium must rely on observation of behavioral presentation and there is considerable overlap between delirium behaviors and nonverbal pain behaviors. Although there is limited research in this area, one study showed that physicians and nurses were likely to misinterpret agitated delirium as an expression of pain in patients whose pain was well controlled before and after the delirium episode (Bruera, Fainsinger, Miller, & Kuehn, 1997).

Pain assessment in older adults with delirium is extremely challenging and is discussed further in the Pain Assessment section.

## Recognizing Painful Conditions in Those Who Cannot Communicate

Many factors affect the ability of the critically ill older adult to communicate pain, including factors that impact patients of all ages (endotracheal intubation, loss of consciousness, sedation, restraints, fatigue, metabolic disorders) (Shannon & Bucknall, 2003), but there are also factors that are unique to the aged person (cognitive impairment, sensory impairment). To overcome these challenges, it is imperative that health care professionals caring for critically ill patients be keenly aware of strategies for recognizing pain in those unable to self-report (see Pain Assessment section). Because of challenges in communicating discomfort and pain when critically ill, nurses must be aware of potential causes of pain to anticipate and facilitate proactive management. Sources of pain common in older adults during critical illness include existing medical conditions, traumatic injuries, surgical/medical procedures (and resulting incisions and wounds), and invasive devices (such as catheters and tubes), blood draws, and immobilization (Jacobi et al., 2002; Puntillo et al., 2001, 2004).

Commonly performed nursing procedures also can cause pain, including turning, positioning, endotracheal suctioning, phlebotomy, dressing changes, insertion and removal of catheters and chest tubes. and wound care (Morrison et al., 1998; Puntillo et al., 2001; Tullmann & Dracup, 2000;). In an effort to determine estimated severity of pain from commonly performed procedures to apply to persons unable to communicate pain (such as those with dementia), Morrison and colleagues (1998) determined perceptions of pain intensity caused by common procedures. Puntillo and colleagues (2001) also evaluated patient's perceptions of pain severity related to procedural pain in 5,957 adult patients, noting individual differences in pain intensity and distress across ages and procedures; but they did note that the most painful procedure was turning. This is of particular concern given that turning is performed frequently in the intensive care unit (ICU) and usually without premedication. See Table 18.2 for common conditions and pain-related procedures.

## Advocating for Those Unable to Communicate

Older patients who are critically ill and often unable to communicate their pain and discomfort require astute and compassionate advocacy by health care providers and family members. Critical care nurses are at the forefront of assuring acute pain best practices are implemented and that the older patient's comfort is achieved. Nurses should consider the report of family members as they know the patient well and can support the nurse in the pain-assessment process, for example, by identifying usual and past behaviors (Herr et al., 2006). Nurses are also prepared to identify indicators for quality improvement, direct and lead interdisciplinary teams, and communicate with key parties to negotiate and secure effective pain management (Dawson, 2008). Nurses must be primary advocates to enssure patient's rights to pain relief for older critically ill persons during this challenging time.

## Knowledge and Attitudes

Misbeliefs regarding analgesic use and the risk of addiction and serious adverse effects, such as respiratory depression, are often factors that interfere with effective

| 18.2 Common Conditions and Procedures in ICU Known to Be Painful | |
|---|---|
| **Causes of Pain** | **Examples** |
| Acute Conditions | |
| Surgical events | Incisions, drains, tubes, orthopedic hardware placement |
| Trauma | Fractures, lacerations, bruisings, burns |
| Medical conditions | Pancreatitis, ulcerative colitis, migraine headaches, peritonitis |
| Psychological conditions | Anxiety, depression, insomnia |
| Procedures | Turning, positioning, suctioning, placement or removal of catheters, tubes or drains, paracentesis, wound dressing |
| Immobility | |
| Preexisting chronic pain conditions | |
| Musculoskeletal | Arthritis, low back pain, fibromyalgia |
| Other conditions | Cancer, stroke, diabetic neuropathy, trigeminal neuralgia |

Inspired by: Henneman, E., & Belden, J. (2006). Psychosocial aspects of critical care. In J. Alspach (Ed.), *Core Curriculum for Critical Care Nursing* (6th ed.). St. Louis, MO: Saunders Elsevier.

pain management in older persons. These concerns are present in patients, families, and also in health professionals (Herr, 2004). With careful monitoring, opioid analgesics can be used safely in older persons and are unlikely to cause addiction in persons without a prior history of substance abuse (AGS, 2002; Kirsh & Smith, 2008). Critical care nurses play a pivotal role in identifying concerns that may have an effect on the treatment plan and to educate and work with the patient and family to address misconceptions.

## Technology Challenges

Awareness of the impact of technology on behavioral measures used to detect pain in older critically ill patients is important. Although invasive-line placement may assist with measuring blood pressure and heart rate, which are often indicators of acute pain, the sympathetic responses commonly associated with pain have been shown to be unreliable and often blunted in persons with dementia (Rainero, Vigletti, Bergamasco, Piness, & Beneditte, 2000; Shannon & Bucknall, 2003). The monitoring system in the critical care setting may itself interfere with patients' behavioral expressions, which are often clues to underlying discomfort.

## Documentation of Pain

A considerable challenge to effective pain assessment and management is the lack of consistent documentation, which is vital in communicating patient information across providers, shifts, and settings. In a study of 52 patients in a critical care setting, Gélinas and colleagues (Gélinas, Fortier, Viens, Fillion, & Puntillo 2004) found that only 1.6% of documented assessments ($n = 183$) used a pain scale and observable indicators, physiologic signs, or behavioral reactions were not documented on a regular basis in a standadized way. Effectiveness of interventions for the management of pain was noted in almost 60% of pain episodes. Accurate and consistent communication of pain assessment and response to treatment is essential in promoting quality pain care.

Many factors affect the ability to assess and treat pain effectively in critically ill older persons. Understanding the unique characteristics of older persons, as well as issues that need to be considered and addressed, contribute to quality pain care.

## Definition and Types of Pain

The International Association for the Study of Pain (IASP) provided an often-cited definition for pain in 1979 that states that pain is an unpleasant sensory and emotional experience associated with actual or potential damage (IASP, 1979). Nursing offered a definition of pain that also has been globally accepted that views pain as "whatever the person experiencing the pain says it is, existing whenever the patient say it does" (McCaffery, 1968, p. 95). Together these definitions convey the complexity of pain, its subjective nature, and the multidimensional components involved, including sensory, affective, cognitive, physiological, and behavioral aspects (McGuire, 1992; Melzack, 1999). Thus, pain is not just a sensation experienced, but includes its unpleasant nature, which can be associated with anxiety, depression and mood state, as well as a cognitive evaluative component that incorporates the meaning of the pain to the individual. Pain is mediated by sensory processes or transmission of stimuli via nociceptors and influenced by many factors that interact in complex ways to produce the total experience of pain.

Because of its subjective nature, the patient's self-report represents the most valid measure of pain and must be obtained as often as possible. Unfortunately, many critically ill patients are unable to provide a self-report of pain because of alterations in their level of consciousness resulting from acute disease, head trauma, and/or sedative agents. Some authors (Anand & Craig, 1996) have proposed an alternative definition for nonverbal patients. They proposed that the behavioral alterations caused by pain are valuable forms of self-report and should be considered as alternative measures of pain. Based on this, pain assessment must be designed to conform to the patient's communication capabilities. Different approaches are described in detail in the Pain Assessment section. Understanding pain conditions and how the type of pain affects assessment and treatment is essential. Following are definitions of pain type to guide the critical care nurse in interpreting assessment findings and recommending intervention approaches that match pain pathology.

## Acute and Chronic Pain

Acute pain has been defined as pain of recent onset and probable limited duration, usually with an identifiable temporal and causal relationship to injury or disease. Chronic or persistent pain is commonly distinguished from acute pain by its persistence beyond the usual time of healing of an injury and by the absence of an identifiable cause of the pain (IASP Task Force on Taxonomy, 1994; Ready & Edwards, 1992). Chronic or persistent pain is typically defined as pain that lasts longer than expected, usually greater than 3 to 6 months (AGS, 2002). However, this traditional acute–chronic pain dichotomy has been challenged by emerging evidence that the biological and physiological foundation for long-term persistent pain is in place within hours of trauma (Carr & Goudas, 1999). Increasingly, acute pain is being viewed as the initiation of an extensive, persistent nociceptive and behavioral cascade triggered by tissue injury that affects the experience and processing of future pain. Thus, aggressive, timely, and effective treatment of acute pain is warranted.

Of most interest to the critical care nurse is acute pain, although many older patients will have underlying chronic conditions. Acute pain is often characterized by activation of signs of increased autonomic activity, including hypertension, tachycardia, vasoconstriction, sweating, increased rate and decreased depth of respiration, skeletal muscle spasm, increased gastrointestinal secretions, decreased intestinal motility and increased sphincter tone, urinary retention, venous stasis and potential for thrombosis, and possible pulmonary embolism (Cousins & Power, 1999). However, although these autonomic responses are often seen in acute pain states, they may be absent, especially in older adults (AGS Panel on Persistent Pain in Older Persons, 2002; Rainero et al., 2000).

## Nociceptive Pain (Somatic, Visceral)

Nociceptive pain is caused by activation of nociceptors (e.g., thermal, chemical, mechanical, or inflammatory) and is primarily related to bone, soft tissue, or internal organ damage and includes both somatic pain (skin and subcutaneous tissue, bone, muscle, blood vessels, and connective tissue) and visceral pain (organs and the linings of body cavities) (AGS, 2002; IASP, 1979; Pasero, 2004). Nociceptive pain is noted as a warning and protection against injury. An example of nociceptive pain is postoperative incisional pain described as moderate to severe sharp stabbing pain localized at the incision site. This pain type typically responds to common analgesics and nonpharmacologic techniques.

## Neuropathic Pain

Neuropathic pain arises from damage and abnormal physiology of the peripheral or central nervous systems and may be unrelated to ongoing tissue damage or inflammation (Dworkin et al., 2003). Neuropathic pain serves no useful purpose and is usually sustained and chronic (Pasero, 2004). An example of neuropathic pain is diabetic peripheral neuropathy that may be described as severe burning in the foot, tingling sensation in the lower calf, and extreme sensitivity to socks or shoes touching the skin of the foot. This type of pain is often complex to treat and adjunct or coanalgesics are the first line of treatment, including anticonvulsants, antidepressants, as well as opioids.

Knowledge of different pain problems that are a result of aging and their common presentations are important tools for critical care nurses as the pain experienced may be related to long-standing persistent pain problems, rather than the acute illness or trauma episode. Table 18.3 presents information on pain types, typical descriptions, and examples of common pain-related conditions associated with aging.

# Physiology of Pain in the Older Patient

## Nociception

Nociception represents the neural and brain activity necessary for a person to feel pain; however, this neural and brain activity alone is not sufficient to cause the experience of pain. Pain is the conscious experience that emerges from nociception, more specifically brain activity (Charlton, 2005). Four processes are involved in nociception: (a) transduction, (b) transmission, (c) perception, and (d) modulation (Carr & Goudas, 1999; McCaffery & Pasero, 1999).

Briefly, transduction refers to mechanical (e.g., surgical incision), thermal (e.g., burn), or chemical (e.g., toxic substance) stimuli that damage tissues. These stimuli lead to the release of neurotransmitters (e.g., prostaglandins, bradykinin, serotonin, histamine, glutamate, and substance P), which stimulate peripheral nociceptive receptors and thus serve to initiate nociceptive transmission. The nociceptive message is then transmitted by nociceptive nerve fibers (A$\delta$ and C) in the dorsal horn of the spinal cord. Large-diameter, myelinated A$\delta$ fibers transmit well-localized sharp pain. Small diameter, unmyelinated C fibers transmit diffuse, dull, and aching pain. In the dorsal horn of the spinal cord and with the liberation of substance P, these fibers then synapse with ascending spinothalamic fibers to reach the central nervous system (CNS), where pain is perceived. Projections to different areas of the CNS allow the patient to express various aspects of the pain experience, for instance: (a) the sensory cortex located in the parietal lobe determines the characteristics of pain (e.g., location, intensity, quality); (b) the limbic system is responsible for the negative emotions associated with pain (e.g., anxiety, fear, anger); (c) the motor cortex—located in the frontal lobe—is responsible for behaviors associated with pain (e.g., facial expressions, body movements). Finally, modulation of pain is mainly the result of liberation of endogenous opioids by the CNS through the descending pathways in the dorsal horn of the spinal cord. These substances link to μ-receptors located on nociceptive fibers, inhibiting the liberation of substance P, thus decreasing or blocking the transmission of the pain sensation.

In summary, nociception is an important physiologic mechanism of pain that can integrate many components that can be used for pain assessment. In transduction, stimuli are sources of pain that should alert the nurse to initiate pain assessment and to ensure a follow-up. Because of the synapsing of nociceptive fibers with motor fibers in the spinal cord, which occurs during transmission, muscular rigidity can appear as a result of a reflex activity (Carr & Goudas, 1999) and can be observed as a behavioral indicator associated with pain. With perception, the patient's self-report of pain can be obtained if the patient is able to communicate with the nurse.

There may be some changes in nociception in the elderly (see Gibson & Farrell, 2004, for a review) The transduction and transmission processes may be affected by advancing age and manifest as a reduction in substance P and a reduction in the density of both myelinated and unmyelinated fibers. These changes may alter the functional integrity of nociceptive nerves, and may slow down nerve-conduction

## 18.3 Types of Pain, Examples, and Treatment

| Type of Pain and Examples | Source of Pain | Typical Description | Effective Drug Classes and Treatment |
|---|---|---|---|
| **Nociceptive: somatic** <br> Arthritis, acute postoperative, fracture, bone metastases | Tissue injury, e.g., bones, soft tissue, joints, muscles | Well localized, constant; aching, stabbing, gnawing, throbbing | Nonopioids, NSAIDs, opioids, physical and cognitive-behavioral therapies |
| **Nociceptive: visceral** <br> Renal colic, bowel obstruction | Visceral | Diffuse, poorly localized, referred to other sites, intermittent, paroxysmal; dull, colicky, squeezing, deep, cramping, often accompanied by nausea, vomiting, diaphoresis | Nonopioids, NSAIDs, Opioids, physical and cognitive-behavioral therapies |
| **Neuropathic** <br> Cervical or lumbar radiculopathy, postherpetic neuralgia, trigeminal neuralgia, diabetic neuropathy, poststroke syndrome, herniated intervertebral disc | Peripheral or central nervous system | Prolonged, usually constant, but can be paroxysmal; sharp, burning, pricking, tingling, squeezing; associated with other sensory disturbances, e.g., paresthesias and dysesthesias; allodynia, hyperalgesia, impaired motor function, atrophy, or abnormal deep tendon reflexes | Tricyclic antidepressants, anticonvulsants, opioids, topical anesthetics, physical and cognitive-behavioral therapies |
| **Undetermined** <br> Myofascial pain syndrome, somatoform pain disorders | Poorly understood | No identifiable pathologic processes or symptoms out of proportion to identifiable organic pathology; widespread musculoskeletal pain, stiffness, and weakness | Antidepressants, antianxiety agents Physical, cognitive-behavioral, and psychological therapies |

Reproduced with permission from Reuben et al. (2008). *Geriatrics at Your Fingertips.* Used with permission American Geriatrics Society.

velocity. Aging also has an impact on the central nervous system but it has not been established yet how those changes may affect nociception. Moreover, the magnitude of the endogenous analgesic response appears to be reduced in older persons, especially with severe pain, which may alter the modulation process. Such changes in nociception may lead to a higher pain threshold, a decreased sensitivity to lower levels of noxious stimuli, but an increased response to higher intensity stimuli (Gibson & Helme, 2001). The critical care nurse should not conclude that older adults experience less pain when they report it. To the contrary, an older person who decides to report pain may present with a greater level of underlying pathology, which should alert the nurse.

## Stress Response

A biological stress response is activated by pain, an obvious stressor (Carr & Goudas, 1999). This stress response involves the nervous, endocrine, and immune systems in the hypothalamo–pituitary–adrenal axis (HPA) (McCance & Huether, 1998; Selye, 1974). The elderly patient is at great risk of presenting with a stress response in critical care units, where stressors, including pain, are numerous.

In the presence of acute pain, the sympathetic nervous system (SNS) is activated. This activation involves the release of norepinephrine and epinephrine. The effects of these stress hormones allow for the observation of physiological responses such as increased blood pressure (BP), heart rate (HR), and respiratory rate (RR), and perspiration, which are common signs of acute pain that have been observed in critically ill patients (Gélinas & Johnston, 2007; Payen et al., 2001; Puntillo et al., 1997).

If pain persists over time or if injuries are located in the bladder or the intestines, the parasympathetic nervous system (PNS) may be dominant. Thus, the BP and HR may decrease rather than increase. In addition, different responses to stressors involving PNS or SNS patterns have been documented (Hurwitz et al., 1993). Thus, the absence of pain-related indicators related to the activation of the SNS does not necessarily imply an absence of pain sensation (Gélinas, Viens, Fortier, & Fillion, 2005; Puntillo et al., 1997).

When the stress response persists, other hormones may be released, including vasopressin, aldosterone, and cortisol. The effects of vasopressin and aldosterone lead to increased sodium and water retention, which result in decreased diuresis, increased blood pressure, and increased cardiac preload (i.e., central venous pressure, pulmonary artery wedge pressure). In addition, cortisol may contribute to multisystemic responses such as infection and hyperglycemia (McCance & Huether, 1998). Therefore, these signs may be associated with pain and can be detected by the critical care nurse.

## Pain Assessment in the Critically Ill Older Adult

Pain assessment is an important part of the quality of care. Because of the nurse's presence at the patient's bedside, the critical care nurse has a unique and important role in pain assessment and management, in collaboration with the patient and his/ her family and the multidisciplinary team.

# Exhibit 18.1

## Description of the PQRSTU

**P (provocative/palliative)**: What causes pain*? What makes pain worse? Better?

**Q (quality)**: What does the pain feel like? (e.g., throbbing, burning, cramping, etc.)

**R (region/radiation)**: Where is the pain? Does it spread anywhere?

**S (severity/signs and symptoms)**: How intense is the pain from 0 (no pain) to 10 (worst possible pain)? Do you feel any other discomforts? The critical care nurse also observes the patient for signs associated with pain.

**T (timing)**: When did the pain first occur? How long did it last? How often did it occur?

**U (understand)**: What do you think it means? The patient who had a similar experience before or is suffering from a chronic pain problem knows himself well.

* Other terms besides "pain" may be used with the elderly to facilitate the interview. † A pain map (e.g. drawings of the human body) may be used to establish the location and extent of pain.

## Verbal and Cognitively Intact Older Adults

Because pain is first recognized as a subjective experience, the patient's self-report of pain represents the most valid measure of pain and must be obtained whenever possible (Herr et al., 2006). A comprehensive pain interview must be done on admission or at the onset of a new pain. It can be obtained by questioning the patient using the mnemonic PQRSTU (see Exhibit 18.1). Older patients may use different terms, such as "discomfort," aching," "hurting," or "soreness" to describe their pain experience. Therefore, it is important to determine the patient's preferred terminology prior to the interview (Herr & Garand, 2001).

After the pain experience has been well described, the nurse routinely monitors the intensity of the pain, which can be measured by various scales (see Figure 18.1) such as the numeric rating scale (e.g., NRS 0–10), the visual analog scale (VAS), the verbal descriptor scale (VDS; Herr, Spratt, Mobily, et al., 2004), or the faces pain scale (e.g., FPS-R; Hicks, von Baeyer, Spafford, van Korlaar, & Goodenough, 2001). It has been noted that the use of a vertical pain intensity scale is easier to use for elderly patients because it reminds them of a thermometer (Herr & Mobily, 1993). Although the NRS and VDS are recommended for the assessment of pain intensity among seniors who are cognitively intact and able to self-report (Hadjistavropoulos et al., 2007), previous studies have shown that pain scales including faces are preferred by acutely and critically ill adults (Carey et al., 1997; Gélinas, 2007b; Stuppy, 1998). The Faces Pain Thermometer (FPT) is a newly developed tool that was tested in postoperative ICU adults, including older persons (Gélinas, 2007b). Higher pain intensity scores with the FPT during a nociceptive procedure (e.g., turning) were obtained compared to rest periods, and FPT scores were highly correlated with the VDS. Thus,

# 18.1

**Pain intensity scales: (A) Numeric rating scale, (B) verbal descriptive scale, (C) faces pain thermometer, (D) Iowa Pain scale.**

NRS (AHCPR, 1992) VDS (Gélinas et al., 2006), Faces (Gélinas, 2007b), Thermometer (Keela Herr, University of Iowa).

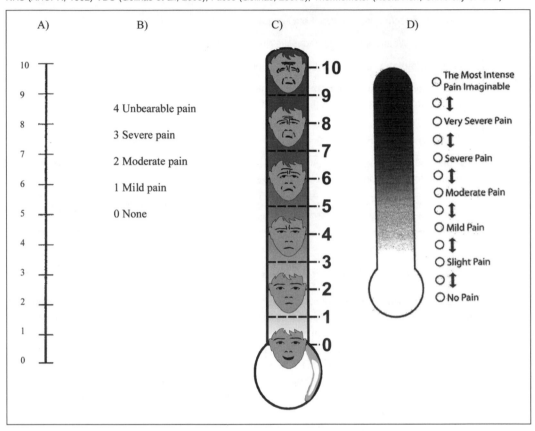

the FPT appears to be an additional scale to consider in the critically ill population. In any case, the use of a pain intensity scale must take into account the patient's preference, and the same tool should be used consistently.

The nurse should be aware of the presence of any sensory deficits (e.g., hearing, vision) and ensure that the older adult's sensory-assistive devices are working properly. Pain intensity scales may be adjusted to accommodate patients' sensory deficits (e.g., use a larger size, provide with written and oral instructions) (Hadjistavropoulos et al., 2007). The use of warm colors such as yellow, red, and orange are also easier for the elderly to distinguish (Matteson & McConnell, 1988). The FPT was developed in a large size (4″ x 14″) and the color red was used to facilitate its use in the elderly patient.

# Exhibit 18.2

## Recommendations for Obtaining of Self-Report of Pain in Critically Ill Patients

1. Start by asking the patient if he/she has pain or not. The critically ill patient who is mechanically ventilated may answer by head nodding or other signs (e.g., blinking, gripping the nurse's hand).
2. Focus on pain intensity initially. If no specific tool is recommended in your institution, select a tool appropriate for the patient and most feasible to use.
3. Make the environment as quiet as possible and allow sufficient time for the patient to respond. Three attempts should be made before concluding that the patient is unable to self-report the pain.
4. Use the same scale each time the patient's pain is assessed.
5. Pain intensity should be assessed on a regular basis, before and after pain management interventions.
6. Pain must be recorded and its documentation easily accessible.

From Kwekkeboom and Herr (2001).

Mechanical ventilation should not be a barrier for critical care nurses in document-ing patients' self-reports of pain. Indeed, many mechanically ventilated patients with a stable condition can use pain scales by pointing to them (Puntillo, 1994; Puntillo & Weiss, 1994; Puntillo et al., 2001). However, pain assessment may be difficult to complete because of the patient's change in communication, a lack of concentration secondary to sedation therapies, and the life/death immediacy of many actions in the critical care environment. In a recent study by Gélinas and Johnston (2007), in a sample of 30 mechanically ventilated patients with unstable conditions, only 10% of them were able to rate their pain level with a scale. To guide the nurses in obtaining the self-report of pain in critically ill patients, recommendations have been made (Kwekkeboom & Herr, 2001; see Exhibit 18.2).

The use of multidimensional pain questionnaires is more time consuming and may be difficult to administer in critical care settings (Graf & Puntillo, 2003). However, the McGill Pain Questionnaire-Short Form (MPQ-SF) has been used for research purposes in critical care, and positive correlations were found with the VAS and the NRS in critically ill patients able to self-report (Berthier et al., 1998; Puntillo & Weiss, 1994). This type of questionnaire has not been studied yet in older adults with cogni-tive impairment.

## Older Adults With Cognitive Deficits

Many seniors with mild to moderate cognitive impairments, and even some with severe impairment, are able to use pain intensity scales (Bjoro & Herr, 2008; Hadjista-vropoulos et al., 2007). Elderly patients with impaired cognition should receive repeated instructions and be given sufficient time to respond (AGS, 2002). Most scales including the NRS, VDS, and FPS-R have showed acceptable reliability and validity in patients with cognitive deficits. The VAS is the less preferred tool by many older adults and shows the highest failure rate (Herr, Spratt, Garand, & Li, 2007; Wynne, Ling, & Remsbourg, 2000). The FPS-R has been found to be the preferred scale in some cognitively impaired patients, particularly African Americans and Hispanics

(Ware, Epps, Herr, & Packard, 2006). However, results have suggested that the FPS-R may measure a broader pain construct, including sensory and affective components. The Iowa Pain Thermometer (IPT; see Figure 18.1) is another available tool that was tested in younger and older patient groups experiencing chronic joint pain, and was identified as the preferred scale in both groups (Herr et al., 2007). The IPT demonstrated the lowest failure rate compared with the VAS and the NRS; the VAS and the NRS had higher failure rates relative to cognitive impairment. According to pain location, the use of a pain chart or asking the patient to point to the body part that hurts has been shown to be an effective approach in cognitively impaired elderly patients (Weiner, Peterson, & Keefe, 1998; Wynne et al., 2000).

Surrogate reporting should be used with caution. In fact, both physicians and nurses tend to underestimate the intensity of the patient's pain, whereas family caregivers tend to overestimate it (Herr & Decker, 2004). On the other hand, family members who know the patient well are encouraged to provide information regarding usual behaviors and assist the nurse in identifying changes in behaviors that may indicate the presence of pain (Bjoro & Herr, 2008). Indeed, seniors with dementia may present with a wide range of pain reactions (Fuchs-Labelle & Hadjistavropoulos, 2004), which becomes challenging for the nurse to detect.

When the patient's self-report is impossible to obtain, direct observation of patient behavior is highly recommended (Hadjistavropoulos et al., 2007; Herr et al., 2006). The American Geriatrics Society Panel on Persistent Pain in Older Adults has compiled a list of common pain behaviors (see Table 18.4) that may be observed in cognitively impaired older persons (AGS, 2002). Pain assessments should be performed during movement or activity so as to identify the presence of pain, as well as before and after the administration of an analgesic to evaluate the efficacy of the intervention, which should lead to the reduction of pain behaviors. Many behavioral tools were developed for older persons with limitations in ability to communicate caused by cognitive deficits (see Aubin, Giguère, Hadjistavropoulos, & Verreault, 2007; Bjoro & Herr, 2008, for a review). The PACSLAC (Fuchs-Labelle & Hadjistavropoulos, 2004), and Doloplus-2 (Wary & Doloplus, 1999; Wary, Serbouti, & Doloplus, 2001) are promising tools and are recommended by experts (Aubin et al., 2007; Hadjistavropoulos et al., 2007; Zwakhalen, Hamers, Abu-Saad & Berger, 2006). However, it must be noted that the validation of the PACSLAC was based on nurses' retrospective reports, and that the English version of the Doloplus-2 is still underway.

Delirium is a form of transient cognitive impairment and is highly prevalent in older adults in the ICU (McNicoll et al., 2003). The challenge with delirium is that there is considerable overlap between delirium behaviors and pain-related behaviors. It still remains unclear whether pain-related behavioral tools may assist the nurse in the detection of pain of older adults who experienced an episode of delirium during episodes of delirium. So far, only one pain assessment tool, the PATCOA, has been developed for this specific population, and was tested in cognitively intact older adults who experienced an episode of delirium during the postoperative phase (Decker & Perry, 2003). Further research is required in elderly patients with cognitive impairment. The critical care nurse should also keep in mind that pain is a modifiable factor of delirium that can be controlled with adequate pain management (Graf & Puntillo, 2003).

| 18.4 | Comprehensive List of Pain Behaviors in Cognitively Impaired Older Adults | |
|---|---|---|
| **Behavior** | **Examples** | |
| Facial expressions | Slight frown, sad, frightened face Grimacing, wrinkled forehead, closed or tightened eyes Any distorted expression Rapid blinking | |
| Verbalizations, vocalizations | Sighing, moaning, groaning Grunting, chanting, calling out Noisy breathing Asking for help Verbal abusiveness | |
| Body movements | Rigid, tense body posture, guarding Fidgeting Increased pacing, rocking Restricted movement Gait or mobility changes | |
| Changes in interpersonal interactions | Aggressive, combative, resists care Decreased social interactions Socially inappropriate, disruptive Withdrawn | |
| Changes in activity patterns or routines | Refuses food, appetite change Increase in rest periods Sleep, rest pattern changes Sudden cessation of common routines Increased wandering | |
| Mental status changes | Crying or tears Increased confusion Irritability or distress | |

Reproduced with permission.
American Geriatrics Society Panel on Persistent Pain in Older Adults. (2002). The management of persistent pain in older persons. *Journal of the American Geriatrics Society, 50*, S211. Available at http://www.americangeriatrics.org/products/positionpapers/JGS5071.pdf

## Nonverbal Intubated/Unconscious Patient

It is not rare for the critically ill patient to be unable to communicate. Indeed, many critically ill patients are unable to provide a self-report of pain because of alterations in their level of consciousness due to acute disease, head trauma, and/or sedative agents. Besides the patient's self-report of pain, the critical care nurse can rely on observation of behavioral and physiological indicators that may be associated with pain. Again, these should not be substituted for a self-report as long as the patient is able to communicate in any way. However, when the patient is unable to communicate, these indicators become unique information for pain assessment (Aslan, Badir, & Selimen, 2003; Kwekkeboom & Herr, 2001). The critical care nurse must be aware that behavioral and physiological indicators are not specific to pain. They can indicate other problems, such as anxiety and discomfort (Carroll et al., 1999; Frazier et al., 2002), or can be influenced by different pharmacological therapies. However, an absence of these indicators does not necessarily mean the absence of pain (Gélinas et al., 2005; Puntillo et al., 1997).

Some efforts have been made for the development of pain assessment tools in the critically ill patient, such as: "Post-Anesthesia Care Unit Behavioral Pain Rating Scale" (PACU BPRS; Mateo & Krenzischek, 1992), "Pain Assessment and Intervention Notation" (PAIN; Puntillo et al., 1997), "Behavioral Pain Scale" (BPS; Payen et al., 2001), "Nonverbal Adult Pain Assessment Scale" (NVPS; Odhner, Wegman, Freeland, Steinmetz, & Ingersoll, 2003) and "Critical-Care Pain Observation Tool" (CPOT; Gélinas, Fillion, Puntillo, Viens, & Fortier, 2006). All these tools have been tested in critically ill adults, including older persons during the postoperative phase or nociceptive procedures. A critical review of those pain assessment tools was recently done (Li, Puntillo, & Miaskowski, 2008). Although these tools show some limitations and may require further validation, the BPS and the CPOT have demonstrated acceptable reliability and validity and are suggested by experts (Li et al., 2008; Sessler, Grap, & Ramsey, 2008). These tools may help support pain assessment in critical care especially in nonverbal patients. The PAIN is also an interesting tool as it provides the nurse with behavioral and physiological indicators, and an algorithm for pain management in the ICU (Puntillo, Stannard, Miaskowsi, Kehrle & Gleeson, 2002; see Exhibit 18.3). It must be noted that the measurements of the PAIN indicators are not standardized and are based on the nurse's clinical judgment, which may lead to different perceptions related to the nurse's experience.

According to the CPOT, it is a recent tool that includes four behaviors: (a) facial expression, (b) body movements, (c) muscle tension, and (d) compliance with the ventilator for intubated patients or vocalization for other patients (see Table 18.5). Items are rated on a scale from 0 to 2 for a possible total score ranging from 0 to 8. It must be emphasized that the CPOT provides a score of the intensity of behavioral reactions, rather than a pain intensity score per se. The items of the CPOT were derived from previously described pain-assessment instruments (Mateo & Krenzischek, 1992; Payen et al., 2001; Puntillo et al., 1997), a chart review of 52 critically ill patients' medical files (Gélinas et al., 2004), and nine focus groups with 48 critical care nurses and interviews of 12 physicians (Gélinas et al., 2005). Also, the instrument demonstrated good interrater reliability and validity in both its French and its English versions (Gélinas et al., 2006; Gélinas & Johnston, 2007). For instance, associations were found between the patients' self-reports of pain and the CPOT scores. Patients in pain obtained higher CPOT scores compared to patients with no pain or less pain. Moreover, higher CPOT scores were obtained during positioning when pain could be higher compared to rest periods.

The CPOT may be used in the following manner. The patient must be observed at rest for a minute to obtain a baseline value for the CPOT. Then, the patient should be observed during nociceptive procedures (e.g., turning, endotracheal suctioning, wound dressing) to detect any changes in the patient's behavior to pain. The patient should be evaluated before and at the peak effect of an analgesic agent to assess whether the treatment was effective in relieving pain (see Table 18.5). For the rating

# Exhibit 18.3

## P.A.I.N. Tool

**STEP 1: Assess Pain**

A. Are Potential Pain-Related Behaviors Present?

| Yes | No | Movements |
|-----|-----|-----------|
| | | No movement |
| | | Slow, decreased, hesitant, cautious |
| | | Restlessness |
| | | Seeking attention through movements |
| | | Vocalization |
| Yes | No | Facial Cues |
| | | Grimacing, frowning, wincing |
| | | Drawn around mouth and eyes |
| | | Teary/Crying |
| | | Wrinkled forehead |
| Yes | No | Posturing/Guarding |
| | | Rigid |
| | | Splinting |
| | | Tense, Stiff |

Based on the behaviors you've noted above, what number would you assign to the pain behavior indicator scale?

| 0 | 1 | 2 | 3 | 4 | 5 | 6 | 7 | 8 | 9 | 10 |
|---|---|---|---|---|---|---|---|---|---|----|
| Patient has no pain | | | | | | | | | | Patient has worst pain imaginable |

*(continued)*

**Exhibit 18.3** *(continued)*

| B. Are Potential Physiological Pain Indicators Present? | | |
|---|---|---|
| Yes | No | Physiological Indicators |
| | | Increased HR |
| | | Decreased HR |
| | | Increased blood pressure |
| | | Decreased blood pressure |
| | | Increased respiratory rate |
| | | Decreased respiratory rate |
| | | Perspiration |
| | | Pallor |

Based on the behaviors you've noted above, what number would you assign to the pain behavior indicator scale?

| 0 | 1 | 2 | 3 | 4 | 5 | 6 | 7 | 8 | 9 | 10 |
|---|---|---|---|---|---|---|---|---|---|---|
| Patient has no pain | | | | | | | | | | Patient has worst pain imaginable |

Nurse's Overall Assessment of Pain Intensity

Based on your observations above, what number do you believe best indicates your assessment of how intense the patient's pain is ? (Circle a number)

| 0 | 1 | 2 | 3 | 4 | 5 | 6 | 7 | 8 | 9 | 10 |
|---|---|---|---|---|---|---|---|---|---|---|
| Patient has no pain | | | | | | | | | | Patient has worst pain imaginable |

Patient has no pain                                        Patient's Self-Report of Pain Intensity

Nurse asks patient, "On a scale of 1–10, where 0 = No Pain, and 10 = Worst Pain Imaginable, tell me or show me how much pain you're having right now."

| 0 | 1 | 2 | 3 | 4 | 5 | 6 | 7 | 8 | 9 | 10 |
|---|---|---|---|---|---|---|---|---|---|---|
| Patient has no pain | | | | | | | | | | Patient has worst pain imaginable |

*(continued)*

**Exhibit 18.3** *(continued)*

| STEP 2: Assess for Potential Problems Influencing Opioid Administration |
| --- |

A. Sedation Level per Ramsay Scale *(check one, below)*
_____ 1. Patient anxious and agitated or restless or both
_____ 2. Patient cooperative, orientated, and tranquil
_____ 3. Patient responds to commands only
_____ 4. Brisk response after light glabellar tap or loud auditory stimulus
_____ 5. Sluggish response to #4, above
_____ 6. No response to #4, above

*There should be no problem with sedation if sedation level is 1 or 2. There is a potential problem if sedation level is 3, there's an actual problem if sedation level is 4, 5, or 6*

B. Hemodynamic and Respiratory Status

What is patient's preop blood pressure? _____ / _____

| YES | NO | |
| --- | --- | --- |
| | | Is patient's systolic blood pressure approx. 20 mmHg less than preop? |
| | | Do you consider patient's present blood pressure to be a problem for pain management? |

What is patient's pre-op heart rate? _____

| YES | NO | |
| --- | --- | --- |
| | | Is patient's heart rate 10–20 beats/min. slower than preop? |
| | | Do you consider patient's heart rate to be a problem for pain management? |

What is patient's current respiratory rate?_____

| YES | NO | |
| --- | --- | --- |
| | | Is patient mechanically ventilated at present? |
| | | Is respiratory rate (i.e., the sum of IMV rate plus patient's spontaneous rate) less than 8/minute? |
| | | Do you consider patient's respiratory rate to be a problem for pain management? |
| | | Is most recent $pCO_2$ level available? |
| | | If available, what is it? |
| | | Do you consider patient's $pCO_2$ to be a problem for pain management? |

*(continued)*

## Exhibit 18.3 *(continued)*

---

**STEP 3: Analgesic Treatment Decision**

---

Patient's standing analgesic order (fill in):

DECISION #1: No Problem. If no potential problems with sedation, BP, HR, RR, noted and patient requires med, then:

*Circle One*

1. If patient's pain intensity score is between 0 and 5, then give lowest dose ordered.
2. If patient's pain intensity score is between 4 and 6, then give midrange dose ordered.
3. If patient's pain intensity score is between 7 and 10, then give highest dose ordered.

NOTE: Other decisions made:

Record: Doses given: _____

Time given: _____

DECISION #2: If Problems

*Check Which*

(1) If sedation level is 3 and patient's pain intensity score is between 3 and 10 and patient requires pain med, then start with lowest dose.
(2) If problem with BP and/or HR and patient's pain intensity score is between 3 and 10 and patient requires pain med, then confer with colleagues about patient management. (Also, consider other potential patient problems, e.g., volume depletion.)
(3) If problem with respirations and/or $PCO_2$, and patient's pain intensity score is between 3 and 10 and patient requires pain med, then confer with colleagues about patient management. (Also, consider possibility that changes in ventilator settings may help respiratory status. If patient is being ventilated and is not being weaned, is respiratory status still a pain management problem?)

NOTE: Other decisions made:

Record: Drug, dose & route: _____

Time given: _____

---

From: Puntillo, K. A., Stannard, D., Miaskoski, C., Kehrle, K., & Gleeson, S. (2002). Use of a pain assessment and intervention notation (P.A.I.N.) tool in critical care nursing practice: Nurses' evaluations. *Heart & Lung, 31*(4), 303–314. Fig. 1-3.

---

of CPOT, the patient should be attributed the highest score observed during the observation period. The patient should be attributed a score for each behavior included in the CPOT and muscle tension should be evaluated last, especially when the patient is at rest, because the stimulation of touch (passive flexion and extension of the arm) may lead to behavior reactions.

In terms of observable indicators, behaviors have received more attention in research than physiological indicators. Indeed, behaviors have been included in all tools developed for critically ill adults. In the few tools in which physiological indicators were included (Odhner et al., 2003; Puntillo et al., 1997), their evaluation was

## 18.5 Description of the Critical-Care Pain Observation Tool (CPOT)

| Indicator | Score | | Description |
|---|---|---|---|
| **Facial expression** | Relaxed, neutral | 0 | No muscle tension observed |
| | Tense | 1 | Presence of frowning, brow lowering, orbit tightening and levator contraction or any other change (e.g., opening eyes or tearing during nociceptive procedures) |
| | Grimacing | 2 | All previous facial movements plus eyelids tightly closed (the patient may present with mouth open or biting of the endotracheal tube) |
| **Body movements** | Absence of movements or normal position | 0 | Does not move at all (doesn't necessarily mean absence of pain) or normal position (movements not aimed toward the pain site or not made for the purpose of protection) |
| | Protection | 1 | Slow, cautious movements, touching or rubbing the pain site, seeking attention through movements |
| | Restlessness | 2 | Pulling tube, attempting to sit up, moving limbs/ thrashing, not following commands, striking at staff, trying to climb out of bed |
| **Compliance with the ventilator (intubated patients)** | Tolerating ventilator or movement | 0 | Alarms not activated, easy ventilation |
| | Coughing but tolerating | 1 | Coughing, alarms may be activated but stop spontaneously |
| | Fighting ventilator | 2 | Asynchrony: blocking ventilation, alarms frequently activated |
| **Vocalization (extubated patients)** (Mateo & Krenzischek, 1992) | Talking in normal tone or no sound | 0 | Talking in normal tone or no sound |
| | Sighing, moaning | 1 | Sighing, moaning |
| | Crying out, sobbing | 2 | Crying out, sobbing |

*(continued)*

**Table 18.5** *(continued)*

| Indicator | Score | | Description |
|-----------|-------|---|-------------|
| **Muscle tension** | Relaxed | 0 | No resistance to passive movements |
| | Tense, rigid<br>Evaluation by passive flexion<br>and extension of upper limbs<br>when patient is at rest or<br>evaluation when patient is<br>being turned | 1 | Resistance to passive movements |
| | Very tense or rigid | 2 | Strong resistance to passive movements,<br>incapacity to complete them |
| TOTAL | _____ / 8 | | |

Adapted from Gélinas, C., Fillion, L., Puntillo, K., Viens, C., & Fortier, M. (2006). Validation of a Critical-Care Pain Observation Tool in adult patients. *American Journal of Critical Care, 15*(4), 420–427. Reproduced with permission.

based on the nurses' judgment. Objective values of physiological indicators in the context of pain in critically ill adults have been documented in few studies so far. Vital signs (PAM [mean arterial pressure], HR, and RR) were found to increase when critically ill patients were exposed to nociceptive procedures (Gélinas & Johnston, 2007; Payen et al., 2001; Young, Siffleet, Nikoletti, & Shaw, 2006). However, these vital signs have not been associated with the patients' self-reports of pain, which limits their validity in pain assessment (Gélinas & Johnston, 2007). Moreover, vital signs may be influenced by many other factors besides pain, including physiologic conditions, homeostatic changes, and medications. Therefore, the critical care nurse should not rely on changes in vital signs as primary indicators but rather consider them as a cue for further assessment of pain (Herr et al., 2006).

Even if behavioral reactions represent more valid indicators for pain assessment, there are situations in the ICU in which the patient cannot express any behavior especially if the patient is heavily sedated, under the effects of blocking agents, or suffering from paralysis. In such situations, the only indicators that remain available are physiologic ones. Tearing and diaphoresis represent autonomic responses to discomfort and can be detected by the critical care nurse (Herr et al., 2006). Also, as technology is evolving, new technologies have been developed and some have been implemented in critical care settings for research purposes. The Near-Infrared Spectroscopy (SPIR) or the Bispectral Index (BIS) are available technologies that may be used for the measurement of the cortical responses to pain. The SPIR have been examined in the neonatal intensive care unit (NICU), and significant increases in cortical responses of the somatosensory cortex were found when infants underwent venipuncture or heel lance (Bartocci, Bergqvist, Lagercrantz, & Anand, 2006; Slater et al., 2006). A pilot study has just been completed in which the NIRS was explored in adults who underwent cardiac surgery, including older persons, and increased cerebral oxygenation was found when patients were exposed to common nociceptive procedures in the operating room (Gélinas et al., in press). Regarding the BIS, which measures cortical arousability, increases in BIS values were found in critically ill sedated adults undergoing a nociceptive procedure, that is, endotracheal suctioning or turning (Li, Miaskowski, Burkhardt, & Puntillo, in press). Further studies on these innovative measures should be conducted in critically ill adult and elderly patients to examine their validity for the detection of pain.

# Pharmacological Methods of Pain Management in the Critically Ill Older Adult

The pharmacological management of pain has infinite variety and is widely used in the critical care unit. In the elderly, physiological decline in renal or hepatic function can affect the pharmacology of analgesics. For instance, increased body fat and reduction in total body water are associated with increasing age. These changes lead to alterations in the volume of distribution of drugs such as an increase for lipophilic drugs (e.g., fentanyl), and a decrease for hydrophilic drugs (e.g., morphine). Also, the reduction in hepatic or renal function affects the metabolism and elimination of drugs. Moreover, older persons are more susceptible to drug side effects. Thus, dosage reductions or longer dosing intervals and monitoring of creatinine clearance are required in the elderly to prevent the accumulation of drugs and the risk of toxicity (AGS, 2002; Pergolizzi et al., 2008).

## Opioid Analgesics

Agonist opioids (see Table 18.6) such as morphine, hydromorphone, and fentanyl have been the most widely used analgesics in the ICU (Jacobi et al., 2002). These agents are recommended for the treatment of severe pain, which is widely experienced by critically ill patients. Because of its water solubility morphine has a slower onset of action and a longer duration compared with fentanyl, which is a lipid-soluble opioid. This makes fentanyl and hydromorphone the preferred opioids for intermittent therapy. Morphine may be particularly problematic in the hypovolemic patient as it can lead to peripheral vasodilatation due to histamine release. On the other hand, fentanyl and hydromorphone lead to minimal histamine release and are the preferred agents in hemodynamically unstable patients. Fentanyl is also recommended in renal-impaired patients as its metabolites are largely inactive and nontoxic, which makes it an effective and safe opioid. Meperidine and codeine are less potent and have limited use in the management of severe pain. A major concern with meperidine is its metabolite, normeperidine, which may cause central nervous system toxicity (irritability, muscle spasticity, tremors, delirium, and seizures), so it is not recommended for repetitive use, and should be avoided in the elderly patient (McCaffery & Pasero, 1999).

### Delivery Methods

In critically ill patients, the intravenous route is the most widely used as it is easy to titrate and it allows continuous infusion of drugs. For these reasons, the intravenous route makes it easier to achieve adequate and proper pain relief in the critically

## 18.6 Pharmacological Agents Used for the Management of Pain

| Analgesic Category | Mechanism of Action | Nociception | Side Effects | Specificity in the Elderly |
|---|---|---|---|---|
| Opioid agonists (e.g., morphine, fentanyl, hydromorphone, codeine, meperidine) | Bind to μ-opioid receptors in the central nervous system (CNS) to:<br><br>1) inhibit the release of excitatory neurotransmitters (substance P) at the dorsal root ganglion of the spinal cord (transmission)<br>2) activate descending inhibitory pathways (modulation)<br>3) alter limbic system activity (perception) | Transmission Perception Modulation | Sedation Confusion Respiratory depression Nausea and vomiting Constipation Pruritus (itching) Urinary retention | Start low, go slow Side effects may be exacerbated Close monitoring of respiratory depression Prophylactic bowel regimen should be initiated Meperidine should be avoided |
| Nonopioid—Acetaminophen | Inhibit prostaglandin synthesis in the CNS | Perception | None if recommended dosage is used (4000 mg/day) Hepatic toxicity in patients suffering from hepatic failure or alcohol abuse (recommended dosage 2000 mg/day) | Safer dosing should not exceed 3000mg/day (Polomano, 2002 in Graf & Puntillo, 2003) |
| Nonopioid—Antiinflammatory agents (NSAIDs) COX-1 and 2 (e.g., aspirin, ibuprofen, naprosyn, ketorolac) COX-2 (e.g., celecoxib, rofecoxib) | Inhibit the enzyme cyclooxygenase (COX-1 and COX-2), which blocks prostaglandin synthesis | Transduction Perception | COX-1 and 2 Gastrointestinal effects Bleeding (by suppressing platelet aggregation) Renal failure COX-2 Not recommended in some patients because of the risk of developing cardiovascular disease (long-term use) | Side effects are high Close monitoring of gastrointestinal bleeding COX-2 are preferred to nonselective COX inhibitors |

(continued)

**Table 18.6** *(continued)*

| Analgesic Category | Mechanism of Action | Nociception | Side Effects | Specificity in the Elderly |
|---|---|---|---|---|
| Adjuvants—Local and systemic anesthetics (e.g., lidocaine, bupivacaine) | Block sodium channels and inhibit the generation of abnormal impulses (local) or suppress aberrant electrical activity in structures associated with pain (systemic) | Transduction (local) Transmission (systemic) | Allergic reaction (topical agent, e.g., EMLA) Parenteral routes (e.g., IV, epidural): CNS toxicity (dizziness, drowsiness, tremors) Cardiovascular effects (arrhythmias) | Careful evaluation of systemic side effect before use |
| Adjuvants—Antidepressants (e.g., amitriptyline, paroxetine, venlafaxine) | Block the reuptake of serotonin and norepinephrine in the CNS, which increases the activity of endogenous opioids (modulation process) | Modulation | Sedation Hypotension Anticholinergic effects (dry mouth, blurred vision, photophobia, constipation, urinary retention, tachycardia) | Significant risk of adverse effects (anticholinergic effects) |
| Adjuvants—Anticonvulsants (e.g., carbamazepine, gabapentin, phenytoin) | Possible mechanism: Block sodium channels and inhibit the generation of abnormal impulses | Transduction | Sedation Dizziness Ataxia Nausea and vomiting | Safer; should be preferred to tricyclic antidepressants |

Adapted from JCAHO (2001), Lehne (2004) McCaffery and Pasero (1999), Melzack and Wall (2003).

ill. Accordingly, analgesics should be administered on a continuous or scheduled intermittent basis with additional bolus doses as required (Jacobi et al., 2002).

Patient-controlled analgesia (PCA) is another method of intravenous delivery that was found to result in stable drug concentrations, a good quality of analgesia, less sedation, less opioid consumption, and fewer adverse effects. However, its use in critically ill patients may be limited based on the importance of patient selection. Indeed, alterations in the level of consciousness or mentation preclude the patient understanding the use of the equipment. Also, the very elderly or patients with renal or hepatic insufficiency may require careful screening.

The epidural route may sometimes be used in the critical care unit after major abdominal surgery, nephrectomy, thoracotomy, and major orthopedic procedures (Puntillo, 1994). Drugs delivered epidurally may be bolused or continuously infused. Again, certain conditions preclude the use of this pain-delivery method: systemic infection, anticoagulation, and increased intracranial pressure. Epidural delivery of opiates provides longer lasting pain relief with less dosing of opiates.

## Monitoring and Managing Opioid Side Effects

The critical care nurse plays a major role in monitoring the patient's pain and opioid side effects, more specifically respiratory depression, which is life-threatening. The older adult may be at higher risk for respiratory depression because it is assumed that sensitivity to CNS-active drugs increases with age (AGS, 2002). The nurse should monitor sedation level and respiratory status at least every 2 hours for the first 24 hours and every 4 hours thereafter, in stable patients. As this technology is more easily available in critical care units, the use of capnography should also be considered in high-risk patients (those with sleep apnea, chronic obstructive pulmonary disease, the very young, or the very old patient) receiving parenteral therapy (Pasero, Manworren, & McCaffery, 2007). As pulse oximeters are widely used in critical care units, they may also support the monitoring of the patient.

Critical respiratory depression can be readily reversed with the administration of the opiate antagonist naloxone. The benefits of reversing respiratory depression with naloxone must be carefully weighed against the risk of a sudden onset of pain and the difficulty of achieving pain relief. To prevent this from occurring, it is important to provide a nonopioid medication for pain management (Pasero & McCaffery, 2000). Moreover, the use of naloxone is not recommended after prolonged analgesia, because it can induce withdrawal and may cause nausea and cardiovascular complications (e.g., arrhythmias) (Jacobi et al., 2002).

Older patients may be at higher risk for other opioid side effects, including constipation and neurotoxicity. Indeed, elderly patients often have reduced intestinal motility, which is the reaosn that constipation may be exacerbated. This side effect must be prevented with prophylactic use of laxatives and other bowel-treatment regimens. Opioid neurotoxicity (i.e., hallucinations, confusion, loss of cognition) is more frequent in dehydrated, severely ill patients with renal impairment. The use of lower starting doses, a close monitoring, and titration may help to reduce the risk of this side effect (Pergolizzi et al., 2008).

## Equianalgesia

When a modification of an opioid is considered, the nurse must be aware of equianalgesic dosages. The goal of equianalgesia is to provide equal analgesic effects with a new agent when opioid replacement is required. Morphine is the standard for the conversion of opioids (see Table 18.7). Prescribed dosages must take into account the patient's age (e.g., infants and elderly patients will usually receive lower dosages of opioids than adult patients) and the patient's health condition (e.g., pain severity, diseases affecting the pharmacokinetics of opioids) (McCaffery & Pasero, 1999). The critical care nurse must have access to a chart for easy referral on the unit to administer the correct dose of opioids to critically ill patients.

# Nonopioid Analgesics

The use of nonopioids (acetaminophen, nonsteroidal antiinflammatory drugs [NSAIDs]; see Table 18.6) in combination with an opioid is now recommended in selected critical care patients. Nonopioids may reduce opioid requirement and provide greater analgesic effect through their action at the peripheral and central levels. Acetaminophen should be maintained at less than 2 g per day for patients with significant

## 18.7  Equianalgesic Chart for Some Common Opioids

### Equianalgesic Dosages

| Opioid | Oral | Parenteral |
|---|---|---|
| Morphine | 30 mg | 10 mg |
| Codeine | 200 mg NR | 130 mg |
| Fentanyl* | — | 100 µg/h (0.1 mg) is equal to 2-4 mg/h morphine IV |
| Hydromorphone | 4–6 mg | 1.5-2 mg |
| Meperidine | 300 mg NR | 75-100 mg |
| Methadone | 20 mg | 10 mg |
| Hydrocodone | 30 mg | — |
| Oxycodone | 15–20 mg | — |

Note: For comparison, a dosage of 10 mg of parenteral morphine is established.
NR = not recommended.
*Fentanyl is also available in the transdermal route (Duragesic).

Adapted from JCAHO (2001), Lehne (2004), McCaffery and Pasero (1999), Melzack and Wall (2003), Warfield and Bajwa (2004).

history of alcohol consumption or malnutrition status. Also, special care must be taken to avoid hepatotoxic doses in patients with hepatic dysfunction.

The use of NSAIDs is indicated in the patient with acute musculoskeletal and soft-tissue inflammation. Some patients, including the elderly, those with hypovolemia, or with preexisting renal impairment may be more susceptible to NSAID-induced renal failure. Also, the persistent use of NSAIDs is associated with a high rate of gastrointestinal bleeding in frail older patients. The use of COX-2 selective drugs appears to be safer than nonselective COX inhibitors in terms of gastrointestinal morbidity and antiplatelet effects, however risks with long-term use remains (AGS, 2009). Ketorolac is the only parenteral NSAID and is often used in the critical care setting, especially for postoperative pain (Summer & Puntillo, 2001). It should not be used more than 5 days, however, as its prolonged use has been associated with an increase in renal failure and bleeding (Jacobi et al., 2002). Therefore, a cautious use of this drug is required in the elderly.

## Adjuvants

Adjuvants (see Table 18.6) are sometimes used in preemptive analgesia, especially in the preoperative context, to prevent the establishment of peripheral and central sensitization of pain. Also, patients suffering from chronic pain may receive adjuvants in their treatment. A careful history of medications and doses is important at the admission of the patient in the intensive care unit (Hamill-Ruth & Marohn, 1999). For instance, a patient taking large doses of opioids on a long-term basis will be relatively tolerant to the effects of opioids administered in the ICU. Also, this patient may show withdrawal if analgesia is inadequate. The use of adjuvants (e.g., anticonvulsivants, antidepressants) for the treatment of chronic pain must also be considered, especially for neuropathic pain. For instance, discontinuing antidepressants may lead to withdrawal such as agitation and altered mental status in the patient. The use of anticonvulsivants (e.g., gabapentin) with relatively low side effect profiles may provide a better choice compared with traditional antidepressants in the older adult (AGS, 2009). The management of pain in patients with chronic pain must be discussed with the multidisciplinary team so that proper pain relief can be achieved for these patients in the ICU.

# Nonpharmacological Methods of Pain Management in the Critically Ill Older Adult

For older patients, a combination of pharmacologic and nonpharmacologic interventions have been shown to improve pain control, decrease analgesic use, increase activity and function, and decrease depression and anxiety (AGS, 2002, 2009; Farrell & Gibson, 1993; Good et al., 1999; Luskin et al., 2000; Rakel & Frantz, 2003). Studies demonstrate that older persons benefit from nonpharmacological approaches and these should be considered as part of the overall treatment plan (AGS, 2002; Herr et al., 2006; Veterans Health Administration/Department of Defense, 2002). However, not all nonpharmacological practices have been thoroughly evaluated in older persons and response to these interventions may vary. For acute postoperative pain, these approaches can be used to supplement analgesic treatment but are not intended to replace analgesics (Pasero, Rakel, & McCaffery, 2005). Nonpharmacological interventions have a place in critical care, but must be evaluated to determine appropriateness for a given patient. Use of nonpharmacological methods must be tailored to the patient's unique circumstances, taking into consideration pain etiology, patient preferences, cognitive ability, and physical capabilities.

Basic comfort measures also contribute to the older person's ability to cope with the pain experience. Assuring the least stressful environment, (e.g, decreased lighting and noise, privacy, limited visitors per patient desire), assuring rest and immobilization as needed, and promoting sleep can all support the older person's overall comfort and response to pain (Bowman, 1997; Miller & Talerico, 2002). Table 18.8 provides information on selected nonpharmacological methods that are useful in pain management for older persons.

## Cognitive-Behavioral Methods

Cognitive-behavioral approaches are often used to manage pain in older persons because of the concerns regarding long-term use of pain medications in this population (Gloth, 2000; Keefe et al., 2002). A variety of cognitive-behavioral methods are available, although appropriateness for the critically ill older adult must be carefully evaluated. Ability of older adults to use these methods is dependent on biological factors (medical comorbidities, sensory changes, cognitive changes), psychological factors (depression,

## 18.8 Selected Nonpharmacologic Interventions for Pain Management in Older Persons

| Intervention | Special Considerations |
|---|---|
| **Physical Methods** | |
| Superficial Heat (hot packs, heating pads, chemical gel packs) | ■ Protect skin and monitor regularly.<br>■ Older patients often prefer heat over cold |
| Superficial Cold (ice packs, chemical gel packs, terry cloth chilled in ice water) | ■ Protect skin and monitor regularly; gradual layering for cold pack that conforms to body contours<br>■ Cold should be avoided in patients with peripheral vascular disease, such as Raynaud's disease<br>■ Older patients often prefer heat and are reluctant to use cold; providing blankets or additional clothing may protect patient from generalized chilling |
| Massage | ■ Determine preference for touch/massage<br>■ Involve family in use<br>■ Back and shoulders, feet and hands usually preferred<br>■ Do not massage over painful extremities or open skin |
| Transcutaneous Electrical Nerve Stimulation (TENS) | ■ Contraindicated in patients with on-demand pacemaker<br>■ Determine patient characteristics that may diminish effect on pain (e.g., obesity, neuroticism, long-term opioid use)<br>■ Alternate electrode sites regularly to prevent skin breakdown |
| Vibration | ■ May be used as substitute for TENS; however, limited evidence<br>■ Often preferred for older adults<br>■ Do not use vibrating devices over areas of thrombophlebitis, over sites where skin has been injured or with migraine or other movement- or noise-exacerbated headaches |
| Mobilization/Immobilization | ■ Determine position of comfort<br>■ ROM to maintain joint function<br>■ Use supports appropriate to the situation (e.g, splinting, traction, positioning techniques) |
| **Cognitive-behavioral** | |
| Distraction (music, humor, movement/rhythm, visiting, television, praying, tapping a rhythm) | ■ Obtain information from patient and family regarding sources of distraction preferred<br>■ Identify music preferences to tailor music therapy<br>■ Be aware that patients distracted from their pain may not look like they are in pain, but this would be incorrect interpretation |
| Relaxation (progressive muscle relaxation, rhythmic breathing) | ■ Use of deep breathing exercises may be helpful<br>■ Consider Jacobson Jaw relaxation technique<br>■ Attempt lighting and noise reduction to promote relaxation |
| Imagery | ■ Determine interest in attempting imagery<br>■ Allow additional time for older adults to create and manipulate images<br>■ Avoid imagery in patients with severe cognitive impairment or psychosis |
| Education | ■ Increases sense of control |

Adapted from Herr et al. (2006). *Evidence-based Guideline for Acute Pain Management in Older Adults*. Iowa City, IA: The University of Iowa.

anxiety, fear of pain, helplessness, cognitive distortions, self-efficacy), and social factors (social support, access to treatment) (Waters, Woodward, & Keefe, 2005). Evidence from uncontrolled and randomized controlled studies suggests that older adults are likely to obtain benefits from these methods (Fry & Wong, 1991; Ersek, Turner, McCurry, Gibbons, & Kraybill, 2003; Reid, Otis, Barry, & Kerns, 2003). For critically ill older adults, the complexity of formal cognitive-behavioral approaches may limit their usefulness, and simpler cognitive approaches described in the text that follows may be more appropriate.

Distraction, including listening to music, watching a video or television, and talking with visitors, can be used as an adjunct to analgesic therapy that may distract from pain. Audiocassettes, with headphones, can be useful to provide individualized music therapy (Good et al., 2000). Music has been shown to improve sleep and to distract from pain after surgery (McCaffery & Good, 2000; Zimmerman, Nieveen, Barnason, & Schmaderer, 1996). Matching the music type used in the intervention to the music type preferred by the older adult increase effectiveness.

Relaxation is a good option as an adjunct therapy to control pain; it has been shown to give the patient a sense of control and to reduce muscle tension and anxiety (Houston & Jesurum, 1999; Miller & Perry, 1990). A simple deep-breathing exercise can be effective in creating relaxation (Good et al., 1999). Guided imagery has been effective in many older adults with pain (Antall & Kresevic, 2004; Deisch, Soukup, Adams, & Wild, 2000), however, some older adults express difficulty understanding the abstract tasks described.

## Physical Methods

Physical treatment approaches can be passive or active. Passive treatment includes superficial and deep-heating modalities, ultrasound, transcutaneous electrical nerve stimulation (TENS), acupuncture, joint mobilization, and soft-tissue massage (Scudds & Scudds, 2005). Active approaches include exercises aimed at increasing strength, endurance, flexibility, and balance. In the critical care setting, passive approaches are more relevant although the scientific evidence to support intervention benefits is greater for active approaches. The discussion that follows focuses on selected physical approaches that can be used with older persons with acute and/or persistent pain in the critical care setting.

Application of heat or cold may reduce sensitivity to pain and reduce muscle spasms (Titler & Rakel, 2001). Superficial heat is a common modality applied over the area of pain either as dry heat, such as an electric heating pad, or as moist heat. Application of heat in older persons requires precautions because of altered pain perception and increased pain thresholds (Gibson & Helme, 2001). Educating the patient or caregiver regarding monitoring for skin integrity and careful observation by staff is necessary.

TENS has been used in older individuals as an adjunct to pharmacologic therapy and involves electrical current passed through the skin via electrodes attached to the surface of the skin. TENS reduces pain by interfering with the gate control of peripheral pain sensations and by stimulating the endogenous opioid system (Sluka, Christy, Peterson, Rudd, & Troy, 1999). TENS has been most effective for acute postoperative pain, whereas controlled studies for management of persistent pain are inconsistent (Rakel & Herr, 2004; Scudds & Scudds, 2005). The use of TENS in the critical care setting may be limited because of contraindication in some patients with pacemakers or automatic implantable defibrillators. Special considerations when applying TENS with older adults are recommended (Johnson, 2002) (See Table 18.8).

Superficial massage has been shown to decrease pain in older persons presumably by relaxing muscles (Hattan, King, & Griffiths, 2000; Piotrowski et al., 2003; Wang & Keck, 2004), and has been found to be effective in critically ill patients (Richards, Gibson, & Overton-McCoy, 2000). It is thought to reduce pain through relaxation and by increasing blood flow to a painful area that may correspond with vasoconstriction, although effects on older adults with chronic pain are unclear. Long, slow strokes to the back and shoulders, or hands and feet, using a warm lubricant are recommended.

## Family-Caregiver Education/Support

Patient and family education is important and includes providing information on the nature of pain, how to use assessment instruments, medications, and nonpharmacologic management strategies (AGS, 2000). Specifically, fears and misbeliefs related to effective pain management must be addressed with the patient and especially the family/caregiver. Resistance to the treatment plan may result if concerns and misbeliefs are not identified and openly discussed. Of particular concern are the misbeliefs that opioids are too strong for older persons and that use of opioids will cause addiction (Herr, 2004; Kirsh & Smith, 2008). As noted earlier, use of opioids in older adults is safe if used according to recommendations that account for changes in aging that affect dosing and adverse reactions (AGS, 2000). Risk of respiratory depression is rare in persons experiencing pain, who are not opioid naïve, and who are monitored closely for sedation. Addiction is a form of psychological dependence on the drug that persists after discontinuation of the drug. It is unlike physical dependence in which the body develops a tolerance to the effects of the drug and responds with a withdrawal reaction if the drug is stopped without tapering (Arnstein, 2004). Although fear of addiction to opioids is a common concern, patients and families should be reassured that it is not likely to occur when treating pain in the critically ill older adult (Miyoshi & Leckband, 2001). In the critical care setting, patients and families require education regarding pain management options, discussion of any fears/concerns regarding analgesic use and side effects, and assurance that patients are monitored closely for any signs of adverse response to opioid therapy.

## Summary

Pain is very complex, especially in the critically ill elderly. Sources of pain in the critical care setting are multiple, and the effects of unrelieved acute pain may have a significant impact on the patient's recovery. To be accurately relieved, pain must first be adequately assessed. Pain assessment is a vital part of critical care nursing practice. Whenever possible, the patient's self-report of pain must be obtained, even if physical barriers such as the endotracheal tube alter the patient's ability to communicate. However, when the patient is unable to communicate in any way, behavioral indicators represent alternative measures of pain assessment. Some tools have been developed for the cognitively impaired and the critically ill population. The critical care nurse must use the appropriate tools to adequately assess the patient's pain. He/she must accurately assess the patient's pain to participate, with the multidisciplinary team, in the development of the patient's pain management plan. To do so, the critical care nurse must also be familiar with analgesia and other therapies, and should consider including nonpharmacological methods to achieve proper pain relief.

# References

Agency for Health Care Policy and Research (AHCPR). (1992). *Acute pain management: Operative or medical procedures and trauma.* Rockville, MD: AHCPR, Public Health Service, U.S. Department of Health and Human Services.

American Geriatrics Society Panel on Persistent Pain in Older Persons (AGS). (2002). The management of persistent pain in older persons. *Journal of the American Geriatrics Society, 50,* S205–S274.

American Geriatrics Society Panel on the Pharmacological Management of Persistent Pain in Older Persons (AGS). (2009). The management of persistent pain in older persons. *Journal of the American Geriatrics Society, 57,* 1331–1346.

American Pain Society. (2003). *Principles of analgesic use in the treatment of acute pain and chronic cancer pain* (4th ed.). Glenville.

American Psychiatric Association (APA). (2000). *Diagnostic and statistical manual of mental disorders* (4th ed., text rev), Washington DC: American Psychiatric Press.

Anand, K. J. S., & Craig, K. D. (1996). New perspectives on the definition of pain. *Pain, 67,* 3–6.

Angus, D. C., Kelley, M. A., Schmitz, R. J., White, A., & Popovich, J. (2000). Current and projected workforce requirements for care of the critically ill and patients with pulmonary disease. *Journal of the American Medical Association, 284*(21), 2762–2770.

Antall, G. F., & Kresevic, D. (2004). The use of guided imagery to manage pain in an elderly orthopaedic population. *Orthopaedic Nursing, 23*(5), 335–340.

Ardery, G., Herr, K., Hannon, B. J., & Titler, M. G. (2003). Lack of opioid administration in older hip fracture patients (ce). *Geriatric Nursing, 24*(6), 353–360.

Ardery, G., Herr, K. A., Titler, M. G., Sorofman, B. A., & Schmitt, M. B. (2003b). Assessing and managing acute pain in older adults: A research base to guide practice. *MEDSURG Nursing, 12*(1), 7–19.

Arnstein, P. (2004). Chronic neuropathic pain: Issues in patient education. *Pain Management Nursing, 5*(4), 34–41.

Aslan, F. E., Badir, A., & Selimen, D. (2003). How do intensive care nurses assess patients' pain? *Nursing in Critical Care, 8*(2), 62–67.

Aubin, M., Giguère, A., Hadjistavropoulos, T., & Verreault, R. (2007). L'évaluation systématique des instruments pour mesurer la douleur chez les personnes âgées ayant des capacités réduites à communiquer. *Pain Research & Management, 12* (3), 195–203.

Bartocci, M., Bergqvist, L. L., Lagercrantz, H., & Anand, K. J. S. (2006). Pain activates cortical areas in the preterm newborn brain. *Pain, 122,* 109–117.

Bernabei, R., Gambassi, G., Lapane, K., Landi, F., Gatsonis, C., Dunlop, R., et al. (1998). Management of pain in elderly patients with cancer. *JAMA: Journal of the American Medical Association, 279*(23), 1877–1882.

Berthier, F., Potel, G., Leconte, P., Touze, M. D., & Baron, D. (1998). Comparative study of methods of measuring acute pain intensity in an ED. *American Journal of Emergency Medicine, 16,* 132–137.

Bjoro, K., & Herr, K. (2008). Assessment of pain in the nonverbal or cognitively impaired older adult. *Clinics in Geriatric Medicine, 24,* 237–262.

Bowman, A. M. (1997). Sleep satisfaction, perceived pain and acute confusion in elderly clients undergoing orthopaedic procedures. *Journal of Advanced Nursing, 26*(3), 550–564.

Brown, J. C., Klein, E. J., Lewis, C. W., Johnston, B. D., & Cummings, P. (2003). Emergency department analgesia for fracture pain. *Annals of Emergency Medicine, 42*(2), 197–205.

Bruera, E., Fainsinger, R. L., Miller, M. J., & Kuehn, N. (1992). The assessment of pain intensity in patients with cognitive failure: A preliminary report. *Journal of Pain & Symptom Management, 7*(5), 267–270.

Carey, S. J., Turpin, C., Smith, J., Whatley, J., & Haddox, D. (1997). Improving pain management in an acute care setting: The Crawford Long Hospital of Emory University experience. *Orthopaedic Nursing, 16* (4), 29–36.

Carr, D. B., & Goudas, L. C. (1999). Acute pain. *Lancet, 353*(9169), 2051–2058.

Carroll, K. C., Atkins, P. J., Herold, G. R., Mlcek, C. A., Shively, M., Clopton, P., et al. (1999). Pain assessment and management in critically ill postoperative and trauma patients: A multisite study. *American Journal of Critical Care, 8*(2), 105–117.

Charlton, J. E. (2005). *Core curriculum for professional education in pain* (3rd ed.). International Association for the Study of Pain. Seattle: IASP Press.

Cousins, M. J., & Power, I. (1999). Acute and postoperative pain. In P. D. Wall & R. Melzack (Eds.), *Textbook of pain* (4th ed., pp. 447–491). Edinburgh: Churchill Livingston.

Dawson, K. A. (2008). Palliative care for critically ill older adults: Dimensions of nursing advocacy. *Critical Care Nursing Quarterly, 31*(1), 19–23.

Decker, S. A., & Perry, A. G. (2003). The development and testing of the PATCOA to assess pain in confused older adults. *Pain Management Nursing, 4*, 77–86.

Deisch, P., Soukup, M., Adams, P., & Wild, M. C. (2000). Guided imagery: Replication study using coronary artery bypass graft patients. *Nursing Clinics of North America, 35*(2), 417–425.

Desbiens, N. A., Wu, A. W., Broste, S. K., Wenger, N. S., Connors, A. F., Jr., Lynn, J., et al. (1996). Pain and satisfaction with pain control in seriously ill hospitalized adults: Findings from the support research investigations. For the support investigators. Study to understand prognoses and preferences for outcomes and risks of treatment. *Critical Care Medicine, 24*(12), 1953–1961.

Dracup, K., & Bryan-Brown, C. W. (1995). Pain in the ICU: Fact or fiction? *American Journal of Critical Care, 4*(5), 337–339.

Dunn, K. S., & Horgas, A. L. (2004). Religious and nonreligious coping in older adults experiencing chronic pain. *Pain Management Nursing, 5*(1), 19.

Dworkin, R. H., Backonja, M., Rowbotham, M. C., Allen, R. R., Argoff, C. R., Bennett, G. J., et al. (2003). Advances in neuropathic pain: Diagnosis, mechanisms, and treatment recommendations. *Archives of Neurology, 60*(11), 1524–1534.

Ersek, M., Turner, J. A., McCurry, S. M., Gibbons, L., & Kraybill, B. M. (2003). Efficacy of a self-management group intervention for elderly persons with chronic pain. *Clinical Journal of Pain, 19*(3), 156–167.

Feldt, K. S., Ryden, M. B., & Miles, S. (1998). Treatment of pain in cognitively impaired compared with cognitively intact older patients with hip-fracture. *Journal of the American Geriatrics Society, 46*(9), 1079–1085.

Feldt, K. S., Warne, M. A., & Ryden, M. B. (1998). Examining pain in aggressive cognitively impaired older adults. *Journal of Gerontological Nursing, 24*(11), 14–22.

Frazier, S. K., Moser, D. K., Riegel, B., McKinley, S., Blakely, W., Kim, K. A., et al. (2002). Critical care nurses' assessment of patients' anxiety: Reliance on physiological and behavioral parameters. *American Journal of Critical Care, 11*(1), 57–64.

Fry, P. S., & Wong, P. T. P. (1991). Pain management training in the elderly: Matching interventions with subjects' coping styles. *Stress Medicine, 7*, 93–98.

Fuchs-Labelle, S., & Hadjistavropoulos, T. (2004). Development and preliminary validation of the Pain Assessment Checklist for Seniors with Limited Ability to Communicate (PACSLAC). *Pain Management Nursing, 5*(1), 37–49.

Gélinas, C. (2007a). Management of pain in cardiac surgery ICU patients: Have we improved over time? *Intensive and Critical Care Nursing, 23*, 298–303.

Gélinas, C. (2007b). Le thermomètre d'intensité de douleur : Un nouvel outil pour les patients adultes en soins critiques [the Faces Pain Thermometer: A new tool for critically ill adults]. *Perspective infirmière, 4*(4), 12–20.

Gélinas, C., Choinière, M., Ranger, M., Denault, A., Deschamps, A., Johnston, C. (in press). *Towards a new approach for the detection of pain in adults: The near-infrared spectroscopy* (NIRS)–A pilot study. Heart & Lung.

Gélinas, C., Fillion, L., Puntillo, K., Viens, C., & Fortier, M. (2006). Validation of a Critical-Care Pain Observation Tool in adult patients. *American Journal of Critical Care, 15*(4), 420–427.

Gélinas, C., Fortier, M., Viens, C., Fillion, L., & Puntillo, K. (2004). Pain assessment and management in critically ill intubated patients: A retrospective study. *American Journal of Critical Care, 13*(2), 126.

Gélinas, C., & Johnston, C. (2007). Pain assessment in the critically ill ventilated adult: Validation of the Critical-Care Pain Observation Tool and physiological indicators. *Clinical Journal of Pain, 23*(6), 497–505.

Gélinas, C., Viens, C., Fortier, M., & Fillion, L. (2005). Les indicateurs de la douleur en soins critiques [Pain indicators in critical care]. *Perspective Infirmière, 2*(4), 12–22.

Gibson, S. J., & Farrell, M. (2004). A review of age differences in the neurophysiology of nociception and the perceptual experience of pain. *Clinical Journal of Pain, 20*(4), 227–239.

Gibson, S. J., & Helme, R. D. (2001). Age-related differences in pain perception and report. *Clinics in Geriatric Medicine, 17*(3), 433–456.

Glasson, J. C., Sawyer, W. T., Lindley, C. M., & Ginsberg, B. (2002). Patient-specific factors affecting patient-controlled analgesia dosing. *Journal of Pain & Palliative Care Pharmacotherapy, 16*(2), 5–21.

Gloth III, F. M. (2000). Geriatric pain. *Geriatrics, 55*(10), 46–48.

Good, M., Picot, B. L., Salem, S. G., Chin, C., Picot, S. F., & Lane, D. (2000). Cultural differences in music chosen for pain relief. Five pain studies. *Journal of Holistic Nursing, 18*(3), 245–260.

Good, M., Stanton-Hicks, M., Grass, J. A., Cranston Anderson, G., Choi, C., Schoolmeesters, L. J., et al. (1999). Relief of postoperative pain with jaw relaxation, music and their combination. *Pain, 81*(1–2), 163–172.

Graf, C., & Puntillo, K. A. (2003). Pain in the older adult in the intensive care unit. *Critical Care Clinics, 19*, 749–770.

Groeger, J. S., Guntupalli, K. K., Strosberg, M., Halpern, N., Raphaely, R. C., Cerra, F., et al. (1993). Descriptive analysis of critical care units in the United States: Patient characteristics and intensive care unit utilization. *Critical Care Medicine, 21*(2), 279–291.

Hadjistavropoulos, T., Herr, K., Turk, D., Fine, P. G., Dworkin, R. H., Helme, R., et al. (2007). An interdisciplinary expert consensus statement on assessment of pain in older persons. *Clinical Journal of Pain, 23*(Suppl. 1), S1–S43.

Hamill-Ruth, R. J., & Marohn, M. L. (1999). Evaluation of pain in the critically ill patient. *Critical Care Clinics, 15*(1), 35–54, v–vi.

Hattan, J., King, L., & Griffiths, P. (2002). The impact of foot massage and guided relaxation following cardiac surgery: A randomized controlled trial. *Journal of Advanced Nursing, 37*(2), 199–207.

Herr, K. (2004). Persistent pain in older adults—We can do better! *New Zealand Family Physician, 3*(2), 68–71.

Herr, K., Coyne, P. J., Key, T., Manworren, R., McCaffery, M., Merkel, S., et al. (2006). Pain assessment in the nonverbal patient: Position statement with clinical practice recommendations. *Pain Management Nursing, 7*(2), 44–52.

Herr, K., & Decker, S. (2004). Assessment of pain in older adults with severe cognitive impairment. *Annals of Long-Term Care, 12*(4), 46–52.

Herr, K. A., & Garand, L. (2001). Assessment and measurement of pain in older adults. *Clinics in Geriatric Medicine, 17*(3), 457–478.

Herr, K.A., & Mobily, P.R. (1993). Comparison of selected pain assessment tools for use with the elderly. *Applied Nursing Research, 6* (1), 39–46.

Herr, K., Spratt, K. F., Garand, L., & Li, L. (2007). Evaluation of the Iowa Pain Thermometer and other selected pain intensity scales in younger and older adult cohorts using controlled clinical pain: A preliminary study. *Pain Medicine, 8*(7), 585–600.

Herr, K., Spratt, K., Mobily, P., & Richardson, G. (2004). Pain intensity assessment in older adults: Use of experimental pain to compare psychometric properties and usability of selected scales in adult and other population. *Clinical Journal of Pain, 20*(4), 207–219.

Hicks, C. L., von Baeyer, C. L., Spafford, P. A., van Korlaar, I., & Goodenough, B. (2001). The Faces Pain Scale–Revised: Toward a common metric in pediatric pain measurement. *Pain, 93*, 173–183.

Horgas, A. L., & Tsai, P. F. (1998). Analgesic drug prescription and use in cognitively impaired nursing home residents. *Nursing Research, 47*(4), 235–242.

Houston, S., & Jesurum, J. (1999). The quick relaxation technique: Effect on pain associated with chest tube removal. *Applied Nursing Research, 12*(4), 196–205.

Hurwitz, B. E., Nelesen, R. A., Saab, P. G., Nagel, J. H., Spitzer, S. B., Gellman, M. D., et al. (1993). Differential patterns of dynamic cardiovascular regulation as a function of task. *Biological Psychology, 36*, 75–95.

International Association for the Study of Pain, Subcommittee on Taxonomy (IASP). Pain terms: A list with definitions and notes on usage. *Pain, 6* 249–252.

IASP Task Force on Taxonomy. (1994). *Classification of chronic pain*. Seattle, WA: IASP Press.

Jacobi, J., Fraser, G. L., Coursin, D. B., Riker, R. R., Fontaine, D., Wittbrodt, E. T., et al. (2002). Clinical practice guidelines for the sustained use of sedatives and analgesics in the critically ill adult [corrected] [published erratum appears in *Critical Care Medicine*, 2002 30(3), 726]. *Critical Care Medicine, 30*(1), 119–141.

Johnson, M. (2002). Transcutaneous electrical nerve stimulation (tens). In S. Kitchen (Ed.), *Electrotherapy: Evidenced-based practice* (11th ed., pp. 259–286). Edinburgh: Churchill Livingstone.

Joint Commission on Accreditzation of Healalthcare Organizations. (JCAHO). *Pain: Curent understanding of assessment, management, and treatments*. Oakbrook Terrace, IC: Author.

Keefe, F. J., Buffington, A. L. H., Studts, J. L., Smith, S. J., Gibson, J., & Caldwell, D. S. (2002). Recent advances and future directions in the biopsychosocial assessment and treatment of arthritis. *Journal of Consulting & Clinical Psychology, 70*(3), 640–655.

Kirsh, K. L., & Smith, H. S. (2008). Special issues and concerns in the evaluation of older adults who have pain. *Clinics in Geriatric Medicine, 24*(2), 263–274, vi.

Kwekkeboom, K. L., & Herr, K. (2001). Assessment of pain in the critically ill. *Critical Care Nursing Clinics of North America, 13* (2), 181–194.

Lay, T. D., Puntillo, K. A., Miaskowski, C. A., & Wallhagen, M. I. (1996). Analgesics prescribed and administered to intensive care cardiac surgery patients: Does patient age make a difference? *Progress in Cardiovascular Nursing, 11*(4), 17-24.

Li, D. T. Y., Miaskowski, C. A., Burkhardt, D. H., & Puntillo, K. A. (in press). Physiologic and behavioral responses associated with noxious procedures in sedated critically ill patients. *Journal of Critical Care.*

Li, D., Puntillo, K., & Miaskowski, C. (2008). A review of objective pain measures for use with critical care adult patients unable to self-report. *Journal of Pain, 9*(1), 2–10.

Luskin, F. M., Newell, K. A., Griffith, M., Holmes, M., Telles, S., DiNucci, E., et al. (2000). A review of mind/body therapies in the treatment of musculoskeletal disorders with implications for the elderly. *Alternative Therapies in Health Medicine, 6*(2), 46-56.

Manfredi, P. L., Breuer, B., Wallenstein, S., Stegmann, M., Bottomley, G., & Libow, L. (2003). Opioid treatment for agitation in patients with advanced dementia. *International Journal of Geriatric Psychiatry, 18*(8), 700–705.

Mateo, O. M., & Krenzischek, D. A. (1992). A pilot study to assess the relationship between behavioral manifestations and self-report of pain in postanesthesia care unit patients. *Journal of Post Anesthesia Nursing, 7*(1), 15–21.

Matteson, M. A., & McConnell, E. S. (1988). *Gerontological nursing: Concepts and practice.* Philadelphia: W. B. Saunders.

McCaffery, M. (1968). *Nursing practice theories related to cognition, bodily pain, and man-environment interactions.* Los Angeles: University of California.

McCaffery, M., & Pasero, C. (1999). *Pain: Clinical manual* (2nd ed.). St. Louis: Mosby.

McCaffrey, R. G., & Good, M. (2000). The lived experience of listening to music while recovering from surgery. *Journal of Holistic Nursing, 18*(4), 378–390.

McCance, K. L., & Huether, S. E. (1998). *Pathophysiology: The biologic basis for Disease in adults and children* (3rd ed.). St. Louis: Mosby.

McGuire, D. B. (1992). Comprehensive and multidimensional assessment and measurement of pain. *Journal of Pain & Symptom Management, 7*(5), 312.

McNicoll, L., Pisani, M. A., Zhang, Y., Ely, E. W., Siegel, M. D., & Inouye, S. K. (2003). Delirium in the intensive care unit: Occurrence and clinical course in older patients. *Journal of the American Geriatrics Society, 51*(5), 591–598.

Meehan, D. A., McRae, M. E., Rourke, D. A., Eisenring, C., & Imperial, F. A. (1995). Analgesic administration, pain intensity, and patient satisfaction in cardiac surgical patients. *American Journal of Critical Care, 4*(6), 435–442.

Melzack, R. (1999). From the gate to the neuromatrix. *Pain,* (Suppl. 6), S121–S126.

Melzack, R., & Wall, P. D. (2003). *Handbook of pain management.* Edinburgh: Churchill Livingston.

Miller, K. M., & Perry, P. A. (1990). Relaxation technique and postoperative pain in patients undergoing cardiac surgery. *Heart & Lung, 19*(2), 136–146.

Miller, L. L., & Talerico, K. A. (2002). Pain in older adults. In *Annual review of nursing research* (Vol 20, pp. 63–88), New York: Springer Publishing Company.

Miyoshi, H. R., & Leckband, S. G. (2001). Systemic opioid analgesics. In J. D. Loeser, S. H. Butler, R. C. Chapman & D. C. Turks (Eds.), *Bonica's management of pain* (3rd ed., pp. 1682–1709). Philadelphia: Lippincott, Williams & Wilkins.

Moore, A. R., & Clinch, D. (2004). Underlying mechanisms of impaired visceral pain perception in older people. *Journal of the American Geriatrics Society, 52*(1), 132–136.

Morrison, R. S., Ahronheim, J. C., Morrison, G. R., Darling, E., Baskin, S. A., Morris, J., et al. (1998). Pain and discomfort associated with common hospital procedures and experiences. *Journal of Pain & Symptom Management, 15*(2), 91–101.

Morrison, R. S., Magaziner, J., Gilbert, M., Koval, K. J., McLaughlin, M. A., Orosz, G., et al. (2003a). Relationship between pain and opioid analgesics on the development of delirium following hip fracture. *Journal of Gerontology Series A Biological Sciences and Medical Sciences, 58*(1), 76-81.

Morrison, R. S., Magaziner, J., McLaughlin, M. A., Orosz, G., Silberzweig, S. B., Koval, K. J., et al. (2003b). The impact of post-operative pain on outcomes following hip fracture. *Pain, 103*(3), 303–311.

Morrison, R. S., & Siu, A. L. (2000). A comparison of pain and its treatment in advanced dementia and cognitively intact patients with hip fracture. *J Pain Symptom Manage, 19*(4), 240-248.

Odhner, M., Wegman, D., Freeland, N., Steinmetz, A., & Ingersoll, G. L. (2003). Assessing pain control in nonverbal critically ill adults. *Dimensions of Critical Care Nursing, 22*(6), 260–267.

Pasero, C. (2004). Pathophysiology of neuropathic pain. *Pain Management Nursing, 5*(47), 3–8.

Pasero, C., Manworren, R. C. B., & McCaffery, M. (2007). IV opioids range orders for acute pain management. *American Journal of Nursing, 107* (2), 62–69.

Pasero, C., & McCaffery, M. (2000). Reversing respiratory depression with naloxone. *American Journal of Nursing, 100*(2), 26.

Pasero, C., Rakel, B., & McCaffery, M. (2005). Postoperative pain management in the older adult. In S. Gibson & D. Weiner (Eds.), *Pain in older persons. Progress in pain research and management* (Vol. 35, pp. 377–401). Seattle, WA: IASP Press.

Payen, J. F., Bru, O., Bosson, J. L., Lagrasta, A., Novel, E., Deschaux, I., Lavagne, P., & Jacquot, C. (2001). Assessing pain in the critically ill sedated patients by using a behavioral pain scale. *Critical Care Medicine, 29* (12), 2258–2263.

Pergolizzi, J., Böger, R. H., Budd, K., Dahan, A., Erdine, S., Hans, G., et al. (2008). Opioids and the management of chronic severe pain in the elderly: Consensus statement of an international expert panel with focus on the six clinically most often used world health organization step III opioids (Buprenorphine, Fentanyl, Hydromorphone, Methadone, Morphine, Oxycodone). *Pain Practice, 8*(4), 287–313.

Piotrowski, M. M., Paterson, C., Mitchinson, A., Kim, H. M., Kirsh, M., & Hinshaw, D. B. (2003). Massage as adjuvant therapy in the management of acute postoperative pain: A preliminary study in men. *Journal of the American College of Surgeons, 197*(6), 1037–1046.

Pooler-Lunse, C., & Price, P. (1992). Pain and the critically ill. *Canadian Nurse, 88*(7), 22–25.

Puntillo, K. A. (1990). Pain experiences of intensive care unit patients. *Heart & Lung, 19*(5 part 1), 526–533.

Puntillo, K. A. (1994). Dimensions of procedural pain and its analgesic management in critically ill surgical patients. *American Journal of Critical Care, 3*(2), 116–122.

Puntillo, K. A., Miaskowski, C., Kehrle, K., Stannard, D., Gleeson, S., & Nye, P. (1997). Relationship between behavioral and physiological indicators of pain, critical care self-reports of pain, and opioid administration. *Critical Care Medicine, 25* (7), 1159–1166.

Puntillo, K. A., Morris, A. B., Thompson, C. L., Stanik-Hutt, J., White, C. A., & Wild, L. R. (2004). Pain behaviors observed during six common procedures: Results from Thunder Project II. *Critical Care Medicine, 32*(2), 421–427.

Puntillo, K. A., Rietman, L., Morris, A. B., Stanik-Hutt, J., Thompson, C. L., & White, C. (2002). Practices and predictors of analgesic interventions for adults undergoing painful procedures. *American Journal of Critical Care, 11*(5), 415–429.

Puntillo, K. A., Stannard, D., Miaskowski, C., Kehrle, K., & Gleeson, S. (2002). Use of a pain assessment and intervention notation (P.A.I.N.) tool in critical care nursing practice: Nurses' evaluations. *Heart & Lung, 31*(4), 303-314.

Puntillo, K., & Weiss, S. J. (1994). Pain: Its mediators and associated morbidity in critically ill cardiovascular surgical patients. *Nursing Research, 43*(1), 31–36.

Puntillo, K.A., White, C., Morris, A.B., Perdue, S.T., Stanik-Hutt, J., Thompson, C.L.,et al. (2001). Patients' perceptions and responses to procedural pain: Results from Thunder Project II. *American Journal of Critical Care, 10*(4), 238–251.

Rainero, I., Vigletti, S., Bergamasco, B., Piressi, L., & Beneditte, F. (2000). Autonomic responses and pain perception in Alzheimer's disease. *European Journal of Pain, 4*(3), 267–274.

Rakel, B., & Frantz, R. (2003). Effectiveness of transcutaneous electrical nerve stimulation on postoperative pain with movement. *Journal of Pain, 4*(8), 455–464.

Rakel, B., & Herr, K. (2004). Assessment and treatment of postoperative pain in older adults. *Journal of PeriAnesthesia Nursing, 19*(3), 194–208.

Reuben, D., Herr, K., Paeala, J., Pollack, B., Potter, J., & Semla, T. (2009). *Geratrics at Your Fingertips: 2009* (II PL ed.). New York: American Geratrics Society.

Ready, L. B., & Edwards, W. T. (Eds.). (1992). *Management of acute pain: A practical guide. Taskforce on acute pain.* Seattle, WA: IASP Publications.

Reid, M. C., Otis, J., Barry, L. C., & Kerns, R. D. (2003). Cognitive-behavioral therapy for chronic low back pain in older persons: A preliminary study. *Pain Medicine, 4*(3), 223–430.

Richards, K. C., Gibson, R., & Overton-McCoy, A. L. (2000). Effects of massage in acute and critical care. *AACN Clinical Issues Advanced Practice in Acute Critical Care, 11*(1), 77–96.

Scudds, R. J., & Scudds, R. A. (2005). Therapy approaches to the management of pain in older adults. In S. J. Gibson & D. K. Weiner (Eds.), *Pain in older persons* (pp. 223–237). Seattle, WA: IASP Press.

Selye, H. (1974). *Stress without distress.* Philadelphia: J.B. Lippincott.

Sessler, C. N., Grap, M. J., & Ramsey, M. A. E. (2008). Evaluating and monitoring analgesia and sedation in the intensive care unit. *Critical Care, 12.* Available at http://ccforum.com/content/12/S3/S2.

Shannon, K., & Bucknall, T. (2003). Pain assessment in critical care: What have we learnt from research. *Intensive & Critical Care Nursing, 19*(3), 154.

Slater, R., Cantarella, A., Gallella, S., Worley, A., Boyd, S., Meek, J., & Fitzgerald, M. (2006). Cortical pain responses in human infants. *e Journal of Neuroscience, 26*(14), 3662–3666.

Sluka, K. A., Christy, M. R., Peterson, W. L., Rudd, S. L., & Troy, S. M. (1999). Reduction of pain-related behaviors with either cold or heat treatment in an animal model of acute arthritis. *Archives of Physical Medicine Rehabilitation, 80*(3), 313–317.

Stanik-Hutt, J. A., Soeken, K. L., Belcher, A. E., Fontaine, D. K., & Gift, A. G. (2001). Pain experiences of traumatically injured patients in a critical care setting. *American Journal of Critical Care, 10*(4), 252–259.

Stein-Parbury, J., & McKinley, S. (2000). Patients' experiences of being in an intensive care unit: A select literature review. *American Journal of Critical Care, 9*(1), 20–27.

Stuppy, D. J. (1998). The Faces Pain Scale: reliability and validity with mature adults. *Applied Nursing Research, 11* (2), 84–89.

Summer, G. J., & Puntillo, K. A. (2001). Management of surgical and procedural pain in a critical care setting. *Critical Care Nursing Clinics of North America, 13* (2), 233–242.

SUPPORT Investigators. (1995). A controlled trial to improve care of seriously ill hospitalized patients: The Study to Understand Prognoses and Preferences for Outcomes and Risks of Treatments (SUPPORT), *Journal of the American Medical Association, 274*, 1591–1598.

Titler, M. G., & Rakel, B. A. (2001). Nonpharmacologic treatment of pain. *Critical Care Nursing Clinics of North America, 13*(2), 221–232.

Tittle, M., & McMillan, S. C. (1994). Pain and pain-related side effects in an ICU and on a surgical unit: Nurses' management. *American Journal of Critical Care, 3*(1), 25–30.

Tullmann, D. F., & Dracup, K. (2000). Creating a healing environment for elders. *AACN Clinical Issues: Advanced Practice in Acute & Critical Care, 11*(1), 34–50.

United States Census Bureau. (2008). *United States census, 2000.* Retrieved June 30, 2008, from http://www.census.gov/main/www/cen2000.html

Wang, H., & Keck, J. F. (2004). Foot and hand massage as an intervention for postoperative pain. *Pain Management Nursing, 5*(2), 59–65.

Ware, L., Epps, C. D., Herr, K., & Packard, A. (2006). Evaluation of the Revised Faces Pain Scale, Verbal Descriptor Scale, Numeric Rating Scale, and Iowa Pain Thermometer in older minority adults. *Pain Management Nursing, 7*(3), 117–125.

Wary, B., & Doloplus, C. (1999). Doloplus-2, a scale for pain measurement. *Soins Gérontologiques, 19*, 25–27.

Wary, B., Serbouti, S., Doloplus, C. (2001). Doloplus 2: Validation d'une échelle d'évaluation comportementale de la douleur chez la personne âgée. *Douleurs, 1*, 35–38.

Waters, S. J., Woodward, J. T., & Keefe, F. J. (2005). Cognitive-behavioral therapy for pain in older adults. *Progress in Pain Research and Management, 35*, 239–262.

Weiner, D., Peterson, B., & Keefe, F. (1998). Evaluating persistent pain in long term care residents: What role for pain maps? *Pain, 76*, 249–257.

Wynne, C. F., Ling, S. M., & Remsbourg, R. (2000). Comparison of pain assessment instruments in cognitively intact and cognitively impaired nursing home residents. *Geriatric Nursing, 21*, 20–23.

Young, J., Siffleet, J., Nikoletti, S., & Shaw, T. (2006). Use of a Behavioural Pain Scale to assess pain in ventilated, unconscious and/or sedated patients. *Intensive and Critical Care Nursing, 22*, 32–39.

Zimmerman, L., Nieveen, J., Barnason, S., & Schmaderer, M. (1996). The effects of music interventions on postoperative pain and sleep in coronary artery bypass graft (CABG) patients. Including commentary by Miaskowski C. *Scholarly Inquiry for Nursing Practice, 10*(2), 153–174.

Zwakhalen, S. M. G., Hamers, J. P. H., Abu-Saad, H. H., & Berger, M. P. F. (2006). Pain in elderly people with severe dementia: A systematic review of behavioural pain assessment tools. *BMC Geriatrics, 6*(3), 1–15

# Part IV

# Approaches to Complex Clinical Issues in Critically Ill Older Adults

# Pressure Ulcer Prevention and Management

# 19

Tom Defloor
Katrien Vanderwee
Carol Dealey

## Introduction

The cost of pressure ulcers is high, both in terms of suffering caused to the patient and the financial burden on society and the patient (Bennett, Dealey, & Posnett, 2004; Edwards, 1994; Hopkins, Dealey, Bale, Defloor, & Worboys, 2006; Langemo, Melland, Hanson, Olson, & Hunter, 2000; Nixon et al., 2006; Thomson & Brooks, 1999). Pressure ulcer prevalence ranges from 2.3 to 28% in long-term-care facilities (Coleman, Martau, Lin, & Kramer, 2002; Lahmann, Halfens, & Dassen, 2005). Incidence figures on intensive care wards vary between 8 and 40% (National Pressure Ulcer Advisory Panel, 2001). Prevention of pressure ulcers is important from the viewpoint of the patient, care provider, and society.

According to a report from the Dutch Health Council, pressure ulcers are responsible for 1.3% of the total costs of Dutch health care and for this reason rate among the top four illnesses as far as costs are concerned. In this study no account has been taken of the nonmedical costs (paid by the patient) and productivity costs (costs of absenteeism as a result of poor health) (Health Council of the Netherlands, 1999; Severens, Habraken, Duivenvoorden, & Frederiks, 2002).

The American Healthcare Cost and Utilization Project reported a mean length of stay for hospitalizations specifically for pressure ulcers of 13 days, and an average

# 19.1

Conceptual model.

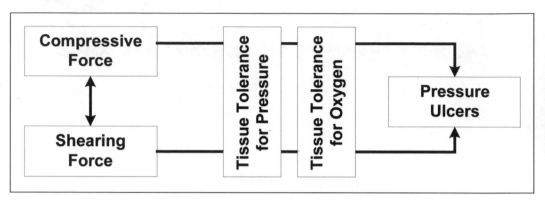

charge of $37,800 (Russo & Elixhauser, 2006). The lowest possible incidence of pressure ulcers in geriatric care can only be achieved if an effective prevention policy is carried out well. This requires a coordinated approach in which account is taken of both effectiveness and the practical feasibility of the preventative measures.

## Pathogenesis

A pressure ulcer is a degenerative change of tissue that originates from a deficiency of oxygen arising from pressure and shearing force (Defloor, 1999; European Pressure Ulcer Advisory Panel, 1999). These forces inhibit the blood supply to the tissue through pressure closing and/or shear closure of the blood vessels (see Figure 19.1). Whether this will eventually result in a deficiency of oxygen in the tissue cells is influenced by the duration and intensity of the pressure and shearing force and by the tolerance of the tissue to these forces. Compressing force is defined as a force that places a vertical load onto the tissue, whereas shearing force is a force that places a parallel force on the tissue.

## Compressing Force

A compressing force higher than the capillary pressure will curb the flow in the capillaries and lymphatic vessels, resulting in, on the one hand, an insufficient oxygen and nutrition supply and, on the other hand, an inadequate drainage of waste products. Perpendicular forces exerted on the skin above a bone part unite in a small area of the subcutaneous fat and muscular tissue just above the bone part. The pressure exerted on the skin becomes greater by a factor of 3 to 5 in the tissue at the bony projection (Welch, 1990). The pressure thus increases with the depth of the tissue. It is smallest on the skin and greatest at the underlying bone tissue. This is one of the reasons why extensive damage can occur in deep tissues, without the skin being affected. This effect is stimulated further by the fact that the skin is mechanically stronger than the deeper lying tissues and in a better state to withstand periods of ischemia.

## Shearing Force

Shearing force is a mechanical burden that is exerted through forces parallel to the surface. Shearing forces occur from a half-sitting position in a bed or armchair. The skeleton and the deep fascia slide downward here because of gravity; the skin and superficial fascia do not slide along with it because of the higher friction coefficient of seat or mattress. This movement of two tissue layers in relation to each other leads to stretching, kinking, and possible tearing of the perforated veins in the subcutaneous tissues, through which a deep necrosis can originate.

## Tissue Tolerance

Compressing force and shearing force is not sufficient to explain the origination of pressure ulcers completely. Other factors (tissue tolerance) also appear to play a role in this process. Tissue tolerance contains a number of risk factors that are known or suspected of influencing the individual's risk of getting pressure ulcers, without being directly influenced by the magnitude or duration of the compressing force and/or shearing force (Defloor, 1999).

The extent to which the exerted pressure will be enough to cause the occurrence of pressure ulcer injury is influenced by the tissue tolerance for pressure. Decrease in the tissue's capacity to dissipate pressure is linked to increased age, dehydration, protein and vitamin deficiency, and stress. Because of the presence of more of these factors, for example, age, diminished skin elasticity, cardiovascular problems, multipathology, decreased mobility, the older adult has an increased risk of the development of pressure ulcers: Specific risk factors for the critical care population are duration of surgery and number of operations, fecal incontinence and/or diarrhea, low preoperative protein and albumin concentrations, disturbed sensory perception, moisture of the skin, impaired circulation, use of inotropic drugs, diabetes mellitus, too unstable to turn, decreased mobility, high APACHE II score, history of vascular disease, intermittent hemodialysis, continuous veno-venous hemofiltration, mechanical ventilation (Keller, Will, van Ramshorst, & van der Werken 2004; Nijs et al., 2009).

So long as the supply of oxygen to the tissue meets its needs, no pressure ulcer occurs. If, however, either the oxygen supply drops, or the tissue's oxygen needs increase, an oxygen deficiency can occur and the risk of pressure ulcer increases. Tissue tolerance to changes in oxygen concentration will be determined by whether the oxygen deficiency can be neutralized or not.

## Observation of Pressure Ulcers

The observation and correct classification of pressure ulcers is important in deciding whether to start prevention and treatment in good time or to intensify it.

# Classification of Pressure Ulcers

Classifying pressure ulcers is done, on the one hand, by evaluating the seriousness of a pressure ulcer injury and, on the other hand, by being able to determine if a skin injury is a pressure ulcer injury or not. A classification system contains a number of grades (or stages). This numerical classification is done on the basis of the gravity of the tissue damage. The higher the grade the greater the tissue damage.

## Historic Classification

There are many classifications of pressure ulcers (David et al., 1983; Haalboom et al., 1997; Panel for the Prediction and Prevention of Pressure Ulcers in Adults,1992; Shea, 1975: Torrance, 1983). Some classification systems are so extensive that, in practice, they are difficult to manage and do not lead to a uniformly correct classification of pressure ulcer injuries. In 1975 Shea, an orthopedic surgeon, first published a pressure ulcer classification system. He divided pressure ulcers into five stages based on the damage to the various tissue layers and the depth.

Most classification systems are based on Shea's work and employ four to five stages (Maklebust & Sieggreen, 1995; Reid & Morison, 1994; Shea 1975). A few systems distinguish six stages, in which still further subgradations are used. The most complex system was Stirling's, which has four stages, in which for each stage up to four subcategories were defined (Lowthian, 1987; Reid & Morison, 1994; Yarkony et al., 2007).

In the United States, NPUAP's (National Pressure Ulcer Advisory Panel's) classification is employed (Panel for the Prediction and Prevention of Pressure Ulcers in Adults, 1992). In Europe, the most frequently used classification system is that of the EPUAP (European Pressure Ulcer Advisory Panel, 1999). Both classifications distinguish four grades or stages. The definitions differ from each other to a minimal extent and are almost identical.

In 2007 the NPUAP confirmed the four stages and added in its staging system a new type of pressure ulcer: the "suspected deep tissue injury" (DTI) (NPUAP, 2007). This is defined as a purple or maroon localized area of discolored intact skin or blood-filled blister caused by damage of underlying soft tissue from pressure and/or shear. The area may be preceded by tissue that is painful, firm, mushy, boggy, warmer, or cooler as compared to adjacent tissue. DTI may be difficult to detect in individuals with dark skin tones. Evolution may include a thin blister over a dark wound bed. The wound may further evolve and become covered by thin eschar. Evolution may be rapid, exposing additional layers of tissue even with optimal treatment.

## Classification Systems

When, after a period of pressure load, the pressure is removed, there is a reactive hyperemia or pressure-related blanchable erythema. This increased blood flow to the tissue is a protective autoregularization mechanism that corrects the deficiency of oxygen in the tissue (Bliss, 1998; Michel & Gillot, 1992; Nixon & McGough, 2001). This redness is called pressure-related blanchable erythema because it becomes white when pressed with the finger or with a transparent disk. Pressure-related blanchable erythema is not considered to be a pressure ulcer. Pressure ulcers are classified into four grades or stages on the basis of the seriousness of the injury (see Figure 19.2):

# 19.2

**Stage 1: Pressure-related nonblanchable erythema.**

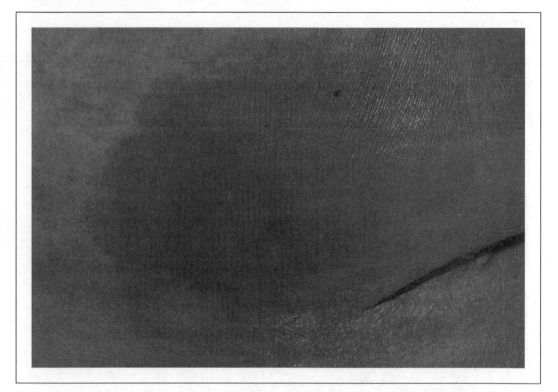

pressure related-nonblanchable erythema (stage 1), blister or abrasion (stage 2; see Figure 19.3), superficial pressure ulcer (stage 3; see Figure 19.4), and deep pressure ulcer (stage 4; see Figure 19.5) (European Pressure Ulcer Advisory Panel, 1999).

A stage 1 (pressure-related nonblanchable erythema) is redness that does not become white when pressed and matches the discoloration of the skin, has warmth, edema, or hardening of the tissue. Pressure-related nonblanchable erythema is easy to observe and is generally considered the most important symptom of a stage 1 pressure ulcer in Caucasians. In patients with dark skin, other symptoms become more important (Panel for the Prediction and Prevention of Pressure Ulcers in Adults, 1992).

In people with a pale complexion this is clinically visible as a marked area of permanent redness. In people with darker skin it can be seen as a marked area of permanent red, blue, or purple tints. This is, however, much more difficult to see. This color change is also coupled with a change in one or more other symptoms such as skin temperature (higher or lower than the surrounding skin), tissue consistency (firm or flaccid), and/or sensitivity (pain, itch) (Panel for the Prediction and Prevention

## 19.3

**Stage 2: Blister.**

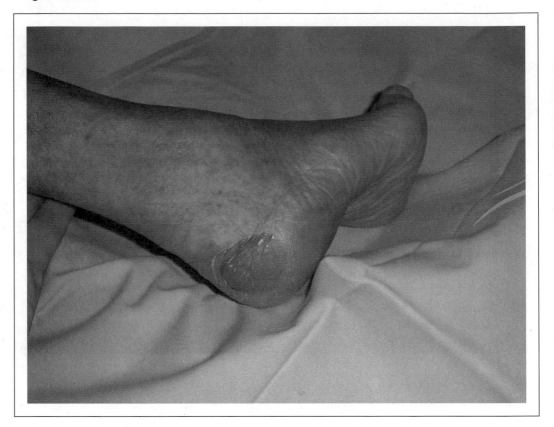

of Pressure Ulcers in Adults, 1992). In principle, pressure-related nonblanchable ery-thema is reversible when pressure and shear force are removed immediately after its occurrence (Halfens, Bours, & Van Ast, 2001: Maklebust, 1987; Smith, 1995; Vanderwee, Grypdonck, DeBaquer, & Defloor, 2006). Pressure-related nonblanchable erythema is an alarm signal, a time at which prevention must certainly begin (Vanderwee, Grypdonck, & Defloor, 2007). The EPUAP advises health care providers to report pressure-related nonblanchable erythema separately in prevalence measurements and not to just add them in with the other stages of pressure ulcer (Defloor et al., 2005).

A stage 2 (blister or abrasion) is a degeneration of the skin (partial skin swelling), including dermis, epidermis, or both. The injury is superficial and is clinically observable as an abrasion or blister. A burst blister is also catalogued as stage 2.

A stage 3 (superficial pressure ulcer) is an injury to the skin (complete skin swelling), including damage or necrosis of the subcutaneous tissue. The injury can extend up to (but not through) the underlying fascia. Clinically it is visible as a deep crater, whether or not with undermining of the adjacent tissue.

A stage 4 (deep pressure ulcer) is an injury to the skin (complete skin swelling) with extensive destruction; tissue necrosis; or damage to muscle, bone, or supporting

# 19.4

**Stage 3: Superficial pressure ulcer.**

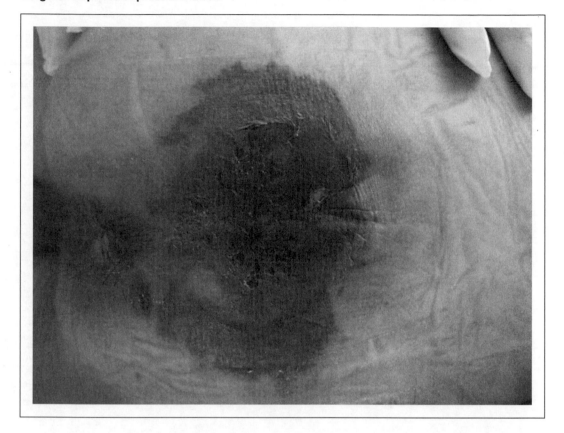

tissue (e.g., tendon or joint capsule). Undermining of the tissue or formation of infected injury is possible The various grades or stages are regarded as manifestations of pressure ulcers, and not as phases that necessarily follow each other. Pressure ulcer can, in some patients, start as a blister, a superficial, or even deep pressure ulcer. Sometimes a blister can evolve directly into a black necrosis spot (deep pressure ulcer).

## Sites of Pressure Ulcers

Pressure ulcers in principle can occur on all parts of the body. Obviously pressure ulcers occur mostly around those areas that have the following characteristics:

- Bone tissue close under the skin surface;
- A relatively thin layer of fat and muscular tissue or a thick layer of fat tissue between bone tissue and skin surface;
- The surfaces of the human body.

In practice pressure ulcers occurs most frequently at the coccyx and the heels because the pressure on those locations is very high and the limited thickness of the tissue does not allow distribution of the pressure.

## 19.5

**Stage 4: Deep pressure ulcer.**

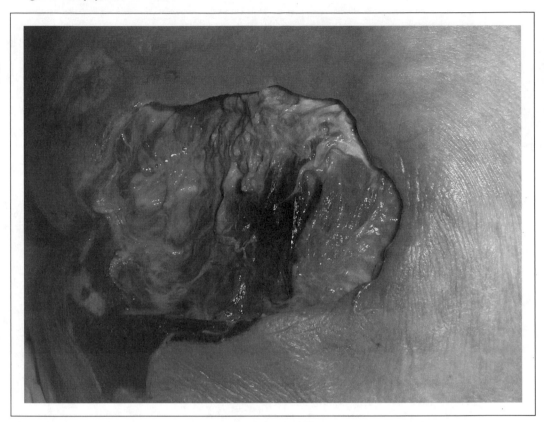

## Observation Methods for Pressure-Related Blanchable and Nonblanchable Erythema

There are two methods to differentiate between pressure-related blanchable and non-blanchable erythema: the finger pressure method and one using a disk. The classic method of determining pressure blanching by redness is the finger-pressure method. With this method, pressure is carefully exerted with the finger or thumb on the red skin site. If the red skin site goes white, this is classified as pressure-related blanchable erythema (Maklebust, 1987). The microcirculation has remained intact and there is no sign of tissue damage. To discern the difference between pressure-related blanchable and nonblanchable erythema, a transparent disk (see Figures 19.6 and 19.7) can be used (Halfens et al., 2001; Vanderwee et al., 2006). A disk is a transparent rounded-off piece of plastic with a diameter of approximately 5 cm. It allows pressure to be exerted on the skin and at the same time to observe whether the skin can be pressed white or not.

# 19.6

**Transparent disk.**

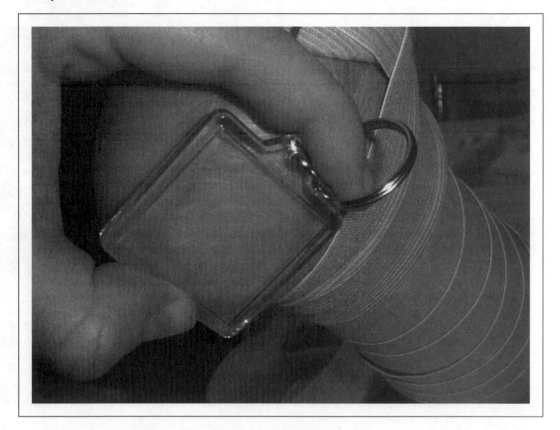

The dynamic process of the blanching of the redness is visible through the transparent disk. This makes observation easier on patients on whom the whitening is only briefly visible after the removal of pressure because the blood vessels fill up quickly. More pressure points with pressure-related nonblanchable erythema can be detected using a transparent disk than using the finger method (Vanderwee et al., 2006).

## Risk Determination

### Definition and Principle

Pressure ulcer prevention starts with detecting patients who run the risk of developing pressure ulcers. The importance of this detection is the need to provide suitable care to meet the specific needs of the patient. Moreover good risk assessment leads to the

## 19.7

**Transparent disk.**

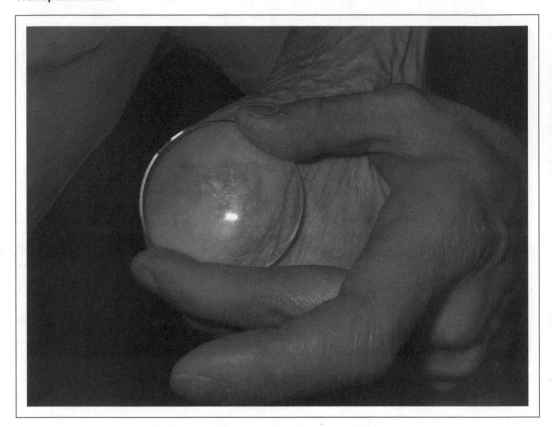

allocation of a well-considered remedy for both patient and society (Lyder, Shannon, Empleo-Frazier, McGeeHee, & White, 2002). This assessment of risk can be made on the basis of a risk scale, clinical observation, and early recognition of pressure-related nonblanchable erythema.

## Risk Scale

A risk scale is a scientifically based measurement in which indicators and factors are recorded, with the aim of identifying patients who run the risk of developing pressure ulcers (Edwards, 1994). The most extensively researched and frequently used risk scale is the Braden scale (See Table 19.1) (Bergstrom, Braden, Kemp, Champagne, & Ruby, 1998). The Braden scale consists of six items: sensory observation, activity,

## 19.1  The Braden Scale

| Sensory Perception | Moisture | Activity |
|---|---|---|
| 1. completely limited<br>2. very limited<br>3. slightly limited<br>4. no impairment | 1. constantly moist<br>2. very moist<br>3. occasionally moist<br>4. rarely moist | 1. bedfast<br>2. chairfast<br>3. walks occasionally<br>4. walks frequently |

| Mobility | Nutrition | Friction and Shear |
|---|---|---|
| 1. completely immobile<br>2. very limited<br>3. slightly limited<br>4. no limitation | 1. very poor<br>2. probably inadequate<br>3. adequate<br>4. excellent | 1. problem<br>2. potential problem<br>3. no apparent problem |

Note: From Braden and Bergstrom (1994), used with permission.

mobility, moistness, nutritional situation, and friction/shearing force (see Figure 19.4). Scores can vary between 6 and 23. The most used cut-off point is 17 (a patient with a score lower than 17 is considered to be an at-risk patient). A low score is associated with a greater risk of pressure ulcer (Bergstrom et al., 1985; Bergstrom, Braden, Laguzza, & Holman, 1987; Braden & Bergstrom, 1987).

Cubbin and Jackson developed a risk-assessment scale for intensive care patients. This scale is based on age, weight, general skin condition, mental condition, mobility, hemodynamic status, respiration, nutrition, incontinence, and hygiene (Jackson, 1999). This scale has had limited testing and the validation procedures used were not very adequate (Shanin et al., 2007). Shanin et al. concluded in their review on intensive care risk assessment that no effective risk assessment scales are described in the literature. Risk scales, however, often fail to predict the development of pressure ulcers adequately (Bergquist, 2001; Bergquist & Frantz, 2001; Boyle & Green, 2001; Chaplin, 1999; Defloor & Grypdonck, 2004; Galvin, 2002; Lindgren, Unosson, Krantz, & Ek, 2002; Perneger et al., 2002; Schoonhoven et al., 2002; Van Marum et al., 2000; Vap & Dunaye, 2002; Wellard & Lo, 2000). Therefore, risk scales have to be combined with clinical expertise and painstaking observation of the skin. This will reduce the number of false positives (the patients at risk based on the risk score, but who are not at risk in reality) and false negatives (the patients not at risk based on the risk score, but who are at risk in reality) (Defloor & Grypdonck, 2004). If pressure-related nonblanchable erythema is observed at pressure points, preventative measures should be started directly, even though the patient is not a risk patient according to a risk scale. It is not recommended to base the risk determination and allocation of preventive material exclusively on risk score lists (Panel for the Prediction and Prevention of Pressure Ulcers in Adults, 1992).

## Clinical Expertise

Combining risk scales with the clinical expertise by the nurse is recommended (CBO, 2002; National Collaborating Centre for Nursing and Supportive Care, 2003). This "clinical expertise" is a judgment by the nurse about the risk of pressure ulcers for an individual patient, based on many years' experience and common sense. The nurse "sees" or "knows" when a patient is at risk.

According to Van Marum, Germs, and Ribbe (1992), nurses consider a patient to be at risk when he is immobile and not at risk when he has a good general physical condition. In tests where clinical expertise is compared to the use of risk scales, the results are variable (Hergenroeder, Mosher, & Sevo, 1992; Salvadalena, Snyder, & Brogdon, 1992; VandenBosch, Montoye, Satwicz, Durkee, & Boylan, 1996).

## Early Recognition of Pressure-Related Nonblanchable Erythema

Observing the patient carefully on a daily basis, with prevention begun as soon as possible after a pressure-related nonblanchable erythema appears is a viabale nursing alternative to using risk scales. By definition, when prevention is started on patients who develop pressure-related nonblanchable erythema, only patients at real risk get prevention (pressure-related nonblanchable erythema points to a risk of development of pressure ulcer injuries). With this method of risk determination, fewer patients are considered as at risk than when using the classic risk scales. From research in geriatric medical and surgical-nursing units it appears that with the observation-only assessment, the number of pressure ulcer injuries stage 2 and higher did not increase as compared to using the classic risk scales (Vanderwee et al., 2007). Of course, the observation method requires that patients are observed very thoroughly and regularly (at least daily), and that immediate prevention is started on the appearance of pressure-related nonblanchable erythema.

## Principles of Prevention

Pressure ulcer prevention is important but not always easy to achieve. Effective preventive measures directly influence the causes of pressure ulcers. These measures reduce the size and/or the duration of the pressure and shearing force. Measures that solely influence tissue tolerance can only be supportive measures. They can reduce the risk of pressure ulcers in limited measure, but whether they can prevent pressure ulcers in high-risk patients is rather doubtful. For effective prevention it is important that continuity of the preventive measures is guaranteed. This means that for an at-risk patient, 24 hours per day, 7 days per week preventive measures must be taken. Thus, prevention must occur both when the patient is lying in bed and when he or she is sitting up in a (wheel) chair, during transfers, and during an operation. If this does not happen, the chance is great that the patient will still develop pressure ulcers.

## Preventive Measures

A distinction can be made depending on the aim of the preventive measures:

- Measures aimed at pressure
- Measures aimed at shearing force

■ Measures aimed at tissue tolerance
■ Other measures

## Preventive Measures Aimed at Pressure

Preventive measures can focus on decreasing the duration of the pressure or decreasing the magnitude of the pressure.

### Reducing the Magnitude of Pressure

The magnitude of pressure is dependent on the size of the supportive surface. If the supportive surface is enlarged, then the magnitude of the pressure that the tissue undergoes is reduced as well. Weight-spreading mattresses enlarge the support surface. The posture also has an influence on the size of the pressure (Defloor, 2000).

### Postures

The pressure is lowest when a patient lies in a semi-Fowler position of 30°. In this position the head is raised up 30° and the foot of the bed 30°. In pressure ulcer prevention this position thus takes preference. The lowest pressure in lying on one's side is measured in a 30° position. In this dorso-lateral position the patient is turned at a 30° angle to the mattress and supported in the back with a cushion that produces a 30° angle. It is important to check that the sacrum is pressure free. The hand must be able to be placed between the lower layer and the sacrum and the buttock must be free.

The higher the head is raised, the greater the pressure becomes. In a 90° upright sitting position the pressure is the greatest. The pressure surface is then at it's smallest, which results in higher pressure thereby increasing the chance of pressure ulcers occurring. When a patient needs to sit upright in bed, (for a meal, for example), a half-sitting position (60°) is recommended. When the patient is sitting the pressure is higher than while lying and the chance of pressure ulcers is great (Defloor & Grypdonck, 1999, 2000). The best position for a patient in an armchair is to have him or her sit back positioning the chair with the legs supported on a footrest. In this position the lowest pressure is measured. It is important that the heels are not supported on the footrest. Otherwise the pressure at the heels is great and pressure ulcers can originate there. If the armchair cannot be tipped backward, the pressure is lowest in an upright sitting position with the feet on the ground.

If a patient slips down in the seat or is sitting askew, the pressure increases sharply. Regular checking on this sitting position and the use of positioning cushions must be a part of every pressure–ulcer-prevention policy.

### Pressure-Redistributing Mattress Systems

The pressure-redistributing system's purpose is to enlarge the pressure surface (contact area between patient and system). There are two groups of pressure-redistributing systems: the static and dynamic systems. Static-pressure-redistributing systems will assume the shape consistent with the pressure exerted on it by the patient's body surface. Examples of this type of mattress are foam and air mattresses. The dynamic-pressure-redistributing systems are electrically driven and change form through external factors (e.g., air pump). The most important dynamic-pressure-reducing systems are the "air-fluidized" beds and the "low air-loss" systems.

## Static-Pressure–Redistributing Systems

Foam mattresses are static-pressure–redistributing systems that consist of viscoelastic or flexible foam. Viscoelastic foam is foam with a "slow memory" (slow foam or viscoelastic foam). This foam tries to adapt its original shape to weight and, in this way, achieve better pressure reduction. The effect is comparable to sitting on a balloon filled with sand: the sand will redistribute itself and take on a new form. The pressure reduction that viscoelastic foam mattresses achieve is real, but insufficiently large to function as the only preventive means for risk patients (Gunningberg, Lindholm, Carlsson, & Sjoden, 2000). Changing position remains necessary, albeit less frequently than on an elastic foam mattress (Defloor, Herremans, et al., 2005). Elastic foam tries to return to its original shape when weight is placed on it. Here the effect is comparable to sitting on a balloon filled with water: the water strives to go back to its original shape. A pressure reduction of 20 to 30% was observed when a subject was laid on a viscoelastic foam mattress compared with an elastic foam mattress (Defloor, 2000; Fontaine, 2000; Willems, 1995). Viscoelastic foam is also recommended for use on stretchers in emergency departments. Prevention has to start as soon as possible. If no preventive measures are taken in the ambulance and in the emergency ward, a patient may already have developed a pressure ulcer prior to being admitted to the intensive care unit. The use of viscoelastic foam on the stretchers in the emergency ward and even in the ambulance would help to reduce the pressure-ulcer risk.

Although a water mattress has a pressure-reducing effect (Neander & Birkenfeld, 1991; Sideranko, Quinn, Burns, & Froman, 1992; Sloan, Brown, & Larson, 1977; Wells & Geden, 1984), this mattress still cannot be recommended. The water mattress hampers the patient's spontaneous position changes. It takes a lot more effort to change position or to be moved. Because of this the duration of immobilization is extended and the risk of pressure ulcers increases. Other known disadvantages of the water mattress are the weight of the mattress and the drop in temperature that it causes (Groen, Groenier, & Schuling, 1999).

## Dynamic-Pressure–Redistributing Systems

The air-fluidized beds consist of a tub, a casing, and a pump system. The mattress is constructed out of silicone granules that are surrounded by a synthetic material cover (Brienza & Geyer, 2000). When warm air (28 to 35° C) is blown through the silicone granules, the silicone granules behave like a liquid. Resulting in the body being, as it were, immersed into the mattress by which means the area of body contact to the mattress is maximized. This can be described as a "quicksand" effect. Pressure redistributing is responsible for a decrease in the magnitude of pressure and shearing force. If the elasticity of the cover is too limited, the pressure-reducing capacity of the air-fluidized bed is decreased. The cover is permeable to bodily fluid, by which means the bodily fluids can simply pass into the tub with the silicone granules.

The "low-air–loss" systems consist, just like the air-fluidized bed, of a pump and a mattress (Brienza & Geyer, 2000). The mattress is made out of various compartments surrounded by an air-permeable cover. A continuous stream of warmed air is blown through the compartments, which is necessary to compensate for any loss of air through the cover. The patient is immersed into the mattress, thus enlarging the contact surface. This can be described as the "hovercraft-effect."Just like air-fluidized beds, the magnitude of pressure and shearing force is reduced. The watertight cover is (micro)-permeable to air. The less elastic the cover, the more the pressure-reducing capacity of the mattress is diminished.

## Pressure-Redistributing–Cushion Systems

In the sitting position, pressure is very great at the contact surface (the bottom) (Bale, Price, Rees-Matthews, & Harding,2001; Garber, Krouskop, & Carter, 1978; Souther, Carr, & Vistnes, 1974; Sprigle, Chung, & Brubaker, 1990; Vandewalle, 1994). To lessen pressure in the sitting position, antipressure ulcer cushions are used to distribute the existent pressure, as evenly as possible, over a large contact surface (a larger surface than when no cushion is used). In this way the tissue at pressure points is less distorted (Kahmann, 1991). The use of cushions is not enough to prevent pressure ulcers. They must be combined with a painstaking observation of the skin and changes of position.

There are several types of cushions available. Based on interface pressure measurements and clinical trials, air cushions reduce pressure better than foam, gel, gel and foam, hollow-fiber, water cushions, or sheepskin (Defloor & Grypdonck, 2000; Shechtman, Hanson, Garrett, & Dunn, 2001; Yuen & Garrett, 2001) in the upright, lolling, or slumped-in-the-chair sitting positions (Defloor & Grypdonck, 1999). With thin air cushions, however, a "bottoming-out" effect (see Figure 19.8) occurs more quickly than with thick air cushions. The patient is then no longer supported by the cushion, but is resting on the underlying surface. Because of this there is high maximum-contact pressure (Defloor & Grypdonck, 1999, 2000; Krouskop, Williams, Noble, & Brown, 1986).

The pressure-reducing capability of viscoelastic foam cushions is, for upright-sitting persons, comparable with that of air cushions (Apatsidis, Solomonidis, & Michael, 2002; Defloor & Grypdonck, 2000; Rosenthal et al., 1996). In a slumped or lolling sitting position, the pressure-reducing capability of the viscoelastic foam cushions is less beneficial than that of air cushions (Defloor & Grypdonck, 1999). Gel and water cushions have either no effect or a limited one (Bar, 1991; Defloor & Grypdonck, 1999, 2000; Souther et al., 1974).

# Decrease of the Duration of Pressure

## Changing Position

Changing position means placing someone into a different position, in which all the points on which the body is supported (the pressure points) are changed. Changing position is only useful if this process is strictly applied, day and night, 7 days a week. The interval between position changes may never be longer than 4 hours if a patient is lying on a pressure-reducing mattress and 2 hours if this is not the case (Defloor, Clark, et al., 2005). Changing position also needs to occur during sitting periods and then with an even greater frequency than while the critically ill older adult is lying down (Panel for the Prediction and Prevention of Pressure Ulcers in Adults, 1992). Although it is recommended that a position is changed for someone lying on a nonpressure-reducing mattress every 2 hours, changing position should occur more frequently, for example every hour, while the patient is sitting. The use of pressure-reducing cushions will allow patients to have their position changed less frequently.

## 19.8

**Bottoming-out effect.**

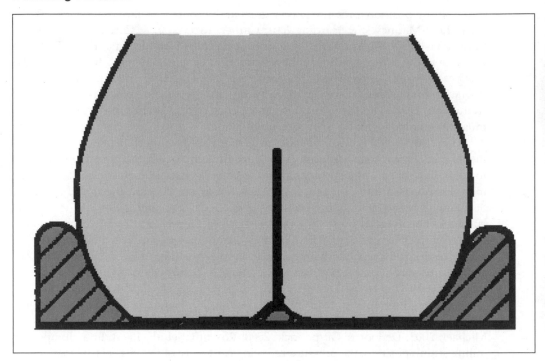

## Alternating Systems

The aim of alternating systems is to decrease the length of time that the tissue is compressed by pressure, by alternating the load to various pressure points of the body. The cells/compartments of the mattress are alternately slowly inflated and slowly deflated or pumped out. Some alternating systems can be placed directly on the bedframe (mattress-replacing systems) or are integrated into the bed. Others need to be placed on top of the mattress (lay-on systems). Both systems are equally effective (Nixon et al., 2006). Alternating systems are useful for pressure-ulcer prevention (Cullum, McInnes, Beller-Syer, & Legood, 2006). Patients who lie on an alternating mattress do not need to have their positions changed (Vanderwee, Grypdonck, & Defloor, 2005). Heel pressure ulcers remain a problem, however. Even on alternating mattresses, a cushion has to be placed under the lower legs so that the heels are not supported on the mattress (floating heels), otherwise many patients develop heel pressure ulcers (Vanderwee et al., 2005).

## Measures Aimed at Shearing Force

On lifting up a slumped patient, the risk is great that traction will be exerted on the skin and the underlying tissues at the sacrum. The tissue gets folded over or is subjected to shearing force (certainly if patients are dragged and not lifted). Any raising action, even sideways tilting (or lifting), can help to ensure that both the skin and underlying tissues are no longer subject to shearing force. Turning or changing the sheets of patients can help to prevent shearing force too (Goode & Allman, 1989). Correct positioning of the sitting attitude, to prevent slumping in the chair or tilting sideways, will greatly reduce shearing force and thus the risk of decubitus.

## Measures Aimed at Tissue Tolerance

Measures aimed at tissue tolerance have only a limited support function and are insufficiently robust to prevent decubitus. The most important measures aimed at tissue tolerance are nourishment interventions. Pressure ulcers are more frequently observed in patients in a poor nutritional state. It is not known if a causal link exists between nutrition and the origination of decubitus. Optimizing the nutritional situation of risk patients can be an element of prevention policy (EPUAP, 2003). It is to be expected that the effect will be to postpone the occurrence of decubitus forming.

# Pressure Ulcer Treatment

Ideally, pressure ulcers should be prevented, however, this is not always possible. It is therefore important to have effective treatment strategies that promote healing. As with any wound, such strategies need to consider both the patient and the wound. Keast, Parslow, Houghton, Norton, and Fraser (2006) suggest that this can be usefully addressed by:

- Identifying and treating the cause of the pressure ulcer;
- Addressing patient-centred concerns;
- Providing local wound care;
- Providing organizational support.

## Identify and Treat the Cause of the Pressure Ulcer

A basic principle of pressure ulcer management is to identify both the patient factors and the circumstances that resulted in the formation of the ulcer and, wherever possible, remove the cause. Healey (2006) suggests that a root-cause-analysis approach can be useful to gather and map information, identify and analyze the problems and to develop solutions to deal with the pressure ulcer. In the acutely ill elderly patient it is important to recognize that tissue resilience is generally reduced as a result of muscle wasting and loss of skin elasticity with aging (Dealey, 2005) and the added impact of acute illness can have major consequences. A full assessment of the patient will identify specific factors, for example, immobility, that have contributed to forma-tion of the pressure ulcer. A common example is that of an elderly person falling at home and lying undetected for many hours, thus resulting in prolonged pressure. This may be exacerbated by incontinence, dehydration, and hypothermia. Another cause of immobility may be major surgery lasting many hours, resulting in prolonged pressure over bony prominences. In both these examples, pressure ulcers developed as a result of a critical incident. However, some patients may have very limited mobility and then develop an acute illness, increasing their existing vulnerability to pressure-ulcer development. Once the assessment has identified the factors relating to the pressure-ulcer development, a plan should be developed to alleviate them, where possible.

## Reduced Mobility

Most acutely ill are bedfast for the majority of the time and they may have limited ability to move within the bed. The management plan should include a strategy for pressure redistribution by repositioning the patient and the use of specialized mat-tresses and beds. As discussed earlier, the use of the $30°^0$ tilt position is useful, particularly so for potentially unstable patients as it requires little movement to get the patient into position. However, patients with breathing difficulties are likely to have difficulty remaining in this position (Young, 2004).

The use of dynamic-pressure-redistribution systems is common for critically ill patients as the majority are deemed to be at high risk of pressure-ulcer development. However, there is insufficient evidence to determine the most appropriate system to promote healing (National Institute for Health and Clinical Excellence, 2005). A pragmatic approach is taken in the Registered Nurses Association of Ontario (RNAO) guidelines (2007), which suggest that selection of equipment should be based on the overall goals of treatment, bed mobility, ease of use, and so on. It is important to note that the guidelines stress the need for ongoing evaluation of patient needs, rates of healing, and monitoring of other bony prominences for incipient pressure ulcers (RNAO). If a patient who previously had a prevention plan in place develops a pressure ulcer, then that plan should be deemed inadequate and must be reviewed. This may include upgrading the pressure-redistribution device in use to a more sophisticated system. For the critically ill elderly patient a continuous low-pressure system (low air loss or air-fluidized) may well be the most appropriate. Care should be taken to ensure adequate pressure relief for the heels as not all mattresses or beds provide this pressure relief adequately (RNAO).

## Poor Nutritional Status and Dehydration

The role of nutrition in the development and healing of pressure ulcers is not absolutely clear. A systematic review of the literature found enteral nutritional support could significantly reduce the risk of pressure ulcers and may promote their healing (Stratton et al., 2005). A randomized study published after the review found improved pressure ulcer healing in a long-term-care facility in elderly patients who had received a protein supplement in addition to standard diet (Lee, Posthauer, Dorner, Redovian, & Maloney, 2006). Bergstrom et al. (2005) undertook a 12-week observational study of elderly patients with pressure ulcers and found that adequate nutritional support for those with stage-3 and stage-4 ulcers (NPUAP staging) was a strong predictor of healing.

An observational study of acutely ill patients with and without wounds who were being tube-fed showed that patients with wounds generally require more protein than those without wounds and that many failed to receive enough protein to meet their needs (Pompeo, 2007). Alix et al. (2007) found that the energy intake of acutely ill elderly patients was low and suggested that 24 to 30 kcal/kg body weight/day would be appropriate and possibly should be higher for those with a low body mass index. Part of the overall assessment of the patient should include a nutritional assessment and identification of any deficits. Loss of fluids and poor intake can also result in dehydration. Advice from a dietician and/or nutrition team can assist in establishing an appropriate regime relevant for the patient's condition. For patients with severe pressure ulcers (grades 3 and 4) the multidisciplinary team should consider their basal energy expenditure and pay particular attention to the increased fluid loss through such wounds (EPUAP, 2003).

### Incontinence

Incontinence of either urine or feces poses a challenge when managing pressure ulcers on the sacrum or buttocks as there is considerable likelihood of the ulcer becoming contaminated. There is also the risk of further skin breakdown as moist skin is more susceptible to friction and shearing forces (Keast et al., 2006). Barrier creams are widely used to protect the skin from incontinence-associated dermatitis (Gray, 2007), but they can interfere with the adherence of dressings over an ulcer. Beitz (2006) has reviewed the management of fecal incontinence in acutely and critically ill patients and provides a range of practical solutions, which are summarized in Table 19. 2. However, she also stresses the importance of identifying the causes of diarrhea and making dietary changes before using other methods such as pharmacotherapy.

### Poor Tissue Perfusion

Poor tissue perfusion is common in the critically ill (Webster, 1999) and the focus of care is to ensure an adequate blood supply to the vital organs, often at the expense of the peripheral blood supply, especially to the lower limbs. Potentially, this may be an issue for the older patient, as one in five suffer from some degree of peripheral arterial disease (Meijer et al., 1998). The two factors combined result in a lower than normal capillary closing pressure at the periphery and can result in the development of heel ulcers. Although it may not be possible to address either of these issues when treating pressure ulcers on the heel, it is important to alleviate the pressure to promote healing.

## Patient-Centered Concerns

Any assessment should identify factors of importance to the patient, including pain, quality of life, and psychosocial issues.

## Pain

The symptom of pain related to pressure ulcers can be seen as an emerging clinical issue (Girouard, Harrison, & VanDenKerfof, 2008). Several qualitative studies have

| 19.2 Management of Fecal Incontinence | |
| --- | --- |
| **Intervention** | **Comments** |
| Containment | ■ Absorbent products such as pads or diapers are widely used. They should be changed when soiled.<br>■ Fecal collectors can be useful to manage loose or liquid feces. They are fixed externally and have a closed system. |
| Skin protection | ■ Skin cleansers and skin protectors can be used with diapers to provide additional skin protection, but there is limited research to identify the best combination. |
| Indwelling drainage devices | ■ Bowel management systems comprising a soft catheter and collection bag can be used for bedbound, immobilized patients. These are relatively new devices and further research is required into their use.<br>■ Rectal catheters are generally contraindicated because of problems with their use. |
| Pharmaceutical agents | ■ Agents should complement other management methods.<br>■ Selection depends on underlying etiology.<br>■ Bulking agents can help to decrease fecal incontinence.<br>■ Antidiarrheal agents can slow peristalsis and transit time, but should NOT be used for infectious diarrhea.<br>■ Antibiotics may be required for infectious diarrhea. |

*Note:* From Beitz (2006).

identified pain as a major factor in patients' experiences of pressure ulcers (Hopkins et al., 2006; Langemo et al., 2000; Spilsbury et al., 2007). Szor and Bourguignon (1999) found that 87% of the 32 patients with pressure ulcers whom they studied experienced pain at dressing change and 84% had pain at rest. Günes (2008) used the McGill Pain Questionnaire and the Faces Rating Scale—Revised (FRS-R) to assess the pain of 47 patients with pressure ulcers of stages 2 to 4 (NPUAP classification). Forty-four (94.6%) patients complained of pain, but the severity of the pain increased with the severity of the ulcer. The study also found that there was a high correlation between the pain scales, indicating that the FRS-R could be of use for patients unable to verbalize their level of distress. This type of pain-assessment scale is of particular relevance to critically ill patients who may be unable to communicate verbally for a variety of reasons. Several pain-assessment tools have been developed for use in the critical care unit, however, a review by Li, Puntillo, and Miaskowski (2008) suggest that although some have good validity and reliability, they have not been adequately tested to determine which should come into standard use. Ahlers et al. (2007) warn that observer-based assessment often underestimates the level of pain suffered. In patients unable to communicate verbally it is a challenge to identify the causes of pain and to differentiate pain specific to the pressure ulcer. However, whatever the cause of the pain, adequate analgesia should be given and its effectiveness monitored. Management of pain related to dressing change will be discussed later.

## Quality of Life and Psychosocial Issues

There is no doubt that pressure ulcers affect the quality of life of the sufferer both emotionally and socially (Hopkins et al., 2006; Spilsbury et al., 2007). However, for critically ill patients with pressure ulcers, their illness generally has a much greater impact during the acute stage. Once this phase passes then the situation may change and the pressure ulcer will be seen as an impediment to recovery (Hopkins et al., 2006; Spilsbury et al., 2007).

# Local Wound Care

## Assessing the Wound

Accurate assessment is the cornerstone of any treatment plan. When assessing a pressure ulcer the following needs to be taken into consideration:

- Grade/stage
- Wound bed appearance
- Presence of undermining
- Exudate
- Surrounding skin
- Pain
- Documentation

### Grading / Staging

Grading of pressure ulcers has been discussed. Consideration of the severity of a pressure ulcer should be a factor in selecting a suitable pressure-redistributing device.

### Wound Bed Appearance

The terms commonly used to describe the wound bed are necrotic, infected, sloughy, granulating, or epithelialzing (Dealey, 2005).

*Necrotic Tissue.* Necrotic tissue presents as a hard black eschar and as it starts to debride it becomes a grey/black slough as shown in Figure 19.5, stage 4 pressure ulcer. There is no exudate with the eschar, but as the necrotic tissue softens and starts to debride there is an offensive exudate, which can become quite heavy.

*Infected Wounds.* Infected wounds of critically ill patients may be particularly vulnerable to infection and, depending on concomitant disease processes, may have reduced signs of infection (Gardener, Franz, & Doebelling, 2001). The early signs of a wound infection are often increased pain and heavier exudates, which may have an offensive odor. The color and smell of the exudate will vary depending on the bacteria infecting the wound.

*Sloughy Tissue.* Sloughy tissue is white or yellow in color and may present as patchy areas on the wound surface. Provided a moist environment is maintained on the

| 19.3 | A Scoring System for Wound Exudate | |
|---|---|---|
| 1 | Minimal | Dressings last at least a week |
| 2 | Moderate | Dressings changed every 2–3 days |
| 3 | Heavy | Dressings changed at least daily |

wound surface, the macrophages will gradually remove slough from the wound and it will disappear as healing progresses (Dealey, 2005).

*Granulation Tissue.* Granulation tissue has a red granular appearance and will gradually fill any wound cavities. It is highly vascularized and easily damaged.

*Epithelial Tissue.* Once the wound bed is filled with granulation tissue, epithelial cells on the wound margin will start to proliferate and cover the wound surface.

## Presence of Undermining

Undermining of the wound edges is commonly seen in pressure ulcers once they are debrided. This can pose an additional challenge to achieving healing as it means that the wound margins are fragile and vulnerable to further breakdown.

## Exudate

The quantity of exudate will, in part, be determined by the size of the pressure ulcer as well as the type of tissue present in the wound bed (World Union of Wound Healing Societies, 2007). Assessment should include identifying the color, consistency, and odor as well as the quantity. The discarded dressing can provide useful information about the quantity and color of exudate, but there are no validated tools for measuring exudate. One pragmatic proposal by Falanga (2000) is to score the exudate level as shown in Table 19.3.

## Surrounding Skin

Wound margins can provide further useful information about exudate levels. For example, the presence of maceration could indicate a heavy level of exudate that is being inadequately managed by the existing dressing regime. Erythema may indicate the presence of infection, but it could also be an early sign of further pressure damage.

## Pain

As discussed earlier, pain is a major factor for pressure ulcers. Dressing change may exacerbate already existing pain and assessment should include any increase in pain at this time (Briggs & Torra i Bou, 2002). Pain may be caused by all stages of the dressing change: removal of the old dressing, cleansing of the wound, and even dressing application.

## Documentation

Maintaining a record of the size of an ulcer makes it possible to monitor healing progress. There are various methods for measuring a wound, all of which have limitations (Dealey, 2005). The simplest method is to measure the greatest length and the greatest width, ensuring that the second measurement is perpendicular to the first. For wounds with a cavity, the greatest depth should also be recorded. It is also useful to make a simple sketch of the wound shape and indicate the measurement points. These types of measurements are of limited value unless used with the full assessment described previously. Dealey suggests that chronic wounds should be measured every 2 to 4 weeks.

# Providing Organizational Support

The principles of wound bed preparation (WBP) provide some useful guidance for the aims of treatment (Shultz et al., 2003):

- Debridement of necrotic tissue,
- Management of exudates,
- Resolution of bacterial imbalance,
- Undermined epithelial edge.

A comprehensive assessment will identify the specific requirements of an ulcer and guide the health care professional to an appropriate plan of care for the individual patient. It should also be noted that healing may not be the goal of care for the terminally ill and treatment should be modified to ensure patient comfort and dignity (RNAO, 2007).

## Debridement of Necrotic Tissue

There are a number of ways of achieving debridement, but not all are suitable for every wound. Sharp debridement is the fastest method, but it should only be undertaken by a practitioner who has been especially trained to undertake the procedure (RNAO, 2007). It can be painful for the patient and analgesia may be required.

Biosurgery or larval therapy involves the use of sterile maggots from the fly *Lucilia sericata* to break down necrotic tissue and then ingest it (Thomas, 2001). This process is not effective on hard necrotic eschar. Although very popular in the United Kingdom, it is used less widely elsewhere.

Enzymatic preparations can be used to separate necrotic tissue by cleaving through the collagen holding it to the wound bed (Douglass, 2003). Autolytic debridement is achieved by dressings maintaining a moist environment at the wound/dressing interface thus enabling macrophages to phagocytoze the necrotic tissue. Examples of suitable dressings are hydrogels and hydrocolloids and also alginates if there is already moisture in the wound bed (Dealey, 2005).

## Management of Exudate

Determining a strategy for exudate management depends on whether the goal is to increase, maintain, or reduce the level of wound moisture (World Union of Wound

Healing Societies, 2007). Management of heavy exudate can be challenging for the nurse and failure to contain exudate is very distressing for the patient. It may be necessary to use a more absorbent dressing, such as an alginate or an absorbent foam, or to increase the frequency of dressing change. If more moisture is required the dressing choice should be one that donates moisture to the wound, such as a hydrogel.

## Resolution of Bacterial Imbalance

Infected pressure ulcers may result in complications such as bacteremias or osteomylitis and can be fatal. Management can be complex, particularly in the critically ill patient. The European Wound Management Association (EWMA) has produced a useful position document on the subject that can provide guidance to the practitioner (EWMA, 2006). Topical antimicrobials, such as cadexomer iodine or silver, in a variety of formats are commonly used and can be effective, but there is no clear evidence of the most effective dressing to use on infected pressure ulcers (Moore & Romanelli, 2006). Systemic antibiotics may also be required, especially for the immunocompromised or if cellulitis, bacteraemia or osteomylitis is present (Moore & Romanelli).

## Epithelial Edge

The aim of treatment is to achieve a clean granulating wound with a healthy wound margin and clear signs of epithelialization. In the vast majority of pressure ulcers if the cause is identified and removed where possible, adequate pressure relief is provided, adequate nutrition is provided, and the wound bed effectively prepared, this aim will be achieved. The goal should then be to protect the wound until healing is completed.

## Pain at Dressing Change

Factors that cause or increase pain will have been identified at assessment and allow appropriate strategies to be developed for the individual. Strategies could include provision of analgesia prior to dressing change; selection of a dressing that is easy to remove, such as the silicone dressings; select a dressing that can remain in place for several days to reduce the frequency of dressing change (Briggs & Torra i Bou, 2002). Two small studies have also considered the effect of combining diamorphine with a hydrogel for appication to painful pressure ulcers of terminally ill patients (Abbas, 2004; Flock, 2003). Both studies showed an improvement in pain control, but further research is required into this mode of application.

## General Comments on Dressing Selection

There is a very broad range of wound-management products available but limited evidence to guide appropriate selection. A systematic review by Bouza, Saz, Munoz, and Amate (2005) found that although there was evidence to show that hydrocolloid dressings were more effective than saline-soaked gauze in healing pressure ulcers, there was insufficient evidence to determine the effectiveness of other dressing types because many of the studies were too small and used poor methodologies.

# Summary

For the most part pressure ulcers can be prevented provided that effective preventive measures are taken early. On admission to the emergency ward or intensive care unit, pressure-ulcer risk should be assessed and prevention—if needed—should be started. To determine the risk, risk scales can be used in combination with clinical expertise. On the appearance of pressure-related nonblanchable erythema, preventative measures need to be started immediately.

The most effective measures focus on pressure reduction and pressure-point variation. Although older intensive care patients are often high-risk patients, adequate prevention can decrease the pressure-ulcer incidence significantly, resulting in less pain and discomfort, a shorter length of stay in the hospital, and decreased costs.

Determination of an adequate preventive approach is not easy and must be adapted to suit the needs of each patient individually. Or as George Bernard Shaw would say: "The golden rule is that there is no golden rule." Finding the best solution is, not surprisingly, a creative nursing task.

## Case Study

## Intensive Care Patient

Mister X, aged 85, was admitted to hospital last week via the Medical Emergency Admissions Unit complaining about progressive shortness of breath on exertion. The patient had no other complaints but was found to weigh 110 kg. He was admitted to the respiratory ward. During the night, he suddenly developed progressive dyspnea and orthopnea and the resuscitation team was called as he needed fast intubation to aid his breathing. Clinical examination showed respiratory crepitations and wheezing. His blood pressure was 180/88 mmHg and heart rate 88/min. A chest X-ray showed a butterfly-formed lung edema and an echocardiogram showed a severe aortic valve stenosis. He was transferred to the intensive care unit. The patient was ventilated at $FIO_2$ (fraction of inspired oxygen) of 50%, with a breathing frequency of 14 and a Tidal Volume of 700 mL. An arterial catheter and a central venous catheter were inserted and the patient was found to have a blood pressure of 101/43 mmHG and a central venous pressure measurement of 14 mmHG. Following treatment (medication and examinations), the patient became hemodynamically stable and he had a good diuresis. The patient had no neurological damage; his score on the Glasgow Coma Scale was 5. The patient received 2 L Glucose 5% / 24 hrs with 2 gr NaCl (sodium chloride). The patient was sedated.

The patient was considered as being at risk of developing pressure ulcers for the following reasons:

- Lack of mobility and activity
- Patient was ventilated
- Patient receiving sedating medication
- Pulmonary disorder

■ Restricted intake of food and fluids
■ Advanced age

When assessing the patient it is important to note that the patient is totally bedfast and cannot be repositioned because he is being ventilated. In addition, the patient is in a semirecumbent position to prevent ventilator-associated pneumonia. On examination he was found to have nonblanchable erythema on his left heel.

To prevent further skin damage, the patient was provided with a low-air–loss mattress. An alternating-air–pressure mattress is not recommended for a patient of this weight as it may bottom out when the patient is seated. The patient's heels are kept pressure-free by means of a heel cushion.

## Pressure-Ulcer–Related Web Sites

■ European Pressure Ulcer Advisory Panel: www.epuap.org
■ National Institute for Health and Clinical Excellence (Guidelines United Kingdom): www.nice.org.uk
■ (American) National Pressure Ulcer Advisory Panel: www.npuap.org
■ Pressure Ulcer Guideline Project of the EPUAP and NPUAP: www.pressureulcerguidelines.org
■ Pressure ulcer classification (Ghent University): www.puclas.ugent.be
■ Scottish Intercollegiate Guidelines Network (Scottish Guidelines): www.sign.ac.uk

## References

Abbas, S. Q. (2004). Diamorphine-Intrasite dressings for painful pressure ulcers. *Journal of Pain & Symptom Management, 28*(6), 532–534.

Ahlers, S. J. G. M., van Gulik, L., van der Veen, A. M., van Dongen, H. P. A., Bruins, P., Belitser, S. V., et al. (2008). Comparisons of different pain scoring systems in critically ill patients in a general ICU. *Critical Care*; Retrieved July 24, 2008, from.http://ccforum.com/content/12/1/R15

Alix, E., Berrut, G., Boré, M., Bouthier-Quintard, F., Buia, J. M., Chlala, A., et al. (2007). Energy requirements in hospitalised elderly people. *Journal of the American Geriatrics Society, 55*(7), 1085–1089.

Apatsidis, D. P., Solomonidis, S. E., & Michael, S. M. (2002). Pressure distribution at the seating interface of custom-molded wheelchair seats: Effect of various materials. *Archives of Physical Medicine and Rehabilitation, 83,* 1151–1156.

Bale, S., Price, P., Rees-Mathews, S., & Harding, K. G. (2001). Recognizing the feet as being at risk from pressure damage. *British Journal of Nursing, 10,* 1320–1326.

Bar, C. A. (1991). Evaluation of cushions using dynamic pressure measurement. *Prosthetics and Orthotics International, 15,* 232–240.

Beitz, J. M. (2006). Faecal incontinence in acutely and critically ill patients: Options in practice. *Ostomy & Wound Management, 52*(12), 56–66.

Bennett, G., Dealey, C., & Posnett, J. (2004). The cost of pressure ulcers in the UK. *Age & Ageing, 33,* 230–235.

Bergquist, S. (2001). Subscales, subscores, or summative score: Evaluating the contribution of Braden Scale items for predicting pressure ulcer risk in older adults receiving home health care. *Journal of Wound, Ostomy, and Continence Nursing, 28*(6), 279–289.

Bergquist, S., & Frantz, R. (2001). Braden Scale: Validity in community-based older adults receiving home health care. *Applied Nursing Research, 14,* 36–43.

Bergstrom, N., Braden, B. J., Laguzza, A., & Holman, V. (1987). The Braden Scale for predicting pressure sore risk. *Nursing Research, 36,* 205–210.

Bergstrom, N., Braden, B., Kemp, M., Champagne, M., & Ruby, E. (1998). Predicting pressure ulcer risk: A multisite study of the predictive validity of the Braden Scale. *Nursing Research, 47,* 261–269.

Bergstrom, N., Braden, B., Laquzza, A., & Holmar, V. (1985). The Braden scale for predicting pressure sore risk: Reliability studies. *Nursing Research, 34,* 383.

Bergstrom, N., Horn, S. D., Smout, R. J., Bender, S.A., Ferguson, M. L., Taler, G., et al. (2005). The national pressure ulcer long-term care study: Outcomes of pressure ulcer treatments in long-term care. *Journal of the American Geriatrics Society, 53,* 1721–1729.

Bliss, M. R. (1998). Hyperaemia. *Journal of Tissue Viability, 8*(4), 4–13.

Bouza, C., Saz, Z., Munoz, A., & Amate, J. M. (2005). Efficacy of advanced dressings in the treatment of pressure ulcers: a systematic review. *Journal of Wound Care, 14*(5), 193–199.

Boyle, M., & Green, M. (2001). Pressure sores in intensive care: Defining their incidence and associated factors and assessing the utility of two pressure sore risk assessment tools. *Australian Critical Care, 14,* 24–30.

Braden, B., & Bergstrom, N. (1987). A conceptual scheme for the study of the etiology of pressure sores. *Rehabilitation Nursing, 12,* 8–12.

Braden, B. J., & Bergstrom, N. (1994). Predictive validity of the Braden Scale for pressure sore risk in a nursing home population. *Research in Nursing & Health, 17*(6), 459–470.

Brienza, D. M., & Geyer, M. J. (2000). Understanding support surface technologies. *Advances in Skin & Wound Care, 13,* 237–244.

Briggs, M., & Torra i Bou, J. E. (2002). Pain at dressing changes: A guide to management. In *EWMA position document: Pain at wound dressing changes.* London: MEP.

CBO. (2002). *Richtlijn Decubitus Tweede Herziening.* [Pressure ulcer guideline, 2nd rev.] Utrecht, The Netherlands: Author.

Chaplin, J. (1999). Pressure sore risk assessment in palliative care. *Journal of Tissue Viability, 10,* 27–31.

Coleman, E. A., Martau, J. M., Lin, M. K., & Kramer, A. M. (2002). Pressure ulcer prevalence in long-term nursing home residents since the implementation of OBRA '87. Omnibus Budget Reconciliation Act. *Journal of the American Geriatrics Society, 50*(4), 728–732.

Cullum, N., McInnes, E., Beller-Syer S, E. M., & Legood, R. (2006). Support surfaces for pressure ulcer prevention (Cochrane Review). *The Cochrane Library.* Oxford, UK: Update Software.

David, J., Chapman, R., & Chapman, E. J. (19830. *An investigation of the current methods used in nursing for the care of patients with established pressure sores:* Harrow: Nursing Practice Research Unit.

Dealey, C. (2005). *Care of wounds* (3rd ed.). Oxford, UK: Blackwell Science.

Defloor, T. (1999). The risk of pressure sores: A conceptual scheme. *Journal of Clinical Nursing, 8,* 206–216.

Defloor, T. (2000). The effect of position and mattress on interface pressure. *Applied Nursing Research, 13,* 2–11.

Defloor, T., Clark, M., Witherow, A., Colin, D., Lindholm, C., Schoonhoven, L., et al. (2005). EPUAP statement on prevalence and incidence monitoring of pressure ulcer occurrence 2005. *EPUAP Review, 6*(3), 74–80.

Defloor, T., & Grypdonck, M. H. F. (1999). Sitting posture and prevention of pressure ulcers. *Applied Nursing Research, 12,* 136–142.

Defloor, T., & Grypdonck, M. (2000). Do pressure relief cushions really relieve pressure? *Western Journal of Nursing Research, 22,* 335–350.

Defloor, T., & Grypdonck, M. (2004). Validation of pressure ulcer risk assessment scales: A critique. *Journal of Advanced Nursing, 48*(6),613–621.

Defloor, T., Grypdonck, M., & De Bacquer, D. (2005). The effect of various combinations of turning and pressure reducing devices on the incidence of pressure ulcers. *International Journal of Nursing Studies, 42,* 37–46.

Defloor, T., Herremans, A., Grypdonck, M., De Schuijmer. J., Paquay, L., Schoonhoven, L., et al. (2005). *Belgische Richtlijn voor Decubituspreventie 2005.* [Belgian pressure ulcer guideline]. Gent, Belgium: Story Scientia.

Douglass, J. (2003). Wound bed preparation: A systematic approach to chronic wounds. *British Journal of Community Nursing 8*(6), (Suppl.), S26–S34.

Edwards, M. (1994). The rationale for the use of risk calculators in pressure sore prevention, and the evidence of the reliability and validity of published scales. *Journal of Advanced Nursing, 20,* 288–296.

European Pressure Ulcer Advisory Panel. (1999). Guidelines on treatment of pressure ulcers. *EPUAP Review, 1,* 31–33.

European Pressure Ulcer Advisory Panel. (2003). Guideline on nutrition in pressure ulcer prevention and treatment. *EPUAP Review, 5*(3), 80–82

European Wound Management Association. (2006). *EWMA position document: Management of wound infection.* London: MEP Ltd.

Falanga, V. (2000). Classification for wound bed preparation and stimulation of chronic wounds. *Wound Repair & Regeneration, 8*(5), 347–352.

Flock, P. (2003). Pilot study to determine the effectiveness of diamorphine gel to control pressure ulcer pain. *Journal of Pain & Symptom Management, 25*(6), 547–554.

Fontaine, R. (2000). Investigating the efficacy of a nonpowered pressure-reducing therapeutic mattress: A retrospective multi-site study. *Ostomy Wound Management, 46*, 34–43.

Galvin, J. (2002). An audit of pressure ulcer incidence in a palliative care setting. *International Journal of Palliative Nursing, 8*, 214–221.

Garber, S. L., Krouskop, T. A., & Carter, R. E. (1978). A system for clinically evaluating wheelchair pressure-relief cushions. *American Journal of Occupational Therapy, 32*, 565–570.

Gardener, S. E., Franz R. A., & Doebelling B. N. (2001). The validity of the clinical signs and symptoms used to identify localised chronic wound infection. *Wound Repair & Regeneration, 9*(3), 178–186.

Girourd, K., Harrison, M. B., & Van Den Kerfof, E. (2008). The symptom of pain with pressure ulcers: A review of the literature. *Ostomy & Wound Management, 54*(5), 30–42.

Goode, P. S., & Allman, R. M. (1989). The prevention and management of pressure ulcers. *Medical Clinics of North America, 73*(6), 1511–1524.

Gray, M. (2007). Incontinence-related skin damage: Essential knowledge. *Ostomy & Wound Management, 53*(12), 28–32.

Groen, H. W., Groenier, K. H., & Schuling, J. (1999). Comparative study of a foam mattress and a water mattress. *Journal of Wound Care, 8*, 333–335.

Günes, U. Y. (2008). A descriptive study of pressure ulcer pain. *Ostomy & Wound Management, 54*(2) 56–61.

Gunningberg, L., Lindholm, C., Carlsson, M., & Sjoden, P. O. (2000). Effect of visco-elastic foam mattresses on the development of pressure ulcers in patients with hip fractures. *Journal of Wound Care, 9*, 455–460.

Haalboom, J. E. R., van Everdingen, J. J. E., & Cullum, N. (1997). Incidence, prevalence and classification. In L. C. Parish, J. A. Withkowski, & J. T. Crissey (Eds.), *The decubitus ulcer in clinical practice.* London: Springer.

Halfens, R. J. G., Bours, G. J. J. W., & Van Ast, W. (2001). Relevance of the diagnosis 'Stage 1 pressure ulcer': An empirical study of the clinical course of stage 1 ulcers in acute care and long-term care hospital populations. *Journal of Clinical Nursing, 10*, 748–757.

Healey, F. (2006). Root cause analysis for tissue viability incidents. *Journal of Tissue Viability, 16*(1), 12–15.

Health Council of the Netherlands. (1999). *Pressure ulcers* (publication no. 1999/23). The Hague: Author.

Hergenroeder, P., Mosher, C., & Sevo, D. (1992). Pressure ulcer risk assessment—Simple or complex? *Decubitus, 5*, 47–52.

Hopkins, A., Dealey, C., Bale, S., Defloor, T., & Worboys, F. (2006). Patient stories of living with a pressure ulcer. *Journal of Advanced Nursing, 56*, 345–353.

Jackson, C. (1999). The revised Jackson/Cubbin pressure area risk calculator. *Intensive and Critical Care Nursing, 15*(3), 169–175.

Kahmann, L. R. M. (1991). *Stand van zaken. Ligondersteuning.* [State of the art. Lying support surfaces, (2 ed.)]. Amsterdam: Gemeenschappelijke Medische Dienst.

Keast, D., Parslow, N., Houghton, P. E., Norton, L., & Fraser, C. (2006). Best practice recommendations for the prevention and treatment of pressure ulcers: Update 2006. *Wound Care Canada, 4*(1), R19–R29.

Keller, P .B., Will, J., van Ramshorst, B., & van der Werken, C. (2004). Pressure ulcers in intensive care patients: A review of risks and prevention. *Intensive Care Medicine, 28*(10), 1379–1388.

Krouskop, T. A., Williams, R., Noble, P., & Brown, J. (1986). Inflation pressure effect on performance of air-filled wheelchair cushions. *Archives of Physical Medicine and Rehabilitation, 67*, 126–128.

Lahmann, N. A., Halfens, R. J., & Dassen, T. (2005). Prevalence of pressure ulcers in Germany. *Journal of Clinical Nursing, 14*(2), 165–172.

Langemo, D. K., Melland, H., Hanson, D., Olson, B., & Hunter, S. (2000). The lived experience of having a pressure ulcer: A qualitative analysis. *Advances in Skin & Wound Care, 13*, 225–235.

Lee, S. K., Posthauer, M. E., Dorner, B., Redovian, V., & Maloney, M. J. (2006). Pressure ulcer healing with a concentrated, fortified, collagen protein hydrolysate supplement: A randomised controlled trial. *Advances in Skin & Wound Care, 19*(2) 92–96.

Li, D., Puntillo, K., & Miaskowski, C. (2008). A review of objective pain measures for use with critical care adult patients unable to self report. *Journal of Pain, 9*(1), 2–10.

Lindgren, M., Unosson, M., Krantz, A. M., & Ek, A. C. (2002). A risk assessment scale for the prediction of pressure sore development: Reliability and validity. *Journal of Advanced Nursing, 38*, 190–199.

Lowthian, P. (1987). The classification and grading of pressure sores. *Care—Science and Practice, 5*, 5–9.

Lyder, C. H., Shannon, R., Empleo-Frazier, O., McGeHee, D., & White, C. (2002). A comprehensive program to prevent pressure ulcers in longterm care: Exploring costs and outcomes. *Ostomy Wound Management, 48*, 52–62.

Maklebust, J., & Sieggreen, M. (1995). *Pressure ulcers: Guidelines for prevention and nursing management.* Springhouse, PA: Springhouse Corporation.

Maklebust, J. (1987). Pressure ulcers: etiology and prevention. *Nursing Clinics of North America, 22,* 359–377.

Meijer, W. T., Hoes, A. W., Rutgers, D., Bots, M. L., Hofman, A., & Grobbee, D. E. (1998). Peripheral arterial disease in the elderly. *Arteriosclerosis, Thrombosis & Vascular Biology, 18,* 185–192.

Michel, C. C., & Gillot, H. (1992). Microvascular mechanism in stasis and ischaemia. In D. L. Bader (Ed.), *Pressure sores: Clinical practice and scientific approach* (pp. 153–163). London: MacMillan.

Moore, Z., & Romanelli, M. (2006). Topical management of grade 3 and 4 pressure ulcers. In *EWMA position document: Management of wound infection.* London: MEP Ltd.

National Collaborating Centre for Nursing and Supportive Care. (2003. Oct.) *The use of pressure-relieving devices (beds, mattresses and overlays) for the prevention of pressure ulcers in primary and secondary care.* London (UK): Author.

National Institute for Health and Clinical Excellence. (2005). *The prevention and treatment of pressure ulcers.* London: NICE.

National Pressure Ulcer Advisory Panel (NPUAD). (2001). Pressure ulcers in America; Prevalence, incidence and implications for the future. An executive summary of the National Pressure Ulcer Advisory Panel monograph [see comment] [erratum appears in *Advances in Skin Wound Care (2002), 15*(6), E1–E3; author reply E-3 PMID: 12477982). *Advances in Skin & Wound Care, 14*(4), 208–215.

Neander, K. D., & Birkenfeld, R. (1991). The influence of various support systems for decubitus ulcer prevention on contact pressure and percutaneous oxygen pressure. *Intensive Care Nursing, 7,* 120–127.

Nijs, N., Toppets A., Defloor, T., Bernaerts, K., Milisen, K., Van den Berghe, G. (2009). Incidence and risk factors for pressure ulcers in the intensive care unit. *Journal of Clinical Nursing, 18*(9), 1258–1266.

Nixon, J., & Mc Gough, A.(2001). The pathophysiology and aetiology of pressure ulcers. In M. Morison (Ed.), *The prevention and treatment of pressure ulcers* (pp. 17–36). Edinburgh: Mosby.

Nixon, J., Nelson, E. A., Cranny, G., Iglesias, C. P., Hawkins, K., Cullum, N. A., et al. (2006). Pressure relieving support surfaces: A randomised evaluation. *Health Technology Assessment, 10,* iii–x, 1.

NPUAP. (2007).*Pressure ulcer stages revised by NPUAP.* Washington, DC: Author. Retrieved July 10, 2008, from http://www.npuap.org/pr2.htm

Panel for the Prediction and Prevention of Pressure Ulcers in Adults. (1992). *Pressure ulcers in adults: Prediction and prevention. Clinical practice guideline number 3.* AHCPR Publication No. 92-0047. Rockville, MD: Agency for Health Care Policy and Research, Public Health Service, U.S. Department of Health and Human Services.

Perneger, T. V., Rae, A. C., Gaspoz, J. M., Borst, F., Vitek, O., & Heliot, C. (2002). Screening for pressure ulcer risk in an acute care hospital: Development of a brief bedside scale. *Journal of Clinical Epidemiology, 55,* 498–504.

Pompeo, M. (2007). Misconceptions about protein requirements for wound healing: Results of a prospective study. *Ostomy & Wound Management, 53*(8), 30–44.

Registered Nurses Association of Ontario. (2007). *Assessment & management of stage I to IV pressure ulcers.* Toronto: Author.

Reid, J., & Morison, M. (1994). Towards a consensus: Classification of pressure sores. *Journal of Wound Care, 3*(3), 157–160.

Rosenthal, M. J., Felton, R. M., Hileman, D L., Lee, M., Friedman, M., & Navach, J. H. (1996). A wheelchair cushion designed to redistribute sites of sitting pressure. *Archives of Physical Medicine and Rehabilitation, 77,* 278–282.

Russo, C. A., & Elixhauser, A. (2006). *Hospitalizations related to pressure sores, 2003.* Rockville, MD: Agency for Healthcare Research and Quality. Retrieved July 10, 2008, from http://www.hcup-us.ahrq.gov/reports/statbriefs/sb3.pdf

Salvadalena, G. D., Snyder, M. L., & Brogdon, K. E. (1992). Clinical trial of the Braden Scale on an acute care medical unit. *Journal of ET Nursing, 19*(5), 160–165.

Schoonhoven, L., Haalboom, J. R. E., Bousema, M. T., Algra, A., Grobbee, D. E., Gyrpdonck, M. H., et al. (2002). Prospective cohort study of routine use of risk assessment scales for prediction of pressure ulcers. *British Medical Journal, 325,* 797–800.

Severens, J. L., Habraken, J. M., Duivenvoorden, S., & Frederiks, C. M. (2002). The cost of illness of pressure ulcers in the Netherlands. *Advances in Skin & Wound Care, 15,* 72–77.

Shahin, E., Dassen, T., & Halfens, R. (2007). Predictive validity of pressure ulcer risk assessment tools in intensive care patients. *World of Critical Care Nursing, 3,* 75–79.

Shea, J. D.(1975). Pressure sores: Classification and management. *Clinical Orthopaedics and Related Research, 112,* 89–100.

Shechtman, O., Hanson, C. S., Garrett, D., & Dunn, P. (2001). Comparing wheelchair cushions for effectiveness of pressure relief: A pilot study. *Occupational Therapy Journal of Research, 21,* 29–48.

Shultz, G. S., Sibbald, G. R., Falanga, V., Ayello, E. A., Dowsett, C., Harding, K., et al. (2003). Wound bed preparation: A systematic approach to wound management. *Wound Repair & Regeneration, 11*(2) (Suppl.), S1–S28.

Sideranko, S., Quinn, A., Burns, K., & Froman, R. D. (1992). Effects of position and mattress overlay on sacral and heel pressures in a clinical population. *Research in Nursing and Health, 15,* 245–251.

Sloan, D. F., Brown, R. D., & Larson, D. L. (1977). Evaluation of a simplified water mattress in the prevention and treatment of pressure sores. *Plastic and Reconstructive Surgery, 60,* 596–601.

Smith, D. M. (1995). Pressure ulcers in the nursing home. *Annals of Internal Medicine, 123,* 433–442.

Souther, S., Carr, S. D., & Vistnes, L. M. (1974). Wheelchair cushions to reduce pressure under bony prominences. *Archives of Physical Medicine and Rehabilitation, 55,* 460–464.

Spilsbury, K., Nelson, A., Cullum, N., Iglesias, C., Nixon, J., & Mason, S. (2007). Pressure ulcers and their treatment and effects on quality of life: Hospital in-patient perspectives. *Journal of Advanced Nursing, 57*(5), 494–504.

Sprigle, S., Chung, K. C., & Brubaker, C. E. (1990). Reduction of sitting pressures with custom contoured cushions. *Journal of Rehabilitation Research and Development, 27,* 135–140.

Stratton, R. J., Ek, A. C., Engfer, M., Moore, Z., Rigby, P., Wolfe, R., et al. (2005). Enteral nutritional support in prevention and treatment of pressure ulcers: A systematic review and meta-analysis. *Ageing Research Reviews, 4*(3), 422–450.

Szor, J. K., & Bourguignon, C. (1999). Description of pressure ulcer pain at rest and at dressing change. *Journal of Wound, Ostomy & Continence Nursing, 26*(3), 115–120.

Thomas, S. (2001). Sterile maggots and the preparation of the wound bed. In G. W. Cherry, K. G. Harding, & T. J. Ryan (Eds.), *Wound bed preparation.* London: Royal Society of Medicine.

Thomson, J. S., & Brooks, R. G. (1999). The economics of preventing and treating pressure ulcers: A pilot study. *Journal of Wound Care, 8,* 312–316.

Torrance, C. (1983). *Pressure sores etiology, treatment and prevention.* Beckenham, UK: Croom Helms.

Van Marum, R. J., Germs, P., & Ribbe, M. W. (1992). De risicoscoring voor decubitus volgens Norton in een verpleeghuis. [The risk assessment according to Norton in a nursing home]. *Tijdschrift voor Gerontologie en Geriatrie, 23,* 48–53.

Van Marum, R. J., Ooms, M. E., Ribbe, M. W., & van Eijk, J. T. (2000). The Duth pressure sore assessment score or the Norton Scale for identifying at-risk nursing home patients? *Age & Ageing, 29*(1), 63–68.

VandenBosch, T., Montoye, C., Satwicz, M., Durkee, L. K., & Boylan, L. B. (1996). Predictive validity of the Braden Scale and nurse perception in identifying pressure ulcer risk. *Applied Nursing Research, 9*(2), 80–86.

Vandewalle, E. (1994). *Het drukredvcerend effect van rolstoelkussens.* [Pressure reducing effect of a wheel-chair cushion]. Master's thesis, Catholique University of Leuven.

Vanderwee, K., Grypdonck, M, & Defloor, T. (2005). The effectiveness of alternating pressure air mattresses for the prevention of pressure ulcers. *Age & Ageing, 34,* 261–267.

Vanderwee, K., Grypdonck, M., & Defloor, T. (2007). Non-blanchable erythema as an indicator for the need for pressure ulcer prevention: A randomized-controlled trial. *Journal of Clinical Nursing, 16,* 325–335.

Vanderwee, K., Grypdonck, M. H., De Baquer, D., & Defloor, T. (2006). The reliability of two observation methods of nonblanchable erythema, Grade 1 pressure ulcer. *Applied Nursing Research, 19,* 156–162.

Vap, P., & Dunaye, T. (2002). Pressure ulcer risk assessment in long-term care nursing. *Journal of Gerontological Nursing, 26,* 37–45.

Webster, N. R. (1999). Monitoring the critically ill. *Journal of the Royal College of Surgeons (Edinburgh), 44*(6), 386–393.

Welch, C. B. (1990). Preventing pressure sores. *British Medical Journal, 300,* 1401.

Wellard, S., & Lo, S. K. (2000). Comparing Norton, Braden and Waterlow risk assessment scales for pressure ulcers in spinal cord injuries. *Contemporary Nurse, 9,* 155–160.

Wells, P., & Geden, E. (1984). Paraplegic body support on convoluted foam, waterbed and standard mattresses. *Research in Nursing & Health, 7,* 127–133. Willems, P. (1995). *Het drukredvcerend effect van schvimrubber matrassen.* [Pressure-reducing effect of foam mattresses. Master's thesis, Catholique University of Leuven.

World Union of Wound Healing Societies. (2007). *Principles of best practice: Wound exudate and the role of dressings. A consensus document.* London: MEP Ltd. Retrieved September 15, 2001, from http://wuwhs.org/dates/2 V4/concensus exudate ENG Final.pdf

Yarkony, G. M., Kirk, P. M., Carlson, C., Roth, E. J., Lovell, L., Heinemann, A., et al. (2007). *Classification of pressure ulcers. Archives of Dermatology, 126*(9), 1218–1219.

Young, T. (2004). The 30 degree tilt position vs. the 90 degree lateral and supine positions in reducing the incidence of non-blanching erythema in a hospital inpatient population: A randomized controlled trial. *Journal of Tissue Viability, 14,* 88–96.

Yuen, H. K., & Garrett, D. (2001). Comparison of three wheelchair cushions for effectiveness of pressure relief. *American Journal of Occupational Therapy, 55*(4), 470–475.

# Wound Healing in the Elderly

# 20

Courtney H. Lyder

## Introduction

Healing wounds is a complicated process and an understanding of the normal function of the skin layers and wound-healing cascade is vital to good outcomes. As people age, changes occur to the skin layers as well as to wound-healing phases that delay or impede the healing process. Complicating the wound-healing process is the fact that a large number of hospitalized elderly will be diagnosed with one or more medical conditions that will also affect wound healing. The combination of these skin layer and wound-healing phase changes in the elderly coupled with medical conditions, including cardiac and respiratory illnesses and diabetes makes it very difficult or impossible to heal chronic wounds such as pressure, arterial, venous, and diabetic ulcers.

This chapter lists the demography of the elderly and the background and significance of wounds. A description of normal skin layers and functions along with the changes that occur as people age follows. The normal wound-healing cascade and changes that occur with the elderly population are then presented. Finally, the influences of poor tissue perfusion, malnutrition, and infection on wound healing are described.

## Background and Significance

The treatment of chronic wounds costs Americans billions of dollars annually and a 10% increase in cost for the treatment of chronic wounds is projected per year (Administration on Aging, 2003). Millions of people are affected by one or more chronic wounds each year (Mustoe, O'Shaughnessy, & Kloesters, 2006; Pittmam, 2007). Pressure ulcers, venous stasis ulcers, and diabetic ulcers comprise most of the chronic wounds (Mustoe et al., 2006). The prevalence of chronic wounds is a concern. One hundred and twenty of 100,000 persons between the ages of 45 and 64, 150 of 100,00 persons between the ages of 65 and 74, and 800 of 100,000 persons over the age of 75 have a chronic wound (Pittman, 2007). Three and a half percent of the population 65 years and older have a venous stasis ulcer. The reoccurrence rate of venous stasis ulcers is approximately 70% (Hess & Kirsner, 2003). Seventeen million people have been diagnosed with diabetes. Approximately 15% of those diagnosed with diabetes will develop a diabetic ulcer (Hanft, Temar, & Williams, 2002; Hess & Kirsner). A lower extremity amputation will be necessary in 15 to 20% of those who have a diabetic ulcer and these numbers are predicted to increase as more people are diagnosed with diabetes (Hanft et al.; Hess & Kirsner).

The most common ulcer to occur in the critical care elder is pressure ulcers. The National Pressure Ulcer Advisory Panel (NPUAP) suggests incidence rates of hospital-acquired pressure ulcers range within 0.4 to 38% (NPUAP, 2001). However, the higher incidence rates of 20 to 38% are found in the critical care areas of the hospital. These elders are most vulnerable because of their comorbid conditions. Moreover, there is ample evidence to suggest these ulcers occur very early (within 72 hours) during the critical care stay. The NPUAP suggests that mortality rates are as high as 60% for elders with pressure ulcers within 1 year of hospital discharge. It should be noted that the ulcer may not cause the demise of the elder, but rather is an indicator of the decline in health status posthospitalization.

The prevalence of facility-acquired pressure ulcers reported by the NPUAP in acute-care facilities ranges from 10 to 18%. Patients over the age of 70 account for 70% of hospital-acquired pressure ulcers (Thomas, 2001). Estimated costs of treating patients with pressure ulcers in 2004 dollars are $9.1 to $11.6 billon annually (Zulkowski, Langemo, Posthauer, & NPUAP, 2005. Treatment cost per pressure ulcer was $20,900 to $151,700 dollars (Zulkowski et al.). As of October 1, 2008, the Centers for Medicare and Medicaid Services will no longer pay for any hospital-acquired stage III or stage IV pressure ulcer. Thus, it will be imperative for hospitals to identify and heal these ulcers early in their development.

## Skin Layers and Function

The skin is the body's largest organ; it forms a protective barrier from the external environment and at the same time maintains internal homeostasis (Wysocki, 2007). The thickness of skin varies from 0.5 mm to 6 mm (Wysocki). Skin weighs approximately 6 pounds or is equal to 15% of the entire body mass for an adult (Wysocki). The skin has several functions, including: (a) protection against pathogens, (b) protection against trauma, (c) protection against ultraviolet radiation, (d) thermoregulation, (e) skin immune system, (f) sensation, (g) metabolism of vitamin D, (h) communication, (i) regeneration of new skin cells, (j) elimination of waste products, and (k) expression

## 20.1  Functions of the Epidermis Layers

| Epidermis Layers | Description and Function |
|---|---|
| Stratum corneum | Top layer (.02 mm to .5 mm)<br>Composed of dead keratinocytes<br>Flat cells without nuclei<br>Cells shed continually<br>Cells consist of keratin (a tough, fibrous, insoluable protein)<br>Protects from external stimulus entering the body<br>Averts water loss |
| Stratum lucidum | Established in thick epidermis of the palms of the hands and soles of the feet<br>One to five cells deep<br>Transparent layer<br>Cells are nonviable<br>Consists of prekeratin filament and protein<br>Protects from friction by the toughness of the layer |
| Stratum granulosum | Granular layer<br>One to five cells deep<br>Diamond shaped not flattened<br>Contains proteins to help organize the keratin filament |
| Stratum spinosum | Spinous layer<br>Contains the desmosome, which is a cell–cell junction<br>Polyhedral<br>Produces involucrin (precursor to cornified envelopes)<br>Contains new keratin filaments |
| Stratum germinativum | Basal layer<br>Single layer of basal keratinocytes<br>Respond to extracellular matrix, growth factors, hormones, and vitamins<br>As cells leave the basal layer differentiation begins<br>Consists of Rete ridges that assist in the adherence of the epidermis to the dermis<br>Melanocytes for skin pigmentation |

of emotions (Allwood & Curry, 2000; Doughty & Sparks-DeFriese, 2007; Langemo & Brown, 2006). The skin is divided into three main layers known as the epidermis, dermis, and subcutaneous. The epidermis and dermis layers are separated by the basement membrane.

The epidermis is avascular and receives oxygen and nourishment by diffusion. Langerhans cells are found in the epidermis and are responsible for identification, uptake, development, arrangement of soluble antigens, and sensitization of T lymphocytes (Wysocki, 2007). The epidermis contains glucose, carbohydrates, and enzymes for energy (Allwood & Curry, 2000). The body's ability to access this energy is crucial to wound healing. The epidermis contains five layers, including: (a) stratum corneum, (b) stratum lucidum, (c) stratum granulosum, (d) stratum spinosum, and (e) stratum germinativum (Allwood & Curry; Wysocki). The description and function of the epidermis layers are listed in Table 20.1 (Allwood & Curry; Wysocki).

## 20.2    Cell Type and Function

| Cell Type | Function |
| --- | --- |
| Fibroblast | ■ Most abundant cell<br>■ Forms connective tissue<br>■ Secretes growth factors |
| Macrophage | ■ Derived from tissue monocytes from bone marrow precursor cells<br>■ Most important cell due to their adaptability<br>■ Secrete growth factors, cytokines, and immune molecules<br>■ Antibacterial effects<br>■ Coagulation<br>■ Angiogenesis<br>■ Tissue remodeling<br>■ Phagocytosis of debris and foreign bodies<br>■ Vital in reabsorption and recycling of tissue and their components<br>■ Participate in immune response<br>■ Critical in wound healing |
| Mast cell | ■ Found surrounding vascular connective tissue<br>■ Mainly in the papillary layer and subcutaneous tissue<br>■ Secrete proteins<br>■ Responsible for the release of histamines with injury, infection, and exposure to allergens<br>■ Numerous in subacute and chronic inflammatory diseases<br>■ Phagocytosis |

The dermis layer is the thickest part of the skin ranging from 2 mm to 4 mm deep (Wysocki, 2007). The dermis contains cells, nerves, skin appendages, and blood vessels. The dermis layer is divided into two layers known as the papillary dermis and reticular layer. The papillary dermis is responsible for the nourishment and oxygenation of the viable cells of the epidermis (Allwood & Curry, 2000; Wysocki). The reticular layer contains hair follicles, nerve sensory endings, sweat glands, and sebaceous glands. The reticular layer of the dermis is accountable for the skin's sturdiness and strength (Allwood & Curry).

Two primary proteins found in the dermis are collagen and elastin. Collagen is a structural protein that is matured by secreted tropocollagen from dermal fibroblasts and an extracellular course (Allwood & Curry, 2000; Wysocki, 2007). The dermis consists of type I fiber-forming collagen, which provides the skin's tensile strength (Wysocki). Elastin is a protein that is fiber forming, which provides elastic recoil to the skin (Allwood & Curry; Wysocki). Elastin forms structures similar to a coil or spring that can be stretched and returned to its original shape (Wysocki).

Three main cell types found in the dermis are fibroblasts, macrophages, and mast cells. Their functions are listed in Table 20.2 (Allwood & Curry; Wysocki).

The subcutaneous layer contains loose connective tissue. This layer connects the dermis to the muscle (Allwood & Curry, 2000). This layer provides vascularization, insulation, energy stores, mobility of the skin, and cushioning for underlying structures (Wysocki, 2007).

## Skin Layer Function Changes in the Elderly

All three of the skin layers are present as people age but changes occur within these layers that affect wound healing. The changes to the epidermis, dermis, and subcutaneous layer begin in the third decade of life and these changes continue over many years (Allwood & Curry, 2000; Doughty & Sparks-DeFriese, 2007). Some of these changes are visible in the second decade of life as a result of excessive exposure to sunlight (Montagna & Carlisle, 1979). Major changes are evident at approximately 70 years old (Doughty & Sparks-DeFriese). The epidermal and dermal junction flattens, which increases shear-injury risk (Pittman, 2007). Changes that occur within the three skin layers are described in Table 20.3 (Allwood & Curry; Baranoski, 2001; Gosain & DiPietro, 2004; Doughty & Sparks-DeFriese; Johnson, 1996; Montagna & Carlisle; Pittman; Roberts, 2007; Vohra & McCollum, 1994; Witkowski & Parish, 2000).

## Repair Mechanisms

Repair occurs by two different mechanisms. The first mechanism is regeneration, which is tissue repair. The second mechanism is scar tissue formation or connective tissue repair. The mechanism for repair depends on the depth of the tissue damage. Partial thickness, which involves the epidermis and dermis layers, heals by regeneration. Full thickness, which extends past the dermis layer, heals by connective tissue repair.

## Normal Wound-Healing Cascade

The normal wound-healing cascade is a complex process that is activated the instant damage occurs to the skin. Knowledge of normal wound-healing phases is essential for the clinician in order to understand the changes that occur as people age. The normal wound-healing cascade and the cell functions will be described in the following sections.

### Homeostasis

Some literature combines the vascular response and inflammatory phase because homeostasis occurs simultaneously with the inflammatory phase (Ayello et al., 2004). Homeostasis is achieved when vasoconstriction of the blood vessels occurs and platelets arrive at the wound. A blood clot is formed by the platelets to hinder blood loss Hess & Kirsner, 2003). Blood clotting is started by commencement of a proteolytic cascade that produces thrombin and fibrin (Knighton, Fiegel, Doucette, Fylling, & Cerra, 1989; Shultz & Mast, 1998). Thrombin works together with platelets to create alpha granule release of platelet growth factors (Knighton et al.). Fibrin creates the blood clot, which consists of fibrin, red blood cells, and platelets (Knighton et al.,

## 20.3 Skin Changes in the Elderly

| Skin Layer | Changes |
|---|---|
| Epidermal layer | ■ Epidermal turnover time increases, which delays wound healing time<br>■ The barrier protection function is deceased, which increases the risk for irritation and breakdown of the skin<br>■ A decrease in the amount of Langerhans cell production increases the risk of cancer and infection<br>■ A decrease in Langerhans cell production decreases immunity properties of the skin<br>■ Melanocytes are decreased as well as an abnormal production of melanocytes, which decrease protection against ultraviolet radiation<br><br>Reduction in sensation, which increases the risk for trauma and injury |
| Dermal layer | ■ Dermis decreases in thickness and appears flatter and thinner<br>■ Decrease in the number of sweat glands: hypothermia and heat stoke are more likely<br>■ Decreased vascular components, approximately 35% of vertical capillary loops<br>■ Blood vessels are more pronounced<br>■ Skin elasticity decreases, which is related to age and sun damage<br>■ Collagen appears to be unwinding and elastin appears to be lysing<br>■ Wrinkling and sagging occur<br>■ Decreased skin turgor is apparent<br>■ Structure is irregularly shaped<br>■ Dehydration of skin<br>■ Decreased macrophage production<br>■ Decreased inflammatory response<br>■ Decrease in mast cells and melanocytes, which affects allergic reactions<br>■ Healing time is delayed<br>■ Bruising and purpura are evident |
| Subcutaneous layer | ■ Decreased amount of subcutaneous fat<br>■ Decrease in thermoregulation<br>■ Decreased insulation to extremities<br>■ Decreased skin fold breadth |

Shultz & Mast). The blood clot is a new matrix that seals the wound and protects it from bacterial invasion and water loss (Mast & Schultz, 1996). Following this initial response, vasodilatation and increased capillary permeability occur, which causes leakage of plasma (Ayello et al., Schultz et al., 2003).

Platelet degranulation provides the first signals to begin the wound-healing cascade. Alpha granule of the platelets contain growth factors, which are: (a) platelet derived growth factors (PDGF), (b) insulin-like growth factor-1 (IGF-1), (c) epidermal growth factors (EGF), (d) fibroblast growth factor (FGF), and (e) transforming growth factor-B (TGF-B) (Schultz et al., 2003). These growth factors are released from platelets and leave the wound, migrating into the surrounding tissue and blood vessels (Mast & Schultz, 1996). Growth factors release signals to inflammatory cells as a response to injured cells (Hess & Kirsner, 2003). Growth factors stimulate production, movement, and delineation of wound cells that include epithelial cells, fibroblasts, and endothelial

## 20.4   Growth Factors and Functions

| Growth Factor | Function |
| --- | --- |
| Platelet derived growth factors (PDGF) | Derived from platelets, fibroblasts, keratinocytes, and macrophages<br>■ Deposition of extracellular matrix<br>■ Angiogenesis<br>■ Fibroblast and immune cell initiation<br>■ Increases collagen synthesis<br>■ Increases TIMP synthesis<br>■ Decreases MMP synthesis |
| Insulin-like growth factor-1 (IGF-1) | Derived from fibroblasts, neutrophils and macrophages<br>■ Stimulation of keratinocytes and fibroblasts<br>■ Initiation of endothelial cell<br>■ Angiogenesis<br>■ Collagen synthesis<br>■ Deposition of extracellular matrix<br>■ Metabolism of cells |
| Epidermal growth factors (EGF) | Derived from fibroblasts, keratinocytes and macrophages<br>■ Stimulation and movement of keratinocytes<br>■ Deposition of extracellular matrix |
| Fibroblast growth factor (FGF) | Derived from fibroblasts, endothelial cells, and macrophages<br>■ Deposition of extracellular matrix<br>■ Angiogenesis<br>■ Initiation of endothelial cell<br>■ Stimulation and movement of keratinocytes |
| Transforming growth factor-B (TGF-B) | Derived from platelets, fibroblasts, and macrophages<br>■ Chemoattractant to fibroblasts<br>■ Deposition of extracellular matrix<br>■ Increases collagen synthesis<br>■ Increases TIMP synthesis<br>■ Decreases MMP synthesis |

cells (Ayello et al., 2004). This begins the inflammatory phase of wound healing, which is catabolic. Growth factors and functions are described in Table 20.4 (Morykwas & Argenta, 1997; Okan, Woo, Ayello, & Sibbald, 2007; Woo, Ayello, & Sibbald, 2007).

## Inflammatory Phase

The first cells to arrive to the wound and initiate phagocytosis are polymorphonuclear neutrophils (PMN) (Hess & Kirsner, 2003). These are blood-borne cells that protect the host from bacteria and infection. Neutrophils release tumor necrosis factor-α (TNF-α) and interleukins IL-2 and Il-4, which are proinflammatory cytokines that work at the site of injury (Mast & Schultz, 1996). Neutrophils also release matrix metalloproteinase eight (MMP-8), which consists of neutrophil elastase and neutrophil collagenase

(Schultz & Mast, 1998). The purpose of MMP-8 is to remove the damaged extracellular matrix, which is replaced with new extracellular matrix (Schultz & Mast). This action allows for the wound-healing cascade to continue in a proper sequence. The number of neutrophils present decreases dramatically within 72 hours after the initial injury has occurred.

Monocytes are crucial in the inflammatory phase. Monocytes are blood-borne cells that are attracted to the wound by complement-derived peptides (C5a), degradation products from fibronectin, and TGF-B (Knighton et al., 1989). Monocytes mature into macrophages within 24 to 48 hours after the injury has occurred (Hess & Kirsner, 2003; Knighton et al.).

Macrophages are considered the most important of the wound cells because they are involved in all phases of wound healing (Frenkel et al., 2002). Macrophages replace neutrophils in the wound and are responsible for several actions during the inflammatory phase. They initiate phagocytosis, which breaks down dead cells and the damaged matrix (Hess & Kirsner, 2003). Macrophages are bactericidal and promote angiogenesis (Ayello et al., 2004).

Macrophages secrete more growth factors and signal for additional macrophages and monocytes to respond to the wound as a result of their chemoattractant properties (Schultz et al., 2003). Macrophages secrete proinflammatory cytokines that attract inflammatory cells into the wound from the surrounding blood vessels (Frenkel et al., 2002). The proinflammatory cytokines are TNF-á and interleukins IL-1, IL-6, and IL-8. IL-1 and TNF-á rouse vascular endothelial cells to express cell bonding (Schultz & Mast, 1998). The IL-1 and TNF-á are mitogenic with fibroblasts, MMP expression is up regulated, and tissue inhibitors of metalloproteinases (TIMPs) are down regulated (Schultz & Mast). The vascular cells construct IL-8 as a response to IL-1 and TNF-á to express cell bonding on the inflammatory cells (Schultz & Mast). IL-6 is responsible for fibroblast production and protein synthesis (Schultz et al., 2003). Amino acids and sugars are converted from macromolecules by macrophages for wound healing (Hess & Kirsner, 2003).

Mast cells are derived from the dermis. One function of these cells is local inflammation, which increases the sensation of pain. Another function of the mast cell is to increase vascular permeability. Histamines, prostaglandins, leukotrienes, and enzymes are released by mast cells.

## Proliferative Phase

The next phase of wound healing is the proliferative phase or the connective tissue phase, which is anabolic. This phase can last for several weeks (Hess & Kirsner, 2003). During the proliferative phase, the number of inflammatory cells decreases and is replaced by fibroblasts, endothelial cells, and keratinocytes (Ayello et al., 2004). Macrophages are mediators for the initiation of the proliferative phase (Frenkel et al., 2001). The proliferative phase is initiated by the stimulation of the movement of fibroblasts, epithelial cells, and vascular endothelial cells to begin the healing of the wound by the formation of granulation tissue (Schultz et al., 2003). Cell movement and production persist as a temporary matrix is created, which contains fibrin and fibronectin (Ayello et al.; Schultz et al.). Granulation tissue replaces the temporary matrix as it fills the wound cavity. Granulation tissue provides a moist surface for cell migration. A decrease in wound dimension occurs as the wound edges contract together, lessening the wound-surface dimension as the wound fills with granulation tissue. Granulation tissue is vastly vascular and damage to this tissue occurs easily. Granulation tissue contains fibroblasts, keratinocytes, macrophages, immature collagen, endothelial cells, and new blood vessels (Hess & Kirsner, 2003).

Approximately 5 days after injury fibroblasts arrive to the wound. Fibroblasts secrete PDGF, IGF-1, bFGF, TGF-â, and keratinocyte growth factor (KGF). Fibroblasts stimulate production of cells, creation of extracellular proteins, and formation of new blood vessels (Ayello et al., 2004; Schultz & Mast, 1998). Fibroblasts produce and release collagen, a major connective tissue protein, as well as elastin and proteoglycans molecules (Ayello et al.). Fibroblasts initiate the production of collagen, which gives the tissue strength and composition (Hess & Kirsner, 2003). Fibroblasts do not perform phagocytosis so dead cells and a damaged matrix impede the migration of these cells.

Keratinocytes are the main cells of the epidermal layer and travel from the wound edges for epithelialization (Hess & Kirsner, 2003; Woo et al., 2007). Epithelialization is the last step in the proliferative phase. Keratinocytes form scar tissue as they travel and reproduce across the wound bed only with the existence of healthy granulation tissue (Hess & Kirsner). Growth factors and cytokines synthesized by keratinocytes are TGF-â, TNF-á, and Il-1/A, which stimulate cell production, extracellular protein formation, and angiogenesis (Mast & Schultz, 1996). Keratinocyte's five main functions are to (a) assist with proliferation of cells, (b) attract other cells to the wound, (c) provide antibacterial properties, (d) initiate epithelialization, and (e) signal transduction activity (Woo et al., 2007).

Endothelial cells promote development of new blood vessels quickly, which are necessary for nutrition for the new tissue. These cells stimulate fibrinolysis, breaking down the temporary matrix so fibroblast movement and collagen synthesis can occur. The growth factors synthesized by endothelial cells are vascular endothelial growth factors (VEGF), bFGF and PDGF (Mast & Schultz, 1996).

## Maturation Phase

The final phase is the maturation phase or the remodeling phase. This phase can take months to years and is catabolic. Collagen fibers are the main substance in the wound and fiber collection increases creating a thick collagenous arrangement. Fibroblasts, MMPs, TIMPs, and TGF are vital to organizing, remodeling, and maturing the collagen fibers (Hess & Kirsner, 2003). Fibroblasts stimulate production of collagen, elastin, proteoglycans, MMPs, and TIMPs (Mast & Schultz, 1996). This action persists until the tensile strength of scar tissue is approximately 80% of normal tissue (Hess & Kirsner). Apoptosis or programmed cell death decreases fibroblast and capillary density (Ayello et al., 2004). Scar tissue decreases and the appearance of the scar tissue becomes less red and flat over time (Ayello et al.). This is known as the remodeling of the scar.

## Wound-Healing Cascade Changes in the Older Adult

Changes in the rate of healing time have been reported in the literature among the fetus, children, adults, and the elderly (Stotts & Wipke-Tevis, 2001). The wound-healing process is greatly affected when elders have one or more medical conditions.

As a person ages, wounds heal slower as well as become chronic because of a delayed inflammatory phase when one or more chronic diseases are present (Stotts & Wipke-Tevis). This can be attributed to changes within the wound-healing cascade as well as the influence of chronic disease and medications that affect tissue perfusion (Gusenoff, Redett, & Nahabedian, 2002; Langemo & Brown, 2006; Stotts & Wipke-Tevis). Malnutrition and infection contribute to impeded wound healing in the elderly (Gusenoff et al.; Stotts & Wipke-Tevis).

Wound-healing studies are limited with human subjects for ethical reasons. Researchers have established that changes occur during the wound-healing cascade, which include (a) an increase of adherence of the platelets to the endothelium; (b) increase of the release of alpha-granules by platelets; (c) a decreased amount of nitric acid by endothelial cells; (d) a decrease of neutrophils; (e) decrease in the response from keratinocytes, fibroblasts, and endothelial cells; and (f) a decrease in collagen (Allwood & Curry, 2000; Doughty & Sparks-DeFriese, 2007). The existence of a direct correlation between animal models and human models is unknown (Swift, Burns, Gray, & DiPietro, 2001). However, three studies using animal models describe changes that occur within the wound-healing cascade, these are described in Table 20.5 (Ashcroft, Horan, & Ferguson, 1997; Quirinia & Viidik, 1991; Swift et al.). Other researchers have observed that injecting activated monocytes/macrophages into wounds increases the healing rate of pressure ulcers in the elderly and spinal cord injured (Frenkel et al., 2001, 2002).

The most important factor in aiding the wound-healing process in elders in critical care is increasing tissue perfusion. This can be incredibly challenging for critically ill elders who have hemodynamic challenges. The wound cannot heal without sufficient blood supply. Intrinsic factors such as anemia, diabetes, cardiovascular disease, hypotension, chronic obstructive pulmonary disease, low blood protein levels, high temperature, and smoking can increase demand for oxygen and the metabolic rate (Doughty & Sparks-DeFriese, 2007; Grey, Harding & Enoch, 2006; Stotts & Wipke-Tevis, 2001). Severe anemia affects tissue perfusion, which decreases the oxygen transportation capability of the blood (Langemo & Brown, 2006; Phillips, 1999; Stotts & Wipke-Tevis). Macrovascular and microvascular changes in the circulatory system in diabetic patients reduce tissue perfusion (Baranoski, 2006; Phillips, 1999). Patients with cardiovascular disease who have low ejection fractions have a reduction in tissue perfusion and low capillary closing (Calianno, 2000). An elevation of 1 degree in body temperature increases oxygen demand and metabolic rate by 10% (Andrychuk, 1998).

Oxygen requirements vary depending on the wound-healing phase. The inflammatory phase has the highest requirement (Doughty & Sparks-DeFriese, 2007). Bactericidal activity is more effective with higher oxygen levels (Doughty & Sparks-DeFriese). Improved collagen synthesis and tensile strength are reported with higher levels of oxygen (Doughty & Sparks-DeFriese). The proliferative phase requires lower oxygen levels (Doughty & Sparks-DeFriese). A degree of hypoxia in the wound can enhance angiogenesis (Doughty & Sparks-DeFriese).

Certain medications that are prescribed to treat chronic diseases can affect the skin layers and wound-healing cascade (Doughty & Sparks-DeFriese, 2005). Corticosteroids impede regeneration of the epidermis and collagen synthesis (Allwood & Curry, 2000; Baranoski, 2006; Tashkin, Murray, Skeans, & Murray, 2004; Torres & Stadelmann, 2006). Antibiotics, corticosteroids, and hormones can change the skin's protective barrier function. The inflammatory response is affected by other medications such as analgesics, antihistamines, and nonsteroidal antiinflammatory agents (Doughty &

## 20.5   Wound Healing Alterations in Animal Models

| Study | Findings |
|---|---|
| Ashcroft, Horan, and Ferguson (1997) | Rate of healing is dependent on the cause, depth, and site of injury |
| | Absence or presence of comorbidities affects wound healing |
| | Age-related changes were noted in the rate and quality of wound healing |
| | A delay in inflammatory response was noted due to monocytes/macrophage and B-lymphocyte migration |
| | Decrease in the number of cytokines released or a damaged migration response |
| | Decreased action of macrophages |
| | Decrease in plasma fibronectin, which could affect attachment and migration of cells |
| | A delay of epithelialization was observed |
| Quirinia and Viidik (1991) | Ischemia affects wound healing more significantly in older rats then younger rats |
| | Repair of vascular components should be a priority intervention |
| | Ischemia is more harmful during the beginning stages of wound healing |
| | Ischemic wounds are more susceptible to infections that impair the inflammatory phase |
| Swift, Burns, Gray, and DiPietro (2001) | Neutrophil migration was unchanged in excisional wounds but macrophage migration was significant |
| | Increase in the number of macrophages but the action of the macrophages was decreased |
| | A reduction in phagocytosis as well as the amount of damaged matrix that was affected |
| | Reduction of signaling from cell surface |
| | Macrophage secretion of VEGF for angiogenesis was reduced |
| | T-cell migration is delayed as well as altered actions of the cells |
| | Inflammatory and proliferative responses are significantly reduced with chemokine-production alterations |

Sparks-DeFriese). Antihypertension, vasoactive medications and diuretics may cause hypotension and dehydration of the skin (Andrychuk, 1998). Chemotherapy medications may interrupt the cell cycle and production of cells (Andrychuk).

Malnutrition and a lack of hydration impede wound healing (Cutting & Cardiff, 1994; Ratliff & Bryant, 2004; Stotts & Wipke-Tevis, 2001). Low protein serum levels are linked with delayed wound healing (Calianno, 2000; Grey et al., 2006). Collagen synthesis is reduced with low blood protein levels so tissue is thinner, which impedes wound healing (Phillips, 1999; Torres & Stadelmann, 2006). Functions of protein include reproduction of cells, construction of antibodies, alteration of the wound, creation of blood vessels, and promotion of collagen synthesis (Andrychuk, 1998). Adequate intake of protein, calories, fat, vitamins, and minerals are vital for suitable nutrition for wound healing (Stechmiller, 2003; Stotts & Wipke-Tevis, 2001). Dehydration is also correlated with wound healing because of drying of the skin (Post-hauer, 2006).

Bacteria from surrounding skin contaminate the wound within 24 hours (Mustoe et al., 2006). High levels of bacteria in wounds can delay or impede wound healing (Cutting & Cardiff, 1994; Ovington, 2001). Chronic wounds are contaminated with bacteria (McGuckin, Goldman, Bolton, & Salcido, 2003; Ovington, 2002). Patients can present with fevers; tachycardia, hypotension, delirium, leukocytosis, or high glucose levels, which affect tissue perfusion and oxygen demands (McGuckin et al.). High quantities of bacteria are found in chronic wounds, which result in a prolonged inflammatory phases (Dow, Browne, & Sibbald, 1999). Inflammatory cells are constantly released, neutrophils continue to migrate to the wound, and thrombosis and vasoconstriction persist (Dow et al.; Falanga, 2002). A reduction in oxygen in a wound results in production of bacteria, damage of tissue, and reduction of platelets (Dow et al). Infected wounds have increased drainage, which alters the production and function of wound cells (Falanga). Extracellular matrix proteins are damaged by proteases that are found in the exudate (Falanga). Copious amounts of drainage can affect growth factors as well as fibroblasts and keratinocytes, which are necessary for wound healing (Falanga).

The management principles to consider in healing wounds in critical care are multifactorial. Thus, you have to understand the unique needs of the critically ill older adult. Assessing the patient as a whole and not simply the whole in the patient is critical. However, several management principles should be considered in wound healing in older adults (Brem & Lyder, 2004). The use of support surfaces to offload pressure (alternating air mattresses, low-air-loss mattresses or air-fluidized mattresses) is critical. Further, the use of frequent turning (every 1 to 2 hours) is beneficial. The removal of debris and/or necrotic tissue in the wound bed, as this may lead to wound infection is necessary. If infection is noted, it is imperative to use silver dressings or to implement IV antibiotics. The use of cleansing solutions or debridement may be very helpful in removing wound debris and/or necrotic tissue. Meeting the nutritional requirements for the critically ill older adults is important as wounds heal with a positive nitrogen balance. If too much protein is lost healing will be delayed as low protein stores lead to negative nitrogen balance, which will further delay healing. Finally, the principle of moist wound healing should be employed. Wounds heal faster when they are moist. Too much exudate may macerate surrounding tissue and if the wound is too dry, granulation tissue will not proliferate.

The following case studies highlight some of the challenges of wound healing for the critically ill older adult.

## Case Study

CC and HPI: A 79-year-old White male was resuscitated by emergency medical technicians at a local grocery store after complaining of chest pain and passing out. Previous medical history: Myocardial infarction (in 1999), hypertension, coronary artery disease, high cholesterol, diabetes, chronic renal insufficiency.

PSH: coronary artery bypass of three vessels (1999), right total knee replacement (1996)

SH: occasional alcohol intake, quit smoking in 1999 (20 PPD), no substance abuse.

Patient arrived at the emergency room unconscious, ventilated with an ambu bag, and intravenous fluid infusing. His heart rate was 40 to 50 with a blood pressure of 70/30 and POX of 88%. He was placed on a ventilator at 100% oxygen and vasopressors were started. Within 12 hours of admission the nursing staff in the intensive care unit identified a purple area on his sacrum that was intact. A wound care consult was obtained. The patient could be turned every 2 hours per protocol. He was on an Atmos air mattress. He had an indwelling catheter and no stool was reported. Patient was NPO (nothing by mouth).

Initial assessment (length, width, and depth) of the sacral area revealed a deep tissue injury pressure ulcer 9 cm x 5 cm x 0 cm. The area had different hues of purple tissue with areas of epidermis sloughing off revealing red tissue. The ulcer was shallow, indurated, and warm. There was no odor or drainage. Although a small area of tissue was visible, it should be noted that the purple area in devitalized tissue needs to be protected.

Treatment orders included an enzyme debridement applied every 12 hours, continue to turn every 2 hours, use of a low-air-loss bed with his head of bed less than 30 degrees as tolerated. A nutritional consult was obtained (see Figure 20.1).

Resuscitation attempts failed when the patient went asystole 3 days after admission.

## Case Study

CC and HPI: A 70-year-old White male arrives at the emergency room with chest pain

PMH: hypertension, high cholesterol.

PSH: none

SH: no alcohol, tobacco, or substance abuse

Cardiac catheterization revealed coronary artery disease and a VAD pump was placed. He had many episodes of hypotension and was on vasopressors. He was on a ventilator for 3 weeks and was weaned to trach color. Patient was placed on the heart transplant list. He had a nasogastric tube for nutrition. He was incontinent of loose stools once or twice a day. An indwelling catheter was in place. He was on a low-air-loss mattress and was turned every 2 hours. There was a period of time during which the patient was unable to be turned because of hypotension. He had an episode of sepsis with fevers of 103 degrees F and was on intravenous antibiotics. He spent 4 weeks in intensive care, where he developed a stage IV pressure ulcer (see Figure 20.2).

## 20.1

**Deep tissue injury pressure ulcer.**

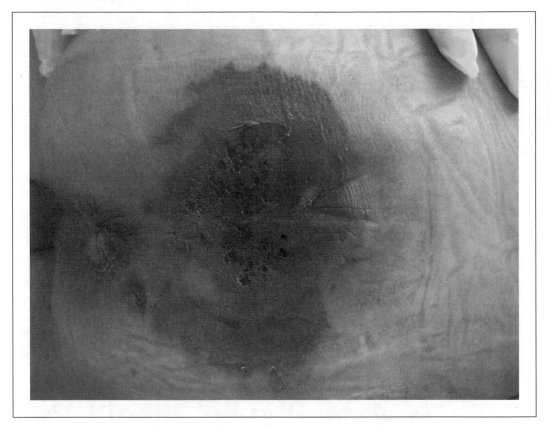

Assessment of the pressure ulcer in the intensive care unit revealed a 5 cm x 5 cm x 0 cm ulcer with a thick yellow brown necrotic area. There was no odor or drainage. The edges were not demarcated. The periulcer tissue was indurated with erythema

Initial treatment included chemical and sharp debridement of thick yellow brown tissue. Bone was revealed in the base of the wound and osteomyelitis was diagnosed. The tissue in the base of the wound was pale pink with edema. Negative pressure wound therapy was started with silver foam dressing once the necrotic tissue was removed and antibiotic therapy was initiated. Patient had a myocutaneous flap placed 2 weeks later.

The patient was unable to receive his heart transplant until the sacral pressure ulcer healed. He eventually received the heart transplant and was discharged home.

# 20.2

**Stage IV pressure ulcer.**

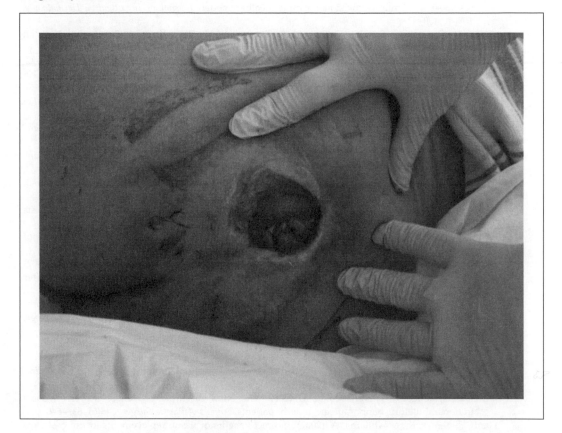

## Summary

Wound healing is a complex process that is affected as people age. Researchers have shown that changes occur within the skin layers and wound-healing cascade that can slow the healing process. These changes can be complicated by chronic disease, medications, nutrition, and infection, which makes it very difficult or impossible to heal chronic wounds such as pressure, arterial, venous, and diabetic ulcers. It is critical for clinicians caring for critically ill older adults to understand the wound-healing processes to optimize treatment.

## References

Administration on Aging. (2003). U.S. Department of Health and Human Services. *A profile of older Americans: 2003*. Retrieved May, 10, 2008, from http://www.infectioncontroltoday.com

Andrychuk, M. (1998). Pressure ulcers: Causes, risk factors, assessment, and intervention. *Orthopaedic Nursing, 4,* 65–81.

Allwood, J., & Curry, K. (2000). Normal and altered functions of the skin. In B. Bullock & R. Henze (Eds.), *Focus on pathophysiology* (pp. 838–844). Baltimore, MD: Lippincott Williams & Wilkins.

Ashcroft, G., Horan, M., & Ferguson, M. (1997). Aging is associated with reduced deposition of specific extracellular matrix components, an upregulation of angiogenesis, and an altered inflammatory response in a murine incisional wound healing model. *Journal of Investigative Dermatology, 108*(4), 430–437.

Ayello, E., Dowsett, C., Schultz, G., Sibbald, R., Falanga, V., Harding, K., et al. (2004). Time heals all wounds. *Nursing 2004, 34*(4), 36–42.

Baranoski, S. (2001). Skin tears: Guard against this enemy of frail skin. *Nursing Management, 32*(8), 25–32.

Baranoski, S. (2006). Raising awareness of pressure ulcer prevention and treatment. *Advances in Skin and Wound Care, 19,* 398–407.

Brem, H., & Lyder, C. (2004). Protocol for successful treatment of pressure ulcers. *American Journal of Surgery, 188,* 9–17.

Calianno, C. (2000). Assessing and preventing pressure ulcers. *Advances in Skin & Wound Care, 13*(5), 244–246.

Cutting, K., & Cardiff, K. (1994). Criteria for identifying wound infection. *Journal of Wound Care, 3*(4), 198–201.

Doughty, D., & Sparks-DeFriese B. (2007). Wound-healing physiology. In R, Bryant & D. Nix (Eds.), *Acute and chronic wounds: Current management concepts* (3rd ed., 56–81). St. Louis: Mosby.

Dow, G., Browne, A., & Sibbald, R. (1999). Infection in chronic wounds: Controversies in diagnosis and treatment. *Ostomy Wound Management, 45*(8), 23–40.

Falanga, V. (2002). Wound bed preparation and the role of enzymes: A case for multiple actions of therapeutic agents. *Wounds: A Compendium of Clinical Research and Practice, 14*(2), 47–57.

Frenkel, O., Shani, E., Ben-Bassat, I., Brok-Simoni, F., Rozenfeld-Granot, G., Kajakaro, G., et al. (2002) Activated macrophages for treating skin ulceration: Gene expression in human monocytes after hypo-osmotic shock. *Clinical and Experimental Immunology, 128,* 59–66.

Frenkel, O., Shani, E., Ben-Bassat, I., Brok-Simoni, F., Shinar, E., & Danon, D. (2001). Activation of human monocytes/macrophages by hypo-osmotic shock. *Clinical and Experimental Immunology, 124,* 103–119.

Gosain, A., & DiPietro, L. (2004, Feb.). Aging and wound healing. *World Journal of Surgery* (online journal).

Grey, J., Harding, K., & Enoch, S. (2006). ABC of wound healing: Pressure ulcers. *British Medical Journal, 332*(4), 472–475.

Gusenoff, J., Redett, R., & Nahabedian, M. (2002). Outcomes for surgical coverage of pressure sores in nonambulatory, nonparaplegic, elderly patients. *Annals of Plastic Surgery, 48*(6), 633–640.

Hanft, J., Temar, K., & Williams, A. (2002). Indirect benefits of tissue replacements justify costs. *Bio Mechanics, IX* (12).

Hess, C., & Kirsner, R. (2003). Orchestrating wound healing: Assessing and preparing the wound bed. *Advances In Skin & Wound Care, 16*(5), 257–259.

Johnson, M. (1996). Skin poblems of older adults. In A. Luggen (Ed.), Core curriculum for gerontological nursing (pp. 540–563). St Louis: Mosby.

Knighton, D., Fiegel, V., Doucette, M., Fylling, C., & Cerra, F. (1989). The use of topically applied platelet growth factors in chronic nonhealing wounds; A review. *Wounds: A Compendium of Clinical Research and Practice, 1,* 71–78

Langemo, D., & Brown, G. (2006). Skin fails too: Acute, chronic, and end-stage skin failure. *Advances in Skin & Wound Care, 19*(4), 206–212.

Mast, B., & Schultz, G. (1996). Interactions of cytokines, growth factors, and proteases in acute and chronic wounds. *Wound Repair and Regeneration, 4,* 411–420.

McGuckin, M., Goldman, R., Bolton, L., & Salcido, R. (2003). The clinical relevance of microbiology in acute and chronic wounds. *Advances In Skin & Wound Care, 16,* 12–25

Montagna, W., & Carlisle, K. (1979). Structural changes in aging human skin. *Journal of Investigative Dermatology, 73,* 47–53.

Morykwas, M., & Argenta, L. (1997). Nonsurgical modalities to enhance healing and care of soft tissue wounds. *Journal of the Southern Orthopaedic Association, 6*(4), 279–288.

Mustoe, T., O'Shaughnessy, K., & Kloeters, O. (2006). Chronic wound pathogenesis and current treatment strategies: A unifying hypothesis. *Plastic and Reconstructive Surgery, 117* (7S), 35S–41S.

National Pressure Ulcer Advisory Panel (NPUAP). (2001). Pressure ulcers in America: Prevalence, incidence, and implications for the future. An executive summary of the National Pressure Ulcer Advisory Panel monograph [see comment][erratum appears in *Advances in Skin & Wound Care*, (2002). *15*(6):E1–3; author reply E-3; PMID: 12477982]. *Advances in Skin & Wound Care, 14*(4), 208–215.

Okan, D., Woo, K., Ayello, E., & Sibbald, R. (2007). The role of moisture balance in wound healing. *Advances In Skin & Wound Care, 20*, 39–53.

Ovington, L. (2001) Battling bacteria in wound care. *Home Heath Care Nurse, 19*(10), 622–630.

Ovington, L. (2002) Dealing with drainage: The what, why, and how of wound exudate. *Home Heath Care Nurse, 20*(6), 368–374.

Phillips, L. (1999). Pressure ulcers—Prevention and treatment guidelines. *Nursing Standard, 14*(12), 56–62.

Pittman, J. (2007). Effect of aging on wound healing: Current concepts. *Journal of Wound, Ostomy, Continence Nursing, 34*(4), 412–417.

Posthauer, M. (2006). Hydration: Does it play a role in wound healing? *Advances in Skin & Wound Care, 19*(2), 97–102.

Quirinia, A., & Viidik, A. (1991). The influence of age on the healing of normal and ischemic incisional skin wounds. *Mechanisms of Aging and Development, 58*, 221–232.

Ratliff, C., & Bryant, D. (2004). Preemptive strike: Use new WOCN guideline to prevent wounds. *SUCCESS in Home Care, 3*, 20–24.

Roberts, M. (2007). Preventing and managing skin tears: A review. *Journal of Wound, Ostomy and Continence Nursing, 34*(3), 256–259.

Shultz, G., & Mast, B. (1998). Molecular analysis of the environment of healing and chronic wounds: Cytokines, proteases, and growth factors. *Wounds: A Compendium of Clinical Research and Practice, 10*(Suppl. F), 1F–9F.

Schultz, G., Sibbald, R., Falanga, V., Ayello, E., Dowsett, C., Harding, K., et al. (2003). Wound bed preparation: A systemic approach to wound management. *Wound Repair and Regeneration, 11*, 1–28.

Stechmiller, J. (2003). Early nutritional screening of older adults: Review of nutritional support. *Journal of Infusion Medicine, 26*(3), 170–177.

Stotts, N., & Wipke-Tevis, D. (2001). Co-factors in impaired wound healing. In D. Krasner, G, Rodeheaver, & G. Sibbald (Eds.), *Chronic wound care: A clinical source book for healthcare professionals* (3rd ed., pp. 265–272). Malvern, PA: HMP Communications.

Swift, M., Burns, A., Gray, K., & DiPietro, L. (2001). Age-related alterations in the inflammatory response to dermal injury. *Journal of Investigative Dermatology, 117*(5), 1027–1035.

Tashkin, D., Murray, E., Skeans, M., & Murray, R. (2004). Skin manifestation of inhaled corticosteroids in COPD patients: Results from Lung Health Study II. *Chest 2004, 126*(4), 1123–1133.

Thomas, D. R. (2001). Prevention and treatment of pressure ulcers: What works? What doesn't? *Cleveland Clinic Journal of Medicine, 68*(8), 704–707.

Torres, J., & Stadelmann, W. (2006).*Wound healing, chronic wounds*. E-medicine. Retrieved October 9, 2008, from http://emedicine.medsurg.com/article/1293452-oveview

Vohra, R., & McCollum, C. (1994). Fortnightly review: Pressure sores. *British Medical Journal, 309*(6958), 853–857.

Witkowski, J., & Parish, L. (2000). The decubitus ulcer: Skin failure and destructive behavior. *International Journal of Dermatology, 39*(12), 894–895.

Woo, K., Ayello, E., & Sibbald, R. (2007). The edge effect: Current therapeutic options to advance the wound edge. *Advances In Skin & Wound Care, 20*(2), 99–117.

Wysocki, A. (2007). Anatomy and physiology of skin and soft tissue. In R. Bryant & D. Nix (Eds.), *Acute and chronic wounds: Current management concepts* (3rd ed., pp. 39–55). St. Louis: Mosby

Zulkowski, K., Langemo, D., Posthauer, M. E., & National Pressure Ulcer Advisory Panel. (2005). Coming to consensus on deep tissue injury. *Advances in Skin & Wound Care, 18*(1), 28–29.

# Substance Abuse and Withdrawal

Marc Sabbe
Joris Vandenberghe

**21**

## Substance Use, Abuse, and Dependence: Terminology and Definitions

The use of psychoactive substances occurs in all times, ages, and cultures. Different categories of chemical substances are consumed to affect the central nervous system and change mental functioning. In general, these psychoactive effects can be summarized as inhibiting, excitatory, hallucinatory, or overlapping. To produce a mind-altering effect, a sufficiently large dose of any drug must reach the brain. Inhalation, injection, ingestion, or snuffing are common routes of administration.

The distinction between substance use and abuse is complex and determined by factors such as substance properties; frequency and quantity of use; personal sensitivity for substance effects; medical condition and potential therapeutic effects of the substance used; attitude toward the substance and psychological dynamics; social, religious, legal, and cultural aspects; context and health; and mental, occupational, relational, social, and societal consequences of substance use. Substance use can evolve to substance abuse and substance abuse can develop into substance dependence or addiction, in which dimensions such as tolerance, withdrawal, and craving (a strong desire for the substance or its effects) are central. These dimensions will be explored further in this chapter.

Substance abuse and dependence as clinical diagnoses are defined in the *Diagnostic and Statistical Manual of Mental Disorders, Fourth Edition, Text Revision, (DSM-IV-TR*; American Psychiatric Association [APA], 2000), as listed in Exhibit 21.1. The *International Statistical Classification of Diseases and Related Health Problems* (*ICD-10*; World Health Organization [WHO], 2007) uses a similar definition for substance-dependence syndrome:

> *A cluster of behavioral, cognitive, and physiological phenomena that develop after repeated substance use and that typically include a strong desire to take the drug, difficulties in controlling its use, persisting in its use despite harmful consequences, a higher priority given to drug use than to other activities and obligations, increased tolerance, and sometimes a physical withdrawal state. (WHO).*

For substance abuse, however, *DSM-IV-TR* (APA) and *ICD-10* (WHO) disagree on terminology and definition. *ICD-10* (WHO) prefers the broader term "harmful use," which is defined as follows: "A pattern of psychoactive substance use that is causing damage to health. The damage may be physical (as in cases of hepatitis from the self-administration of injected psychoactive substances) or mental (e.g. episodes of depressive disorder secondary to heavy consumption of alcohol)" (WHO). Harmful use as defined in *ICD-10* (WHO) includes psychoactive substance abuse. A scientific attempt to assess the harmfulness of different substances, as determined by their potential for physical harm, dependence, and social harm, resulted in the following order, from most harmful to least harmful: heroin, cocaine, barbiturates, street methadone, alcohol, ketamine, benzodiazepines, amphetamines, tobacco, buprenorphine, cannabis, solvents, 4-methylthioamphetamine (4-MTA), LSD (lysergic acid diethylamide), methylphenidate, anabolic steroids, gammahydroxybutyraat (GHB), ecstasy, alkyl nitrates, and khat (Nutt, King, Saulsbury & Blakemore, 2007).

The substances of abuse, doping agents, or medicinal drugs can be categorized based on chemical properties. However, from a clinical point of view, they should be grouped in terms of their effects on mental functioning. Three major groups can be recognized. First are substances that have dose-dependent inhibitory properties, such as opioids (heroin and others) and benzodiazepines. The inhibitory properties manifest clinically as calming effects—anxiolysis, analgesia, relaxation, sedation, and/or sleep—and can be accompanied by a deep feeling of well-being with euphoria or a feeling of encapsulation and altered perception of time and distance. The second group consists of the central nervous system stimulants, such as cocaine and amphetamines. These induce feelings of power; hypersexuality and increased sexual performance; increased energy, attention and concentration, and reduced fatigue; as well as an increased feeling of self-confidence. The third group is comprised of hallucinogens such as LSD, mescaline, and psilocybine.

Many substances have a combination of some of these three effects and sometimes they are dose dependent. For instance, cannabis can have inhibitory and hallucinogenic properties, and ecstasy excitatory and hallucinogenic properties. The effects vary by individual and instance, whereas others such as alcohol are dose dependent. In small doses, alcohol stimulates the brain; in large doses, alcohol is inhibitory. Psychoactive medication, used in daily medical practice, can have the same effects on mental functioning (e.g., psycholeptics, psychoanaleptics and psychodysleptics) (Tournier,

# Exhibit 21.1

## *DSM-IV-TR* Substance Abuse and Dependence Criteria

### *DSM-IV Substance-Abuse Criteria*

Substance abuse is defined as a maladaptive pattern of substance use leading to clinically significant impairment or distress as manifested by one (or more) of the following, occurring within a 12-month period:

1. Recurrent substance use resulting in a failure to fulfill major role obligations at work, school, or home (such as repeated absences or poor work performance related to substance use; substance-related absences, suspensions, or expulsions from school; or neglect of children or household).
2. Recurrent substance use in situations in which it is physically hazardous (such as driving an automobile or operating a machine when impaired by substance use).
3. Recurrent substance-related legal problems (such as arrests for substance-related disorderly conduct).
4. Continued substance use despite having persistent or recurrent social or interpersonal problems caused or exacerbated by the effects of the substance (for example, arguments with spouse about consequences of intoxication and physical fights).

Note: The symptoms for abuse have never met the criteria for dependence for this class of substance. According to the *DSM-IV-TR*, a person can be abusing a substance or dependent on a substance but not both at the same time (APA, 2000, p. 199).

### *DSM-IV-TR Substance-Dependence Criteria*

Substance dependence is defined as a maladaptive pattern of substance use leading to clinically significant impairment or distress, as manifested by three (or more) of the following, occurring any time in the same 12-month period:

1. Tolerance, as defined by either of the following:
   (a) A need for markedly increased amounts of the substance to achieve intoxication or the desired effect or
   (b) Markedly diminished effect with continued use of the same amount of the substance.
2. Withdrawal, as manifested by either of the following:
   (a) The characteristic withdrawal syndrome for the substance or
   (b) The same (or closely related) substance is taken to relieve or avoid withdrawal symptoms.
3. The substance is often taken in larger amounts or over a longer period than intended.
4. There is a persistent desire or unsuccessful efforts to cut down or control substance use.
5. A great deal of time is spent in activities necessary to obtain the substance, use the substance, or recover from its effects.
6. Important social, occupational, or recreational activities are given up or reduced because of substance use.
7. The substance use is continued despite knowledge of having a persistent physical or psychological problem that is likely to have been caused or exacerbated by the substance (for example, current cocaine use despite recognition of cocaine-induced depression or continued drinking despite recognition that an ulcer was made worse by alcohol consumption).

*Note*: From American Psychiatric Association. (2000). *Diagnostic and statistical manual of mental disorders* (4th ed., text rev., pp. 197–198). Washington DC: American Psychiatric Press.

Grolleau, Cougnard, Molimard, & Verdoux, 2009). Depending on the drug, physical or mental dependency, tolerance, abstinence reactions, and withdrawal effects can occur.

## Dependence

Substance dependence is a diagnosis, as described in *ICD-10* (WHO, 2007) and *DSM-IV-TR* (APA, 2000), but there is also a clinical dimension of substance use. As a clinical dimension, mental and physical dependency are distinguished.

Mental dependence results from the pleasant substance-induced effects. Compared to those experiences, daily life during drug-free periods is considered uninteresting. Individuals who experienced unpleasant effects of a particular drug rarely continue their drug intake. The rehabilitation process to overcome mental dependence is long and difficult. Physical dependence can be explained on a cellular level and often accompanies mental dependency. Specific cellular processes "demand" the presence of the substance. Physical dependence is connected with the abstinence reactions.

Patients with a mental or physical dependence for a specific drug might develop a tendency to manipulate professionals and family to receive the substance of abuse or a substance producing similar desired or cellular effects. The nature of the substance is an important factor in determining whether or not dependency will develop. Cocaine and opioids are considered to have severe dependency-developing properties, followed by nicotine, alcohol, and benzodiazepines. Besides the nature of the substance, the individual susceptibility for dependence is another mediating factor influencing dependency. This susceptibility is multifactorial and probably partially genetically mediated. The reward deficiency syndrome might be a central concept linking genotype and phenotype in substance dependency. This syndrome is described as an at least partly inherited decreased capacity to experience pleasant feelings of reward (for instance, safety, warmth, a full stomach, or rewarding social interactions) as a result of daily experiences. In reward deficiency syndrome, stronger stimuli such as psychoactive substances are needed to induce these pleasant feelings of reward or to alleviate the negative emotions that arise from continuing deprivation of reward-associated feelings (Blum et al., 2000; Comings & Blum, 2000).

## Tolerance

Tolerance is defined as a decrease in response to a dose of a psychoactive substance that occurs with continued use (WHO, 2007). Both physiological and psychosocial factors may contribute to tolerance. Tolerance may be physical, behavioral, or psychological (Isaac, Janca, & Sartorius, 1994). Physical tolerance results from a "down regulation" of the specific receptors stimulated by the substance, resulting in the need for increasing doses of the substance to experience the same effect. Tolerance is best known for opioids, but also exists for alcohol, benzodiazepines, and barbiturates (Dupen, Shen, & Ersek, 2007). The number and sensitivity of the opioid receptors diminishes and more substance is needed to occupy the same number of receptors, and thus to induce the same inhibitory effect. Clinically, this effect is relevant if medicinal drugs of the same category are needed because a dose increase is then necessary. For instance, a patient with heroin addiction needing opioid analgesia will require a larger dose to reach a sufficient analgesic effect. Tolerance and dependency are related but possess distinguishable dimensions.

## Abstinence Reactions and Withdrawal

Withdrawal is defined as a group of physical and psychological symptoms of variable clustering and degree of severity that occur on the cessation or reduction of use of a psychoactive substance that has been taken repeatedly, usually for a prolonged period and/or in high doses (WHO, 2007). Withdrawal state is one of the indicators of substance dependence. The onset and course of the syndrome are time-limited and are related to the type of substance and the dose being taken immediately prior to the cessation or reduction of use (Isaac et al., 1994). Abstinence or withdrawal reactions often present a mirror image of the acute substance effects. Withdrawal from an inhibitory substance such as opioids, benzodiazepines, barbiturates, or high doses of alcohol presents as an excitatory state, with restlessness and motor, behavioral, mental, and autonomic hyperactivity. Withdrawal from stimulants will often result in apathy and depressive feelings.

On a physiological level, withdrawal states can be understood as a result of tolerance and down regulation of receptors that the substance involved has affinity for. In the absence of the substance, the effects of the endogenous ligands will be minimal because of receptor down regulation and the balance between inhibition and excitation will shift in the opposite direction of the substance effect. Some withdrawal symptoms as, for instance, disturbed sleep, unpleasant feelings, irritability, and restlessness can be seen in all substance-withdrawal states.

## Substance Abuse in a Geriatric Population in Critical Care: Prevalence and Consequences

Illegal drug use is relatively rare among older adults, but there is a growing problem of abuse of prescription drugs. Psychoactive medications with abuse potential, such as benzodiazepines and opioids, are used by at least one in four older adults, and such use is likely to grow as the population ages. The present population of older adults consumes two to three times more psychoactive medications than younger age groups (Sheahan, 2000). It is estimated that up to 11% of older women misuse prescription drugs. Factors associated with drug abuse in older adults include female sex, social isolation, history of a substance-use or mental health disorder, and medical exposure to prescription drugs with abuse potential (Culberson & Ziska, 2008; Simoni-Wastila & Yang, 2006). However, little is known about the epidemiology of abuse in older adults, mainly because of research undersampling. Even problematic use of prescription drugs by older adults is usually unintentional. In addition, older adults present clinical and functional problems caused by limited substance abuse, such as drowsiness, sedation, confusion, memory loss, or other impairment of cognitive function, falls or other accidents, leading to hospitalization or institutionalization. In conclusion, the problem of substance abuse in an older population cannot be underestimated.

Alcohol abuse is another important problem in the geriatric population. Up to 16% of the elderly have alcohol-use disorders (Johnson, 2000; Menninger, 2002). Approximately 20% of medical and surgical hospital patients (Sander et al., 2006) and 10% of patients in intensive care units (Moss & Burnham, 2006) demonstrate an alcohol-use disorder. An important proportion of these patients are elderly, given the high prevalence of alcohol use disorders in older adults and their overrepresentation in hospitalizations. Up to 25% of hospitalized older adults are estimated to abuse alcohol (Ondus, Hujer, Mann, & Mion, 1999) and 14% of elderly patients in emergency departments (O'Connell, Chin, Cunningham, & Lawlor, 2003). Among elderly people, sociodemographic factors associated with alcohol use disorders include being male, socially isolated, single, and separated or divorced (O'Connell et al.). Alcohol abuse can appear for the first time late in life. One third of older people who abuse alcohol develop a problem with alcohol in later life, whereas the other two thirds grow older with the medical and psychosocial sequelae of early-onset alcoholism (Pierucci-Lagha, 2003). In addition, the effects of alcohol and substance abuse in older adults are influenced by physical, developmental, and psychosocial changes that occur with aging. Identification of alcohol and substance abuse presents a challenge for health care providers as older adults often present with atypical symptoms.

Finally, smoking is another quite prevalent form of substance abuse in the elderly. In Europe and in the United States, daily smoking among older adults (65 years of age and older) ranges from 8 to 20%, but this has declined over the past decades (Christensen, Low, & Anstey, 2006; Husten et al., 1997). Because substance abuse in older adults is mainly a problem of psychoactive medications, tobacco, and alcohol, the rest of this chapter will focus on these substance disorders.

In *critical care*, a term that is used to refer to intensive care and emergency medicine, several problems might arise in relation to substance abuse in the elderly: intoxication, withdrawal, delirium, behavioral problems, acute (e.g., respiratory depression) and chronic (e.g., liver cirrhosis) medical consequences, diagnostic problems (e.g., assessing consciousness in patients taking inhibitory substances) and therapeutic problems (e.g., relative insensitivity to sedating or analgesic effects of currently used medications in critical care). To anticipate and adequately deal with these problems, adequate detection of substance abuse in the elderly in a critical care setting is imperative. Underdetection and undermanagement of substance abuse has significant implications for patient outcomes and resource use. Especially among the older population, substance misuse is largely overlooked and underreported. Many factors contribute to this, not least the fact that presentation may be atypical and hence easily missed by health care providers (McGrath, Crome, & Crome, 2005). Alcohol-related problems may also be misinterpreted as normal consequences of aging. However, alcohol is a commonly abused substance among older adults, and age-related changes predispose these patients to a greater sensitivity to its effects (Letizia & Reinbolz, 2005). Clinical guidance is sparse, except for alcohol withdrawal. Early detection of the potential problem is the first step in adequate management.

## Case Study

A 73-year-old man who lived alone in his own home was admitted to the emergency department (ED) after being found in his bed by a social worker. He had not been seen by his neighbors for several days, and when found he was lying in his excreta, suggesting he had not been able to get out of bed for days. He was disoriented; physical examination noted high fever and auscultation of the lungs suggested pneumonia. He was a known alcoholic. Initially, the focus of care in the ED was to treat the pneumonia, a potentially life-threatening condition in an older person. His condition, however, deteriorated over time. His oxygen saturation decreased, although oxygen was adminis-tered; he became more and more restless, disoriented, hypertensive, and his body temperature further increased. His respiratory status also deteriorated. Beside the decreased saturation, his respiratory rate increased and he demonstrated the beginning of respiratory muscle fatigue. The potential need for mechanical ventilation was sug-gested. However, an experienced colleague suggested that the initial treatment with oxygen had contributed to exacerbating an existing withdrawal syndrome. He also suggested that the increased body temperature was a result of withdrawal, which also explained the respiratory distress as increased body temperature is correlated with an increase in $CO_2$ production and ventilation. The therapeutic options were mechanical ventilation and/or withdrawal therapy. It was decided to first treat the withdrawal syndrome by titrating intravenous doses of benzodiazepines until his restlessness disap-peared, and, if still necessary, mechanical ventilation would be started at that time. As the withdrawal syndrome was treated, oxygen consumption and $CO_2$ production dramatically decreased. Work of breathing also declined and there was no further indication for mechanical ventilation. [Note: typically in situations such as this, the immediate treatment in the ED focuses on correcting the underlying condition that is life threatening; however, this scenario highlights how a life-threatening condition can be caused by or exacerbated by substance withdrawal.]

## Intoxication

Intoxication by excessive intake of psychoactive substances results in a specific toxi-drome and is not limited to patients with substance abuse or dependence. Intoxication can be intentional or accidental. Intentional intoxication can be driven by the desire to experience strong substance effects or by suicidal intent. Substance abuse is a known risk factor for suicidality, which is high in a geriatric population. If several substances are combined, a complex and hard-to-diagnose toxidrome may present. Accidental intoxication can be the result of a mistake, confusion, forgetfulness or concentration, or memory problems that are more prevalent in old age (Zermansky et al., 2006).

## Withdrawal

Withdrawal is the most important problem in critical care for geriatric substance-abuse patients because of its danger and negative impact on prognosis, morbidity, and mortality (DeWit et al., 2008; Li, Sun, Puri, Marsh, & Anis, 2007). A substantial proportion (18%) of older patients develop drug withdrawal and drug withdrawal increases the odds of requiring mechanical ventilation almost threefold. In addition, critical illness and hospital admission often implies a forced cessation of all substances, including tobacco, alcohol, and psychotropic medication exceeding medical prescrip-tion. Withdrawal can be delayed if critical patients receive opioids, benzodiazepines, or other sedatives during their stay in the intensive care unit. It can lead to agitation, aggression, delirium, and seizures. Withdrawal from opioids, benzodiazepines, and nicotine is discussed in more detail at the end of this chapter.

## Delirium

The most evident cause of delirium in critical care is severe withdrawal of alcohol or benzodiazepines (substance-withdrawal delirium in the *DSM-IV-TR* classification of delirium [APA, 2000]). On the other hand, acute intoxication might also provoke delirium (substance-intoxication delirium). A history of substance abuse, old age, and the medical consequences of prolonged substance abuse (e.g., brain damage, organ dysfunction, among others) are all predisposing factors for delirium because of general medical condition and delirium resulting from multiple etiologies. Taken together, a high index of suspicion for delirium in geriatric substance-abuse patients is justified, and preventive strategies for withdrawal and delirium are imperative in this patient population (Tetrault, & O'Connor, 2008). Delirium is dealt with in more detail in chapter 26 of this text.

## Behavioral Problems

The mixture of shame and craving might drive substance-abuse patients to secretive, dishonest, and manipulative behavior to obtain (or obtain higher doses of) the substance of abuse. For example, patients might disregard unit rules about leaving the unit, smoking in places where it is prohibited. Acute substance intoxication can be accompanied with severe behavioral disruption with disinhibition, loss of decorum, apathy, and so on. Withdrawal is often accompanied by irritability, resulting in uncooperative attitudes, agitation, or even aggression. Delirium will often lead to the most problematic behavioral changes with wandering behavior, agitation, aggression, and motor restlessness with a tendency to remove (often vital) catheters or tubes. In the presence of neurodegenerative disorders, behavioral problems in elder substance-abuse patients can be more prominent or atypical.

## Acute Medical Consequences of Substance Abuse

Acute medical consequences are related mostly to substance intoxication or caused by the combination of the substance of abuse and comorbidity or medication. Alcohol, benzodiazepines, and opioids or combinations of these substances can induce impaired consciousness (up to coma) and respiratory depression or aspiration of gastric content, with risk for hypoventilation and carbon dioxide retention. In addition, COPD predisposes to respiratory insufficiency and is more frequent in a geriatric population and in patients with a history of tobacco abuse. Drugs may acutely precipitate respiratory failure by compromising respiratory pump function and/or by causing pulmonary pathology. Polysubstance overdoses are common, and clinicians should anticipate complications related to multiple drugs. Impairment of respiratory pump function may develop from central nervous system (CNS) depression (suppression of the medulla oblongata, stroke, or seizures) or respiratory muscle fatigue (increased respiratory workload, metabolic acidosis). Drug-related respiratory pathology may result from parenchymal (aspiration-related events, pulmonary edema, hemorrhage, pneumothorax, infectious and noninfectious pneumonitis), airway (bronchospasm and hemorrhage), or pulmonary vascular insults (endovascular infections, hemorrhage, and vasoconstrictive events). Alcohol, cocaine, amphetamines, opiates, and benzodiazepines are the most commonly abused drugs that may induce events leading to acute respiratory failure (Wilson & Saukkonen, 2004). Antidotes (naloxon for opioids and flumazenil for benzodiapzepines) should be considered, especially when respiratory failure is primarily caused by CNS depression. However, the short half-life of these antagonists often urges for repeated or continued administration. Acute withdrawal symptoms or adrenergic overstimulation can be seen with the use of antagonists in a sensitive population (Mintzer & Griffiths, 2005; Mintzer, Stoller, & Griffiths, 1999; van Dorp, Yassen, & Dahan, 2007; Weinbroum, Flaishon, Sorkine, Szold, & Rudick, 1997).

Geriatric patients are more vulnerable in general, but also more vulnerable to psychotropic substance effects in specific. Other examples of acute medical problems related to substance abuse in critical care patients are acute myocardial pump failure; acute pancreatitis; rhabdomyolysis, especially after acute intoxication resulting in immobilization or coma; and infections (Al-Sanouri, Dikin, & Soubani, 2005). Also, some medical treatments for alcohol abuse as (for instance, disulfiram [Antabuse]) can cause acute medical problems if combined with alcohol. In severe reactions, there may be respiratory depression, cardiovascular collapse, arrhythmias, myocardial infarction, acute congestive heart failure, unconsciousness, convulsions, and death. The intensity of the reaction may vary with each individual but is generally proportional to the amount of disulfiram and alcohol ingested. Older adults are more sensitive to the impact of disulfiram–alcohol interactions.

## Chronic Medical Consequences of Substance Abuse

During intensive care or emergency service hospitalization, physicians are often confronted with the more chronic consequences of substance abuse. Alcohol may cause or worsen chronic illnesses or symptoms such as insomnia, depression, and hypertension (Pierucci-Lagha, 2003). Older alcohol misusers and abusers are at excess risk for myriad physical problems and premature death because alcohol interacts with the natural aging process in negative ways (Dowling, Weiss, & Condon, 2008) to increase risks for injuries, cardiomyopathy, cardiac dysrhythmic events, hypotonic circulatory dysregulation, immune suppression, cancers, gastrointestinal problems, bleeding, neurocognitive deficits and bone loss (Jenkins, 2000; Sander et al., 2006; Stevenson, 2005). Low-volume and reduced daily alcohol consumption appear to be protective against blood clots in the coronary and brain vessels, bone loss and falls, and cognitive decline compared with current abstainers. At higher levels, alcohol has the opposite effect (Stevenson).

Significant adverse effects that may be associated with benzodiazepine use in the elderly include falls, cognitive impairment, sedation, and impairment of driving skills, all of which are particularly related to the long half-life of benzodiazepines. Age-related pharmacokinetic and pharmacodynamic changes increase the potential for certain side effects in the elderly (Madhusoodanan & Bogunovic, 2004).

## Diagnostic Problems

The diagnosis of substance abuse or withdrawal is often problematic, but substance abuse itself can also interfere with the diagnosis of other medical problems in geriatric critical care patients. A toxidrome or withdrawal state can mask other medical problems or blur assessment or follow-up of parameters such as consciousness, pulse, respiration, and so on. Intoxication, withdrawal, or delirium states might complicate diagnostic procedures such as RX, scanners, EEG (electroencephalograph), punctures (venous, arterial or lumbar) among others. However, as mentioned previously, the incidence of substance abuse in an older population and its large representation in the hospitalized population means that suspicion for substance abuse or withdrawal must always be present. Prophylactic therapy may confirm the suspicion of abuse and prevent limited cooperation with diagnostic interventions.

## Therapeutic Problems and Increased Risk of Complications

Substance abuse might interfere with the treatment for other medical problems. Tolerance resulting from abuse of inhibitory substances can lead to relative insensitivity to sedating, hypnotic, or analgesic effects of currently used medications in critical care. Higher doses than usual might be required. Behavioral problems related to intoxication, withdrawal, or delirium might also interfere with therapeutic interventions such as endotracheal intubation, assisted ventilation, catheters, and others. Many older adults drink alcohol and take medications that may interact negatively with alcohol. Some of these interactions result from age-related changes in the absorption, distribution, and metabolism of alcohol and medications. Others are caused by disulfiram-like reactions, (e.g., respiratory depression, cardiovascular collapse, arrhythmias, myocardial infarction, acute congestive heart failure), as described earlier, which are observed with some medications, exacerbation of therapeutic effects and adverse effects of medications when combined with alcohol, and alcohol's interference with the effectiveness of some medications (Moore, Whiteman, & Ward, 2007).

In alcohol abusers, bleeding complications are increased twofold during and after surgery. Immune suppression results in an increased incidence of infectious complications like pneumonia, wound infection, and urinary tract infection. In particular, septic encephalopathy is often misinterpreted as alcohol withdrawal syndrome. Because of the fact that patients abusing alcohol show a two- to fivefold higher rate of postoperative complications, they require increased attention to avoid latency of treatment and the development of multiple organ failure (Sander et al., 2006).

## Detection of Substance Abuse in a Geriatric Population in Critical Care

Early detection of potential substance abuse in hospitalized patients is of extreme importance. Beside the immunosuppressive effects of specific drugs, the clinical presentation of abstinence or withdrawal induces increased morbidity and mortality, results in a longer hospital stay, and complicates patient care. Today, for each patient, suspicion of any substance abuse is justified and appropriate. Active clinical and guided chemical survey should be considered as a routine preventive measure.

### History

The patient may report substance abuse. However, one should be careful not to put too much emphasis on a negative substance history obtained from the patient. Patients often minimize or deny substance abuse. More often, family members may provide information about an older patient's substance abuse; however, family is rarely approached for such information. One caveat is that information from direct relatives can also be misleading. The patient may hide the substance abuse from relatives. Furthermore, direct relatives sometimes share the same abuse or may provide the patient with the substance to keep a relative social peace at home. In summary, a negative history has only limited relevance. A positive history is meaningful, but quite often the frequency, dose, and kind of substances is minimized. The patient's health record, previous hospitalizations, and medical problems, and actual or past use of prescription or psychoactive medications with abuse potential might also alert the clinician for potential substance abuse.

## Drugs or Attributes

Each substance has its specific attributes, depending on the substance itself and mode of administration. For instance, to inject heroin most often syringes, a lighter, and a spoon can be found. Or the drug and attributes can be present on the body of the patient, or these can be found in the vicinity of the patient within the hospital.

## Clinical Examination

External clinical signs may indicate previous or recent substance abuse. Damage to mucous membranes and tissues of the nasal cavity, which may cause a dripping nose or nasal bleeding, swallowing difficulties or throat infections, may betray cocaine use. Puncture signs or thrombophlebitis may suggest intravenous heroin use.

Clinical signs as well as mental and physical indicators may demonstrate the presence of a specific toxidrome. Dissociation between usually paired physiological changes, such as increased pulse rate and increased blood pressure versus increased pulse rate and decreased blood pressure may also indicate substance abuse. In addition, a cluster of symptoms and signs may be another finding in the clinical examination. Increased pulse rate, blood pressure, body temperature combined with irritability or restlessness may be the result of intoxication with a stimulant such as cocaine. On the other hand, these clinical signs may also indicate the presentation of alcohol or benzodiazepine withdrawal. It is important to mention that the absence of a toxidrome does not mean that there is no poisoning. Multiple compound ingestion, simultaneous disorders, symptom-free intervals, or missing signs may obscure a specific toxidrome but do not exclude that toxidrome. Specific clinical signs, such as spider nevi, may indicate specific chronic substance abuse.

## Laboratory Findings

Anemia, thrombocytopenia, and abnormal liver enzyme activity are typical biochemical signs specific for alcohol abuse, although these are not always present. Based on a combination of history, clinical signs, and biochemical indices, toxicology screening might be performed to detect the abused substances or its metabolites in urine or blood.

## Screening Instruments

No validated screening or assessment instruments are available for identifying or diagnosing drug abuse in the older population (Simoni-Wastila & Yang, 2006). General screening instruments might be used. Specific scores, such as the CAGE score (acronym for cut down, annoyed by criticism, guilty about drinking, eye-opener drinks) (Buchsbaum, Buchanan, Centor, Scholl, & Lawton, 1991), have been evaluated to help in detecting alcohol use (see Exhibit 21.2) and appear useful in geriatric patients (Beullens & Aertgeerts, 2004). The CAGE is the most consistent brief screening instrument, but its threshold may need to be adjusted in the elderly (Conigliaro, Kraemer, & McNeil, 2000). One limitation of the CAGE questionnaire is its inability to differentiate between current and former alcohol abuse (Moss & Burnham, 2006). Furthermore, using the CAGE score might be problematic in geriatric critical care patients because of a combination of sedation, serious illness, possible cognitive or perceptual impairment, and potential impaired communication. Other screening assessments have been recommended for use with older adults, such as the Michigan Alcohol Screening Test-Geriatric version (MAST-G; Beullens & Aertgeets, 2004; instrument can be found at http://findarticles.com/p/articles/mi_m0FSS/is_4_14/ai_n17210418), Alcohol-Related Problems Survey, and the Alcohol Use Disorders Identification Test (AUDIT; Sorocco & Ferrell, 2006). The MAST-G is also available and validated in a short version, the SMAST-G. Interestingly, different screening instruments might capture different aspects of unsafe drinking. The CAGE is most valuable when screening for dependence, whereas instruments such as the SMAST-G and the AUDIT are more sensitive for detecting harmful and hazardous drinking in the elderly. In a study by Moore and colleagues (Moore, Seeman, Morgenstern, Beck, & Reuben, 2002), fewer than half of all persons screening positive on either the CAGE or the SMAST-G screened positive on both measures. Combining complementary screening instruments as the CAGE and the SMAST-G is probably the most effective and sensitive screening method (Moore et al.; Sorocco & Ferrell).

# Withdrawal

It is of clinical importance that we distinguish withdrawal from sedatives such as alcohol and benzodiazepines, from withdrawal of substances such as opioids and nicotine.

## Alcohol and Benzodiazepine Withdrawal

The incidence of alcohol and benzodiazepine abuse is clearly underestimated. Up to 20% of older critically ill patients are at risk for a certain degree of withdrawal. There are four stages of alcohol withdrawal. The first stage is the result of an autonomic hyperactivity that appears within hours of the last drink and peaks within 48 hours. Although the patient is fully responsive, tremulousness, sweating, anxiety, and insomnia are the most prominent symptoms. Most symptoms resolve, but many patients progress to more severe stages. The second stage is dominated by hallucinations, which are usually visual and may last for a week. The third stage is neuronal excitation, accompanied by seizure activity. The last stage is delirium tremens characterized by

# Exhibit 21.2

## CAGE Questionnaire

**Have you ever felt you should** *c*ut down on your drinking?

Yes

No

**Have people** *a*nnoyed you by criticizing your drinking?

Yes

No

**Have you ever felt bad or** *g*uilty about your drinking?

Yes

No

**Have you ever had a drink first thing in the morning (as an** "*e*ye opener") to steady your nerves or get rid of a hangover?

Yes

No

    The CAGE is scored by allocating 1 point for each "yes" answer. Total scores of 2 or above are thought to be clinically significant and may indicate alcohol dependence.

    The CAGE questionnaire was developed by Dr. John Ewing, founding director of the Bowles Center for Alcohol Studies, University of North Carolina at Chapel Hill. CAGE is an internationally used assessment instrument for identifying problems with alcohol. "CAGE" is an acronym formed from the italicized letters in the questionnaire (cut–annoyed–guilty–eye).

    The exact wording that can be used in research studies can be found in: J. A. Ewing (1984). Detecting Alcoholism: The CAGE Questionnaire. *Journal of the American Medical Association, 252*, 1905–1907.

disorientation, confusion, impaired attention, and all of the previous-stage symptoms. Attention must be paid so that alcohol-withdrawal syndrome is not confused with other neurologic complications of alcohol abuse, such as Wernicke's or hepatic encephalopathy. In Wernicke's encephalopathy—caused by thiamine (vitamin $B_1$) deficiency mostly in the context of chronic alcoholism combined with unbalanced diet—confusion is accompanied by ataxia, nystagmus, and ophthalmoplegia. Hepatic encephalopathy is caused by increased plasma ammonia and other neurotoxic substances, and is found mostly in the context of liver failure. In hepatic encephalopathy, confusion is often accompanied by flapping tremor (asterixis) and bodily signs of liver failure,

The diagnosis of alcohol withdrawal should be considered if alcohol abuse is suspected in combination with a poor nutritional state and with clinical signs of auditory and tactile disturbances; of adrenergic stimulation such as tachycardia, hypertension, and hyperthermia; and of behavior ranging from restlessness to seizures. It has been suggested that these effects result from a reduction of neurotransmission in the $GABA_A$ (gamma-aminobutyric acid) pathways and an overstimulation of the glutamate pathways (Follesa et al., 2005).

## Prevention

Regarding prevention, there are two major ongoing discussions. First, is there still a place for intravenous alcohol administration? Second, should the preventive administration of alcohol or benzodiazepines be symptom triggered or a fixed-schedule therapy?

The administration of alcohol for the prevention of alcohol withdrawal syndrome has long been performed with widespread recommendations. The arguments were that it provided effective management without excessive sedation and limited risk of respiratory depression compared with preventive benzodiazepine administration. Generally, if well titrated, the patient remains cooperative to participating in all aspects of patient care. However, studies have not demonstrated any advantage of using alcohol infusions over benzodiazepines but rather indicated a higher morbidity. Because of the paucity of well-designed clinical trials, and because of intravenous ethanol's questionable efficacy, inconsistent pharmacokinetic profile, hepatic toxicity, and relatively narrow therapeutic index, routine use of this drug is not recommended in critically ill patients who have alcohol withdrawal syndrome or are at risk for it (Hodges & Mazur, 2004).

A recent systematic review (Stead, Perera, Bullen, Mant, & Lancaster, 2008; *Cochrane Database* 2005 CD005063) considered benzodiazepine therapy as the gold standard if started early and in sufficient doses. Benzodiazepines with a slow onset of action are preferred to minimize dependency on benzodiazepines. Long-acting benzodiazepines (e.g., diazepam b.i.d.) in gradual tapering doses are preferred because the plasma level decreases gradually and slowly after intake, avoiding secondary withdrawal. However, in the presence of impaired liver function, as is often seen in alcoholic liver cirrhosis, short-acting benzodiazepines without active metabolites and with renal clearance and minimal hepatic metabolization (e.g., lorazepam) are preferred: however, more frequent administration (t.i.d. or q.i.d.) and very gradual dose decreases are then necessary to avoid secondary withdrawal.

Many other medicinal drugs have been used and studied, few of them have added value (Ntais, Pakos, Kyzas, & Ioannidis, 2005). Neuroleptics, such as haloperidol, have been used frequently. Although they reduce the severity of symptoms, they are less effective in preventing delirium or seizures. Beta blockers and centrally acting adrenergic agonists such as clonidine ameliorate symptoms, but do not reduce the risk of delirium or seizures. As anticipated, anticonvulsant agents have been advocated. Beside pure symptom management, no beneficial effects could be demonstrated.

It is important to note that although the scientific literature is clear on the preventive use of benzodiazepines, the discussion remains whether fixed therapeutic strategies should be preferred over a symptom-triggered approach. The best prevention with less medication required is early titration of the benzodiazepines triggered by withdrawal symptoms. Although the detoxification process is faster, such a symptom-triggered strategy requires an adequate and frequent monitoring policy and early detection of withdrawal symptoms. In settings less experienced in or equipped for withdrawal evaluation and frequent monitoring, a fixed dose of benzodiazepines is advisable to prevent withdrawal, delirium, and seizures. However, a fixed therapeutic strategy still requires bedside evaluation of breakthrough withdrawal symptoms to adjust dose or add symptom-triggered benzodiazepine administration on top of the fixed doses. Interindividual variation in the doses needed to prevent withdrawal, delirium, and seizures is high and depends on body weight, recent alcohol and benzodiazepine intake, other abuse, patient history, and other parameters. If a fixed therapeutic strategy is chosen, oversedation has to be avoided, first because it may mask important neurologic information, and second because it can prolong or complicate the ICU stay (Petignat, 2005).

In addition to prevention of withdrawal, supportive care must be added. Special attention must be given to glucose plasma levels, acidosis, and to the classic vitamin deficiencies that chronic alcohol abusers have, specifically vitamin B and folic acid insufficiency (Moss & Burnham, 2006). Thiamine (vitamin $B_1$ must be given to the patient before (or simultaneously with) any glucose infusion is given intravenously to prevent neuronal damage (Wernicke's encephalopathy). Supplements of electrolytes such as magnesium and sodium may be necessary as deficiencies are often observed in chronic alcohol consumers. Therapy for pulmonary infection (*Serratia, H. influenzae,* and *S. pneumoniae*) and pancreatitis need to be considered.

### Treatment of Alcohol and Benzodiazepine Withdrawal

An acute exacerbation occurs if alcohol abuse was not suspected or the preventive benzodiazepine titration was insufficient. Aggressive benzodiazepine administration and supportive therapy such as reducing hyperthermia is necessary, but quite often requires extra oxygen or ventilatory support. Specifically in the intensive care setting, there is some direct evidence for the use of benzodiazepines. As adjunctive treatment with benzodiazepines, clonidine was most effective, but an add-on of haloperidol instead of clonidine showed superior safety in patients with cardiac or pulmonary risk (Spies et al., 1996).

## Withdrawal From Opioids

The clinical presentation of opioid withdrawal can be as vague as a severe case of influenza, up to severe withdrawal symptoms. The onset of symptoms depends on the half-life of the abused opioid(s). Sympathetic and adrenergic hyperactivity are responsible for the clinical symptoms and signs of opioid withdrawal. Symptoms ranging from restlessness, agitation, and anxiety up to seizures can occur, but cognitive and mental functioning remain unaffected. Nausea, vomiting, diarrhea, and abdominal cramps are common. Diffuse myalgia and signs of piloerection (erection of the hair of the skin), yawning, lacrimation, and rhinorrhea are frequent. The cornerstone of the therapy is preventive substitution with a long-acting opioid. However, it depends on the health care setting as to how such programs are set up. In the hospital, if opioid analgesia is needed, dose adjustment is warranted. If no opioid analgesia is needed, oral methadone or buprenorphine can be given if oral administration is possible. Otherwise, intravenous substitution is indicated. Benzodiazepines, clonidine, antidepressants, or other drugs can be added. Most of these drugs are considered safe to add but no therapeutic effectiveness has been demonstrated (Amato et al., 2008; Tetrault, & O'Connor, 2008).

## Withdrawal From Nicotine

Tobacco products are highly addictive and successful cessation is not simple. Smokers acutely admitted to the hospital, or an intensive care unit, are forced to stop smoking. Nicotine replacement therapy has been promoted in ambulatory settings. However, in critical care setting certain questions have been proposed. Does nicotine replacement therapy in the critically ill patient influence the cardiovascular system and myocardial oxygen consumption in such a way that it has a negative effect on outcome? When prescribing nicotine in the critically ill, one needs to weigh the risks and benefits; it is difficult to determine the exact incidence of nicotine withdrawal in critically ill smokers. One should be aware of the potential adverse effects of nicotine replacement therapy before initiating such treatment in critically ill patients. Recent studies demonstrated increased hospital mortality in critically ill patients following such nicotine replacement therapy (Stead et al., 2008).

## Long-Term Management

The objective is to taper and stop benzodiazepines or opioids (if medically possible) before discharge to avoid iatrogenic abuse or dependence. Long-term planning beyond the acute presentation should be part of the overall treatment protocol and implies a multidisciplinary approach, including psychiatric assessment and motivational strategies (Tetrault & O'Connor, 2008). Medication to reduce craving should be considered in patients without contraindications to its use. Participation in individual, group, and family therapy and attendance at self-help group meetings such as AA (Alcoholics Anonymous) should be encouraged (Sattar, Petty, & Burke, 2003). The evidence to date suggests that older people may respond at least as well as younger people to treatment if interventions are specifically targeted to that age group (McGrath et al., 2005; Stevenson, 2005).

## Summary

In summary, substance abuse in the elderly is predominantly a problem of alcohol abuse and abuse of prescription drugs such as benzodiazepines and opioids. Detection is difficult and a high index of suspicion is warranted, ideally combined with the use of screening instruments. Intoxication as well as withdrawal can pose serious problems and interfere with somatic illness and medical management. Specific interventions for intoxication and withdrawal are mandatory to reduce morbidity and mortality. Long-term management of the substance-abuse or dependence problem should follow the acute care.

# References

Al-Sanouri, I., Dikin, M., & Soubani, A.O. (2005). Critical care aspects of alcohol abuse. *Southern Medical Journal, 98*(3), 372–381.

Amato, L., Minozzi, S., Davoli, M., Vecchi, S., Ferri, M. M., & Mayet, S. (2008). Psychosocial and pharmacological treatments versus pharmacological treatments for opioid detoxification. *Cochrane Database Systematic Review, 8*(4), CD005031.

American Psychiatric Association. (2000). *Diagnostic and statistical manual of mental disorders* (4th ed., text rev.). Washington DC: American Psychiatric Press

Beullens, J., & Aertgeerts, B. (2004). Screening for alcohol abuse and dependence in older people using DSM criteria: A review. *Aging and Mental Health, 8*(1), 76–82.

Blum, K., Braverman, E. R., Holder, J. M., Lubar, J. F., Monastra, V. J., Miller, D., et al. (2000). Reward deficiency syndrome: A biogenetic model for the diagnosis and treatment of impulsive, addictive, and compulsive behaviors. *Journal of Psychoactive Drugs, 32* (Suppl. i–iv), 1–112.

Buchsbaum, D. G., Buchanan, R. G., Centor, R. M., Scholl, S. H., & Lawton, M. J. (1991). Screening for alcohol abuse using CAGE scores and likelihood ratios. *Annals of Internal Medicine, 115*(10), 774–777.

Christensen, H., Low, L. F., & Anstey, K .J. (2006). Prevalence, risk factors and treatment for substance abuse in older adults. *Current Opinion in Psychiatry, 19*(6), 587–592.

Comings, D. E., & Blum, K. (2000). Reward deficiency syndrome: Genetic aspects of behavioral disorders. *Progress in Brain Research, 126*, 325–341.

Conigliaro, J., Kraemer, K., & McNeil, M. (2000). Screening and identification of older adults with alcohol problems in primary care. *Journal of Geriatric Psychiatry and Neurology, 13*(3), 106–114.

Culberson, J. W., & Ziska, M. (2008). Prescription drug misuse/abuse in the elderly. *Geriatrics, 63*(9), 22–31.

De Wit, M., Gennings, C., Zilberberg, M., Burnham, E. L., Moss, M., & Balster, R. L. (2008). Drug withdrawal, cocaine and sedative use disorders increase the need for mechanical ventilation in medical patients. *Addiction, 103*, 1500–1508.

Dowling, G. J., Weiss, S .R., & Condon, T. P. (2008). Drugs of abuse and the aging brain. *Neuropsychopharmacology, 33*(2), 209–218.

Dupen, A., Shen, D., & Ersek, M. (2007). Mechanisms of opioid-induced tolerance and hyperalgesia. *Pain Management in Nursing, 8*(3), 113–121.

Ewing, J. A. (1984). Detecting alcoholism: The CAGE Questionnaire. *Journal of the American Medical Association, 252*, 1905–1907.

Follesa, P., Biggio, F., Talani, G., Murru, L., Serra, M., Sanna, E., et al. (2005). Neurosteroids, GABA receptors, and ethanol dependence. *Psychopharmacology, 186*(3), 267–280.

Hodges, B., & Mazur, J.E. (2004). Intravenous ethanol for the treatment of alcohol withdrawal syndrome in critically ill patients. *Pharmacotherapy, 24*(11), 1578–1585.

Holbert, K. R., & Tueth, M. J. (2004). Alcohol abuse and dependence. A clinical update on alcoholism in the older population. *Geriatrics, 59*(9), 38–40.

Husten, C. G., Shelton, D. M., Chrismon, J. H., Lin, Y. C., Mowery, P., & Powell, F. A. (1997). Cigarette smoking and smoking cessation among older adults: United States, 1965–94. *Tobacco Control, 6*(3), 175–180.

Isaac, M., Janca, A., & Sartorius, N. (1994). *ICD-10 symptom glossary for mental disorders.* Retrieved March 2009, from http://whqlibdoc.who.int/hq/1994/WHO_MNH_MND_94.11.pdf

Jenkins, D. H. (2000). Substance abuse and withdrawal in the intensive care unit. Contemporary issues. *Surgery Clinics of North America, 80*(3), 1033–1053

Johnson, I. (2000). Alcohol problems in old age: A review of recent epidemiological research. *International Journal of Geriatric Psychiatry, 15*(7), 575–581.

Letizia, M., & Reinbolz, M. (2005). Identifying and managing acute alcohol withdrawal in the elderly. *Geriatric Nursing, 26*(3), 176–183.

Li, X., Sun, H., Puri, A., Marsh, D. C., & Anis, A. H. (2007). Medical withdrawal management in Vancouver: Service description and evaluation. *Addictive Behaviors 32*, 1043–1053.

Madhusoodanan, S., & Bogunovic, O. J. (2004). Safety of benzodiazepines in the geriatric population. *Expert Opinion in Drug Safety, 3*(5), 485–493

McGrath, A., Crome, P., & Crome, I. B. (2005). Substance misuse in the older population. *Postgraduate Medical Journal, 81*(954), 228–231.

Menninger, J. A. (2002). Assessment and treatment of alcoholism and substance-related disorders in the elderly. *Bulletin of the Menninger Clinic, 66*(2), 166–183.

Mintzer, M. Z., & Griffiths, R. R. (2005). Flumazenil-precipitated withdrawal in healthy volunteers following repeated diazepam exposure. *Psychopharmacology (Berlin), 178*(2–3), 259–267.

Mintzer, M. Z., Stoller, K .B., & Griffiths, R .R. (1999). A controlled study of flumazenil-precipitated withdrawal in chronic low-dose benzodiazepine users. *Psychopharmacology (Berlin), 147*(2), 200–229.

Moore, A. A., Seeman, T., Morgenstern, H., Beck, J. C., & Reuben, D. B. (2002). Are there differences between older persons who screen positive on the CAGE questionnaire and the Short Michigan Alcoholism Screening Test-Geriatric Version? *Journal of the American Geriatrics Society, 50*(5), 858–862.

Moore, A. A., Whiteman, E. J., & Ward, K. T. (2007). Risks of combined alcohol/medication use in older adults. *American Journal of Geriatric Pharmacotherapy, 5*(1), 64–74.

Moss, M., & Burnham, E.L. (2006). Alcohol abuse in the critically ill patient. *Lancet, 368*(9554), 2231–2242.

Ntais, C., Pakos, E., Kyzas, P., & Ioannidis J.P. (2005). Benzodiazepines for alcohol withdrawal. *Cochrane Database Systematic Reviews, 20*(3), CD005063.

Nutt, D., King, L. A., Saulsbury, W., & Blakemore, C. (2007). Development of a rational scale to assess the harm of drugs of potential misuse. *Lancet, 369*(9566), 1047–1053.

O'Connell, H., Chin, A. V., Cunningham, C., & Lawlor, B. (2003). Alcohol use disorders in elderly people—Redefining an age old problem in old age. *British Medical Journal, 327*(7416), 664–667.

Ondus, K. A., Hujer, M. E., Mann, A. E., & Mion, L. C. (1999). Substance abuse and the hospitalized elderly. *Orthopedic Nursing, 18*(4), 27–34.

Petignat, P. A. (2005). [The management of the alcohol withdrawal syndrome in the intensive care unit] *Revue Medicale de le Suisse, 1*(45), 2905–2911.

Pierucci-Lagha, A. (2003). [Alcoholism and aging. 1. Epidemiology, clinical aspects and treatment] *Psychologie and Neuropsychiatrie du Vieillissement, 1*(3), 197–205.

Sander, M., Neumann, T., von Dossow, V., Schönfeld, H., Lau, A., Eggers, V., et al. (2006). [Alcohol use disorder: Risks in anesthesia and intensive care medicine]. *Internist (Berlin), 47*(4), 332, 334–336, 338, passim.

Sattar, S. P., Petty, F., & Burke, W. J. (2003). Diagnosis and treatment of alcohol dependence in older alcoholics. *Clinics in Geriatric Medicine, 19*(4), 743–761.

Sheahan, S. L. (2000). Medication use and misuse by the elderly. Reducing health dangers. *Advance for Nurse Practioners, 8*(12), 41–42, 47, 76.

Simoni-Wastila, L., & Yang, H. K. (2006). Psychoactive drug abuse in older adults. *American Journal of Geriatric Pharmacotherapy, 4*(4), 380–394.

Sorocco, K. H., & Ferrell, S. W. (2006). Alcohol use among older adults. *Journal of General Psychology, 133*(4), 453–467.

Spies, C. D., Dubisz, N., Neumann, T., Blum, S., Müller, C., Rommelspacher, H., et al. (1996). Therapy of alcohol withdrawal syndrome in intensive care unit patients following trauma: Results of a prospective, randomized trial. *Critical Care Medicine, 24*(3), 414–422.

Stead, L. F., Perera, R., Bullen, C., Mant, D., & Lancaster, T. (2008). Nicotine replacement therapy for smoking cessation. *Cochrane Database Systematic Reviews, 23*(1), CD000146.

Stevenson, J. S. (2005). Alcohol use, misuse, abuse, and dependence in later adulthood. In J. J. Fitzpatrick, J. Stevenson, & M Sommers (Eds.), *Annual review of nursing research* (Vol. 23, pp. 245–280). New York: Springer Publishing Company.

Tetrault, J. M., & O'Connor, P. G. (2008). Substance abuse and withdrawal in the critical care setting. *Critical Care Clinics, 24*(4), 767–788, viii.

Tournier, M., Grolleau, A., Cougnard, A., Molimard, M., & Verdoux, H. (2009). Factors associated with choice of psychotropic drugs used for intentional drug overdose. *European Archives of Psychiatry and Clinical Neurosciences, 259*(2), 86–91.

van Dorp, E. L., Yassen, A., & Dahan, A. (2007). Naloxone treatment in opioid addiction: The risks and benefits. *Expert Opinion in Drug Safety, 6*(2), 125–132.

Weinbroum, A. A., Flaishon, R., Sorkine, P., Szold, O., & Rudick, V. (1997). A risk-benefit assessment of flumazenil in the management of benzodiazepine overdose. *Drug Safety, 17*(3), 181–196.

Wilson, K. C., & Saukkonen, J. J. (2004). Acute respiratory failure from abused substances. *Journal of Intensive Care Medicine, 19*(4), 183–193.

World Health Organization. (2007). *International statistical classification of diseases 10th revision (ICD-10).* Geneva: Author. Retrieved March 31, 2009, from http://www.who.int/classifications/apps/icd/icd10online/

Zermansky, A. G., Alldred, D. P., Petty, D. R., Raynor, D. K., Freemantle, N., Eastaugh, J., et al. (2006). Clinical medication review by a pharmacist of elderly people living in care homes—Randomised controlled trial. *Age & Ageing, 35*(6), 555–556.

# Urinary Incontinence in Critically Ill Older Adults

# 22

Mary H. Palmer

## Case Study

Mrs. Myers is an 85-year-old woman who had been living independently in her own home until one evening she tripped over her dog, fell, and broke her right hip. She lay on the kitchen floor overnight, for 14 hours, until her son found her the next morning and called 911. While in the emergency room, her urine-soaked clothes were removed and sequential compression devices were applied to both legs to prevent deep venous thrombosis. Low molecular weight heparin (LMWH) was administered. An intravenous line was inserted to optimize fluid management and oxygen therapy via nasal cannula was instituted. Mrs. Myers was cleared for surgery after a medical consult and baseline laboratory tests. Almost 24 hours after she fell, Mrs. Myers underwent intravenous sedation and an indwelling urinary catheter was inserted perioperatively. Her hip fracture was repaired with an open reduction and internal fixation. Surgery lasted for approximately 1 hour and she experienced a brief period of hypotension in the recovery room. After stabilizing her blood pressure, the rest of her stay in the recovery room was uneventful. Intravenous opioid analgesics were ordered for postoperative pain. She was admitted to the intensive care unit for overnight observation and she rested comfortably over night.

During her first full postoperative day, the intravenous fluids and indwelling urinary catheter were discontinued and she was moved to a general medical–surgical unit. Her pain medication was switched to a nonsteroid antiinflammatory drug. By early afternoon she was evaluated by a physical therapist but remained on bedrest because of multiple bruises on her right leg, trunk, and arm. X-ray indicated there were no other broken bones. She refused food, only drank clear liquids, and fretted about her dog all day. During the night, the nursing assistant, Sarah Burnes, assigned to Mrs. Myers found her agitated, trying to get out of bed, and soaked in urine. Ms. Burnes changed Mrs. Myers's soiled bed linens and clothing, put an absorbent pull-up brief on Mrs. Myers, and a disposable incontinence pad on the bed. She left the room and told the nurse that Mrs. Myers needed medication for confusion. She did not mention the incontinent episode to the nurse.

---

# Introduction

Over 317,000 older adults fracture their hips annually ("HCUP facts and figures," 2005) and are hospitalized for medical management and surgical repair. Older adults represent 38% of discharged patients from nonfederal hospitals and have greater risks from hospitalization than younger patients (R. M. Palmer, 2006).

Many of these individuals enter the acute care setting continent of urine but leave incontinent wearing an indwelling catheter, an absorbent product, or both. In a study of hospitalized female hip-fracture patients, 21% of women who were continent prior to their hospitalization for hip-fracture repair became incontinent during hospitalization. The risk factors associated with becoming incontinent in these women were admission from a nursing home, presence of confusion, use of wheelchair or walking device, and prefracture dependence on others for ambulation (M. H. Palmer, Baumgarten, Langenberg, & Carson, 2002).

Urinary incontinence is considered a potentially life-threatening condition (Wilson, 2006). It is associated with frailty (Miles et al., 2001); falls (Brown et al., 2000); depression (van der Vaart, Roovers, de Leeuw, & Heintz, 2007); diabetes mellitus (Smith, 2006); coexisting complaints of fatigue, cough, and fecal incontinence (Stenzelius, Mattiasson, Hallberg, & Westergren, 2004); and long-term care placement (A. Morrison & Levy, 2006). In community-dwelling women urinary incontinence is associated with physical decline measured by walking speed and sit-to-stand speed. Cognitive decline, however, was associated with difficulty in coping with incontinence (Huang, Brown, Thom, Fink, & Yaffe, 2007).

In stroke patients urinary incontinence had a significant impact on long-term functional outcomes. Although the proportion of patients with urinary incontinence decreased over time, incontinent stroke survivors were four times more likely to be institutionalized after their first poststroke year than continent survivors (Kolominsky-Rabas, Hilz, Neundoerfer, & Heuschmann, 2003).

Evidence exists that urinary incontinence can be prevented and effectively treated in older adults, including the frail elderly (Fonda et al., 2005). Little evidence from the acute care setting is available, especially in critically ill older adults, but overwhelming evidence from the community and long-term care settings indicate that the key to effective treatment is prompt and comprehensive assessment (*CMS Manual System* 2005; Fonda et al.). The need for best practices related to urinary elimination in critically ill older adults is especially compelling. Extended use of urinary catheters, that is, beyond 48 hours, in elderly surgical patients in the acute care setting is associated with poor patient outcomes, including urinary tract infections and postoperative mortality (Wald, Epstein, Radcliff, & Kramer, 2008). In an effort to reduce these complications, Medicare will no longer reimburse hospitals for hospital-acquired catheter-associated urinary tract infections after October 1, 2008 (Wald & Kramer, 2007). Nurses caring for critically ill older adults will need to use measures to preserve urinary continence throughout the illness and to provide incontinence treatment that maintains the maximal feasible continence level relative to patient condition and medical management.

The purpose of this chapter is to provide background information about urinary incontinence and to discuss evidence-based approaches meeting the urinary continence needs of critically ill older adults.

# Physiology of Micturition

Micturition, a complex physiologic process that involves the storage and emptying of urine from the bladder, is not completely understood. Neural control of micturition involves the cortex, posterior hypothalamus, midbrain, and pons (Griffiths & Tadic, 2008). In the absence of dysfunction during the storage phase (sympathetic system activation) during which the bladder fills, afferent signals are sent to the sacral cord, to the periaqueductal gray (PAG), located in the midbrain, and to the prefrontal cortex. Through the prefrontal cortex, inhibitory signals are sent back to the PAG, which inhibits the excitation of the pontine micturition center (PMC). As a consequence, the bladder walls remain relaxed, continuing to stretch, and the urinary sphincters remain contracted. At this point, micturition is at an unconscious level. As the bladder continues to fill and the wall to stretch, the intensity of the afferent signals to the spinal cord grows. When the intensity exceeds a threshold, at about 300 to 400 cc of urine in the bladder, the frontal lobe is activated and conscious inhibition of micturition occurs (Vogel, 2001). The individual is aware of the increasing need to void, but continues to inhibit the voiding urge until toilet facilities are located and accessed.

When emptying occurs under conscious control, the prefrontal inhibition of the PAG is removed, thus allowing the PAG to excite the pontine micturition center (Griffiths & Tadic). Consequently, efferent signals are sent to the sacral reflex center, located between S2 and S4. With this parasympathic system activation, the detrusor contracts because of cholinergic/muscarinic stimulation. In coordination with bladder contraction, the bladder outlet and urethra, under alpha-adrenergic stimulation, are relaxed to allow urine to empty. The nucleus of Onuf, located in the sacral ventral horns, innervates the external urinary sphincter via the somatic nerve, causing sphincter relaxation.

| 22.1 Age-Related Changes That Can Contribute to Urinary Incontinence in Frail Elderly People | |
|---|---|
| **Age Related** | **Change: Potential Effects on Continence** |
| 1. **Bladder ultrastructure on electron microscopy**<br>a. Dysjunction pattern<br>b. Muscle and axon degeneration | Bladder overactivity and urge incontinence<br>Impaired bladder contractility, increased residual urine, and decreased functional bladder capacity |
| 2. **Bladder function**<br>a. Decreased capacity<br>b. Increased involuntary detrusor contractions<br>c. Decreased contractility during voiding<br>d. Increased residual urine | Increased likelihood of urinary symptoms and incontinence |
| 3. **Urethra**<br>a. Decreased closure pressure in women | Increased likelihood of stress and urge incontinence |
| 4. **Prostate**<br>a. Increased incidence of benign prostatic obstruction | Increased likelihood of urinary symptoms and incontinence |
| 5. **Decreased estrogen (women)** | Increased incidence of atrophic vaginitis and related symptoms<br>Increased incidence of recurrent urinary tract infections<br>Decreased urethral pressure |
| 6. **Increased nighttime urine production** | Increased likelihood of nocturia and nighttime incontinence |
| 7. **Altered central and peripheral neurotransmitter concentrations and actions** | Increased likelihood of lower urinary tract dysfunction |
| 8. **Altered immune function** | Increased likelihood of recurrent urinary tract infections |

*Note.* From "Incontinence in the Frail Elderly," by D. Fonda, C. E. DuBeau, D. Harari, J. G. Ouslander, M. H. Palmer, & B. Roe, 2005. In *Incontinence, Management Vol. 2.* P. Abrams, L. Cardozo, S. Khoury & A. Wein (Eds.), p. 1170. Paris: Health Publication Ltd. Copyright 2005 by the International Continence Society. Reprinted with permission of the publisher.

## Age-Related Changes That Affect Urinary Continence

Although age does not cause urinary incontinence, some age-related anatomical and physiologic changes to the lower urinary tract can increase vulnerability. These changes include reduced bladder capacity and voided volumes and an increase in the number of uninhibited detrusor contractions (Fonda et al., 2005). In men, benign prostatic hypertrophy increases the incidence of bladder neck obstruction. Decreased circulating estrogen levels in women lead to increased incidence of atrophic vaginitis and decreased urethral pressure (Fonda et al.) (see Table 22.1).

# Bladder Function and Aging

Recent research on aging effects on the female lower urinary tract reveals a decline in detrusor contractility, bladder sensation, and urethral sphincter function. Bladder capacity does not appear to diminish significantly (Pfisterer, Griffiths, Schaefer, & Resnick, 2006). There is little aging effect on 24-hour urine production (mean 1,765 mL) and micturition frequency (8 voids per 24 hours is considered the norm). In addition urethral profile length did not change but the maximum urethral closure pressure declines with age (Pfisterer, Johnson, Jenetzky, Hauer, & Oster, 2007).

Men also experience aging effects on their lower urinary tracts. In a cross-sectional study with men aged 40 to greater than 80 years old, older men experienced an increase in postvoid residual urine volumes, decreased peak flow rate, and voided volume. Although prostate volume increased with age, no significant differences existed in these parameters between obstructed and nonobstructed men (Madersbacher et al., 1998). Impaired contractility seen in older adults, instead of aging, may be caused by myogenic, ischemic, or neurogenic factors and is evidenced by decreased urinary flow rates and elevated postvoid residual urine volumes (about 50 mL or less) (DuBeau, 2006).

Urinary continence is a socially constructed term. It assumes voluntary control of urine and that urination occurs at socially acceptable times and in socially acceptable places. The lack of continence carries a social stigma ("NIH State-of-the-Science Conference," 2007). Many older adults can still relate stories of embarrassment over their own childhood enuresis, and describe feelings of powerlessness over being incontinent in their old age (Hagglund & Ahlstrom, 2007).

Continence should also be viewed as a dignity issue. The United Nations declared dignity as a human right in 1948 ("The universal declaration of human rights: 1948–2008," 2007). On behalf of incontinent nursing home residents, a human rights complaint was filed by the Ontario Federation of Labour to the Human Rights Commission (Walkom, 2008). The case was subsequently dismissed, but it started a new ongoing dialogue about the link between continence and dignity.

In addition, recent changes in the Centers for Medicare and Medicaid Services (CMS) Guidelines related to hospital-acquired catheter-related urinary tract infections emphasize the need to assess at admission the presence of conditions that place the older adult at risk and the need to prevent catheter-related urinary tract infections during a hospital stay (Hess & Rook, 2007). Thus, nurses play a central role in providing proactive assessment and interventions to prevent, treat, and manage urinary incontinence.

# Urinary Incontinence: Definition of Terms

The International Continence Society provides a succinct definition of urinary incontinence: "any complaint of any involuntary leakage of urine" (Abrams et al., 2002, p. 168). Urinary incontinence, a symptom that occurs in the storage phase of micturition, although prevalent in older adults, is not caused by age ("NIH State-of-the-Science Conference," 2007). At the most functional level, incontinence occurs when intravesical pressure exceeds intraurethral pressure. Nurses can assess and identify the type of incontinence their patients are experiencing and use evidence-based interventions to treat or manage incontinence.

Two major types of urinary incontinence are stress urinary incontinence and urge urinary incontinence. A combination of symptoms of both stress and urge urinary incontinence is called mixed incontinence (Abrams et al., 2002). In community-dwelling studies of older adults, women have higher prevalence of urinary incontinence than do men (Goode et al., 2008).

## Stress Urinary Incontinence

Stress urinary incontinence is caused by physical (not emotional) stress, resulting from physical activity or positioning. During the storage phase of normal micturition, the pressure in the bladder (intravesical pressure) remains lower than the pressure within the urethra (intraurethral pressure). When an individual vomits, coughs, sneezes, or laughs intraabdominal pressure rises. This action results in a corresponding increase in intravesical pressure and normally intraurethral pressure will also increase. For individuals with stress urinary incontinence, intraurethal pressure either does not increase or does not increase sufficiently to maintain the pressure gradient. Under conditions when intravesical pressure is greater than the intraurethral pressure, urine escapes from the bladder.

One reason for the failure of the urethral pressure to increase can be that the periurethral muscles surrounding are weak from acquired or congenital factors, see Table 22.2. Stress urinary incontinence occurs more often in women than men (except for men who have had prostate cancer surgery or damage to their pelvic floors from surgery, injury, or disease).

## Urge Urinary Incontinence

Urge urinary incontinence involves bladder function abnormalities, rather than the sphincter function abnormalities found with stress urinary incontinence. Urge urinary incontinence is also a symptom of overactive bladder. Normally the bladder fills passively, and involuntary (uninhibited) bladder contractions are absent or suppressed. However, when there are contractions of a sufficient magnitude that are not inhibited during the filling cycle, involuntary urine loss may occur. Uninhibited bladder contractions may also result from deconditioned voiding reflexes (Wein, 1986). For example, some older adults resort to frequent voiding and maintaining chronic low bladder volume in an attempt to avoid incontinent episodes. This can lead to reduced bladder capacity and, with time, thickening of the bladder wall, aggravating the decreased tone and increasing involuntary bladder contractions.

A cerebral etiology of urge incontinence has been proposed. It is theorized that global impairment of cerebral perfusion and regional underperfusion of the frontal lobes results in urge incontinence and reduced bladder sensation (Griffiths et al., 1994). In detrusor overactivity, the smooth muscle may exhibit abnormal mechanical activity and a reduced response to intrinsic nerve stimulation (Brading, 1997). Brading proposed that changes in the properties of the detrusor allow transmission of local neural activity throughout the bladder wall, resulting in a coordinated detrusor contraction (Brading).

Individuals with urge urinary incontinence often report having a sudden and overwhelming urge to urinate and they may lose urine while attempting to reach the toilet. The prevalence of urge urinary incontinence was higher in community-dwelling

| 22.2 | Definition of Terms for Lower Urinary Tract Symptons (LUTS) | |
|---|---|---|
| **Lower Urinary Tract Symptoms (LUTS)** | **Definition** | |
| Increased daytime frequency | The complaint by the patient who considers that he/she voids too often by day. | |
| Nocturia | The complaint that the individual has to wake at night one or more times to void. | |
| Urgency | The complaint of a sudden compelling desire to pass urine, which is difficult to defer. | |
| Urinary incontinence | The complaint of any involuntary leakage of urine. | |
| Stress urinary incontinence | The complaint of involuntary leakage on effort or exertion, or on sneezing or coughing. | |
| Urge urinary incontinence | The complaint of involuntary leakage accompanied by or immediately preceded by urgency. | |
| Mixed urinary incontinence | The complaint of involuntary leakage associated with urgency and also with exertion, effort, sneezing, or coughing. | |

*Note.* From The Standardisation of Terminology of Lower Urinary Tract Function: Report from the Standardisation Sub-committee of the International Continence Society. *Journal of Neurourology and Urodynamics*, 2002, Vol. *21*, pp. 167–178. Copyright 2002 by the International Continence Society. Printed with permission of the publisher.

older women than older men in one large survey. In women aged 65 to 74 years, 19.1% reported urge incontinence as compared to 8.2% of men in the same age group (Stewart et al., 2003). Urge urinary incontinence was also a significant factor in institutionalization for men (Nuotio, Tammela, Luukkaala, & Jylha, 2003).

## Mixed Urinary Incontinence

The International Continence Society definition of mixed incontinence is, "the complaint of involuntary leakage associated with urgency and also with exertion, effort, sneezing or coughing" (Abrams et al., 2002, p. 168). Mixed urinary symptoms such as problems with storing urine (urinary incontinence and frequency, urgency) and voiding symptoms (incomplete bladder emptying) are prevalent in adults over 75 years of age (Stenzelius et al., 2004).

## Urinary Incontinence Related to Toilet-Access Issues

People with normal bladders and urinary function can still experience functional incontinence. This type of incontinence occurs when an individual has a full bladder but has no access to a toilet. Hospitalized and nursing home residents unable to use the toilet independently may experience functional incontinence if they do not get assistance to the toilet in time.

## Overactive Bladder

Overactive bladder (OAB) is defined as "urgency with or without urge urinary incontinence, usually with frequency and nocturia" (Wein & Rovner, 2002, p. 7). Occurrence of OAB symptoms is unpredictable (Balkrishnan, Bhosle, Camacho, & Anderson, 2006). OAB is reported to have a significant effect on quality of life (Milsom et al., 2001) by decreasing self-esteem and increasing the fear of being incontinent in public (Wein & Rackley, 2006). OAB is characterized by involuntary bladder contractions during the storage of urine, which may be spontaneous or provoked, for example, by a local irritant (i.e., bladder stone or toxin) (J. Morrison et al., 2002).

Impaired contractility in the presence of detrusor hyperactivity (DHIC) was identified by Resnick and Yalla as a cause of urinary incontinence in older adults (Resnick & Yalla, 1987). Recent research on detrusor overactivity reveals a wide range of symptomats including decreased bladder capacity and increased bladder sensation (Pfisterer, Griffiths, Rosenberg, Schaefer, & Resnick, 2006). The relationship between detrusor overactivity and urge urinary incontinence is not clear, and a method to classify severity of detrusor overactivity has been attempted (Miller, DuBeau, Bergmann, Griffiths, & Resnick, 2002).

### Urgency

Urgency is defined as "the complaint of a sudden compelling desire to pass urine, which is difficult to defer" (Abrams et al., 2002). In a 10-year study with an older population, urgency and urge urinary incontinence significantly predicted death in men, after adjusting for socioeconomic status, smoking, and alcohol use (Nuotio et al., 2002).

### Frequency

Frequency is defined as more than eight voids in a 24-hour period (Milsom et al., 2001). In a multicountry study with 16,776 subjects older than 40 years, frequency was the most prevalent symptom (reported by 85% of the sample) (Milsom). Both frequency and urgency increased with age and there was little difference in prevalence in men and women.

### Nocturia

Nocturia, waking from sleep to void one or more times a night, is a prevalent condition that increases with age with 90% of people over the age of 80 years reporting it (Fonda et al., 2005). In a secondary analysis of a longitudinal study Johnson and his colleagues found that hypertension, older age, and diuretic use were associated with two or more episodes of nocturia in community-dwelling older adults (Johnson, Sattin, Parmelee, Fultz, & Ouslander, 2005). In a population-based study older men reported nocturia more frequently than women (Tikkinen, Tammela, Huhtala, & Auvinen, 2006).

Individuals with overactive bladder symptoms are at risk of experiencing incontinent episodes because of their increased need for toilet access. Another urinary symptom that can occur in critically ill older adults is bladder outlet obstruction, which can lead to urinary retention.

## Bladder Outlet Obstruction

According to the International Continence Society, bladder outlet obstruction (BOO) is a lower urinary tract symptom. Obstruction of the bladder outlet may result in obstructive symptoms such as decreased urine flow; hesitancy; sensation of incomplete emptying; and irritative symptoms such as urgency, frequency, nocturia, and dysuria (Dmochowski, 2005). Urinary retention is also a sign of BOO. Griffiths refers to "bladder failure," a condition that exists in older adults whose bladders do not contract adequately to empty the bladder of urine (Griffiths, 2003).

## Urinary Retention

Urinary retention is characterized as being either acute or chronic; pain is present with acute retention, when a person is unable to void. Chronic urinary retention is generally defined as a postvoid residual urine volume greater than 300 mL (Kaplan, Wein, Staskin, Roehrborn, & Steers, 2008). The underlying etiology for urinary retention is not clear but has been postulated as being caused by one or more of the following: (a) mechanical obstruction leading to increased resistance to flow, (b) detrusor sensory or motor innervation disruption, and (c) overdistension of the detrusor (Thomas, Chow, & Kirby, 2004).

The leading cause of acute urinary retention in men is increased prostate gland volume, most commonly caused by benign prostatic hypertrophy (BPH) in which the bladder neck is obstructed and flow is impeded (Kolman, Girman, Jacobsen, & Lieber, 1999). Risk factors for acute urinary retention in men also include increased age and decreased peak urinary flow rates (< 12 ml/sec) (Jacobsen et al., 1997) and medication usage such as those with anticholinergic effects (Meigs et al., 1999). Recent developments in the understanding of detrusor functioning indicate that detrusor underactivity may occur in the absence of bladder outlet obstruction in men (Thomas, Cannon, Bartlett, Ellis-Jones, & Abrams, 2004). Detrusor underactivity is defined as "contraction of reduced strength and/or duration, resulting in prolonged bladder emptying and/ or a failure to achieve complete bladder emptying in a normal time span" (Abrams et al., 2002, p. 175). Performing a transurethral resection to relieve bladder outlet obstruction did not alleviate voiding symptoms for men with detrusor underactivity.

Urinary retention is considered rare in women, although norms for postvoid residual urine volumes for women are not well established. In one study investigating the relationship between postvoid residual volumes and urinary tract infections with 204 postmenopausal women, the mean postvoid residual volume was 53.13 ml. In women with higher postvoid residual urine volumes a higher rate of urinary tract infections was reported (Stern, Hsieh, & Schaeffer, 2004). Evidence also exists that estrogens have a role in detrusor function, and in this study there was a statistically significant relationship between oral estrogen therapy and postvoid residual urine volumes (women on estrogen replacement therapy had lower postvoid residual urine volumes than women not on estrogen replacement therapy). The use of oral estrogen replacement therapy, however, appeared to have no protective effect against recurring urinary tract infections (Stern et al.).

Risk factors for urinary retention have been identified in different clinical populations. For example, urinary retention is prevalent in patients who have had an ischemic stroke. Other correlates included cognitive impairment, diabetes mellitus, aphasia, poor functional status, and urinary tract infections (Kong & Young, 2000). Fecal impaction is often cited in the clinical literature as contributing to urinary retention, yet little evidence has been provided to support this claim. For example, fecal impaction was not a statistically significant factor in either urinary retention or detrusor underactivity in nursing home residents who underwent urodynamic testing (Starer, Likourezos, & Dumapit, 2000). But another study showed that the greatest risks for urinary retention in women were fecal impaction, advanced age, history of diabetes mellitus, and use of medications with anticholinergic effects (Borrie et al., 2001).

Inability to transfer independently, that is, dependence on others to transfer, was found to be directly correlated with fecal impaction and urinary retention, thus leading the authors to conclude a third factor, immobility, may play a key role in both urinary and bowel emptying (Starer et al., 2000). Transfer ability also plays a role in the development of urinary incontinence during the first year of nursing home admission (M. H. Palmer, German, & Ouslander, 1991). It was also found to be an independent predictor of hip fracture (Walter, Lui, Eng, & Covinsky, 2003).

Postoperative urinary retention was noted in 39.5% of patients who underwent orthopedic surgical procedures. Associated factors included increased age and the amount of intravenous fluids infused in the 24-hour postoperative period (Wynd, Wallace, & Smith, 1996). The large amount of fluids infused during the perioperative interval was implicated in high catheterization rates in elderly male veterans undergoing surgery with spinal or general anesthesia (Kemp & Tabaka, 1990). Factors associated with urinary retention in older women admitted to a geriatric rehabilitation center (63% had orthopedic surgery) included cognitive impairment, presence of chronic conditions, impaired mobility, and polypharmacy (Hershkovitz, Manevitz, Beloosesky, Gillon, & Brill, 2003). Concern over instrumentation of the urinary tract and its relation to sepsis has led to calls for identification of patients who may be at risk for developing urinary retention (Wroblewski & del Sel, 1980) and for nonpayment for catheter-associated urinary tract infections (Wald & Kramer, 2007).

Management of urinary retention and the development of urinary tract infections in surgical patients have been the subjects of numerous studies. Straight catheterization in the recovery room, to prevent bladder overdistension, was found to have no benefit in preventing overdistension. The authors, however, found an increase in urinary tract infections in patients who had received straight catheterization (Hozack, Carpiniello, & Booth, 1988). Michelson and colleagues noted that use of indwelling catheters on a short-term basis reduced the incidence of urinary retention in hip and knee replacement patients (Michelson, Lotke, & Steinberg, 1988). Their findings support an earlier study that found indwelling catheters superior to straight catheterization and they did not increase the risk of urinary tract infections (Oishi et al., 1995). Catheterization is often used to preemptively prevent bladder distension or as a response to a patient's inability to empty the bladder after surgery (Knight & Pellegrini, 1996; Kumar, Mannan, Chowdhury, Kong, & Pati, 2006). The strongest correlate for bacterial colonization is duration of catheter use (Cornia, Amory, Fraser, Saint, & Lipsky, 2003). Indwelling catheters are often used in the immediate postoperative period to avoid bladder overdistension, but they can act as a single-point restraint. To prevent urinary tract infections and colonization, the duration of indwelling catheterization is usually limited to 24 to 48 hours (Wald, Epstein, & Kramer, 2005).

Urinary retention is a prevalent problem, especially after orthopedic surgery, but its etiology is not clear and controversy exists over the amount of postvoid residual urine volume that is clinically significant (amounts vary from 50 to 250 ml) (Yarnold, 1999). Thus assessing postvoid residual urine volumes during critical illnesses, especially in individuals with potential for urethral obstruction or incomplete bladder emptying, is a prudent nursing measure. Portable bladder ultrasounds may be used for this purpose to avoid unwarranted catheterization (Newman, 2008).

# Incident Urinary Incontinence

Hospitalized patients, like Mrs. Meyers in the case study, may normally be dry but become incontinent during hospitalization. Other terms used to describe incontinence that occurs in usually continent individuals are *transient incontinence* and *acute-onset incontinence*. These terms are used to imply the potentially reversible nature of incontinence. The underlying assumption is that once the underlying factor or condition is treated, the incontinence will resolve. In critically ill older adults it is difficult to determine if new incontinence is the start of an established pattern of incontinence or transient or acute-onset incontinence. The important point is not to assume incontinence is inevitable or caused by age. An incontinence history and an assessment for the underlying causes of incontinence must be done. Major risk factors for urinary incontinence include both reversible and irreversible factors, including cognitive, functional, infectious, metabolic, and pharmacologic factors.

## Cognitive Factors

Delirium is considered a medical emergency and requires immediate attention (Fernandez, Callahan, Likourezos, & Leipzig, 2008) (see chapter 26 on delirium). Older adults can become confused from medication reactions, infections, or other medical conditions. While they are confused, they may forget how and where to go to the bathroom or even be unaware that they need to empty their bladder.

Urinary incontinence is highly prevalent in patient populations exhibiting cognitive impairment resulting from dementia (Fonda et al., 2005). The proposed mechanisms include cerebral neuropathy, specifically in the frontal lobes (Griffiths et al., 1994), and the inability to carry out activities of daily living independently (Fonda).

Confusion during hospitalization increases the risk of urinary incontinence (M. H. Palmer, Myers, & Fedenko, 1997). Proposed reasons for this finding include inability to toilet independently because of confusion and lack of assistance to toilet in a timely manner. In bivariate analyses men developed urinary incontinence at twice the rate of women recovering from hip-fracture surgery, yet in the presence of dementia no significant differences between men and women in urinary incontinence incidence was detected (M. H. Palmer et al.).

## Functional Factors

Urinary continence is dependent on accessing appropriate toilet facilities in a timely manner. Evidence exists that people with limited mobility and the inability to transfer independently experience higher prevalence and incidence of urinary incontinence than people with unimpaired mobility (Fonda et al., 2005). Incontinent older adults receiving assistance with ambulation often experience improvement in incontinence (Schnelle et al., 2003), indicating that urinary incontinence may often be caused by lack of access or inadequate access to toilet facilities rather than specific pathophysiology. DuBeau noted that impaired mobility posed greater risk for urinary incontinence than cognitive impairment in nursing home residents (DuBeau, 2005). Preexisting dependent ambulation also increases risk of hospital-acquired urinary incontinence in female hip-fracture patients (M. H. Palmer et al., 2002).

Another consequence of immobility is constipation and, if left untreated, fecal impaction. Hard stool blocking the rectum becomes almost impossible to pass without medications or enemas. Impaction is considered a cause of incontinence (Schnelle & Leung, 2004) although the mechanism is unclear. Thus, critically ill older adults on bedrest or unable to access toilet facilities independently are at risk of developing functional decline, fecal impaction, and perhaps, urinary incontinence.

The care plan should reflect information that patients with functional limitations are at risk of becoming incontinent and toilet alternatives and behavioral interventions may be appropriate to use.

## Infectious Factors

Urinary tract infections may irritate the bladder and cause both strong urges to urinate and a sensation of needing to urinate frequently. If a urinary tract infection is suspected, especially in a catheterized patient, it must be treated immediately because of the risk of life-threatening urosepsis. Urinary tract infections are the most frequent cause of bacteremia and they are associated with high mortality (Tal et al., 2005). Because many research reports on urinary tract infections in the elderly do not provide a consistent definition of a urinary tract infection, the prevalence and incidence of urinary tract infection are difficult to determine. In some reports, the presence of 100,000 colonies of a uropathogen per milliliter of urine is considered an indication of a urinary tract infection. Bacteriuria, however, is not considered a urinary tract infection unless symptoms of infection are present (*CMS Manual System,* 2005). Research indicates little correlation between bacteriuria and symptoms of a urinary tract infection in elderly patients (Hedstrom, Grondal, & Ahl, 1999). In a preoperative screening, Johnstone and colleagues found that 14.8% of women had a positive culture ($10^5$ colonies/ milliliter), although it is not reported how many were symptomatic. In another study with hip-fracture patients, 38% had a positive urinary culture on admission to the hospital. The most common bacteria was *Escherichia* coli (45%) (Johansson, Athlin, Frykholm, Bolinder, & Larsson, 2002).

Symptoms of urinary tract infections in noncatheterized older adults include at least three symptoms: (a) increase in temperature of greater than 2 degrees Fahrenheit or single temperature measurement that is greater than 100 degrees Fahrenheit; (b) new or increased burning pain on urination, frequency, or urgency; (c) new flank or suprapubic pain or tenderness; (d) change in the character of the urine (e.g., new bloody urine, foul smell, or amount of sediment) or new pyuria or microscopic hematuria as reported from a laboratory; and (e) worsening cognitive or functional status (e.g., confusion, decreased appetite, unexplained falls, recent-onset incontinence, lethargy or decreased activity). In catheterized patients at least two symptoms are needed to indicate a urinary tract infection (*CMS Manual System,* 2005).

Some urinary tract infections are considered to be a complication of urinary tract instrumentation, specifically catheterization. Catheter-associated urinary tract infections entail additional costs for diagnostic tests and extra medications; median costs for a catheter-associated urinary tract infection was $356 (1998 dollars) (Tambyah, Knasinski, & Maki, 2002). Catheter-related bacteriuria has been associated with increased mortality (Saint & Chenoweth, 2003), but controversy exists over prophylactic antibiotic use to prevent urinary tract infections (Cardosi, Cardosi, Grendys, Fiorica, & Hoffman, 2003). In general, antibiotic use for asymptomatic bacteriuria is not recommended (*CMS Manual System* 2005; Midthun, Paur, Bruce, & Midthun, 2005). The use of silver-coated catheters has been advocated to reduce the prevalence of urinary tract infections (Hashmi, Kelly, Rogers, & Gates, 2003; Kassler & Barnett, 2008; Maki & Tambyah, 2001) although others did not find a reduction in urinary tract infections associated with silver-hydrogel catheter use (Lai & Fontecchio, 2002). A *Cochrane Systematic Review* on symptomatic urinary tract infections in elderly women found studies to be of poor quality and optimal treatment duration could not be determined (Lutters & Vogt, 2002).

After a woman's ovaries stop producing estradiol, estradiol levels decrease in the urogenital tract. As a result urogential tissue atrophies, becoming thin, dry, and susceptible to inflammation. Atrophic vaginitis is inflammation of vaginal tissues and symptoms can include urinary urgency, polyuria, and incontinence (Castelo-Branco, Cancelo, Villero, Nohales, & Julia, 2005). Guidelines for treatment of atrophic vaginitis include topical estrogen and use of water-soluble lubricants, vaginal moisturizers, oral or topical administration of vitamin E, and some Chinese herbs (Castelo-Branco et al.). The role atrophic vaginitis plays in the development of urinary incontinence is not clear but its treatment may relieve urinary symptoms.

## Metabolic Factors

Diabetes mellitus is a known risk factor for urinary incontinence in women and the risk increases as the duration of diabetes increases (Lifford, Curhan, Hu, Barbieri, & Grodstein, 2005). The continence mechanism and detrusor contractibility are impaired because of neuropathy, thus incomplete bladder emptying may occur. In a cross-sectional study with 1,017 postmenopausal women, those with diabetes had more severe urinary incontinence, were less able to completely empty their bladders, and had more discomfort with urination than did women without diabetes (Jackson, Scholes, Boyko, Abraham, & Fihn, 2005). In the presence of heart disease the risk for urinary incontinence for a diabetic is even greater.

An older adult with an abnormally high blood glucose level, which happens with uncontrolled diabetes mellitus, may urinate in frequent large amounts that overwhelm the bladder and thus result in urinary incontinent episodes.

## Pharmacologic Factors

Many medications affect the urinary tract, including diuretics, anticholinergics, beta blockers, alpha adrenergic agonists, and alpha adrenergic antagonists, (see Table 22.3) Polypharmacy and medications that are potentially inappropriate for older adults (see Try This for Beers, available at http://consultgerirn.org/uploads/File/trythis/issue16_2.pdf). Criteria for potentially inappropriate medications for the elderly

## 22.3  Risk and Associated Factors for Urinary Retention

| Risk Factor | Reference |
| --- | --- |
| Cognitive impairment | (Kong & Young, 2000) |
| Diabetes mellitus | (Kong & Young) |
| Poor functional status | (Kong & Young) |
| Urinary tract infections | (Kong & Young) |
| Fecal impaction | (Starer et al., 2000) |
| Advanced age | (Starer et al.) |
| Medications with anticholinergic effects | (Borrie et al., 2001) |
| Immobility | (Starer et al.) |
| Amount of intravenous fluids administered perioperatively | (Wynd, Wallace, & Smith, 1996) |
| Polypharmacy | (Hershkovitz et al., 2003) |
| Presence of chronic conditions | (Hershkovitz et al.) |
| Decreased peak urine flow in men | (Abrams et al., 2002) |
| Ischemic stroke | (Kong & Young) |

(Molony, 2008) should be monitored closely for their impact on urinary function. Older adults may be using multiple medications that share similar pharmacological activity on the bladder that may increase the risk of urinary incontinence (Ruby et al., 2005).

## Assessment

In the long-term care and community settings, assessment includes a comprehensive history and physical examination. Essential components of the history include history of urinary incontinence and past or current treatment of urinary incontinence. Factors that have an impact on neurological status of anatomical structures include: history of pelvic or abdominal surgery, radiation, trauma, back surgery, or trauma. This assessment may not be feasible to conduct with a critically ill older adult, but documentation in the medical record may provide information relevant to urinary function.

Comorbidities, especially those that result in frailty (Miles et al., 2001), difficulty ambulating or transferring (M. H. Palmer et al., 1991), and stroke (Goode et al., 2008) may play a role in the development or worsening of urinary incontinence. As noted earlier, the medication history, especially medications with urologic activity, is essential to creating a care plan to lessen or reverse urinary incontinence.

Useful information from a bladder record is similar to many elements in standard intake and output charts. These include: (a) times and amount of voiding; (b) whether voiding was continent or not; (c) timing of bowel movements; (d) fluid intake, including intravenous fluids and amount of caffeinated beverages ingested. Not only is evidence of the physiologic functioning of the gastrointestinal and urinary tracts obtained, but information about elimination patterns and toileting habits is also provided (Sampselle, 2003). Although a 3- or 7-day bladder record has been recommended in healthy community-based older adults (Locher, Goode, Roth, Worrell, & Burgio, 2001; Tincello, Williams, Joshi, Assassa, & Abrams, 2007), this may not be possible during hospitalizations with a short length of stay. The very act, however, of keeping a bladder record serves as a prompt or cue for caregivers to provide toileting and to create self-awareness in the older adult of the need to void (Sampselle).

Information about patient preference for incontinence treatment is limited. In one study with cognitively intact inpatients, many functionally dependent individuals preferred catheters over medications and scheduled toileting. The authors suggested that these individuals either did not want to be dependent on caregivers for toileting assistance or they had little faith in the ability of the staff to achieve timely toileting (Pfisterer et al., 2007).

## Physical Examination

Postvoid residual volumes should be assessed to rule out urinary retention resulting from incomplete bladder emptying that can occur from peripheral neuropathy secondary to diabetes mellitus (Newman, 2008) or changes in normal voiding stances (i.e., men trying to void while in bed rather than standing next to the bed). Skin should be assessed for incontinence-associated dermatitis (Gray, 2007). Incontinence-associated dermatitis-affected skin exhibits inflammation in skin folds or other areas exposed to urine or feces. The skin may appear bright red and have maculopapular red rash with satellite lesions, indicating cutaneous candidiasis. In addition, the patient may report that the skins itches and burns (Gray). Skin exposed to urine and feces requires special care and protectants to prevent or reduce breakdown. In critically ill older adults with diarrhea or fecal incontinence, a rectal trumpet has been used to manage the collection of fecal material and maintain perineal skin integrity (Grogan & Kramer, 2002). A 32-French nasopharyngeal airway was used as a rectal trumpet and findings revealed that this appliance was effective is containing fecal matter and helping to restore skin integrity. In addition, pressure ulcer prevention measures should be instituted.

For the critically ill older adult able to ambulate or sit up in a chair, an environmental assessment should also be conducted. Capezuti and colleagues (2008) recommend seating height to be approximately 120% of the individual's lower leg length to promote sit-to-stand movements and to prevent falls. For individuals dependent on others for toileting needs, access to call bells or other devices to communicate with caregivers is especially critical.

Gender-specific physical examination includes prostate examination in men to determine presence of prostatic enlargement that may contribute to incomplete emptying, especially when they are unable to assume their normal voiding stance. In women, if their condition permits, urogenital tissue should be examined for atrophic vaginitis, purulent discharge, and evidence of prolapse. This information assists in deciding the course of treatment. For example, behavioral interventions would be ineffective in treating incontinence that is caused by inflammation or obstruction. When prolapse is present, longitudinal evidence suggests that vaginal descent is not associated with stress or urge incontinence (Bradley, Zimmerman, Wang, & Nygaard, 2008).

Information from the assessment must be reviewed and interdisciplinary efforts (e.g., nursing, medicine, pharmacy, physical therapy, etc.) to treat factors that cause incident incontinence (i.e., fecal impaction) and affect urinary tract function (i.e., diabetes mellitus) must occur concurrently with interventions to manage incontinence (i.e., behavioral interventions or urinary collection devices).

## Treatment

Behavioral therapies are the first treatment of choice for incontinence in institutional and community-dwelling adults because of low adverse effects and evidence of their effectiveness. Measurement of the effectiveness of these interventions includes patient satisfaction, and dryness level, that is the number of dry voids divided by the number of total voids multiplied by 100. Bladder records have also been used in the evaluation of treatment (Bryan & Chapple, 2004) but no evidence of their use in the acute care or critical care environment is available.

Despite the lack of evidence in health care settings where critically ill older adults are treated, these preventive measures should still be attempted. As concern over hospital-acquired complications and patient safety increases, the need for nursing measures designed to preserve function, such as urinary continence, and to prevent complications (e.g., falls associated with incontinence, urinary tract infections associated with indwelling catheter use) is compelling.

For example, in the place of a bladder record used in long-term-care settings, critical care nurses can use information already documented on intake and output forms to determine voiding patterns. Further information about factors that affect continence may be revealed when medication sheets that display the type, timing, and amount of administered medications are reviewed for medications that affect the urine storage and emptying functions of the lower urinary tract.

The paucity of evidence for treatment effectiveness is also compounded by the lack of evidence-based outcomes, including quality-of-life measures, for critically ill older adults. Figure 22.1 displays an algorithm to use to guide treatment. Medical justification for inserting and keeping an indwelling catheter in place, that is, the need for a strict intake and output record, may preclude the use of behavioral interventions. However, the need to measure urine volumes may be met with the use of portable bladder ultrasound rather than an indwelling catheter (Newman, 2008).

### Prompted Voiding

Prompted voiding involves caregiver prompting to elicit requests from the older adult for: (a) toileting assistance; (b) efforts to self-toilet; (c) provision of toileting assistance; and (d) social reinforcement from the caregiver for toileting-assistance requests, being continent between toileting episodes, and voiding into the toilet when assistance was provided (M. H. Palmer, 2005). Indicators of success for the intervention include: bladder capacity greater than 200 mL and less than 700 mL, ability to recognize the need to void, maximum voided volume of greater than 150 mL, postvoid residual urine volume less than 100 mL, and ability to void when given assistance to the toilet (Lyons & Specht, 2000). Because prompted voiding requires staff adherence to the

# 22.1

**Critically ill older adults flow chart.**

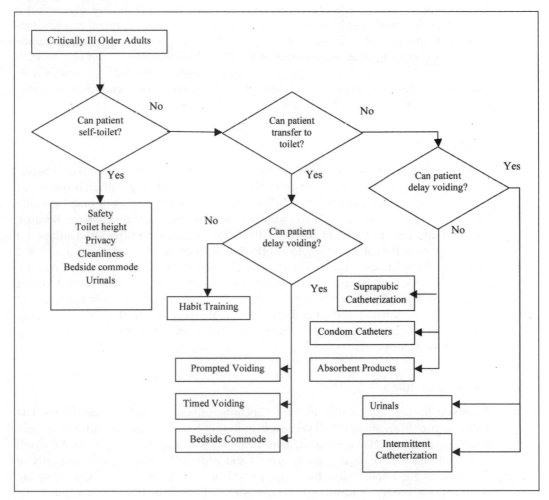

protocol, staff performance models have been developed. One model involved statistical quality control (Schnelle, Cruise, Rahman, & Ouslander, 1998) and the other involved supervisory nurses who observed direct care workers performance of the prompted-voiding intervention (Burgio et al., 1990). Bladder capacity and postvoid residuals are easily measured with bladder ultrasound and if the person is physically able to cooperate with toileting, a trial of prompted voiding should be tried to prevent or treat urinary incontinence. It may take up to 3 days to determine if the older adult responds to prompted voiding by having fewer incontinent episodes, more continent voidings, and increased number of requests for assistance with toileting.

### Timed Voiding

Timed voiding involves a fixed schedule of offering assistance to toilet. Timed voiding is the most commonly used intervention for continence in health care settings (Ostaszkiewicz, Johnston, & Roe, 2004). Not enough evidence exists, for or against, to recommend timed voiding as an effective toileting schedule (Ostaszkiewicz et al.). As with prompted voiding, timed voiding may be effective if the individual cooperates with toileting assistance and there is evidence that the number of incontinent episodes decreases when timed voiding is used.

### Habit Training

Habit training or habit retraining is used when rehabilitating the bladder is unfeasible. Before starting a habit-training program, the individual's voiding pattern is discerned from keeping a 3-day bladder record. The goal is to preempt an incontinent episode by adjusting a toileting schedule according to the individual's voiding pattern. Because the older adult is a passive participant in this intervention, it requires strict adherence by the caregiver for habit training to be effective. A systematic literature review found limited evidence to determine if continence improvement is worthwhile in relation to its labor-intensive nature (Ostaszkiewicz, Chestney, & Roe, 2004). Habit training may be effective with older adults who have a discernable voiding pattern but cannot delay voiding. Nursing staff members consistently assigned to the individual may observe the voiding pattern and be able to preempt an incontinent episode by offering toileting assistance.

### Toilet Substitutes

Toilet substitutes to prevent incontinence include urinals and bedside commodes. The goal is to provide increased toilet access to individuals with limited mobility or energy levels. Several models of female and male urinals are available (Fader, 2003). Although there is little research on the use of urinals and bedside commodes with critically ill older adults, these toilet substitutes may provide the necessary toilet access as healing occurs and as the older adult regains strength to ambulate or transfer to a commode.

## Catheterization

Bladder decompression to prevent or treat urinary retention are major reasons for indwelling catheter use but Jain and colleagues found that indwelling catheters were inappropriately used for the management of urinary incontinence in 21% of the hospitalized medical patients studied (Jain, Parada, Davis, & Smith, 1995). Failing to discontinue an indwelling catheter that does not have a medical justification is considered an indicator of poor care (Landi et al., 2004). Criteria used to justify long-term catheterization include wound contamination from urinary incontinence or fecal incontinence, urinary retention that cannot be managed medically or surgically, terminal illness, and failure of other treatments accompanied by a patient preference for catheterization

(*The Merck Manual of Geriatrics*, 2008). Recommendations exist to use indwelling catheters only for justified medical reasons and for the shortest period of time (Leone et al., 2003).

Physicians are sometimes not aware that their patients have an indwelling catheter. In one study, for example, physicians were unaware of 28% of catheterizations in their patients (Saint et al., 2000). Saint and colleagues (Saint, Lipsky, & Goold, 2002) suggested that indwelling catheters act as a single point restraint. Researchers reporting on a national survey found that 23% of older surgical patients had an indwelling urinary catheter (Wald et al., 2008). Patients discharged to extended-stay facilities with an indwelling catheter had greater odds for rehospitalization for urinary tract infections and for death after adjusting for age and comorbid conditions (Wald et al., 2005). Nonpayment for hospital-acquired catheter-associated urinary tact infections provides hospitals a financial incentive to find other means to manage urinary elimination. In another national survey, 12% and 9% of non-Veterans Administration (VA) hospitals used condom catheters and suprapubic catheterization, respectively. The researchers conducting this study noted that the use of these alternatives can lower bacteriuria rates. Use of systems to monitor which patients have indwelling catheters and to measure the duration of catheterization may also help prevent hospital-acquired urinary tract infections (Saint et al., 2008).

If an indwelling catheter is indicated because of the patient's medical condition or need for close monitoring of intake and output, a silver-coated catheter may reduce catheter-associated urinary tract infections (Kassler & Barnett, 2008). The guideline published by the Centers for Disease Control and Prevention in 1981 to prevent catheter-associated urinary tract infections recommends insertion of the catheter using aseptic technique and a closed drainage system (Centers for Disease Control and Prevention, 1981). In addition, automated reminders to either remove or continue using an indwelling catheter may reduce catheterization duration (Saint et al., 2008).

## Absorbent Products

Urine containment strategies, such as absorbent underpads for beds and wearable products (such as pads and pull-up briefs) should only be used after assessment for the type of incontinence, amount of urine lost, and self-care abilities of the individual. Absorbent products, however, are often employed in the absence of assessment (Connor & Kooker, 1996) because health care providers often lack necessary knowledge about incontinence and its assessment and treatment (Cooper & Watt, 2003) and do not view urinary incontinence as an important clinical condition (Molander, Sundh, & Steen, 2002). In the nursing home setting, 99% of incontinent patients used absorbent products (Watson, Brink, Zimmer, & Mayer, 2003), yet little is known about the short- and long-term effects of the use of absorbent products on patient outcomes and on subsequent follow-up by health care providers to assess and treat urinary incontinence. When absorbent products are indicated, assessment of the most appropriate product should occur (see Exhibit 22.1).

## Medications

Several medications administered orally that have anticholinergic effects are available for urge urinary incontinence. The overall goal of anticholinergic medication use for

## Exhibit 22.1

### Assessment for Absorbent Product Use

Assess individual's functional ability regarding:

> Delaying voiding
>
> Disrobing to use toilet
>
> Use of assistive devices
>
> Level of ability to self-toilet

Assess absorbent product for:

Capacity to contain urinary leakage:

  Does capacity match voided volume for the individual?

  Comfort

> Does it fit at waist and leg openings?
>
> Does it generate heat to the point of discomfort?
>
> Does it chafe?
>
> Is it bulky or noticeable under clothing?

Ease of application/removal:

> Can the individual remove and reapply without help?

*Note.* From *CMS Long Term Care Journal*–Urinary Incontinence, Volume II. (2004, Oct.). Retrieved June 5, 2008, from http://cms.internetstreaming.com/courses/36/handouts/Agenda+UI+10-2004.doc

urge incontinence is to reduce the intensity of detrusor contraction (Roxburgh, Cook, & Dublin, 2007). These medications may be contraindicated for frail older adults, those with multiple chronic conditions, or those taking multiple medications. Evidence exists that the dual use of bladder anticholinergic medications (e.g., oxybutynin or tolterodine) with cholinesterase inhibitors for dementia may actually result in faster rate of functional decline in high-functioning nursing home residents than in those taking cholinesterase inhibitors without use of anticholinergic medications for incontinence (Sink et al., 2008). No medications are currently available in the United States to treat stress urinary incontinence. Medications causing urinary incontinence are listed in Table 22.4; medications used to treat urinary incontinence are listed in Table 22.5.

### Case Study Revisited

Four days after her discharge from the intensive care unit, Mrs. Myers was discharged to a large long-term care facility for rehabilitation. She was wearing an absorbent

| 22.4 | Medications That Can Cause or Contribute to Incontinence in Frail Older Adults and Medication's Effects on Continence | |
|---|---|---|
| **Medications** | **Effects on Continence** | |
| Alpha adrenergic agonists | Increase smooth muscle tone in urethra and prostatic capsule and may precipitate obstruction, urinary retention, and related symptoms | |
| Alpha adrenergic antagonists | Decrease smooth muscle tone in the urethra and may precipitate stress incontinence in women | |
| Angiotensin converting enzyme (ACE) inhibitors | Cause cough that can exacerbate incontinence | |
| Antimuscarinic agents | May cause urinary retention and constipation that can contribute to incontinence | |
| Calcium channel blockers | May cause urinary retention and constipation that can contribute to incontinence | |
| Cholinesterase inhibitors | Increase bladder contractility and may precipitate incontinence | |
| Diuretics | Cause polyuria and precipitate incontinence | |
| Opioid analgesics | May cause urinary retention, constipation, confusion, and immobility–all of which can contribute to incontinence | |
| Psychotropic drugs<br>  Sedatives<br>  Hypnotics<br>  Antipsychotics | May cause confusion and impaired mobility and precipitate incontinence<br>Some agents have anticholinergic effects | |
| Other drugs<br>  Calcium channel<br>  blockers (pyridines)<br>  Gabapentin<br>  Glitazones<br>  Nonsteroidal<br>  antiinflammatory agents | Can cause edema, which can lead to polyuria while supine and exacerbate nocturia and nighttime incontinence | |

*Note*. From "Incontinence in the Frail Elderly,", by D. Fonda, C. E. DuBeau, D. Harari, J. G. Ouslander, M. H. Palmer, & B. Roe, 2005. In *Incontinence, Management Vol. 2*. P. Abrams, L. Cardozo, S. Khoury & A. Wein (Eds.), p. 1177. Health Publication Ltd. Copyright 2005 by the International Continence Society. Reprinted with permission of the publisher.

product and had received no assistance to the toilet during her hospitalization. On admission to the facility a bladder record was instituted and on the first morning after her admission, the nursing assistant assigned to care for Mrs. Myers offered her assistance with transferring to a bedside commode to void. When seated on the commode, Mrs. Myers promptly voided. She also had a bowel movement. The bladder record revealed Mrs. Myers' normal voiding pattern. She voided within 30 minutes on awakening and approximately every 3 hours during the day. She woke once during the night between 1 am and 3 am to void. Mrs. Myers also drank the majority of fluids with her meals and had a glass of milk at bedtime. She had no trouble with moving her bowels regularly.

## 22.5 Medications to Treat Urinary Incontinence

| Medication | Mechanisms | Dose | Comments |
|---|---|---|---|
| **Bladder Outlet Obstruction in Men with Urge or Overflow Incontinence** | | | |
| Alfuzosin | Adrenergic blockage | 10 mg by mouth once/day | Relieve symptoms of male outlet obstruction, may reduce postvoid residual volume and outlet resistance, and may increase urinary flow rate. Effect occurs within days to weeks. Adverse effects include hypotension, fatigue, asthenia, and dizziness. |
| Doxazosin | | 1–8 mg by mouth once/day | |
| Prazosin | | 0.5–2 mg by mouth b.i.d. | |
| Tamsulosin | | 0.4–0.8 mg by mouth once/day | |
| Terazosin | | 1–10 mg by mouth once/day | |
| Dutasteride | 5 alpha-Reductase inhibition | 0.5 mg by mouth once/day | These medications reduce prostate size and obstructive symptoms and make transurethral resection of prostate glands greater than 50 grams, less likely to be needed. |
| Finasteride | | 5 mg by mouth once/day | Adverse effects are minimal and consist of sexual dysfunction (example: decreased libido, erectile dysfunction) |
| **Detrusor Overactivity in Urge Incontinence** | | | |
| Darifenacin | Anticholinergic effects, selective $M_3$ muscarinic antagonism | Extended-release: 7.5 mg by mouth once/day | Adverse effects are similar to those of oxybutynin but because of bladder selectivity may be less severe. |
| Solifenacin | Anticholinergic effects, selective $M_1$ and $M_3$ muscarinic antagonism | Extended-release: 5–10 mg by mouth once/day | Adverse effects are similar to those of oxybutynin, but because of bladder selectivity may be less severe. |
| Imipramine | Tricyclic antidepressant, anticholinergic, and alpha-agonist effects | 25 mg by mouth at night; may increase in increments of 25 mg to a maximum dose of 150 mg | Is useful for the treatment of nocturia |

*(continued)*

**Table 22.5** *(continued)*

| Medication | Mechanisms | Dose | Comments |
|---|---|---|---|
| Oxybutynin | Smooth muscle relaxation, anticholinergic, nonselective muscarinic, and local anesthetic effects<br>Immediate release: 2.5–5 mg by mouth t.i.d. to q.i.d.<br>Extended release: 5–30 mg by mouth once/day<br>Transdermal: 3.9 mg twice/week | Efficacy may increase over time. Adverse effects include anticholinergic effects (example: dry mouth, constipation) that may interfere with adherence and worsen incontinence. Adverse effects are less severe with extended-release and transdermal forms. | |
| Tolterodine | Anticholinergic effects, selective $M_3$ muscarinic antagonism | Immediate release: 1–2 mg by mouth b.i.d.<br>Extended release: 2–4 mg by mouth once/day | Efficacy and adverse effects are similar to those of oxybutynin, but long-term experience is limited. Because $M_3$ receptors are targeted, adverse effects are less severe than those of oxybutynin. Dose reduction is needed in patients with severe renal impairment |
| Trospium | Anticholinergic effects | Immediate release: 20 mg by mouth b.i.d. (20 mg once/day in renal insufficiency) | Adverse effects are similar to those of oxybutnin. Dose reduction is needed in patients with renal impairment. |

Medications with anticholinergic effects should be used judiciously in the elderly.

*Note.* From "Drugs Used To Treat Incontinence", Merck Manuals Online Medical Library for Health Professionals. (2007, August). Retrieved June 8, 2008, from http://www.merck.com/mmpe/print/sec17/ch228/ch228b.html, Table 3; http://www.merck.com/media/mmpe/pdf/Table_228-3.pdf. Copyright 2008 by Merck & Co., Inc. Printed with permission of the publisher.

The nurse in charge of Mrs. Myers's care placed her on a prompted voiding schedule every 3 hours during daytime hours and asked that Mrs. Myers be helped with toileting before retiring at bedtime and that Mrs. Myers be checked during the hours of 1 am to 3 am, and offered help with toileting if she was awake.

Mrs. Myers subsequently regained her urinary continence and ability to ambulate, albeit more slowly than at her prefracture pace. After 20 days of rehabilitation she was discharged to her son's home using a cane for ambulation. She also continued keeping a bladder record, finding it helpful to remind her to seek toilet facilities in a timely way.

# Summary

Despite limited information about evidence-based interventions specifically designed for critically ill older adults, nurses can act to promote urinary continence and protect patient dignity. One common barrier to widespread implementation to these interventions has been resistance to changing behaviors that have traditionally promoted staff convenience, most notably the use of urine containment strategies such as absorbent products or the use of indwelling catheters without medical justification. The standard of care of critically ill older adults should include a comprehensive assessment for urinary elimination needs and the patient's self-care abilities prior to the development of a care plan and initiation of behavioral and other interventions designed to treat or manage urinary incontinence.

Evidence that urinary continence assessment and care planning has occurred could include the documentation of: (a) duration of indwelling catheterization; (b) use of urinary containment measures such as condom catheters, female and male urinals, and absorbent products; (c) incidence and type of hospital-acquired urinary tract infections; (d) incidence and type of hospital-acquired skin complications related to incontinence; (e) self-reported patient and family satisfaction with care; and (f) patients' report of preservation of their sense of dignity.

Typical outcome measures for incontinence interventions have traditionally included wetness levels and quality of life. In critically ill older adults, outcome measures need to be developed to determine if the feasible maximal level of continence is being achieved.

## Resources for Patient Education

National Institute on Aging, Age Page: Urinary Incontinence. To order this Age Page in English or Spanish, visit
www.niapublications.org

American Geriatrics Society Foundation for Health in Aging, Patient Handout: Urinary Incontinence and Its Treatment.
www.healthinaging.org

National Association for Continence
www.nafc.com

Simon Foundation
www.simonfoundation.org

## Resources for Caregiver Education

Hartford Geriatric Nursing Initiative, Try This Series, located at
http://www.hartfordign.org/resources/education/tryThis.html

International Consultation on Incontinence. (2009). Abrams, P., Cardozo, L., Khoury, S., & Wein, A. (Eds.). *Incontinence (4th ed.) Portsmoouth, UK: Health Publications, Ltd. (For more information contact the International Continence Society at www.icsoffice.org)*

## References

Abrams, P., Cardozo, L., Fall, M., Griffiths, D., Rosier, P., Ulmsten, U., et al. (2002). The standardisation of terminology of lower urinary tract function: Report from the Standardisation Sub-committee of the International Continence Society. *Neurourology and Urodynamics, 21*(2), 167–178.

Balkrishnan, R., Bhosle, M. J., Camacho, F. T., & Anderson, R. T. (2006). Predictors of medication adherence and associated health care costs in an older population with overactive bladder syndrome: A longitudinal cohort study. *Journal of Urology, 175*(3 Pt 1), 1067–1071; discussion 1071–1072

Borrie, M. J., Campbell, K., Arcese, Z. A., Bray, J., Hart, P., Labate, T., et al. (2001). Urinary retention in patients in a geriatric rehabilitation unit: Prevalence, risk factors, and validity of bladder scan evaluation. *Rehabilitation Nursing, 26*(5), 187–191.

Brading, A. F. (1997). A myogenic basis for the overactive bladder. *Urology, 50*(6A Suppl.), 57–67; discussion 68–73.

Bradley, C. S., Zimmerman, M. B., Wang, Q., & Nygaard, I. E. (2008). Vaginal descent and pelvic floor symptoms in postmenopausal women: A longitudinal study. *Obstetrics & Gynecology, 111*(5), 1148–1153.

Brown, J. S., Vittinghoff, E., Wyman, J. F., Stone, K. L., Nevitt, M. C., Ensrud, K. E., et al. (2000). Urinary incontinence: does it increase risk for falls and fractures? Study of Osteoporotic Fractures Research Group. *Journal of the American Geriatrics Society, 48*(7), 721–725.

Bryan, N. P., & Chapple, C. R. (2004). Frequency volume charts in the assessment and evaluation of treatment: How should we use them? *European Urology, 46*(5), 636–640.

Burgio, L. D., Engel, B. T., Hawkins, A., McCormick, K., Scheve, A., & Jones, L. T. (1990). A staff management system for maintaining improvements in continence with elderly nursing home residents. *Journal of Applied Behavior Analysis, 23*(1), 111–118.

Capezuti, E., Wagner, L., Brush, B. L., Boltz, M., Renz, S., & Secic, M. (2008). Bed and toilet height as potential environmental risk factors. *Clinical Nursing Research, 17*(1), 50-66.

Cardosi, R. J., Cardosi, R. P., Grendys, E. C., Jr., Fiorica, J. V., & Hoffman, M. S. (2003). Infectious urinary tract morbidity with prolonged bladder catheterization after radical hysterectomy. *Am J Obstetrics & Gynecology, 189*(2), 380–383; discussion 383–384.

Castelo-Branco, C., Cancelo, M. J., Villero, J., Nohales, F., & Julia, M. D. (2005). Management of postmenopausal vaginal atrophy and atrophic vaginitis. *Maturitas, 52* (Suppl. 1), S46–52.

Centers for Disease Control and Prevention. (1981). *Guideline for prevention of catheter-associated urinary tract infections.* Retrieved July 30, 2008, from http://www.cdc.gov/NCIDOD/DHQP/gl_catheter_assoc.html

*CMS Long Term Care Journal.* (2004, Oct.) *Urinary incontinence—Volume II.* Retrieved June 5, 2008, from http://cms.internetstreaming.com/courses/36/handouts/Agenda+UI+10-2004.doc

*CMS Manual System.* (2005). *§483.25(d) Urinary incontinence.* Retrieved April 25, 2008, from http://www.cms.hhs.gov/transmittals/downloads/r8som.pdf

Connor, P. A., & Kooker, B. M. (1996). Nurses' knowledge, attitudes, and practices in managing urinary incontinence in the acute care setting. *Medsurg Nursing, 5*(2), 87–92, 117.

Cooper, G., & Watt, E. (2003). An exploration of acute care nurses' approach to assessment and management of people with urinary incontinence. *Journal of Wound, Ostomy, and Continence Nursing, 30*(6), 305–313.

Cornia, P. B., Amory, J. K., Fraser, S., Saint, S., & Lipsky, B. A. (2003). Computer-based order entry decreases duration of indwelling urinary catheterization in hospitalized patients. *American Journal of Medicine, 114*(5), 404–407.

Dmochowski, R. R. (2005). Bladder outlet obstruction: Etiology and evaluation. *Review in Urology, 7* (Suppl. 6), S3–S13.

DuBeau, C. E. (2005). Improving urinary incontinence in nursing home residents: Are we FIT to be tied? *Journal of the American Geriatrics Society, 53*(7), 1254–1256.

DuBeau, C. E. (2006). The aging lower urinary tract. *Journal of Urology, 175*(3 Pt 2), S11–15.

Fader, M. (2003). Review of current technologies for urinary incontinence: Strengths and limitations. *Proceedings of the Institution of Mechanical Engineers [H], 217*(4), 233–241.

Fernandez, H. M., Callahan, K. E., Likourezos, A., & Leipzig, R. M. (2008). House staff member awareness of older inpatients' risks for hazards of hospitalization. *Archives of Internal Medicine, 168*(4), 390–396.

Fonda, D., DuBeau, C., Harari, D., Ouslander, J. G., Palmer, M. H., & Roe, B. (2005). Incontinence in the frail elderly. In P. Abrams, L. Cardozo, S. Khoury, & A. Wein (Eds.), *Incontinence* (Vol. 2). Paris: Health Publications Ltd.

Goode, P. S., Burgio, K. L., Redden, D. T., Markland, A., Richter, H. E., Sawyer, P., et al. (2008). Population based study of incidence and predictors of urinary incontinence in black and white older adults. *Journal of Urology, 179*(4), 1449–1453; discussion 1453–1444.

Gray, M. (2007). Incontinence-related skin damage: essential knowledge. *Ostomy Wound Management, 53*(12), 28–32.

Griffiths, D., & Tadic, S. D. (2008). Bladder control, urgency, and urge incontinence: Evidence from functional brain imaging. *Neurourology and Urodynamics, 27*(6), 466–474.

Griffiths, D. J. (2003). Editorial: Bladder failure—A condition to reckon with. *Journal of Urology, 169*(3), 1011–1012.

Griffiths, D. J., McCracken, P. N., Harrison, G. M., Gormley, E. A., Moore, K., Hooper, R., et al. (1994). Cerebral aetiology of urinary urge incontinence in elderly people. *Age Ageing, 23*(3), 246–250.

Grogan, T., & Kramer, D. (2002). The rectal trumpet: Use of a nasopharyngeal airway to contain fecal incontinence in critically ill patients. *Journal of Wound, Ostomy and Continence Nursing, 29*(4), 193–201.

Hagglund, D., & Ahlstrom, G. (2007). The meaning of women's experience of living with long-term urinary incontinence is powerlessness. *Journal of Clinical Nursing, 16*(10), 1946–1954.

Hashmi, S., Kelly, E., Rogers, S. O., & Gates, J. (2003). Urinary tract infection in surgical patients. *American Journal of Surgery, 186*(1), 53–56.

*HCUP Facts and Figures: Statistics on Hospital-Based Care in the United States, 2005.* (2005). Retrieved June 5, 2008, from http://www.hcup-us.ahrq.gov/reports/factsandfigures/HAR_2005.pdf

Hedstrom, M., Grondal, L., & Ahl, T. (1999). Urinary tract infection in patients with hip fractures. *Injury, 30*(5), 341–343.

Hershkovitz, A., Manevitz, D., Beloosesky, Y., Gillon, G., & Brill, S. (2003). Medical treatment for urinary retention in rehabilitating elderly women: Is it necessary? *Aging Clinical and Experimental Research, 15*(1), 19–24.

Hess, C. T., & Rook, L. J. (2007). Understanding recent regulatory guidelines for hospital-acquired catheter-related urinary tract infections and pressure ulcers. *Ostomy Wound Management, 53*(12), 34–42.

Hozack, W. J., Carpiniello, V., & Booth, R. E., Jr. (1988). The effect of early bladder catheterization on the incidence of urinary complications after total joint replacement. *Clinical Orthopaedics and Related Research, 231*, 79–82.

Huang, A. J., Brown, J. S., Thom, D. H., Fink, H. A., & Yaffe, K. (2007). Urinary incontinence in older community-dwelling women: The role of cognitive and physical function decline. *Obstetrics & Gynecology, 109*(4), 909–916.

Jackson, S. L., Scholes, D., Boyko, E. J., Abraham, L., & Fihn, S. D. (2005). Urinary incontinence and diabetes in postmenopausal women. *Diabetes Care, 28*(7), 1730–1738.

Jacobsen, S. J., Jacobson, D. J., Girman, C. J., Roberts, R. O., Rhodes, T., Guess, H. A., et al. (1997). Natural history of prostatism: Risk factors for acute urinary retention. *Journal of Urology, 158*(2), 481–487.

Jain, P., Parada, J. P., David, A., & Smith, L. G. (1995). Overuse of the indwelling urinary tract catheter in hospitalized medical patients. *Archives of Internal Medicine, 155*(13), 1425–1429.

Johansson, I., Athlin, E., Frykholm, L., Bolinder, H., & Larsson, G. (2002). Intermittent versus indwelling catheters for older patients with hip fractures. *Journal of Clinical Nursing, 11*(5), 651–656.

Johnson, T. M.II, Sattin, R. W., Parmelee, P., Fultz, N. H., & Ouslander, J. G. (2005). Evaluating potentially modifiable risk factors for prevalent and incident nocturia in older adults. *Journal of the American Geriatrics Society, 53*(6), 1011–1016.

Kaplan, S., Wein, A., Staskin, D., Roehrborn, C., & Steers, W. (2008). Urinary retention and post-void residual urine in men: Separating truth from tradition. *Journal of Urology, 180*(1), 47–54.

Kassler, J., & Barnett, J. (2008). A rehabilitation hospital's experience with ionic silver foley catheters. *Urologic Nursing, 28*(2), 97–100.

Kemp, D., & Tabaka, N. (1990). Postoperative urinary retention: Part II—A retrospective study. *Journal of Post Anesthesia Nursing, 5*(6), 397–400.

Knight, R. M., & Pellegrini, V. D., Jr. (1996). Bladder management after total joint arthroplasty. *Journal of Arthroplasty, 11*(8), 882–888.

Kolman, C., Girman, C. J., Jacobsen, S. J., & Lieber, M. M. (1999). Distribution of post-void residual urine volume in randomly selected men. *Journal of Urology, 161*(1), 122–127.

Kolominsky-Rabas, P. L., Hilz, M. J., Neundoerfer, B., & Heuschmann, P. U. (2003). Impact of urinary incontinence after stroke: Results from a prospective population-based stroke register. *Neurourology and Urodynamics, 22*(4), 322–327.

Kong, K. H., & Young, S. (2000). Incidence and outcome of poststroke urinary retention: A prospective study. *Archives of Physical Medicine and Rehabilitation, 81*(11), 1464–1467.

Kumar, P., Mannan, K., Chowdhury, A. M., Kong, K. C., & Pati, J. (2006). Urinary retention and the role of indwelling catheterization following total knee arthroplasty. *Int Brazilian Journal of Urology, 32*(1), 31–34.

Lai, K. K., & Fontecchio, S. A. (2002). Use of silver-hydrogel urinary catheters on the incidence of catheter-associated urinary tract infections in hospitalized patients. *American Journal of Infection Control, 30*(4), 221–225.

Landi, F., Cesari, M., Onder, G., Zamboni, V., Barillaro, C., Lattanzio, F., et al. (2004). Indwelling urethral catheter and mortality in frail elderly women living in community. *Neurourology and Urodynamics, 23*(7), 697–701.

Leone, M., Albanese, J., Garnier, F., Sapin, C., Barrau, K., Bimar, M. C., et al. (2003). Risk factors of nosocomial catheter-associated urinary tract infection in a polyvalent intensive care unit. *Intensive Care Medicine, 29*(7), 1077–1080.

Lifford, K. L., Curhan, G. C., Hu, F. B., Barbieri, R. L., & Grodstein, F. (2005). Type 2 diabetes mellitus and risk of developing urinary incontinence. *Journal of the American Geriatrics Society, 53*(11), 1851–1857.

Locher, J. L., Goode, P. S., Roth, D. L., Worrell, R. L., & Burgio, K. L. (2001). Reliability assessment of the bladder diary for urinary incontinence in older women. *Journals of Gerontology. Series A, Biological Sciences and Medical Sciences, 56*(1), M32–35.

Lutters, M., & Vogt, N. (2002). Antibiotic duration for treating uncomplicated, symptomatic lower urinary tract infections in elderly women. *Cochrane Database of Systematic Reviews*, (3), CD001535.

Lyons, S. S., & Specht, J. K. (2000). Prompted voiding protocol for individuals with urinary incontinence. *Journal of Gerontological Nursing, 26*(6), 5–13.

Madersbacher, S., Pycha, A., Schatzl, G., Mian, C., Klingler, C. H., & Marberger, M. (1998). The aging lower urinary tract: A comparative urodynamic study of men and women. *Urology, 51*(2), 206–212.

Maki, D. G., & Tambyah, P. A. (2001). Engineering out the risk for infection with urinary catheters. *Emerging Infectious Diseases, 7*(2), 342–347.

Meigs, J. B., Barry, M. J., Giovannucci, E., Rimm, E. B., Stampfer, M. J., & Kawachi, I. (1999). Incidence rates and risk factors for acute urinary retention: The health professionals follow-up study. *Journal of Urology, 162*(2), 376–382.

*The Merck Manual of Geriatrics*. (2008). Retrieved June 8, 2008, from http://www.merck.com/mkgr/mmg/tables/100t2.jsp

Merck Manuals Online Medical Library for Health Professionals. (2007, August). *Drugs used to treat incontinence*. Retrieved June 8, 2008, from http://www.merck.com/mmpe/print/sec17/ch228/ch228b.html, Table 3; http://www.merck.com/media/mmpe/pdf/Table_228-3.pdf

Michelson, J. D., Lotke, P. A., & Steinberg, M. E. (1988). Urinary-bladder management after total joint-replacement surgery. *New England Journal of Medicine, 319*(6), 321–326.

Midthun, S., Paur, R., Bruce, A. W., & Midthun, P. (2005). Urinary tract infections in the elderly: A survey of physicians and nurses. *Geriatric Nursing, 26*(4), 245–251.

Miles, T. P., Palmer, R. F., Espino, D. V., Mouton, C. P., Lichtenstein, M. J., & Markides, K. S. (2001). New-onset incontinence and markers of frailty: Data from the Hispanic Established Populations for Epidemiologic Studies of the Elderly. *Journals of Gerontology. Series A, Biological Sciences and Medical Sciences, 56*(1), M19–24.

Miller, K. L., DuBeau, C. E., Bergmann, M., Griffiths, D. J., & Resnick, N. M. (2002). Quest for a detrusor overactivity index. *Journal of Urology, 167*(2 Pt 1), 578–584; discussion 584–585.

Milsom, I., Abrams, P., Cardozo, L., Roberts, R. G., Thuroff, J., & Wein, A. J. (2001). How widespread are the symptoms of an overactive bladder and how are they managed? A population-based prevalence study. *BJU International, 87*(9), 760–766.

Molander, U., Sundh, V., & Steen, B. (2002). Urinary incontinence, its influence on daily life, and use of continence aids in two cohorts of 85/86-year-old free-living men and women, born 10 years apart. *Archives of gerontology and geriatrics, 35*(3), 275–281.

Molony, S. (2008). *Beers criteria for potentially inappropriate medication use in older adults—Part II: 2002 criteria considering diagnoses or conditions. Try this: Best practices in nursing care to older adults.* Retrieved June 5, 2008, from http://consultgerirn.org/uploads/File/trythis/issue16_2.pdf

Morrison, A., & Levy, R. (2006). Fraction of nursing home admissions attributable to urinary incontinence. *Value Health, 9*(4), 272–274.

Morrison, J., S. W., Brading, A., Blok, B., Fry, C., de Groat, W., Kakizaki, H. (2002). Neurophysiology and neuropharmacology. In P. Abrams, L. Cardozo, S. Khoury, & A. Wein (Eds.), *Incontinence. 2nd International Consultation on Incontinence* (ed. 21, pp. 83–163). Paris: Health Publications Ltd.

Newman, D. K. (2008). *Using the BladderScan for bladder volume assessment*. Retrieved April 21, 2008, from http://www.seekwellness.com/incontinence/using_the_bladderscan.htm

NIH State-of-the-Science Conference. (2007, Feb.). *Prevention of fecal and urinary incontinence in adults*. Retrieved June 5, 2008, from http://www.annals.org/cgi/content/short/148/6/449

Nuotio, M., Tammela, T. L., Luukkaala, T., & Jylha, M. (2002). Urgency and urge incontinence in an older population: Ten-year changes and their association with mortality. *Aging Clinical and Experimental Research, 14*(5), 412–419.

Nuotio, M., Tammela, T. L., Luukkaala, T., & Jylha, M. (2003). Predictors of institutionalization in an older population during a 13-year period: The effect of urge incontinence. *Journals of Gerontology. Series A, Biological Sciences and Medical Sciences, 58*(8), 756–762.

Oishi, C. S., Williams, V. J., Hanson, P. B., Schneider, J. E., Colwell, C. W., Jr., & Walker, R. H. (1995). Perioperative bladder management after primary total hip arthroplasty. *Journal of Arthroplasty, 10*(6), 732–736.

Ostaszkiewicz, J., Chestney, T., & Roe, B. (2004). Habit retraining for the management of urinary incontinence in adults. *Cochrane Database of Systematic Reviews, 2,* CD002801.

Ostaszkiewicz, J., Johnston, L., & Roe, B. (2004). Timed voiding for the management of urinary incontinence in adults. *Cochrane Database of Systematic Reviews, 2,* CD002802.

Palmer, M. H. (2005). Effectiveness of prompted voiding for incontinent nursing home residents. In B. Mazurek Melnyk & E. Fineout-Overholt (Eds.), *Evidence-based practice in nursing & healthcare: A guide to the best practice* (pp. CD 20–30). Philadelphia: Lippincott Williams & Wilkins.

Palmer, M. H., Baumgarten, M., Langenberg, P., & Carson, J. L. (2002). Risk factors for hospital-acquired incontinence in elderly female hip fracture patients. *Journals of Gerontology. Series A, Biological sciences and medical sciences, 57*(10), M672–677.

Palmer, M. H., German, P. S., & Ouslander, J. G. (1991). Risk factors for urinary incontinence one year after nursing home admission. *Research in Nursing Health, 14*(6), 405–412.

Palmer, M. H., Myers, A. H., & Fedenko, K. M. (1997). Urinary continence changes after hip-fracture repair. *Clin Nurs Res, 6*(1), 8–21; discussion 21–24.

Palmer, R. M. (2006). Perioperative care of the elderly patient. *Cleveland Clinic Journal of Medicine, 73* (Suppl. 1), S106–110.

Pfisterer, M. H., Griffiths, D. J., Rosenberg, L., Schaefer, W., & Resnick, N. M. (2006). The impact of detrusor overactivity on bladder function in younger and older women. *Journal of Urology, 175*(5), 1777–1783; discussion 1783.

Pfisterer, M. H., Griffiths, D. J., Schaefer, W., & Resnick, N. M. (2006). The effect of age on lower urinary tract function: A study in women. *Journal of the American Geriatrics Society, 54*(3), 405–412.

Pfisterer, M. H., Johnson, T. M., 2nd, Jenetzky, E., Hauer, K., & Oster, P. (2007). Geriatric patients' preferences for treatment of urinary incontinence: A study of hospitalized, cognitively competent adults aged 80 and older. *Journal of the American Geriatrics Society, 55*(12), 2016–2022.

Resnick, N. M., & Yalla, S. V. (1987). Aging and its effect on the bladder. *Semiars in Urology, 5*(2), 82–86.

Roxburgh, C., Cook, J., & Dublin, N. (2007). Anticholinergic drugs versus other medications for overactive bladder syndrome in adults. *Cochrane Database of Systematic Reviews, 4,* CD003190.

Ruby, C. M., Hanlon, J. T., Fillenbaum, G. G., Pieper, C. F., Branch, L. G., & Bump, R. C. (2005). Medication use and control of urination among community-dwelling older adults. *Journal of Aging and Health, 17*(5), 661–674.

Saint, S., Kowalski, C., Kaufman, S., Hofer, T., Kauffman, C., Olmsted, R., et al. (2008). Preventing hospital-acquired urinary tract infection in the United States: A national study. *CID, 46,* 243–250.

Saint, S., & Chenoweth, C. E. (2003). Biofilms and catheter-associated urinary tract infections. *Infectious Disease Clinics of North America, 17*(2), 411–432.

Saint, S., Lipsky, B. A., & Goold, S. D. (2002). Indwelling urinary catheters: A one-point restraint? *Annals of Internal Medicine, 137*(2), 125–127.

Saint, S., Wiese, J., Amory, J. K., Bernstein, M. L., Patel, U. D., Zemencuk, J. K., et al. (2000). Are physicians aware of which of their patients have indwelling urinary catheters? *American Journal of Medicine, 109*(6), 476–480.

Sampselle, C. M. (2003). Teaching women to use a voiding diary. *American Journal of Nursing, 103*(11), 62–64.

Schnelle, J. F., Cadogan, M. P., Grbic, D., Bates-Jensen, B. M., Osterweil, D., Yoshii, J., et al. (2003). A standardized quality assessment system to evaluate incontinence care in the nursing home. *Journal of the American Geriatrics Society, 51*(12), 1754–1761.

Schnelle, J. F., Cruise, P. A., Rahman, A., & Ouslander, J. G. (1998). Developing rehabilitative behavioral interventions for long-term care: Technology transfer, acceptance, and maintenance issues. *Journal of the American Geriatrics Society, 46*(6), 771–777.

Schnelle, J. F., & Leung, F. W. (2004). Urinary and fecal incontinence in nursing homes. *Gastroenterology, 126*(1 Suppl. 1), S41–47.

Sink, K. M., Thomas, J., 3rd, Xu, H., Craig, B., Kritchevsky, S., & Sands, L. P. (2008). Dual use of bladder anticholinergics and cholinesterase inhibitors: Long-term functional and cognitive outcomes. *Journal of the American Geriatrics Society, 56*(5), 847–853.

Smith, D. B. (2006). Urinary incontinence and diabetes: A review. *Journal of Wound, Ostomy, and Continence Nursing, 33*(6), 619–623.

Starer, P., Likourezos, A., & Dumapit, G. (2000). The association of fecal impaction and urinary retention in elderly nursing home patients. *Archives of Gerontology and Geriatrics, 30*(1), 47–54.

Stenzelius, K., Mattiasson, A., Hallberg, I. R., & Westergren, A. (2004). Symptoms of urinary and faecal incontinence among men and women 75+ in relations to health complaints and quality of life. *Neurourology and Urodynamics, 23*(3), 211–222.

Stern, J. A., Hsieh, Y. C., & Schaeffer, A. J. (2004). Residual urine in an elderly female population: Novel implications for oral estrogen replacement and impact on recurrent urinary tract infection. *Journal of Urology, 171*(2 Pt 1), 768–770.

Stewart, W. F., Van Rooyen, J. B., Cundiff, G. W., Abrams, P., Herzog, A. R., Corey, R., et al. (2003). Prevalence and burden of overactive bladder in the United States. *World Journal of Urology, 20*(6), 327–336.

Tal, S., Guller, V., Levi, S., Bardenstein, R., Berger, D., Gurevich, I., et al. (2005). Profile and prognosis of febrile elderly patients with bacteremic urinary tract infection. *Journal of Infection, 50*(4), 296–305.

Tambyah, P. A., Knasinski, V., & Maki, D. G. (2002). The direct costs of nosocomial catheter-associated urinary tract infection in the era of managed care. *Infection Control and Hospital Epidemiology: The Official Journal of the Society of Hospital Epidemiologists of America, 23*(1), 27–31.

Thomas, A. W., Cannon, A., Bartlett, E., Ellis-Jones, J., & Abrams, P. (2004). The natural history of lower urinary tract dysfunction in men: The influence of detrusor underactivity on the outcome after transurethral resection of the prostate with a minimum 10-year urodynamic follow-up. *BJU International, 93*(6), 745–750.

Thomas, K., Chow, K., & Kirby, R. S. (2004). Acute urinary retention: A review of the aetiology and management. *Prostate Cancer and Prostatic Diseases, 7*(1), 32–37.

Tincello, D. G., Williams, K. S., Joshi, M., Assassa, R. P., & Abrams, K. R. (2007). Urinary diaries: A comparison of data collected for three days versus seven days. *Obstetrics & Gynecology, 109*(2 Pt 1), 277–280.

Tikkinen, K. A., Tammela, T. L., Huhtala, H., & Auvinen, A. (2006). Is nocturia equally common among men and women? A population based study in Finland. *Journal of Urology, 175*(2), 596–600.

*The Universal Declaration of Human Rights: 1948–2008.* (2007, Dec.). Retrieved May 13, 2008, from www.un.org/Overview/rights.html

van der Vaart, C. H., Roovers, J. P., de Leeuw, J. R., & Heintz, A. P. (2007). Association between urogenital symptoms and depression in community-dwelling women aged 20 to 70 years. *Urology, 69*(4), 691–696.

Vogel, S. L. (2001). Urinary incontinence in the elderly. *Ochsner Journal, 3*(4), 214–218.

Wald, H., Epstein, A., & Kramer, A. (2005). Extended use of indwelling urinary catheters in postoperative hip fracture patients. *Medical Care, 43*(10), 1009–1017.

Wald, H., & Kramer, A. (2007). Nonpayment for harms resulting from medical care. Catheter-associated urinary tract infections. *Journal of the American Medical Association, 298*(23), 2782–2784.

Wald, H., Epstein, A., Radcliff, T., & Kramer, A. (2008). Extended use of urinary catheters in older surgical patients: A patient safety problem? *Infection Control and Hospital Epidemiology: The Official Journal of the Society of Hospital Epidemiologists of America, 29*(2), 116–124.

Walkom, T. (2008, Feb.). *Ontario's human rights commission says it's too busy to probe elder care.* Retrieved April 21, 2008, from http://www.thestar.com/News/Canada/article/305913

Walter, L. C., Lui, L. Y., Eng, C., & Covinsky, K. E. (2003). Risk of hip fracture in disabled community-living older adults. *Journal of the American Geriatrics Society, 51*(1), 50–55.

Watson, N. M., Brink, C. A., Zimmer, J. G., & Mayer, R. D. (2003). Use of the Agency for Health Care Policy and Research Urinary Incontinence Guideline in nursing homes. *Journal of the American Geriatrics Society, 51*(12), 1779–1786.

Wein, A., & Rovner, E. S. (2002). Definition and epidemiology of overactive bladder. *Urology, 60* (Suppl. 5A), 7–11.

Wein, A. J. (1986). Physiology of micturition. *Clinics in Geriatric Medicine, 2*(4), 689–699.

Wein, A. J., & Rackley, R. R. (2006). Overactive bladder: A better understanding of pathophysiology, diagnosis and management. *Journal of Urology, 175*(3 Pt 2), S5–10.

Wilson, M. M. (2006). Urinary incontinence: Selected current concepts. *Medical Clinics of North America, 90*(5), 825–836.

Wroblewski, B. M., & del Sel, H. J. (1980). Urethral instrumentation and deep sepsis in total hip replacement. *Clinical Orthopaedics and Related Research 146*, 209–212.

Wynd, C. A., Wallace, M., & Smith, K. M. (1996). Factors influencing postoperative urinary retention following orthopaedic surgical procedures. *Orthopaedic Nursing, 15*(1), 43–50.

Yarnold, B. D. (1999). Hip fracture. Caring for a fragile population. *American Journal of Nursing, 99*(2), 36–40; quiz 41.

# Heart Failure in the Critically Ill Older Patient

# 23

Debra K. Moser
Michael W. Rich

Heart failure (HF) is a clinical syndrome that usually develops after sufficient myocardial cell damage has occurred to impair ventricular contractility or relaxation. To maintain tissue and organ viability, the neurohumoral axis is activated. Neurohumoral activation is adaptive initially; however, with time, sustained neurohumoral activation produces symptomatic and progressive HF. There is no cure for HF, although with recent advances in treatment, prognosis can be improved, hospitalizations prevented, and quality of life enhanced. These improvements, however, are modest in most patients (Cleland et al., 2006; Koelling, Chen, Lubwama, L'Italien, & Eagle, 2004; Shahar & Lee, 2000).

In the 1980s through the 1990s, HF emerged as a significant public health threat that reached epidemic proportions (Garg, Packer, Pitt, & Yusuf, 1993; Ho, Anderson, Kannel, Grossman, & Levy, 1993; McMurray, Petrie, Murdoch, & Davie, 1998; O'Connell, 2000). Since that time, the prevalence of HF has increased (Ni, Nauman, & Hershberger, 1999), and it now afflicts more than 5 million people in the United States (Rosamond et al., 2008) and 30 million of the 1 billion people in the 47 countries represented by the European Society of Cardiology (McMurray & Stewart, 2002). The negative impact of HF is expected to worsen dramatically in coming years (Gambassi et al., 2000; Zannad et al., 1999), amid concerns that HF remains an unchecked epidemic (Butler & Kalogeropoulos, 2008; Fang, Mensah, Croft, & Keenan, 2008).

The worsening HF epidemic is thought to be the product of two major phenomena—the aging of the population and improved survival from the potentially deadly manifestations of cardiac disease (e.g., acute myocardial infarction, dysrhythmias, sudden cardiac death). Heart failure incidence increases dramatically with age (Ahmed, 2007; Thomas & Rich, 2007). This coupled with the rapidly rising number of elderly people in the United States and worldwide, along with increasing longevity will increase both incidence and prevalence of HF. Better treatment, and improved survival from acute cardiac events means that there are more individuals alive with damaged hearts who could later go on to develop HF, which is the final common pathologic endpoint for a number of cardiac conditions and cardiovascular risk factors (e.g., acute myocardial infarction, hypertension, diabetes). Against this backdrop, the purpose of this chapter is to provide an overview of the unique care needs of critically ill older adults hospitalized with HF. Many, if not most, hospitalizations for exacerbations of HF occur because of issues (e.g., failed self-care or inadequate use of evidence-based therapies) related to management of the chronic heart failure patient in the outpatient setting. Critical care nurses are an important link in the chain of education and advocacy that results in better educated patients, and the provision of appropriate care by health care providers. Thus, a portion of this chapter concentrates on chronic outpatient management so as to provide the critical care nurse with the information needed to better educate patients and their families and to advocate for evidence-based therapy.

# Changes With Aging That Predispose Older Adults to Heart Failure

A number of factors associated with aging contribute to the higher incidence and prevalence of HF seen in elderly individuals. These include physiologic changes with aging, the higher incidence of hypertension and coronary artery disease with aging, and the higher rate of multiple comorbidities in elderly individuals (Table 23.1).

## Cardiovascular Aging

Physiology and pathophysiology of aging are covered in depth in chapter 12 of this book. Changes in cardiovascular physiology with aging (Lakatta, 2002, 2003; Lakatta & Levy, 2003a, 2003b) that contribute specifically to development of HF are outlined in Table 23.1.

Briefly, aging is associated with an increase in collagen deposition and cross-linking in arterial walls, a change that predisposes one to increasing arterial stiffness. Aging also is associated with deterioration of elastin fibers in the arterial walls, a change that coupled with increasing collagen deposition, leads to increasing systolic blood pressure. These arterial changes also increase left ventricular afterload, putting increasing stress on the left ventricle. Elevated afterload along with myocardial collagen deposition produces myocardial stiffness. Myocardial stiffness is compounded by myocyte hypertrophy, which occurs to compensate for increasing afterload, myocardial stiffness, and an increase in myocyte apoptosis that occurs with aging. These

## 23.1   Physiologic and Pathophysiologic Changes With Aging That Increase Susceptibility to Heart Failure

| Physiologic or Pathophysiologic Change | Predisposition to Heart Failure |
| --- | --- |
| ■ Normal aging<br><br>  ● Collagen deposition and degeneration of elastin in arterial walls leads to increased arterial stiffness<br>  ● Increased myocardial interstitial collagen deposition leads to myocardial stiffness<br>  ● Increased myocardial hypertrophy in response to increased afterload and increased myocardial apoptosis<br>  ● Reduced responsiveness to beta-adrenergic stimulation<br>  ● Impaired adenosine triphosphate production by mitochondria in response to increased demands<br>  ● Decreased nitric oxide production | ■ Development of systolic hypertension, a major risk factor for heart failure<br>■ Increased left ventricular afterload that can increase cardiac work and reduce cardiac output<br>■ Alterations in left ventricular diastolic filling characterized by decreased early filling and augmented atrial contraction<br>■ Predisposition to diastolic heart failure and atrial fibrillation<br>■ Diminished ability to increase heart rate and contractility<br>■ Impaired beta$_2$-mediated peripheral arterial vasodilation leads to increased afterload<br>■ Decreased ability to increase cardiac output with increased myocardial demand<br>■ Reduced peak coronary blood flow; endothelial dysfunction with increased development of atherosclerosis and myocardial ischemia |
| ■ Increased incidence and prevalence of coronary artery disease<br>■ Increase in myocardial ischemia and infarction<br>■ Increased incidence and prevalence of age-associated cardiac disorders<br>■ Increase in valvular heart disease, dysrhythmias, hypertension<br>■ Coronary artery disease is one of the 2 major cause of heart failure, along with hypertension<br>■ Increased propensity for heart failure development, which is often multifactorial | |
| ■ Increased incidence and prevalence of comorbidities | ■ Predisposition to coronary artery disease<br>■ Pulmonary, renal, hepatic, and gastrointestinal system changes reduce compensatory ability of these organ systems and predispose to fluid overload |
| ■ Declining function of renal, pulmonary, hepatic, gastrointestinal systems | ■ Altered pharmacokinetics and pharmacodynamics predispose to toxicities and side effects |

changes alter diastolic function and provide one reason for the higher prevalence of HF with normal left ventricular ejection fraction seen in older adults.

Other changes that may contribute to the development of HF include a decrease in cardiac and vascular response to beta-adrenergic stimulation with increasing age. This change is associated with a decrease in peak contractility, maximal heart rate, and peripheral vasodilation. These alterations result in a decrease in attainable cardiac output meaning that elderly individuals have an attenuated ability to increase cardiac output when faced with increased demand.

Changes in endothelial function with aging can contribute to ischemia during periods of increased myocardial oxygen demand through two mechanisms. First, the production of nitric oxide decreases with aging, reducing maximum coronary blood flow, as nitric oxide is important for coronary vasodilation and coronary blood flow regulation. Second, endothelial dysfunction can contribute to atherosclerosis, increasing the risk for ischemia.

The changes in endothelial function, beta-adrenergic responsiveness, and arterial and myocardial stiffness produce a progressive decline in maximal cardiac performance and cardiac reserve. This decline in cardiac reserve can be substantial and makes elderly patients susceptible to the development of ADHF (acute decompensated heart failure). Moreover, ADHF develops more easily in the elderly compared to younger individuals in response to physical stressors (e.g., ischemia, volume overload, or surgery).

## Comorbidities and Declining Function of Organ Systems

Given the adverse cardiovascular changes with aging noted previously, it is not surprising that the prevalence of cardiovascular disease increases with age. Ischemic heart disease and hypertension are the two most common causes of HF, and they often coexist in elderly individuals predisposing them to HF and ADHF.

The incidence of diabetes increases with age up to age 80, as does that of chronic obstructive pulmonary disease. Diabetes adversely affects endocrine and renal function, and promotes ischemic heart disease, which contributes to the development of HF and to ADHF. The presence of chronic obstructive pulmonary disease renders pulmonary compensation difficult when fluid overload occurs with ADHF.

In addition to adversely affecting the cardiovascular system, aging affects other systems. Renal function declines with age such that elderly individuals are more prone to fluid overload because the renal system is unable to handle excess fluid and sodium intake. Because of age-related declines in gastrointestinal, hepatic, and renal function, the pharmacokinetics and pharmacodynamics of most drugs are altered in elderly individuals and older adults are more susceptible to side effects and toxicities. Many factors that affect loading condition adversely (e.g., anemia, atrial fibrillation, and hypothyroidism) are more common among elders and predispose them to the expression of symptomatic HF.

In summary, multiple factors conspire to increase the incidence of HF, contribute to the development of ADHF, and render the management of elderly HF patients difficult. Understanding these factors provides perspective to clinicians caring for elderly patients as they work to reduce the increased morbidity and mortality seen in elderly HF patients.

## Case Study

Ms. G.T. is an 83-year-old Caucasian woman with a long history of hypertension, diabetes, and a remote myocardial infarction. She developed HF 5 years ago and has been hospitalized twice during that time with ADHF, thought to be precipitated by taking her medications only intermittently and eating high-salt foods during family celebrations. She is a widow who lives alone, but whose daughter lives nearby. Her daughter checks on her mom daily by phone and visits at least once a week to take her mom shopping and run errands. Ms. G.T. prepares her own meals daily, but eats dinner with her daughter and her family once a week. A neighbor called Ms. G.T.'s daughter to say that she thought Ms. G.T. was having more trouble "getting around and looks kind of pale" during the past month. Ms. G.T.'s daughter called her mom, but her mom says she is just tired, needs some rest, is irritated by the "interference," and says she is doing "just fine." Ms. G.T.'s daughter accepts her mother's assessment as she is really busy with her own family.

## Hospitalization for Heart Failure in Older Adults

Individuals 65 and older account for about 12% of the U.S. population, yet they are responsible for approximately 35% of hospital stays annually (Nagamine, Jiang, & Merrill, 2006). An acute exacerbation of chronic HF is the most common reason Medicare-aged individuals are hospitalized, and has been for at least the past 2 decades (Fang et al., 2008; Nagamine et al.; O'Connell, 2000; Schocken et al., 2008). Thus, most of the estimated $34 billion direct and indirect annual costs for HF (Rosamond et al., 2007) are a result of hospitalizations for acute decompensated HF (ADHF) in elders (Lee, Chavez, Baker, & Luce, 2004; Liao et al., 2006, 2007; Linne, Liedholm, Jendteg, & Israelsson, 2000). Hospitalizations among elderly individuals are thought to be responsible for more than 70% of these annual HF health care costs (Lee et al.). Largely as a result of these hospitalizations, health care costs are higher for elders with HF than for elders without HF (Liao et al.). Moreover, elders hospitalized for ADHF have a substantially higher mortality rate, and higher rehospitalization rates than younger patients hospitalized with ADHF. Since 1980, hospital admissions for HF have doubled (Miller & Missov, 2001). After being discharged from a hospitalization for decompensated HF, 27% of patients are readmitted within 90 days for recurrent HF, whereas 29% of these are readmitted more than once, and 6-month readmission rates across the United States average about 44 to 47% (Kimmelsteil & Konstam, 1995; Krumholz et al., 1997; Miller & Missov; Rosamond et al.). The increasing rates of hospitalization for HF among elders is of particular concern given the need of many elders for additional nursing care after discharge (Croft et al., 1997) and the high risk for rehospitalization and mortality among elderly individuals (Dar & Cowie, 2008).

Data from national registries in the United States (i.e., ADHERE [Acute Decompensated Heart Failure National Registry]) (Adams et al., 2005) and Europe (e.g., Euro-Heart Failure Surveys) (Nieminen et al., 2006) demonstrate that the typical patient admitted for ADHF is older than 70 years of age, equally likely to be a man or woman, and has a history of HF, coronary artery disease, and hypertension (Dar & Cowie, 2008). On average in the United States, patients admitted with ADHF spend a total of about 5 days in the hospital and if admitted to an intensive care unit, they spend about 3 days there (Dar & Cowie). Longer length of stay in elderly HF patients is predicted by female gender and worse functional status (Formiga et al., 2008). Mortality in the hospital is about 4%, whereas it is 10% in the 30 days following discharge, and about 36% in the year following discharge (Dar & Cowie). Higher mortality rates are found in the elderly compared to younger patients. Other indicators of worse prognosis are renal insufficiency, lower hemoglobin level, and use of inotropes during the hospitalization (Dar & Cowie).

## Acute Heart Failure Syndromes

Acute HF is commonly defined as the development of signs and symptoms of cardiac dysfunction that occur as a new presentation of HF or as an acute exacerbation of existing HF (Niemenen et al., 2005). It is useful for clinicians to remember that acute HF is not a homogeneous condition and for that reason, we usually refer to acute HF syndromes to describe the possible presentations and etiologies for ADHF. Hypertensive crisis, pulmonary edema, new acute HF, large myocardial infarction leading to cardiogenic shock, worsening chronic HF, and advanced/end-stage HF are all capable of presenting as acute HF. Of these, worsening chronic HF is the most common cause of hospitalizations in elderly individuals. Acute decompensated HF can be precipitated by a number of factors, including acute coronary syndrome, dysrhythmias, fluid overload, uncontrolled hypertension, nonadherence to prescribed medications or diet or other self-care activities, anemia, infection, pulmonary disease, ingestion of cardiac toxins, or thyroid abnormalities. Of these, the most common causes are acute coronary syndrome, nonadherence to the recommended medication and diet regimen, dysrhythmias—particularly atrial fibrillation, poorly controlled hypertension, and infection (Dar & Cowie, 2008).

## Management of Acute Decompensated Heart Failure

### Case Study

Ms. G.T.'s daughter receives a call at work from Ms. G.T.'s neighbor who says the ambulance just took Ms. G.T. to the hospital. The neighbor called the ambulance after she went to check on Ms. G.T. because she hadn't seen her getting her mail for a few days and found her so short of breath that she couldn't speak or walk to the phone. Ms. G.T. was taken to the nearest emergency department (ED) and had to be resuscitated because she suffered a respiratory arrest when she arrived. She was intubated and placed on assist control mechanical ventilation with positive end-expiratory pressure (PEEP) as she was hypoxic and acidotic. Her chest X-ray revealed cardiomegaly and diffuse pulmonary congestion consistent with pulmonary edema. Her blood pressure was 220/124 and heart rate 122. She was given 120 mg intravenous furosemide, and was placed on a nitroglycerine drip titrated to decrease her blood pressure. The examining physician noted an $S_3$, and marked pitting edema in the feet and ankles. Cardiac enzymes were drawn to rule out infarction and the first set was within normal limits. The electrolyte panel was notable for hyponatremia and mild hyperkalemia. Ms. G.T.'s blood glucose was 465 mg/dl and her HgbA1$_C$ (hemoglobin A1$_c$) was 9.5%. Her b-type natriuretic peptide (BNP) level was 1223 pg/ml. The complete blood count was notable for anemia, liver function was normal, the blood urea nitrogen (BUN) and creatinine levels were elevated, and there was no sign of infection from the urinalysis. The electrocardiogram revealed sinus tachycardia, ventricular hypertrophy, and no evidence of old or acute myocardial infarction.

## Diagnosis of Acute Decompensated Heart Failure

### Symptoms and Signs

Most patients with ADHF are admitted to the hospital from the emergency department, the most common place for elders to present with symptoms (Fonarow & Corday, 2004). Because HF is not a specific disease, but a clinical syndrome, there are no specific diagnostic criteria by which one can make a definitive diagnosis. A history of HF in a patient presenting with symptoms and signs of ADHF is strongly predictive of the diagnosis (Heart Failure Society of America [HFSA], 2006a), but ultimately, the diagnosis of ADHF is based largely on presenting signs and symptoms (Table 23.2) (Allen & O'Connor, 2007).

Dyspnea is the most common symptom of ADHF in both younger and older HF patients. The prevalence of dyspnea on exertion in ambulatory elders is as high as 95% in some studies and dyspnea at rest is present in up to 65% (Ahmed, 2007). Among hospitalized elders with ADHF, 90% have dyspnea at rest (Ahmed). The occurrence of this symptom also makes the diagnosis difficult as dyspnea is a common symptom of a number of respiratory conditions and, in the elderly, acute shortness of breath may also be a manifestation of myocardial ischemia and infarction, pneumonia, pulmonary embolism, or chronic lung disease. Increasing fatigue is another common symptom, but because of its vague nature and the accommodations that elders make when faced with such symptoms, its significance is often missed. The diagnosis of ADHF in elderly patients also is made more difficult because elderly patients present atypically more commonly than do younger patients. Atypical symptoms include confusion or worsening mental status, irritability, somnolence, and anorexia.

The hallmark signs of ADHF are jugular venous distension (the most specific sign of fluid overload in elders) (Ahmed, 2007), $S_3$ gallop, and peripheral edema. In elderly HF patients, these signs can be present in ADHF, but they are also commonly present in other comorbid conditions seen in elders, making a definitive diagnosis of ADHF more difficult in the older adult. Increasing weight is a common sign, but one that is commonly ignored or not measured by patients and thus missed. Ascites and

| 23.2 | Symptoms and Signs That Suggest a Diagnosis of Acute Decompensated Heart Failure in Older Patients |
|---|---|

**Symptoms**

- Escalating dyspnea on exertion, orthopnea, and/or paroxysmal nocturnal dyspnea
- Increasing fatigue, weakness, lethargy, anorexia, altered sensorium
- Increasing edema, weight, or abdominal girth

**Signs**

- Elevated jugular venous pressure
- Edema
- S3 or S4 heart sounds
- Ascites
- Tachycardia
- Diffuse or laterally displaced point of maximal intensity
- Rales
- Tachypnea

hepatomegaly may also be present with long-standing, severe fluid overload. Because HF with preserved ejection fraction is more common among elders (Ahmed), they may present with ADHF without elevated jugular venous pressure or an $S_3$ gallop.

When uncertainty exists about the source of symptoms, measurement of plasma B-type natriuretic peptide (BNP) or N-terminal pro-BNP (NT-pro-BNP) can assist in the determination of the cause of dyspnea (HFSA, 2006a). Although BNP levels rise with increasing age, thus reducing their specificity in elders (Omland, 2008), a normal value in an elderly patient who presents with dyspnea strongly suggests that ADHF is not the cause of the symptom. Although BNP levels are prognostic of outcomes in patients with ADHF, their diagnostic accuracy in the intensive care unit is reduced because many elderly patients in such units have comorbid conditions other than HF that can be associated with elevated BNP levels (i.e., hypoxia, renal failure, shock, and pulmonary hypertension) (Omland). Other diagnostic tools, such as chest radiography and echocardiography, that are useful in HF, have limitations that also must be considered when using them in elderly patients (Table 23.3).

### Diagnostic Tests

Several routine diagnostic tests can assist in the evaluation and management of patients with ADHF (HSFA, 2006a). A chest radiograph is indicated to identify pulmonary congestion, the presence of cardiomegaly, and to rule out other causes of symptoms, such as pneumonia. An electrocardiogram and measurement of at least two sets of cardiac troponin are used to identify ongoing ischemia or new infarction as a cause of ADHF. A complete blood count is used to assess for anemia or infection, whereas

## 23.3 Problems Reducing the Diagnostic Utility of Chest Radiography and Echocardiography in Elderly Acutely Ill Patients

| Test | Problem |
|---|---|
| Chest radiography | Reduced ability to obtain good-quality chest radiograph |
| | ■ patient confusion |
| | ■ poor inspiratory effort |
| | ■ kyphosis of the thoracic spine |
| | Reduced ability to adequately interpret the film |
| | ■ presence of chronic lung disease |
| | ■ scarring |
| | ■ atelectasis |
| Echocardiography | Normal heart size with diastolic heart failure |
| | Presence of heart failure with preserved ejection fraction |
| | Diastolic dysfunction with reversal of amplitude of early and late diastolic filling waves is also a characteristic of normal aging |

serum electrolytes and routine blood chemistry are indicated to determine whether electrolyte imbalances or hyperglycemia are present. Liver and renal function tests will illuminate presence of comorbid liver or renal problems. Thyroid hormone and thyroid-stimulating hormone tests identify hyper- or hypothyroidism as factors contributing to ADHF. A urinalysis is helpful to screen for proteinuria or if there is reason to suspect a urinary tract infection. As discussed previously, BNP or NT-pro-BNP levels are helpful in making the diagnosis of ADHF when the cause of dyspnea is uncertain.

## Case Study

Ms. G.T. experienced a rapid, large diuresis in the ED with improvement of her pulmonary congestion and acidosis, although she remained hypoxic, hypertensive, and tachycardic during early weaning attempts so the decision was made to transfer her to the intensive care unit for closer monitoring and titration of therapy with a diagnosis of ADHF. Events precipitating her decompensation were difficult to determine as Ms. G.T. could not communicate by writing and she had not seen her primary care provider for several months. It was unclear what medications Ms. G.T. was prescribed or routinely took, and what her usual diet, weight, or self-management activities were.

It was hoped that further information could be obtained when the daughter arrived and Ms. G.T. was extubated.

## Treatment Goals

Definition of therapeutic goals is essential in ADHF as the potential for harm or inadequate therapy is high if such goals are not considered during the treatment process. The two paramount goals in the treatment of ADHF are to (a) institute and (b) maintain evidence-based therapies that improve prognosis and enhance quality of life. A major step in achieving these goals in elderly HF patients and one that is often overlooked in the critically ill, is to return patients to their previous state (or to a higher state) of functioning. If this step is not achieved, elderly patients can experience a series of steady declines from each exacerbation that make subsequent exacerbations more likely, increase patients' long-term dependence on others for care, and markedly reduce patients' quality of life. The importance of increasing or maintaining quality of life among symptomatic elderly HF patients cannot be underestimated (Stanek, Oates, McGhan, Denofrio, & Loh, 2000).

Other important steps to achieving the major treatment goals in ADHF include improvement of symptoms and optimization of volume status. Factors precipitating decompensation should be identified and addressed. Chronic outpatient oral drug therapy should be reviewed and optimized. Although polypharmacy may be a necessity in elderly HF patients, careful review of elderly patients' drug regimen by a clinician with expertise in geriatric pharmacology often can reduce the number of extraneous medications, associated adverse reactions, and patient difficulties with adherence (Rich et al., 1995; Rich, Gray, Beckham, Wittenburg, & Luther, 1996). A final vital step in achieving the treatment goals is beginning the vital process of patient and family/caregiver education and counseling and ensuring that it is continued once the patient is transferred out of the intensive care unit and out of the hospital.

In an attempt to operationalize the goals of treatment of ADHF, the European Society of Cardiology published the first set of guidelines devoted exclusively to the treatment of acute HF (Nieminen et al., 2005), although some other organizations have now addressed ADHF within their chronic HF guidelines (HFSA, 2006a). The European Society of Cardiology treatment goals were divided into several categories: *clinical* (reduce symptoms, signs, and body weight while determining underlying causes of ADHF); *laboratory* (normalize electrolytes, blood glucose, BNP, and decrease blood urea nitrogen or creatinine and total bilirubin); *hemodynamic* (decrease pulmonary artery occlusion pressure to <18 mmHg while increasing cardiac output); *outcome* (decrease intensive care unit and hospital length of stay, transition to an outpatient regimen that maintains clinical stability, and increase survival and time to readmission); and *tolerability* (low rate of withdrawal from therapeutic measures and low incidence of adverse effects).

The goals of therapy often are not met in elderly HF patients because of demands for quick turnaround of beds in hospitals, changes in the physician reimbursement system, lack of continuity of care, and time constraints (Fonarow, 2003; Riegel & Moser, 2008). For all of these reasons, it is not uncommon for clinicians to fail to make the coordinated effort necessary to identify and manage the underlying cause of the exacerbation or to undertake all of the necessary steps to optimize patient outcomes.

This failure can lead to inadequate management and discharge of elderly patients while they are still highly vulnerable to readmission (Moser, Doering, & Chung, 2005).

Because the management of ADHF is driven by an episodic, acute care view, attention to all of the details of care necessary to achieve optimal outcomes in elderly HF patients may seem out of the realm of responsibility for nurses caring for critically ill patients. Yet, as the first clinicians to see and manage these patients, nurses have the responsibility to advocate for comprehensive care. Use of a transitional care model that (see chapter 6) acknowledges the chronicity of HF, the need for continuity of care, and employs a case management approach by advanced practice nurses caring for elderly HF patients has been found to be quite effective in avoiding these failures (Naylor et al., 1999). Other successful models of care through which the goals of therapy are met for elderly HF patients include multidisciplinary HF disease management models (Blue et al., 2001; Stewart & Horowitz, 2002; Stromberg et al., 2003). In a meta-analysis of 29 trials of a variety of multidisciplinary management strategies, specially trained HF nurses were identified as one of three crucial elements that should be included to improve patient outcomes (McAllister, Stewart, Ferrua, & McMurray, 2004).

## Case Study

In the intensive care unit, care was taken to attend to each of Ms. G.T.'s comorbidities, and to uncover the cause of her acute exacerbation of HF. She was determined to be markedly fluid overloaded, but to have relatively good perfusion ("wet-warm" profile). Her hyperglycemia was treated with intravenous insulin based on blood sugars. Her hypertension was controlled with careful titration of nitroglycerine, which also helped relieve her pulmonary congestion. She continued to experience diuresis with additional doses of intravenous furosemide, but care was taken to avoid overdiuresis, although it was difficult to determine her true dry weight. Nonetheless, it was clear that she suffered from substantial fluid overload. As her hypertension and pulmonary congestion decreased, her tachycardia also decreased, and she was weaned and extubated. Serial cardiac enzymes revealed no ischemic insult, and serial B-type natriuretic peptide (BNP) levels demonstrated a steady decline in BNP level. Daily weights demonstrated steadily decreasing weight. An echocardiogram was performed as it appeared one had not been done in the past several years. This test confirmed that she had HF from systolic dysfunction. Work-up to determine the source of her anemia was begun, but the initial working diagnosis was anemia related to chronic HF. Her renal insufficiency was thought to be secondary to ADHF and inadequate outpatient drug therapy for her HF.

When Ms. G.T.'s daughter arrived and Ms. G.T. was able to speak, Ms. G.T.'s nurse and physician attempted to determine the factors precipitating her acute exacerbation. Ms. G.T. admitted that she did not follow a low-salt diet as "it tastes horrible" and her primary care provider told her it was unnecessary; she stated that he told her "your water pill will take care of any extra salt you eat." Ms. G.T.'s daughter brought in her medication bottles and also got the medications she was prescribed from the doctor's office. She had been prescribed the following medications by her primary care physician: furosemide 20 mg every day, digoxin 0.125 mg once a day, enalapril 2.5 mg twice a day, diltiazem (dose unreadable), and metformin 850 mg once a day. Ms. G.T, stated that she preferred to save her money rather than spend it on all her medications. She commonly took all her medications only every other day to make them last longer and believed that they were just as effective. She had stopped taking her oral diabetic agent because she said it gave her diarrhea. The HF nurse case manager was called in to assist in the coordination of Ms. G.T.'s care as she made the transitions from critical care to step-down unit and eventually home. She began working with the critical care physician and nurse as they planned to optimize Ms. G.T.'s oral medication regimen and discontinue inappropriate medications in anticipation of discharge. She also is working with the critical care team to begin patient and family teaching to help avoid future exacerbations.

## Monitoring Patients' Progress During Hospitalization

Fluid overload (from a variety of sources) is a common cause of ADHF, and monitoring fluid status in hospitalized patients is essential to properly determine progress in meeting therapeutic goals. The Heart Failure Society of America guidelines recommend monitoring daily weights, fluid balance, renal function, and electrolyte status to assess the effectiveness and potential negative consequences of diuresis (HFSA, 2006a). Possibly because monitoring of fluid status has become so routine, the importance of these data tend to be overlooked by clinicians, and some clinicians express skepticism about the value of weights in monitoring fluid status. In a recent study, Chaudhry and associates demonstrated the strong predictive value for hospitalization of weight gain in the week prior to a hospitalization for ADHF (Chaudhry, Wang, Concato, Gill, & Krumholz, 2007). Moreover, data from thousands of patients enrolled in an acute heart failure registry, ADHERE (Acute Decompensated Heart Failure National Registry), demonstrate that fewer than 50% of patients experience a substantial weight loss ( = 5 pounds) during their hospitalization (Fonarow & Corday, 2004). Thus, attention to daily monitoring of fluid status is warranted and deserves attention from clinicians.

A daily cardiovascular examination is indicated and it is important to assess for improvement in the signs and symptoms that brought the patient to the hospital. Although the clinical signs show improvement at a faster rate than do patients' subjective symptoms, patients are still quite capable of detecting changes in their symptom status on a daily basis and such subjective assessments need to be monitored (Allen et al., 2008). Heart failure symptoms are often not extensively evaluated in the hospital because patients remain relatively inactive. As a consequence, clinicians only assess symptoms at rest. Encouraging patients to walk in the hall and assessing their symptoms during or after this activity provides an opportunity for appropriate evaluation of symptoms. Assessing symptoms while patients are walking may lead to more aggressive management of fluid status during acute care and thereby reduce some of the undertreatment of fluid overload and early readmissions seen, particularly among elders.

Recent evidence suggests that using serial measurements of BNP or N-terminal prohormone B-type natriuretic peptide (NT-pro-BNP) to guide therapy, particularly in the hospitalized patient, may result in earlier discharge and better assessment of a patient's readiness for discharge (Disomma et al., 2008; Gallegos, Maclaughlin, & Haase, 2008; Masson et al., 2008; Miller Hartman, Grill, Burnett, & Jaffe, 2009; Valle et al., 2008). Although a definitive recommendation awaits the results of ongoing large randomized trials of use of serial BNP or NT-pro-BNP to tailor therapy, evidence to date suggests that prognosis is worse in patients whose BNP or NT-pro-BNP fails to decrease with therapy during hospitalization and that outcomes may be improved in patients whose therapy is guided using serial measurements of either of these neurohormones.

## Treatment

Management of ADHF is commonly guided by the results of an assessment of patients' hemodynamic presentation, that is, are they fluid overloaded or not (i.e., "wet" or "dry") and are they suffering from poor perfusion or not (i.e., "cold" or "warm") (Fonarow & Weber, 2004). For patients who are "wet and warm," the recommended therapy includes intravenous (IV) diuretics and IV nesiritide, nitroglycerine, or nitroprusside to reduce fluid overload and filling pressures to relieve symptoms. For patients who are "wet and cold," IV diuretics are supplemented with IV nesiritide, nitroglycerine, or nitroprusside if the patient's systemic vascular resistance (SVR) is thought to be high or with an inotrope or pressor if the SVR is low. Nitroglycerine is the agent of choice in elderly patients with ADHF who need intravenous vasodilators because of the higher likelihood of renal problems with the use of nesiritide or nitroprusside. If the patient presents as "dry and cold" IV inotropes or pressors are indicated as these patients have low blood pressure and cardiac output. As a consequence, they require astute management of fluid status. Patients who are "dry and warm" usually do not require IV therapy or hospitalization and the cause of their symptoms needs to be further investigated.

Elderly patients are managed with these principles, although clinicians need to provide greater attention to precisely determining fluid status in older compared to younger patients to avoid overdiuresis. In addition, vasodilators and inotropes are used in elderly individuals, but greater caution is needed as elders do not tolerate swings in blood pressure as well as younger patients and may require lower doses than younger patients because of their altered renal and liver function.

Particularly important in the management of ADHF in the elderly is optimization of blood pressure; heart rate; blood glucose; cardiac rhythm; and attention to ischemia, anemia, and other conditions that can precipitate acute exacerbations of chronic HF. It is substantially more difficult for elderly individuals to compensate for physiologic insults or to regain homeostasis than it is for younger individuals. As a consequence, it is essential to address physiologic abnormalities early to avoid acute exacerbations from developing, and it is important to correct these abnormalities when an exacerbation does occur.

## Diuretics

Because diuretics increase urinary excretion of fluid, they are useful in the mobilization of excess fluid that contributes to most HF exacerbations. Intravenous diuretics usually provide symptomatic relief when congestion is part of the clinical presentation of

ADHF. Diuretics are appropriate for elders as they are for younger patients, but elders need closer monitoring for the adverse effects associated with diuretic use and care needs to be taken to avoid overdiuresis. Adverse events for which elders need to be monitored include dehydration with associated hypotension and reduced renal function (Domanski et al., 2003). Electrolyte abnormalities, particularly hypokalemia, are also common. In secondary analyses, the use of non-potassium–sparing diuretics has been associated with increased risk of mortality in HF patients, causing some to call for a randomized controlled trial comparing the use of non-potassium–sparing diuretics with that of potassium sparing diuretics (Domanski et al., 2003; Domanski, Tian, Haigney, & Pitt, 2006).

As do younger patients, elderly patients can suffer from so-called diuretic resistance, which is a decreased response or lack of response to administration of diuretic doses that were formerly effective. Many cases of diuretic resistance are thought to be related to lack of adherence to the low-sodium-diet recommendation and continued high-sodium intake. In these cases, working closely with patients to reduce sodium intake may be beneficial. The addition of sequential nephron blocking agents for diuresis can be helpful in some cases. In other cases, the use of IV diuretics is helpful in overcoming diuretic resistance, particularly if gut edema can be reduced. Continuous infusions may also be helpful. An underrecognized cause of diuretic resistance is thiamine deficiency, which can occur in patients who are placed on dose loop diuretics for a prolonged period.

A potential alternative to diuresis in select patients with ADHF is the use of ultrafiltration (Costanzo et al., 2007; Rogers et al., 2008). This option is useful in patients with severe diuretic resistance, renal insufficiency, or need for removal of large amounts of extracellular fluid. This therapeutic option can now be delivered at the bedside without a central line. Findings from the Ultrafiltration versus Intravenous Diuretics for Patients Hospitalized for Acute Decompensated Heart Failure (UNLOAD) trial demonstrated a mean fluid loss at 48 hours with ultrafiltration that was significantly greater than that seen with IV diuresis (Costanzo et al.). On 3-month follow-up, patients who received ultrafiltration had a lower rehospitalization rate and fewer unscheduled clinic visits for ADHF. Ultrafiltration appeared safe and although there were no subgroup comparisons by age, the mean age of participants was 63 years and patients with preserved systolic function were included.

## Vasodilators

The intravenous vasodilators—nitroprusside, nitroglycerine, and nesiritide (a recombinant peptide identical to human BNP)—are commonly used in ADHF to reduce elevated filling pressures and SVR, improve symptoms, and increase cardiac output and organ perfusion. Unlike inotropes, the use of intravenous vasodilators does not produce ischemia or dysrhythmias. Because cardiac output is afterload dependent in HF, vasodilation and reductions in SVR even in normotensive patients can improve cardiac output and maintain blood pressure.

Of these three drugs, nitroglycerine and nesiritide are more commonly used because of the greater potential for toxicity and adverse effects in nitroprusside. Among elderly patients with declining renal function, nitroglycerine may be the best option given the suggestion for declining renal function and increased mortality with nesiritide (Sackner-Bernstein, Kowalski, Fox, & Aaronson, 2005). There are no studies comparing the efficacy of these three drugs, but the Vasodilation in the Management of

Acute CHF (VMAC) study compared intravenous nitroglycerin, nesiritide and placebo (Publication Committee for the VMAC Investigators, 2002). In this trial, 489 hospitalized patients with dyspnea at rest from ADHF were randomized to IV nesiritide, IV nitroglycerin, or placebo, in addition to standard medications. The mean age of patients was 60 to 62 years, patients with preserved systolic function were included, but there were no comparisons among age subgroups. After 3 hours, the placebo group was further randomized to active treatment with nesiritide or nitroglycerin. Hemodynamics improved to a greater extent in the nesiritide group than the other two groups. Nesiritide improved dyspnea at 3 hours compared with placebo but not compared with nitroglycerin. There were greater reductions in filling pressures with nesiritide over time in the hospital, although there was no difference in symptoms. Therefore, it appears that given the possibility for negative impact on renal function in elders and the similarities with nitroglycerine, IV nitroglycerine is the vasodilator of choice in elderly patients.

## Inotropic Agents

Historically, inotropic agents (e.g., dobutamine, dopamine, and milrinone) were used commonly in ADHF, particularly when blood pressure was low. More recently, their use has diminished with data demonstrating their negative effects. Long-term use of inotropes is associated with increased mortality. Even short-term use that improves hemodynamics and blood pressure does not improve number of days hospitalized or in-hospital mortality compared to placebo and is associated with increased risk of atrial fibrillation and hypotension requiring intervention (Cuffe et al., 2002). Moreover, inotropes may be less effective in elderly patients and thus the use of inotropes in ADHF is limited to short-term use in elderly patients who present with cardiogenic shock. Inotropes also are appropriate in the short term in patients with low blood pressure, despite adequate filling pressures, who show no improvement with vasodilators.

## Arginine Vasopressin Receptor Antagonists

Given that fluid overload is the most common cause of acute exacerbations of HF, investigators are examining new approaches to the pharmacologic management of HF using medications that can increase fluid excretion without adversely affecting electrolytes or renal function (Farmakis, Filippatos, Kremastinos, & Gheorghiade, 2008; Oghlakian & Klapholz, 2009). Arginine vasopression (AVP, also known as antidiuretic hormone) is a neurohormone that is increased in patients with HF. AVP causes vasoconstriction and water retention in excess of sodium retention. As a consequence, hyponatremia, a predictor of poor outcomes in patients with HF (Gheorghiade et al., 2007), is common in patients with severe HF and excessive fluid retention. The effects of AVP are mediated by receptors found in the kidneys ($V_2$ receptors) and in vascular smooth muscle and myocardium ($V_{1a}$ receptors). Inhibition of either one or both of these receptors by a class of drugs now commonly known as "vaptins" (for example, conivaptin, satavaptin, lixivaptan) produces excretion of free water (aquaresis) and normalization of serum sodium level. Use of this class of drugs in ADHF is associated with reduction in weight and improved hemodynamics without negative effects on blood pressure, electrolytes, or heart rate. The impact of vaptins on morbidity and mortality outcomes await the results of large-scale clinical trials currently underway.

## Optimization of Chronic Therapy

Despite publication of multiple chronic heart failure guidelines, many patients still do not receive optimal drug therapy and this problem is more prevalent in elderly patients (Setoguchi, Levin, & Winkelmayer, 2008) in part because of the lack of studies that include very elderly patients or that make subgroup comparisons by age. Nonetheless, although practitioners should be cognizant of potential altered pharmacodynamics in elders and their effect on drug therapy, available evidence suggests that guideline-driven therapy that is beneficial in younger HF patients is equally beneficial in older ones (HFSA, 2006a). Thus, in elderly patients with systolic dysfunction, angiotensin converting enzyme (ACE) inhibition and beta-adrenergic blockage is recommended as standard therapy (HFSA). In patients truly intolerant of ACE inhibitors because of cough or angioedema, angiotensin receptor blockers are indicated. Worsening renal function, hypotension, and hyperkalemia occur with equal frequency in ACE inhibitors and angiotensin receptor blockers and are not an appropriate indication for changing from an ACE inhibitor to an angiotensin receptor blocker. Chronic renal insufficiency is common in HF and elders and is not considered a contraindication to ACE inhibitors or angiotensin receptor blockers (Ahmed, Kiefe, & Allman, 2002). Volume status must be considered carefully when starting and uptitrating these medications in elders in whom fluid balance may be more precarious. Starting these medications at low doses and increasing the dose gradually at 2- to 4-week intervals may assist clinicians in helping their elderly patients achieve the target dose (Rich, 2005). In African American elders, the addition of combination hydralazine and isosorbide dinitrate has been shown to decrease mortality (Taylor et al., 2004). This combination also is useful in patients who do not tolerate ACE inhibitors or angiotensin receptor blockers. Elderly patients with congestion should be treated with oral diuretics and usually loop diuretics are necessary. Aldosterone antagonists are considered when patients with an LV ejection fraction of < 30 to 40% remain symptomatic despite optimal therapy on ACE inhibitors and beta-blocking agents. Digoxin is sometimes added to the regimen in patients who remain symptomatic despite treatment with diuretics, an ACE inhibitor, or ARB and beta-blockers (Hunt et al., 2005). There is no survival advantage to using digoxin, but there is a modest reduction in rehospitalization and improvement in symptoms with its use. Initiation of digoxin therapy is not indicated for the treatment of ADHF (Hunt et al.). Digoxin can be used regardless of underlying rhythm, and although it is used for rate control in patients in atrial fibrillation, beta-blockers are more effective in this regard. Combination therapy with hydralazine and isosorbide dinitrate may be useful in patients who remain symptomatic on standard therapy, and such therapy effectively reduces morbidity and mortality (Hunt et al.). African American HF patients particularly may benefit from therapy with this combination of medications. Drugs in each class used in HF are outlined in Table 23.4.

In patients with HF and preserved systolic function, treatment options are less clear owing to the paucity of clinical trials. Based on limited data, consensus guidelines recommend vigilant control of blood pressure in elderly patients with HF and preserved systolic function (HFSA, 2006a). For patients with congestion, loop diuretics are indicated although great care should be taken to avoid overdiuresis. Angiotensin

## 23.4   Medications for Chronic Outpatient Drug Therapy

| Drug | Initial Dose | Maintenance or Maximum Dose |
| --- | --- | --- |
| **Angiotensin-converting enzyme Inhibitors** | | |
| Captopril | 6.25 mg tid | 50 mg tid |
| Enalapril | 2.5 mg bid | 10–20 mg bid |
| Lisinopril | 2.5-5 mg daily | 20–40 mg daily |
| Quinapril | 5 mg bid | 20 mg bid |
| Ramipril | 1.25–2.5 mg daily | 10 mg daily |
| **Angiotensin receptor blocking agents** | | |
| Candesartan | 4–8 mg daily | 32 mg daily |
| Losartan | 25–50 mg daily | 50–100 mg daily |
| Valsartan | 20–40 mg bid | 160 mg bid |
| **Beta-adrenergic blocking agents** | | |
| Carvedilol | 3.125 mg bid | 25 mg bid, or 50 mg bid |
| Carvedilol CR | 10 mg daily | for patients >85 kg |
| Metoprolol CR/XL | 12.5–25 mg daily | 80 mg daily |
| | | 200 mg daily |
| **Diuretic therapy** | | |
| **Loop diuretics** | | |
| Bumetanide | 0.5-1.0 mg daily or bid | 10 mg daily |
| Furosemide | 20–40 mg daily or bid | 400–600 mg daily |
| Torsemide | 10–20 mg daily | 200 mg daily |
| **Thiazides** | | |
| Chlorothiazide | 250–500 mg daily or bid | 1000 mg |
| Chlorthalidone | 25–50 mg daily | 100 mg |
| Hydrochlorothiazide | 25 mg daily or bid | 200 mg |
| Indapamide | 2.5 mg daily | 5 mg |
| Metolazone | 5 mg daily | 20 mg |
| **Sequential nephron blockade** | | |
| Metolazone | 2.5–10 mg once plus loop diuretic | |
| Hydrochlorothiazide | 25–100 mg once or twice plus loop diuretic | |
| Chlorothiazide (IV) | 500–1000 mg once plus loop diuretic | |
| **Aldosterone antagonist therapy** | | |
| Eplerenone | 25 mg daily | 50 mg |
| Spironolactone | 12.5–25 mg daily | 25–50 mg |

*(continued)*

**Table 23.4** *(continued)*

| Drug | Initial Dose | Maintenance or Maximum Dose |
|------|-------------|-----------------------------|
| **Digitalis** Digoxin | 0.125–0.25 mg daily or 0.125 mg daily or every other day in those older than 70, with low body mass or impaired renal function | 0.125–0.25 mg (loading not needed) |

Abbreviations: bid = twice per day; prn = when necessary; tid = three times per day.

Adapted with permission from Riegel, B., & Moser, D. K. Care of patients with chronic heart failure. In D. K. Moser & B. Riegel (Eds.), *Cardiac Nursing: A Companion to Braunwald's Heart Disease*. Philadelphia: Elsevier; 2008:930-950. ©2008 Elsevier Inc.

receptor blockers or ACE inhibitors are recommended for patients with HF and preserved systolic function (HFSA). Beta-blockade is recommended in patients in this group if they have had a myocardial infarction, have hypertension, or have atrial fibrillation and need rate control (HFSA).

## Management of Comorbidities

Much of the high cost of HF hospitalization is related to the presence of comorbidities (Liao et al., 2007), and elderly HF patients commonly have multiple comorbidities that complicate their care. In a study of Medicare beneficiaries, 40% of those with HF had five or more noncardiac comorbid conditions (Braunstein et al., 2003). A comprehensive approach to patient management produces the best outcomes and an important aspect of the comprehensive approach is recognition and treatment of all comorbid conditions. Hospitalization offers an excellent opportunity for optimization of therapy for HF and for any comorbid conditions. All elderly patients should be assessed for the presence of comorbidities and therapy coordinated to avoid adverse effects while optimizing all comorbid conditions. Comorbidities should be actively and vigorously managed as many can contribute to progression or worsening of HF. Diabetes, hypertension, and hyperlipidemia should be controlled using the most recent evidence-based guidelines to manage therapy (HFSA, 2006a; Hunt et al., 2005). Table 23.5 includes common comorbidities and related comments about management.

## Promoting Patient Self-Care

Health care providers commonly think of HF as an acute, episodic condition that requires intense intervention followed by periods of quiet. It is these periods of "quiet" that are the most challenging to patients who in these times are charged with managing all of their care. In fact, the vast majority of care is performed by patients and the informal caregivers who support them (usually family members or friends) in the home setting (HFSA, 2006a). Considering the huge challenge this engenders for many

## 23.5   Common Comorbidities Among Elders With Heart Failure

| Comorbidity | Comments | Key Points |
|---|---|---|
| *Renal dysfunction* | Independent risk factor for morbidity and mortality | ■ Keep fluid status optimized to decrease potential for damage from diuretics and angiotensin-converting enzyme inhibitors<br>■ Data from ADHERE suggest that angiotensin-converting enzyme inhibition may preserve renal function over the long term |
| *Anemia* | Independent risk factor for morbidity and mortality | ■ Beneficial effects of iron and erythropoietin on cardiac function and exercise capacity have been reported, but additional study is needed |
| *Cognitive impairment* | In elders, cognitive impairment is twice as likely to occur in those with than without heart failure | ■ Cognitive impairment adversely affects self-care in multiple dimensions<br>■ Cognitive impairment is associated with increased short-term and long-term mortality |
| *Chronic obstructive pulmonary disease* | One of the most common comorbidities in heart failure patients | ■ Because dyspnea is a presenting symptom of both, diagnostic uncertainty is common; measurement of b-type natriuretic peptide level is helpful to distinguish cardiac and pulmonary causes of dyspnea<br>■ Beta-blockers may exacerbate pulmonary disease; beta-agonists may induce tachycardia and arrhythmias; corticosteroids may promote fluid retention |
| *Sleep-disordered breathing* | May occur in as many as 70% of heart failure patients | ■ Associated with increase in adverse events<br>■ Referral for sleep study and management of sleep disordered breathing may be appropriate |
| *Depression* | As many as 36% of hospitalized heart failure patients meet *DSM-IV* criteria for depression; 20% have major depression and 16% have depressive symptoms | ■ Depression is strongly and independently associated with morbidity and mortality<br>■ Depressed patients have more difficulties with self-care<br>■ Can screen for depression prior to discharge by asking: During the past 2 weeks have you been bothered by (1) little interest or pleasure in doing things or (2) feeling down, depressed, or hopeless<br><br>  ● Score answers to these 2 questions on a scale from 0 = not at all, 1 = several days; 2 = more than half the days; 3 = every day<br>  ● A total score of 3 or greater suggests depression and patient referral for further assessment and treatment should be made |

*(continued)*

**Table 23.5 *(continued)***

| Comorbidity | Comments | Key Points |
|---|---|---|
| *Diabetes* | | |
| *Arthritis* | Highly prevalent in older patients and the leading cause of disability | ■ NSAIDs interfere with diuretics, ACEIs and ARBs promote fluid retention, and may contribute to worsening renal function |
| *Obesity* | Increasingly common in HF patients | ■ Contributes to disability and functional limitations<br>■ Increases risk of hypertension, diabetes, sleep-disordered breathing, venous thromboembolic disease, and skin breakdown |

patients and their families (Moser et al., 2005), it is not surprising that failure of patient self-care is one of the most common causes of rehospitalization. It is tempting for clinicians to blame patients for their poor self-care, but lack of appropriate and effective patient education and counseling on the part of health care providers is a root cause of poor patient self-care.

Heart failure patient self-care requires expertise in a number of relatively complex activities (Exhibit 23.1). Riegel and associates recently examined the characteristics of experts in self-care and discovered that fewer than 10% of heart failure patients could be considered expert (Riegel, Vaughan, Dickson, Goldberg, & Deatrick, 2007). Patients who were considered experts were characterized by their ability to describe their symptoms, link them to HF pathophysiology (even in simple terms), and then had a plan for managing symptoms. Experts also demonstrated an understanding of their treatment and impact, and could verbalize a comprehensive understanding of the medication regimen. Experts were vigilant about their self-care, actively sought information about HF, had good family support and engaged family members. The number of self-care tasks patients must perform and the high level of functioning required to be expert at self-care suggest that our education and counseling strategies need to be much more comprehensive, evidence-based, and extensive than those used in usual practice. Such a discussion is beyond the scope of this chapter, but the Heart Failure Society of America heart failure guideline includes recommendations and advice about appropriate teaching strategies (www.hfsa.org). Exhibit 23.2 also lists some recommended strategies for enhancing adherence.

Patient adherence to the recommended regimen is a major self-care activity that patients often find difficult (Wu, Moser, Chung, et al., 2008; Wu, Moser, Lennie, & Burkhart, 2008; Wu, Moser, Lennie, Peden, et al., 2008). It is never sufficient to simply provide patients with the information that health care providers believe is important for adherence (HFSA, 2006a). Patients must be taught the skills they need to engage in the requested behavior and it is helpful, while teaching, to consider specific critical target behaviors. For example, when teaching patients how to follow a low-sodium diet, one might keep in mind that at the end of teaching the nurse can expect that patient to be able to pick low-sodium foods off a restaurant menu, or to sort foods

# Exhibit 23.1

## Heart Failure Self-Care Activities

■ Medication taking

 Take, don't stop, identify side effects and differentiate them from other effects

  Average of 9–13 pills per day     Complex instructions for some

■ Following a low-sodium diet

  Following a diabetic diet, low-fat diet, others

  Know levels, know how to calculate, shop, cook, follow when not at home, adapt family customs

■ Avoidance of excess fluid intake (no more than 48–64 ounces/day for most patients)

■ Monitoring symptoms of worsening heart failure

  Daily weighing and what to do; symptom recognition and what to do; which symptoms are important,

  which are not; when to act with symptom escalation

■ Physical activity

  How much, how, what if never done, rest?

■ Home monitoring of blood pressure

■ Alcohol restriction and smoking cessation

■ Manage comorbidities, emotional problems, cognitive impairment, functional impairment,

  social isolation, lack of financial resources

■ Flu vaccine, other prevention activities

■ Negotiate the health care system

  Keep appointments, transitions, multiple care providers

into low- and high-sodium categories (HFSA). Consideration of what you expect patients to be able to do guides teaching so that it is more than simple advice to "eat less salt."

Prior to discharge, health care providers should assess patients for the factors known to interfere with self-care and address those factors (Moser & Watkins, 2008). For example, clinicians should address patients' financial barriers to buying medications before discharge. Patients who lack a source of social support upon discharge will need help to mobilize support from friends, relatives, their church or other group, or home health care. Low health literacy, anxiety and depression, cognitive impairment, poor functional status, sensory impairments, lack of social support, and presence of comorbidities (all factors common to aging heart failure patients) can conspire to limit patients' abilities to engage in effective self-care (Moser & Watkins).

# Exhibit 23.2

## Strategies for Improving Adherence in Patients With Heart Failure

- Remember that knowledge is necessary but not sufficient to achieve treatment adherence.
- Assess potential barriers to adherence, such as lack of knowledge, memory problems, and beliefs or values that are inconsistent with self-care behaviors.
- Identify those patients able to self-dose, and teach these patients to use PRN diuretics to manage elevations in weight.
- Use once-daily dosing whenever possible, and tailor medications to patients' daily schedules
- Consider providing pre-prepared pill dispensers.
- Make sure that all pill bottles are labeled in large print with the drug name and dosing regimen.
- Provide patients with an updated medication list at each visit.
- Provide written instructions for medication changes made at each visit.
- Do not assume that patients are taking all of their medicines all the time; be open to hearing about problems and working through solutions ("Lots of patients have trouble taking their water pills on a regular basis. Are you having this problem? Other problems?").
- Ask about any over-the-counter substances taken, such as herbs or vitamins.
- Address potential financial difficulties or problems with access to care during the patient's stay in the hospital.
- Follow up with patients about self-care through e-mails or by phone.
- Consider providing care to patient at worksite.
- Provide patients with take-home material about diet and medication and the importance of treatment adherence.
- Provide scale for daily weights, if needed.
- _____

Adapted with permission from Riegel, B., & Moser, D. K. Care of patients with chronic heart failure. In D. K. Moser& B. Riegel (Eds.), *Cardiac Nursing: A Companion to Braunwald's Heart Disease*. Philadelphia: Elsevier; 2008:930-950. ©2008 Elsevier Inc.

## Case Study

After weaning Ms. G.T. from intravenous nitroglycerine, her doctors and nurses worked to optimize her oral HF drug therapy. They increased her oral furosemide dose to 40 mg every day, began uptitrating her enalapril, added a beta-blocker, and continued the digoxin 0.125 mg once a day. Her oral diabetic agent remained unchanged. The HF nurse continued with teaching Ms. G.T. and her daughter so that they both understood the importance of taking medications daily. She worked to ensure that Ms. G.T. understood her new medication regimen and understood that she should throw away her diltiazem and not refill that prescription as she was now on medications that would better control her blood pressure given her HF. The nurses began teaching Ms. G.T. about following a 2-gram per day sodium diet while working on determining her barriers to following the diet. They also began teaching her about how to monitor for symptoms, including performing daily weights, and what to do about escalating symptoms. Ms. G.T. and her daughter were also seen by the dietician and diabetes educator so they could better understand all aspects of diabetes care and learn how to follow a diet appropriate for both HF and diabetes. Knowing that Ms. G.T. and her daughter were likely to be overwhelmed by all the new information they were receiving they planned to refer Ms. G.T. for visits from a home health nurse for at least 2 weeks after discharge to reinforce their teaching and also to evaluate how well Ms. G.T. managed at home alone. To enhance her regular outpatient care, they referred her to a cardiologist who had a nurse practitioner working with him who specialized in HF and in providing comprehensive HF care.

## Discharge

Premature discharge from a hospitalization for ADHF is one reason for the high readmission rate seen in elders with HF. To address this problem, the Heart Failure Society of America HF guidelines specifically provide criteria for discharge (HFSA, 2006a). Prior to discharge all patients with HF need to (a) have factors precipitating their exacerbation of HF addressed, (b) have optimal fluid status obtained, (c) have achieved the transition from IV to oral diuretic, (d) have patient and family education completed, (e) chronic outpatient drug therapy optimized or near-optimized, and (f) have a follow-up clinic visit scheduled within 7 to 10 days (HFSA). Patients with more advanced HF who have recurrent hospitalizations need to (a) have oral medication regimen stable for 24 hours, (b) have had IV therapy discontinued at least 24 hours prior to discharge,(c) ambulate so that functional status can be assessed, (d) have plans (for example, scale ready for daily weights, home nurse visit, or telephone follow-up within 3 days of discharge) in place for postdischarge management, and (e) be referred to an HF disease management program if available (HFSA).

Additional resources are available from OPTIMIZE-HF to assist in the discharge-planning process. These resources include a (a) heart failure discharge summary checklist; (b) "Dear Doctor Letter" for the referring physician; and (c) take-home packet for patients on what to do if symptoms worsen, dietary information, and advice on reading food labels, and other education information. This resource packet is available at https://www.optimize-hf.org/art/OPT-CombinedToolkit.pdf.

## Summary

The care of patients with ADHF is challenging, particularly so when the patient is elderly. Hospitalization for ADHF is common among elderly adults, but critical care nurses are in a position to assist patients and their families improve aspects of self-care that can substantially reduce the risk of rehospitalization. In addition, they can advocate for delivery of evidence-based care to improve outcomes in this vulnerable patient population.

## References

Adams, K. F., Jr., Fonarow, G. C., Emerman, C. L., LeJemtel, T. H., Costanzo, M.R., Abraham, W. T., et al. (2005). Characteristics and outcomes of patients hospitalized for heart failure in the United

States: Rationale, design, and preliminary observations from the first 100,000 cases in the Acute Decompensated Heart Failure National Registry (ADHERE). *American Heart Journal, 149,* 209–216.

Ahmed, A. (2007). Clinical manifestations, diagnostic assessment, and etiology of heart failure in older adults. *Clinics in Geriatric Medicine, 23,* 11–30.

Ahmed, A., Kiefe, C. I., & Allman, R. M. (2002). Survival benefits of angiotensin-converting enzyme inhibitors in older heart failure patients with perceived contraindications. *Journal of the American Geriatrics Society, 50,* 1659–1666.

Allen, L. A., & O'Connor, C. M. (2007). Management of acute decompensated heart failure. *Canadian Medical Association Journal, 176,* 797–805.

Blue, L., Lang, E., McMurray, J. J., Davie, A. P., McDonagh, T. A., Murdoch, D. R., et al. (2001). Randomised controlled trial of specialist nurse intervention in heart failure. *British Medical Journal, 323,* 715–718.

Braunstein, J. B., Anderson, G. F., Gerstenblith, G., Weller, W., Niefeld, M., Herbert, R., et al. (2003). Noncardiac comorbidity increases preventable hospitalizations and mortality among Medicare beneficiaries with chronic heart failure. *Journal of the American College of Cardiology, 42,* 1226–1233.

Butler, J., & Kalogeropoulos, A. (2008). Worsening heart failure hospitalization epidemic we do not know how to prevent and we do not know how to treat! *Journal of the American College of Cardiology, 52,* 435–437.

Chaudhry, S. I., Wang, Y., Concato, J., Gill, T. M., & Krumholz, H. M. (2007). Patterns of weight change preceding hospitalization for heart failure. *Circulation, 116,* 1549–1554.

Cleland, J. G., Charlesworth, A., Lubsen, J., Swedberg, K., Remme, W. J., Erhardt, L., (2006). A comparison of the effects of carvedilol and metoprolol on well-being, morbidity, and mortality (the "patient journey") in patients with heart failure: a report from the Carvedilol Or Metoprolol European Trial (COMET). *Journal of the American College of Cardiology, 47,* 1603–1611.

Costanzo, M .R., Guglin, M. E., Saltzberg, M. T., Jessup, M. L., Teerlink, J. R., Jaski, B. E., et al. (2007). Ultrafiltration versus intravenous diuretics for patients hospitalized for acute decompensated heart failure. *Journal of the American College of Cardiology, 49,* 675–683.

Croft, J. B., Giles, W. H., Pollard, R. A., Casper, M. L., Anda, R. F., & Livengood, J. R. (1997). National trends in the initial hospitalization for heart failure. *Journal of the American Geriatrics Society, 45,* 270–275.

Cuffe, M. S., Califf, R. M., Adams, K .F., Jr., Benza, R., Bourge, R., Colucci, W. S., (2002). Short-term intravenous milrinone for acute exacerbation of chronic heart failure: A randomized controlled trial. *Journal of the American Medical Association, 287,* 1541–1547.

Dar, O., & Cowie, M. R. (2008). Acute heart failure in the intensive care unit: Epidemiology. *Critical Care Medicine, 36,* S3–8.

Disomma, S., Magrini, L., Pittoni, V., Marino, R., Peacock, W. F., & Maisel, A. (2008). Usefulness of serial assessment of natriuretic peptides in the emergency department for patients with acute decompensated heart failure. *Congestive Heart Failure, 14,* 21–24.

Domanski, M., Tian, X., Haigney, M., & Pitt, B. (2006). Diuretic use, progressive heart failure, and death in patients in the DIG study. *Journal of Cardiac Failure, 12,* 327–332.

Domanski, M., Norman, J., Pitt, B., Haigney, M., Hanlon, S., & Peyster, E., (2003). Diuretic use, progressive heart failure, and death in patients in the Studies Of Left Ventricular Dysfunction (SOLVD). *Journal of the American College of Cardiology, 42,* 705–708.

Fang, J., Mensah, G. A., Croft, J. B., & Keenan, N. L. (2008). Heart failure-related hospitalization in the U.S., 1979 to 2004. *Journal of the American College of Cardiology, 52,* 428–434.

Farmakis, D., Filippatos, G., Kremastinos, D. T., & Gheorghiade, M. (2008). Vasopressin and vasopressin antagonists in heart failure and hyponatremia. *Current Heart Failure Reports, 5,* 91–96.

Fonarow, G. C. (2003). The Acute Decompensated Heart Failure National Registry (ADHERE): Opportunities to improve care of patients hospitalized with acute decompensated heart failure. *Reviews in Cardiovascular Medicine, 4* (Suppl, 7), S21–30.

Fonarow, G. C., & Corday, E. (2004). Overview of acutely decompensated congestive heart failure (ADHF): A report from the ADHERE registry. *Heart Failure Reviews, 9,* 179–185.

Fonarow, G. C., & Weber, J. E. (2004). Rapid clinical assessment of hemodynamic profiles and targeted treatment of patients with acutely decompensated heart failure. *Clinics in Cardiology, 27* (Suppl. V), V1–V9.

Formiga, F., Chivite, D., Manito, N., Mestre, A. R., Llopis, F., & Pulol, R. (2008). Admission characteristics predicting longer length of stay among elderly patients hospitalized for decompensated heart failure. *European Journal of Internal Medicine, 19,* 198–202.

Gallegos, P. J., Maclaughlin, E. J., & Haase, K. K. (2008). Serial monitoring of brain natriuretic peptide concentrations for drug therapy management in patients with chronic heart failure. *Pharmacotherapy, 28*, 343–355.

Gambassi, G., Forman, D. E., Lapane, K. L., Mor, V., Sgadari, A., Lipsitz, L. A., et al. (2000). Management of heart failure among very old persons living in long-term care: Has the voice of trials spread? The SAGE Study Group. *American Heart Journal, 139*, 85–93.

Garg, R., Packer, M., Pitt, B., & Yusuf, S. (1993). Heart failure in the 1990s: Evolution of a major public health problem in cardiovascular medicine. *Journal of the American College of Cardiology, 22*, 3A–5A.

Gheorghiade, M., Rossi, J. S., Cotts, W., Shin, D. D., Hellkamp, A. S., Pina, I. L., . (2007). Characterization and prognostic value of persistent hyponatremia in patients with severe heart failure in the ESCAPE Trial. *Archives of Internal Medicine, 167*, 1998–2005.

Heart Failure Society of America. (2006a). HFSA 2006 Comprehensive Heart Failure Practice Guideline. *Journal of Cardiac Failure, 12*, e86–e103.

Ho, K. K., Anderson, K. M., Kannel, W. B., Grossman, W., & Levy, D. (1993). Survival after the onset of congestive heart failure in Framingham Heart Study subjects. *Circulation, 88*, 107–115.

Hunt, S. A., Abraham, W. T., Chin, M. H., Feldman, A. M., Francis, G. S., Ganiats, T. G., (2005). ACC/AHA 2005 Guideline Update for the Diagnosis and Management of Chronic Heart Failure in the Adult: A report of the American College of Cardiology/American Heart Association Task Force on Practice Guidelines (Writing Committee to Update the 2001 Guidelines for the Evaluation and Management of Heart Failure): Developed in collaboration with the American College of Chest Physicians and the International Society for Heart and Lung Transplantation: Endorsed by the Heart Rhythm Society. *Circulation, 112*, e154–235.

Kimmelstiel, C. D., & Konstam, M. A. (1995). Heart failure in women. *Cardiology. 86*, 304–309.

Koelling, T. M., Chen, R. S., Lubwama, R. N., L'Italien, G. J., & Eagle, K. A. (2004). The expanding national burden of heart failure in the United States: The influence of heart failure in women. *American Heart Journal, 147*, 74–78.

Kroenke, K., Spitzer, R. L., & Williams, J. B. (2003). The Patient Health Questionnaire-2: Validity of a two-item depression screener. *Medical Care, 41*, 1284–1292.

Krumholz, H. M., Parent, E. M., Tu, N., Vaccarino, V., Wang, Y., Radford, M.J., et al. (1997). Readmission after hospitalization for congestive heart failure among Medicare beneficiaries. *Archives of Internal Medicine, 157*, 99–104.

Lakatta, E. G. (2002). Age-associated cardiovascular changes in health: Impact on cardiovascular disease in older persons. *Heart Failure Reviews, 7*, 29–49.

Lakatta, E. G. (2003). Arterial and cardiac aging: major shareholders in cardiovascular disease enterprises: Part III: cellular and molecular clues to heart and arterial aging. *Circulation, 107*, 490–497.

Lakatta, E. G., & Levy, D. (2003a). Arterial and cardiac aging: Major shareholders in cardiovascular disease enterprises: Part I: Aging arteries: a "set up" for vascular disease. *Circulation, 107*, 139–146.

Lakatta, E.G., & Levy, D. (2003b). Arterial and cardiac aging: Major shareholders in cardiovascular disease enterprises: Part II: The aging heart in health: links to heart disease. *Circulation, 107*, 346–354.

Lee, W. C., Chavez, Y. E., Baker, T., & Luce, B. R. (2004). Economic burden of heart failure: A summary of recent literature. *Heart & Lung, 33*, 362–371.

Liao, L., Jollis, J. G., Anstrom, K. J., Whellan, D. J., Kitzman, D. W., Aurigemma, G. P., et al. (2006). Costs for heart failure with normal vs reduced ejection fraction. *Archives of Internal Medicine, 166*, 112–118.

Liao, L., Anstrom, K .J., Gottdiener, J. S., Pappas, P. A., Whellan, D. J., Kitzman, D. W., et al. (2007). Long-term costs and resource use in elderly participants with congestive heart failure in the Cardiovascular Health Study. *American Heart Journal, 153*, 245–252.

Linne, A. B., Liedholm, H., Jendteg, S., & Israelsson, B. (2000). Health care costs of heart failure: Results from a randomised study of patient education. *European Journal of Heart Failure, 2*, 291–297.

Masson, S., Latini, R., Anand, I. S., Bariera, S., Angelici, L., Vago, T., et al. (2008). Prognostic value of changes in N-terminal pro-brain natriuretic peptide in Val-HeFT (Valsartan Heart Failure Trial). *Journal of the American College of Cardiology, 52*, 997–1003.

McAlister, F. A., Stewart, S., Ferrua, S., & McMurray, J. J. (2004). Multidisciplinary strategies for the management of heart failure patients at high risk for admission: A systematic review of randomized trials. *Journal of the American College of Cardiology, 44*, 810–819.

McMurray, J. J. V., & Stewart, S. (2002). The burden of heart failure (supplement). *European Heart Journal, 4*, D50–D58.

McMurray, J. J., Petrie, M. C., Murdoch, D. R., & Davie, A. P. (1998). Clinical epidemiology of heart failure: Public and private health burden. *European Heart Journal, 19* (Suppl.), P9–16.

Miller, L. W., & Missov, E. D. (2001). Epidemiology of heart failure. *Cardiology Clinics, 19,* 547–555.

Miller, W. L., Hartman, K. A., Grill, D. E., Burnett, J. C., Jr., & Jaffe, A. S. (2009). Only large reductions in concentrations of natriuretic peptides (BNP and NT-proBNP) are associated with improved outcome in ambulatory patients with chronic heart failure. *Clinical Chemistry, 55,* 78–84.

Moser, D. K., Doering, L. V., & Chung, M. L. (2005). Vulnerabilities of patients recovering from an exacerbation of chronic heart failure. *American Heart Journal, 150,* 984.

Moser, D. K., & Watkins, J. F. (2008). Conceptualizing self-care in heart failure: A life course model of patient characteristics. *Journal of Cardiovascular Nursing, 23,* 205–218; quiz 219–220.

Nagamine, M., Jiang, J., & Merrill, C. T. (2006). *Trends in elderly hospitalizations, 1997–2004.* Statisticsl brief #14, Agency for Healthcare Research and Quality, Retrieved March 11, 2009, from http://www.hcup-us.ahrq.gov/reports/statbriefs/sb14.pdf

Naylor, M. D., Brooten, D., Campbell, R., Jacobsen, B. S., Mezey, M. D., Pauly, M. V., et al. (1999). Comprehensive discharge planning and home follow-up of hospitalized elders: A randomized clinical trial. *Journal of the American Medical Association, 281,* 613–620.

Ni, H., Nauman, D. J., & Hershberger, R. E. (1999). Analysis of trends in hospitalizations for heart failure. *Journal of Cardiac Failure, 5,* 79–84.

Nieminen, M. S., Brutsaert, D., Dickstein, K., Dexler, H., Follath, F., Harjola, V .P., et al. (2006). EuroHeart Failure Survey II (EHFS II): A survey on hospitalized acute heart failure patients: Description of population. *European Heart Journal, 27,* 2725–2736.

Nieminen, M. S., Bohm, M., Cowie, M. R., Drexler, H., Filippatos, G. S., Jondeau, G., et al. (2005). Executive summary of the guidelines on the diagnosis and treatment of acute heart failure: The Task Force on Acute Heart Failure of the European Society of Cardiology. *European Heart Journal, 26,* 384–416.

O'Connell, J. B. (2000). The economic burden of heart failure. *Clinics in Cardiology, 23,* III6–1120.

Oghlakian, G., & Klapholz, M. (2009). Vasopressin and vasopressin receptor antagonists in heart failure. *Cardiology Reviews, 17,* 10–15.

Omland, T. (2008). Advances in congestive heart failure management in the intensive care unit: B-type natriuretic peptides in evaluation of acute heart failure. *Critical Care Medicine, 36,* S17–S27.

Publication Committee for the VMAC Investigators. (2002). Intravenous nesiritide vs nitroglycerin for treatment of decompensated congestive heart failure: A randomized controlled trial. *Journal of the American Medical Association, 287,* 1531–1540.

Rich, M. W. (2005). Office management of heart failure in the elderly. *American Journal of Medicine, 118,* 342–348.

Rich, M. W., Gray, D. B., Beckham, V., Wittenberg, C., & Luther, P. (1996). Effect of a multidisciplinary intervention on medication compliance in elderly patients with congestive heart failure. *American Journal of Medicine, 101,* 270–276.

Rich, M. W., Beckham, V., Wittenberg, C., Leven, C. L., Freedland, K. E., & Carney, R. M. (1995). A multidisciplinary intervention to prevent the readmission of elderly patients with congestive heart failure. *New England Journal of Medicine, 333,* 1190–1195.

Riegel, B., & Moser, D. K. (2008). *Cardiac nursing: A companion to Braunwald's heart disease* (pp. 930–950). Philadelphia: Elsevier.

Riegel, B., Vaughan Dickson, V., Goldberg, L. R., & Deatrick, J. A. (2007). Factors associated with the development of expertise in heart failure self-care. *Nursing Research, 56,* 235–243.

Rogers, H. L., Marshall, J., Bock, J., Dowling, T. C., Feller, E., Robinson, S., et al. (2008). A randomized, controlled trial of the renal effects of ultrafiltration as compared to furosemide in patients with acute decompensated heart failure. *Journal of Cardiac Failure, 14,* 1–5.

Rosamond, W., Flegal, K., Furie, K., Greenlund, K., Haase, N., Hailpern, S. M., et al. (2008). Heart disease and stroke statistics—2008 update: A report from the American Heart Association Statistics Committee and Stroke Statistics Subcommittee. *Circulation, 117,* e25–146.

Rosamond, W., Flegal, K., Friday, G., Furie, K., Go, A., Greenlund, K., et al. (2007). Heart disease and stroke statistics–2007 update: A report from the American Heart Association Statistics Committee and Stroke Statistics Subcommittee. *Circulation, 115,* e69–171.

Sackner-Bernstein, J. D., Kowalski, M., Fox, M., & Aaronson, K. (2005). Short-term risk of death after treatment with nesiritide for decompensated heart failure: A pooled analysis of randomized controlled trials. *Journal of the American Medical Association, 293,* 1900—1905.

Schocken, D. D., Benjamin, E. J., Fonarow, G. C., Krumholz, H .M., Levy, D., Mensah, G. A., et al. (2008). Prevention of heart failure: A scientific statement from the American Heart Association

Councils on Epidemiology and Prevention, Clinical Cardiology, Cardiovascular Nursing, and High Blood Pressure Research; Quality of Care and Outcomes Research Interdisciplinary Working Group; and Functional Genomics and Translational Biology Interdisciplinary Working Group. *Circulation, 117*, 2544–2565.

Setoguchi, S., Levin, R., & Winkelmayer, W. C. (2008). Long-term trends of angiotensin-converting enzyme inhibitor and angiotensin-receptor blocker use after heart failure hospitalization in community-dwelling seniors. *International Journal of Cardiology, 125*, 172–177.

Shahar, E., & Lee, S. (2007). Historical trends in survival of hospitalized heart failure patients: 2000 versus 1995. *BMC Cardiovascular Disorders, 7*, 2.

Stanek, E. J., Oates, M. B., McGhan, W. F., Denofrio, D., & Loh, E. (2000). Preferences for treatment outcomes in patients with heart failure: Symptoms versus survival. *Journal of Cardiac Failure, 6*, 225–232.

Stewart, S., & Horowitz, J. D. (2002). Home-based intervention in congestive heart failure: Long-term implications on readmission and survival. *Circulation, 105*, 2861–2866.

Stromberg, A., Martensson, J., Fridlund, B., Levin, L. A., Karlsson, J. E., & Dahlstrom, U. (2003). Nurse-led heart failure clinics improve survival and self-care behaviour in patients with heart failure. Results from a prospective, randomised trial. *European Heart Journal, 24*, 1014–1023.

Taylor, A. L., Ziesche, S., Yancy, C., Carson, P., D'Agostino, R., Jr., Ferdinand, K., et al. (2004). Combination of isosorbide dinitrate and hydralazine in blacks with heart failure. *New England Journal of Medicine. 351*, 2049–2057.

Thomas, S., & Rich, M. W. (2007). Epidemiology, pathophysiology, and prognosis of heart failure in the elderly. *Clinics in Geriatric Medicine, 23*, 1–10.

Valle, R., Aspromonte, N., Giovinazzo, P., Carbonieri, E., Chiatto, M., di Tano, G., et al. (2008). B-type natriuretic Peptide-guided treatment for predicting outcome in patients hospitalized in sub-intensive care unit with acute heart failure. *Journal of Cardiac Failure, 14*, 219–224.

Wu, J. R., Moser, D. K., Chung, M. L., & Lennie, T. A. (2008). Predictors of medication adherence using a multidimensional adherence model in patients with heart failure. *Journal of Cardiac Failure, 14*, 603–614.

Wu, J. R., Moser, D. K., Lennie, T. A., & Burkhart, P. V. (2008). Medication adherence in patients who have heart failure: A review of the literature. *Nursing Clinics of North America, 43*,133–153.

Wu, J. R., Moser, D. K., Lennie, T. A., Peden, A. R., Chen, Y. C., & Heo, S. (2008). Factors influencing medication adherence in patients with heart failure. *Heart & Lung, 37*, 8–16, 16 e11.

Zannad, F., Briancon, S., Juilliere, Y., Mertes, P. M., Villemot, J. P., Alla, F., et al. (1999). Incidence, clinical and etiologic features, and outcomes of advanced chronic heart failure: The EPICAL Study. Epidemiologie de l'Insuffisance Cardiaque Avancee en Lorraine. *Journal of the American College of Cardiology, 33*, 734–742.

# Perioperative Care of the Elderly

# 24

Jeffrey H. Silverstein

## Introduction

Although the elderly tend to represent a relatively large percentage of surgery and intensive care (ICU) patients in the United States, there are few randomized controlled trials focused on the perioperative care of elderly patients. Specifically, there is limited 1A level of evidence available to direct the care of the geriatric patient preparing for surgery (for levels of evidence see: http://www.essentialevidenceplus.com/concept/ebm_loe.cfm?show=oxf ord). Thus, much of the evidence used to direct practice is extrapolated from related circumstances. An excellent short reference guide called *Geriatrics At Your Fingertips* is available in a small pocket edition as well as on the Internet (Reuben et al., 2006) (http://www.geriatricsatyourfingertips.org/). Fortunately for our patients, this absence of evidence does not mean that we don't have to take care of them.

Perioperative care of the elderly involves determining the need for surgery, preparing the patient for surgery, transport to and from the operating room (OR), caring for the patient in the OR, managing the immediate postoperative issues of emergence from surgery and anesthesia, and ultimately recovering completely. This chapter assumes that the reader has referred to the many other chapters in this book for detailed information on general issues of aging and for the bedside nursing care of critically ill older adults, and therefore focuses on the immediate perioperative period.

The context of the relationship between the ICU and the operating room comes in two basic forms. Many patients undergo major surgery with a planned admission to the ICU. Most major cardiac surgical cases (coronary artery bypass, major valve surgery), many major neurosurgical procedures, and essentially all liver transplants (which do occur in a few geriatric patients) are followed by ICU admission. In the realm of general surgery, surgeons may plan for patients undergoing major procedures to be admitted to the ICU, occasionally based primarily on the age of the patient. Criteria for admission to the ICU vary tremendously among different institutions, with some admitting many elective patients and others almost never admitting purely elective surgical patients. Frequently, the ICU is called on to admit a patient who has undergone either an elective or emergent surgical procedure who is in need of prolonged intensive care that cannot be managed in a postanesthesia care unit (PACU). Once again, there are huge institutional differences in what constitutes an appropriate use of an ICU versus a PACU bed, with staffing issues being the predominant variable. Finally, many patients who are in the ICU either following surgery or for medical illness require a trip to the operating room for surgery. These patients typically return to the ICU following their procedure.

## Variability in the Elderly

In approaching the elderly as patients, one of the most important concepts to understand is the tremendous variability in how bodies age. Within an individual person, organs are frequently affected differently with age. The changes noted in this and other chapters usually describe what is found on average in elderly patients. Every individual will manifest different changes and could have, for example, a relatively young heart with old kidneys. A good example of the difference between the average changes associated with age and an individual patient is found in our assessment of aging kidney function, which is measured by the glomerular filtration rate (GFR). GFR is reported to decrease by 1 ml/year. Thus, for individuals between the age of 20 to 30, the GFR is about 116 mL/min/1.73m$^2$ and, individuals aged 70 and greater have an average GFR of about 75 mL/min/1.73m$^2$. However, about one third of participants in a large study that defined this change had no change in GFR, whereas other showed much greater decrements (Lindeman, 1993). Thus, it is important to not assume that an 80 year old has a standard type of deterioration but rather to make judgments based on individual evaluation. There are formulas that estimate GFR based on age and serum creatinine levels. (estimated GFR $= 170 \times \text{Creat}^{-0.999} \times \text{Age}^{-0.176} \times \text{BUN}^{-0.170} \times \text{Alb}^{+0.318} \times 0.762$ (if female) $\times 1.80$ (if African American)) but these should be used with caution because the result is frequently inaccurate (Lindeman). The important point of this discussion is to understand that there is so much variability in how patients age, that although all the available data will inform your evaluation, each critical care nurse has to make a complete individual assessment of each patient.

## Outcomes From Surgery in the Elderly

Anyone who cares for the elderly patient eventually confronts the question of the utility of undertaking a surgical procedure in an old person. What we do know about outcomes for elderly patients undergoing surgery is based almost exclusively on elective surgery (Silverstein, 2008). In assessing the value of surgery, it is important to determine what outcomes are important. It is common to measure functionality in the elderly using measures referred to as activities of daily living (ADL) and instrumental activities of daily living (IADL) (Lawton & Brody, 1969). ADLs are those activities required for self-care, whereas IADLs are activities required to live independently. The important outcome for many geriatric patients is to avoid disability and preserve functional status. Even after elective surgery, elderly patients will take on average about 3 months to return to full ADLs and 6 months to return to preoperative levels of IADL (Lawrence et al., 2004). Although the research is scarce, outcomes including ADLs and IADL, and other quality-of-life measures suggest that the elderly who survive the ICU return to reasonable functional status (Kaarlola, Tallgren, & Pettila, 2006; Kleinpell & Ferrans, 2002). ICU staff can legitimately encourage the patient and their families that ICU is worth the effort and pays off in quality survival. Although there is a clear role for palliative end–of-life care in the ICU, it is realistic to approach most elderly ICU admissions as patients likely to be returned to functional health.

Diagnosis in the elderly can be difficult; delayed diagnosis may be associated with a poorer prognosis. Elderly patients, for reasons that are not well understood, frequently present with diminished, muted, or less specific symptoms than younger patients (see case #1). As an example, there is some frequency of diagnosis of cholecystitis in the ICU, but a significant number of patients over the age of 65 do not manifest classic symptoms (Parker, Vukov, & Wollan, 1997). In about one third of patients with peptic ulcer disease the first sign of ulcer disease is perforation (Hilton et al., 2001). Just to make matters more confusing, nurses must keep in mind that acute mesenteric ischemia, a surgical emergency, frequently presents with pain out of proportion to all other physical findings. In general, the lack of symptoms means that by the time an elderly patient with abdominal catastrophe arrives in the ICU he or she is usually sicker than would be the case for younger patients. Although in case #1 the patient began her operation in a stable condition and deteriorated as the systemic infection evolved, this deterioration might not occur until the patient is in the ICU. It is not uncommon for an elderly patient to appear stable and then rapidly deteriorate.

## Case Study 1

An 85-year-old female who was relatively active, volunteered at church and played tennis, was found to have a premalignant polyp on a screening colonoscopy. Her medical history included only hypertension controlled by medication. She underwent a laparoscopic colectomy and was discharged home on postoperative day 2. On postoperative day 8 she is brought to the emergency room (ER) lethargic and hypotensive (80/40). She receives 2 liters of intravenous fluid with good immediate result in that she becomes more alert and her blood pressure rises to 110/80. She has no peritoneal signs but some nonspecific discomfort. She is taken to the OR and is found to have a anastomic breakdown with fecal spoilage of the peritoneum. The patient is admitted to the ICU intubated, ventilated, and with intravenous vasopressor support.

# The Anesthesia Team's Evaluation of the ICU Patient

The anesthesia team may consist of one or more anesthesiologists, certified registered nurse anesthetists (CRNA), anesthesia residents, student nurse anesthetists, and/or anesthesia assistants.

In this section, we discuss the anesthesia perspective on acutely ill patients to assist the ICU nurse in communicating with these members of the team (and perhaps entice you to study nurse anesthesia). Anesthesia can be thought of as the art and science of controlling physiologic processes while the surgeon operates. Clearly the human body would not tolerate most surgeries without anesthesia because of normal compensatory mechanisms (pain and withdrawal, fight or flight, etc.) that are present even in sick ICU patients. Keeping vital signs, such as heart rate and blood pressure within normal limits during surgery should be thought of as maintaining homeostasis. In aging there appears to be a state of *homeostenosis,* in that the range and capacity of homeostatic mechanisms are more limited. This provides a challenge to the ICU and anesthesia teams when working with elderly patients. In developing an anesthetic plan for an older adult, the anesthesia team must be familiar with the effects of aging on multiple organ systems, particularly the brain, lungs, and heart. In addition, the anesthesia team has to understand the physiologic changes of age, such as increase in body fat, decreased glomerular filtration, and reduced hepatic blood flow, which affect anesthetic drug action and duration.

## Preoperative Evaluation

When a member of the anesthesia team sees a patient prior to surgery, what is he or she looking for? The most important goal of preoperative assessment is not risk assessment. During the preanesthesia assessment, we seek to determine the patient's medical status, determine whether anything further can be done to either understand a patient's status or improve that status and plan for the recovery process. Unlike many if not most specialties, the role of the chief complaint is filled by a request for anesthesia services for a specific operation. The anesthesia team starts with the assumption that the diagnosis and need for surgery are correct. The approach used by the anesthesia team was most clearly articulated by Muravchick (1997) who described our approach as a vertical or systems-based approach (see Figures 24.1A and 24.1B). As part of this approach, the anesthesia team does assign an American Society of Anesthesiologists (ASA) physical status classification (see Exhibit 24.1).

The ASA score is a clinician's tool that allows anesthesia team members to communicate with each other. As the ASA score does not incorporate age or type of operation, both significant influences on outcomes, the ASA score is not a good predictor of perioperative risk (Muravchick 1997).

The typical approach to assessing a medical patient starts from the history of the presenting illness. The answer to the question, "Why are you here" is generally the chief complaint. The physician proceeds through the process moving from this chief complaint to a diagnosis.

The anesthesiologist is generally presented with a patient who already has a diagnosis and a planned procedure. Rather than begin with a complaint and conclude by making a diagnosis, we start with the planned procedure and attempt to determine

# Exhibit 24.1

## American Society of Anesthesiologists Physical Status Categories

| | |
|---|---|
| P1 | A normal healthy patient |
| P2 | A patient with mild systemic disease |
| P3 | A patient with severe systemic disease |
| P4 | A patient with severe systemic disease that is a constant threat to life |
| P5 | A moribund patient who is not expected to survive without the operation |
| P6 | A declared brain-dead patient whose organs are being removed for donor purposes |

the physical and mental status of the patient to ultimately assess the reserve of organ systems. For example, a patient coming to the operating room with an acute cholecystitis for a cholecystectomy might have normal cardiac and pulmonary function, but limited renal function. Decreased renal function would alter the approach to fluid administration and monitoring.

Physiologic status is more important than chronological age in understanding the ability of a patient to tolerate anesthesia and surgery. That does not mean that chronological age is unimportant. Chronological age is easy to determine and generally uncontested. Age has repeatedly been found to be associated with an increased risk of morbidity, mortality, and poor surgical outcomes. Nonetheless, age alone is insufficient to predict even short-term surgical outcomes. The number of diseases (disease burden) appears to be the primary determinant of outcomes. Perhaps a useful way to understand aging is that it appears to be an important modifier of disease load. Elderly patients with limited or low disease load have relatively lower risk of postoperative complications. The combination of advanced age and a high disease load is associated with extremely high rates of morbidity and mortality (see Figure 24.2). A careful preoperative evaluation is extremely important in preparing the older adult for surgery. Other physicians may be consulted as part of the preoperative evaluation. Some institutions may require this activity. From a practical perspective, these consultations should cover the perioperative period, including immediate postoperative care. The ICU nurse has a vested interest in the outcomes of these evaluations and can be extremely helpful in acting as an intermediary between the anesthesia team and consulting physicians (see case #2). Statements such as, "the patient has been cleared for surgery" (cleared for ICU care?) or "avoid hypotension and hypoxemia" are of limited value. Much more useful to the anesthesia and surgical teams is a complete overview of the patient's medical condition, recent evaluations, and medications. In an ICU, it is important for the preoperative evaluator to talk to ICU staff. The best plans are based on good communication among the ICU staff, generalist and specialist physicians, the surgical and anesthesia teams, and the patient and family members.

Age and disease load appear to be cofactors in determining major anesthesia complications. In the front row of the figure the blue boxes represent patients with no disease load, advancing age has a limited impact on anesthetic complications. As

# 24.1A

**A vertical or systems-based approach.**

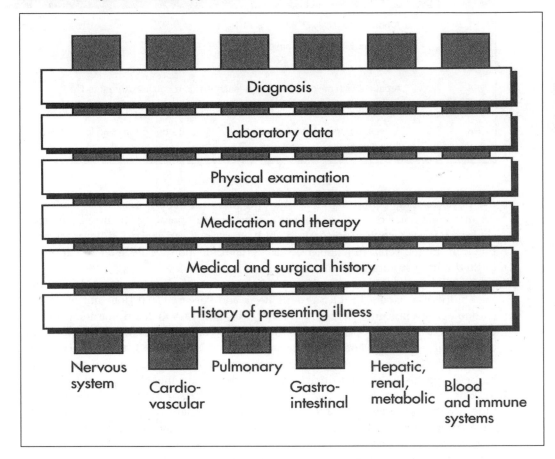

the number of diseases increases, the impact of age becomes apparent. A patient > 74 years of age has an increasing complication rate as disease load increases, so a 75-year-old with three major diagnoses has approximately a 20% chance of having a complication.

Medication management protocols that have been jointly set by all of the important caregivers are often useful. Any requests for additional consultation should clearly define the issues that need to be addressed and the expected role of the consultant.

An undeveloped area of medical care is the involvement of geriatricians in perioperative care in general, and specifically in the ICU. The general sense seems to be that geriatric issues are long-term issues or somehow not relevant in the ICU. There is extensive data to suggest that comprehensive geriatric assessment (CGA) has a place in perioperative care. The most compelling data suggest a significant ability to prevent geriatric-specific postoperative complications such as delirium and pressure ulcers (Marcantonio, Flacker, Wright, & Resnick, 2001).

# 24.1B

**A vertical or systems-based approach.**

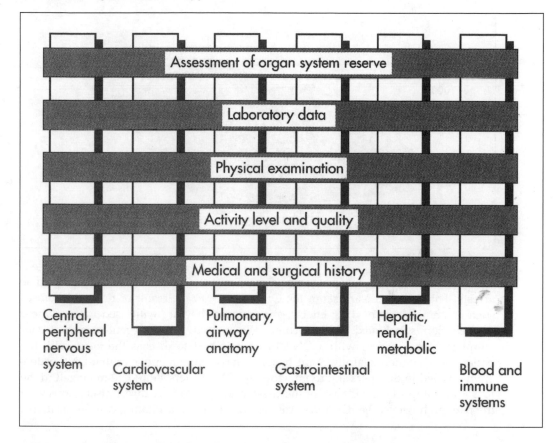

Assessment of organ system reserve

Laboratory data

Physical examination

Activity level and quality

Medical and surgical history

Central, peripheral nervous system

Cardiovascular system

Pulmonary, airway anatomy

Gastrointestinal system

Hepatic, renal, metabolic

Blood and immune systems

All health care institutions require consent for surgery. Some, but definitely not all, require a separate consent for anesthesia services. Many patients already in an ICU do not have the capacity to participate in an informed-consent process. Although beyond the scope of this chapter, the ethical and legal questions regarding who is legally authorized to represent the patient varies greatly from state to state in the United States, so ICU nurses need to know what the local policies and procedures require (see chapter 5, this volume).

"Do not resuscitate" (DNR) orders or other advanced care directives need to be understood in the context of elective or emergency surgery (see chapters 5 and 8). DNR orders frequently indicate that the patient does not want to be intubated or supported by mechanical ventilation. Intubation and mechanical ventilation are standard components of general anesthesia. If the anesthesia staff does not believe the patient can be weaned from mechanical ventilation after a surgical procedure, a DNR order cannot be interpreted to mean that the patient should be actively extubated and allowed to perish. An important distinction is that cardiac arrests in the operating

## 24.2

**Major anesthesia complications per 1000 as a function of age and associated disease.**

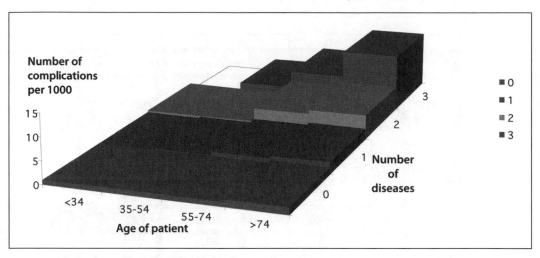

room carry a very favorable prognosis in comparison to even other in-hospital cardiac arrests. This is because arrests in the OR are often to the result of reversible causes such as hemorrhage or drug effects, and because they are witnessed events where resuscitation is instituted within seconds. When elective or emergent surgery is contemplated for a patient with a DNR order it is best to discuss the issue with the patient or the patient's family. Some hospitals have standing policies that DNR orders are rescinded in the operating room. How the DNR orders should be managed in the ICU is also important. It is best for the anesthesiologist to have direct discussions with the patient; however the ICU nurse can be invaluable in facilitating communications.

## Case Study 2

An 85-year-old male with a history of Parkinson's disease and hypertension is scheduled for a whipple procedure and postoperative ICU admission. He is taking Sinemet CR and Eldepryl and he had a deep brain stimulator placed 6 months ago.

Sinemet CR is a controlled-release tablet that is prescribed to relieve the muscle stiffness, tremor, and weakness associated with Parkinson's disease. It may also be given to relieve Parkinson-like symptoms resulting from other medical problems (e.g., encephalitis or carbon monoxide poisoning)

Sinemet CR contains two drugs, carbidopa and levodopa. The drug that actually produces the anti-Parkinson's effect is levodopa. Carbidopa is added to prevent vitamin $B_6$ from destroying levodopa.

Eldepryl (selegiline) prevents the breakdown of dopamine. Low levels of dopamine are associated with Parkinson's disease. Eldepryl is used together with other medicines to treat Parkinosnian symptoms.

Deep brain stimulators (DBS) are like pacemakers, but the electrodes are placed in the brain. When the stimulator is turned on, patient movement is easier and smoother. DBS units, like cardiac pacemakers and debibrillators, could theoretically be activated or altered by the stray electrical current from electrosurgical units. Depending on the type and location of the surgery, the neurologist may elect to reprogram the DBS for surgery.

In the preoperative consultation, the patient's physician(s) should indicate (a) when the Sinemet and Elepryl should be stopped; if it can be taken the morning of surgery, that is ideal. (b)The physician needs to also indicate when to continue the drugs. It is usually best to reinstitute Parkinson's medication as soon as possible after surgery. This medication is only available in oral form, so it may have to be crushed and administered via a nasogastric tube. The management of the DBS should also be clear. Particularly for a patient being weaned from mechanical ventilation, getting the patient's Parkinson's regimen optimized can be extremely important to success. Critical care nurses can play a crucial role in assuring that all parties are communicating about these issues effectively.

In addition to the consultation, nurses and physicians in the ICU need to understand the drug interactions that may affect the patient. Patients receiving eldepryl need to avoid high tyramine foods as this can cause severe hypertension. Some branched chain amino acid total parenteral nutrition formulas may contain tyramine.

# Transportation of the Patient to and From the OR

The transfer of a ventilated patient to the OR creates a number of situations that can be anticipated and managed (see Exhibit 24.2). It is important for the anesthesia staff to understand why the patient needs mechanical ventilation. Does the patient have primary respiratory failure or does the patient require intubation for supportive care, even though there is nothing particularly wrong with the patient's lungs and chest? ICU ventilators are generally more powerful and have more features than the ventilators that are part of anesthesia machines. In part this is because weaning a patient off an anesthesia ventilator usually involves reversing a drug and a short wake-up period, whereas weaning a patient following acute respiratory distress syndrome (ARDS) can make use of more advanced ventilator settings. When transferring a patient to the OR who is on a ventilator, the information regarding the tidal volume, respiratory rate, inspired concentration of oxygen (FiO2), and any PEEP (positive end-expiratory pressure) should be communicated to the anesthesia staff. It is possible to maintain PEEP during transport by adding a PEEP valve to the bag-valve respirator used for ventilation.

The responsibility of transportation of ICU patients will vary from institution to institution. ICU patients should be monitored during transport. The appropriate monitoring should be based on the clinical status of the patient. For most transportation, the most important and useful monitor is the pulse oximeter, which provides both pulse and oxygen saturation. If a patient has been hemodynamically unstable, has been on vasoactive infusions, or has an indwelling arterial catheter, continuous

# Exhibit 24.2

## Checklist for Transport of the Elderly ICU Patient

☐ Obtain a transport monitor

☐ Transport defibrillator

☐ Ensure adequate volumes of IV fluids/infusions

☐ Assess adequate sedation/analgesia

☐ Remove unneeded equipment/linens/supplies from patient's bed

☐ Connect transport monitor

☐ Call porter(s)

☐ Unplug and package equipment

☐ Ensure lines/transducers are orderly and secured to patient

☐ Obtain $O_2$ tank

☐ Ensure tank is full

☐ Obtain transport ventilator or bag-valve device

☐ Connect patient to $O_2$ delivery device

☐ Check monitor

☐ Essential documents

☐ Consent for procedures

☐ Medical record

☐ Review patient's clinical condition before transport

☐ Advise the anesthesia team of any changes in the patient since the preoperative evaluation

monitoring of blood pressure is advisable. Although the electrocardiograph (ECG) is the most common monitor, it is useful primarily in cardiac cases (evolving myocardial infarction [MI], postcardiac surgery) and should be accompanied by the ability to perform defibrillation during transport.

The ultimate goal of transport is not just to move the patient, but to transfer patient care to another group. Critical care nursing should be at the forefront of clear communication with other members of the patient's medical team (see Exhibit 24.3).

## Overview of Anesthesia Methods

Anesthesiologists have developed two major approaches to anesthesia. General anesthesia involves the administration of medications whose principal effects occur in the central nervous system. Sedation can be thought of as a subtype of general anesthesia.

# Exhibit 24.3

## Things the Anesthesia Team Wants to (or Should Want to) Know at Transport

Vital signs: Pulse, blood pressure, respiratory rate, temperature, pain level

❑ Stable or unstable

❑ Ventilatory status:

❑ Oxygen Saturation (pulse oximetry or blood gas)

❑ If on supplementary oxygen

❑ Type of device and percentage of oxygen

❑ If on mechanical ventilation

❑ Respiratory pattern, controlled, intermittent, etc.

❑ Respiratory rate

❑ Tidal volume

❑ Minute volume

❑ Drug infusions

Regional anesthesia, the second major approach, is based on the use of one of the local anesthetic agents to block nerves. In spinal or epidural anesthesia local anesthetic agents are applied in or around the spinal canal. Local anesthetic agents can be injected around peripheral nerves to provide anesthesia to the area of the body covered by that nerve or nerves. These same agents, when injected subcutaneously, block sensation of the skin in that immediate area. The two main forms of anesthesia are neither distinct nor mutually exclusive. A patient undergoing a procedure with spinal anesthesia is likely to receive hypnotic medications in concentrations that produce sedation, whereas a patient undergoing general anesthesia may have a peripheral nerve block to control postoperative pain. Opioids most frequently cross the line between general and local anesthetic agents as they are frequently added into mixtures of local anesthetic agents in epidural analgesia and other forms.

## General Anesthesia

Unconsciousness is the most apparent feature of general anesthesia, but may be the least important in terms of protecting the patient. The features of general anesthesia are (a) lack of consciousness, including amnesia for events that occur under anesthesia; (b) analgesia or absence of pain; (c) lack of movement in response to painful stimuli; and (d) control of the reflex responses to painful stimuli. In discussing anesthesia with patients, anesthesia personnel frequently invoke the idea of sleep, as in "You will go to sleep to have your surgery." Physiologically, the anesthetic state is nothing like natural sleep and patients do not wake up well rested from anesthesia. Although ether was used as the sole anesthetic agent in the early years of anesthesia, modern general anesthesia results from alterations at multiple receptors and multiple drugs are almost always used to produce general anesthesia.

All patients coming to an operating room are monitored with an electrocardiogram, intermittent blood pressure device, and oxygen saturation. It is necessary to monitor end tidal carbon dioxide in all patients requiring endotracheal intubation (or other inserted airway device) and temperature should be monitored for most procedures requiring general anesthesia. An 18-gauge or larger intravenous catheter inserted into a peripheral vein is almost universally desired for the conduct of anesthetic care for major surgery. Longer central venous catheters can be used, understanding that the flow through the catheter is inversely related to the length (fluid flows slower through longer catheters). If a central venous catheter is desired (or if the ICU would prefer that one be placed), this can be done once the patient is under anesthesia.

The beginning of general anesthesia is called induction. In most cases anesthesia is induced by the intravenous injection of hypnotic agents. The most common induction agent in the United States is currently propofol. It is possible to induce anesthesia by inhaling certain volatile anesthetics, but this is an extremely uncommon practice in adult patients. Older patients require less of almost all drugs used during the induction of anesthesia. Following the induction of anesthesia, an endotracheal tube is inserted. In recent years, an alternative airway device called a laryngeal mask airway (LMA) has been used in place of endotracheal tubes for elective surgeries, but would not typically be used for major surgeries or ICU patients.

The center of an anesthesia workstation is an anesthesia machine. The primary parts of an anesthesia machine are controls for gases (oxygen, air, nitrous oxide), vaporizers to administer volatile anesthetics, and a ventilator that includes a manual ventilation bag. In addition, many modern anesthesia machines include the physiologic monitors (ECG, BP, pulse oximetry [$SpO_2$], invasive pressures) as a integral part of the machine. Other monitors commonly used in the operating room include neuromuscular blockade monitors, cerebral oximeters, and processed electroencephalography. As in ICUs, pulmonary artery catheters are becoming rare, whereas echocardiography, particularly transesophageal echocardiography (TEE), is becoming routine during cardiac surgery and common for general surgery in major centers. ICU nurses receiving cases from the cardiac OR should inquire about the last echo exam prior to arrival in the ICU, as this technology provides a clear assessment of cardiac function.

A primary goal during anesthesia is to maintain the blood pressure and heart rate nearly normal during the surgery. As the stimulation from the surgery increases and decreases, the amount of medications needed to achieve stability varies over the course of a case. The level of anesthesia is usually referred to as depth. Light anesthesia may be associated with reactions to pain, movement, or other signs of awakening. Excessively deep may be associated with hypotension.

One of the risks of general anesthesia is awareness or recall under general anesthesia. Recall is rare but can happen. The risk increases when patients are hypotensive for other reasons (e.g., sepsis, heart failure) because this limits the amount of anesthetic agent that can be safely administered. If a patient should indicate that he or she recalled information during surgery, the anesthesia team should be notified to follow up. Recall must be taken seriously and such complaints should never be dismissed.

# Anesthetic Agents

## Volatile Anesthestics

For years, ether was the ultimate anesthetic agent. It produced amnesia, analgesia, muscle relaxation, and it stimulated respiration. Unfortunately, almost all patients became exceptionally nauseated and ether had a tendency to explode and cause fires in the OR. Today, the most common agents are isoflurane, sevoflurane, and desflurane (see Table 24.1). Isoflurane is currently the old agent, which replaced halothane and enflurane in the 1980s. Both sevoflurane and desflurane are more rapidly acting and, more important, more rapidly waning agents that are particularly useful for ambulatory anesthesia. All of these drugs come as a liquid and must be poured into a device called a vaporizer, which adds the agents in small percentages to the gas used to ventilate the patient. Because the patient also exhales these gases, anesthesia ventilators have to have scavenging systems to remove the exhaled gas from the environment. Otherwise, the operating room would rapidly smell of anesthetic gas. These drugs appear to have profound action on GABAergic centers in the brain; however, the mechanism of action of these drugs is unknown. Volatile anesthetics can, and frequently are, used as the only anesthetic agent for a patient's procedure. Isoflurane and desflurane are too pungent to inhale while conscious, but sevoflurane is not so bad and is routinely used to induce anesthesia in children when an IV cannot be easily inserted. Each of these agents has subtle differences of interest to the anesthesia team. For most major surgery, the volatile anesthetics are combined with other agents and used as part of the maintenance regimen (see Exhibit 24.4). By adjusting a dial, the concentration of agent can be increased or decreased. Blood pressure responds to changing levels within 30 to 60 seconds of an adjustment. It is this ability to titrate blood pressure up and down effectively that maintained the popularity of volatile anesthetics. Considerably less volatile anesthesia are needed in the elderly. Extremely ill patients might not tolerate any volatile anesthetic and will require alternative intervention to prevent awareness during anesthesia.

## Narcotics or Opioids

In modern anesthetic practice, the primary narcotic analgesic is fentanyl. This synthetic derivative of morphine provides intense analgesia. Like all related drugs, fentanyl decreases respiratory drive and can cause apnea. During general anesthesia or while mechanically ventilated in an ICU setting, fentanyl can be titrated for effective pain relief. Under general anesthesia, the anesthesia team is primarily observing heart rate and blood pressure to understand when a patient needs additional narcotic during a case. Although individuals may differ significantly, low-dose fentanyl (1–2 ug/kg) can be used for sedation, moderate dose (2–5 ug/kg) is used during general anesthesia, and high-dose (5–20 ug/kg) is used in cardiac surgery and other major invasive procedures. Remientanil is a very rapid acting (and hence rapidly disappearing) narcotic that has become popular in some operating room settings. Although extremely easy to titrate to effect, it is currently very costly and is not routinely used in critical care cases.

## 24.1  Anesthetic Drugs

| Anesthetic/Drug | General Use | Age-Related Changes |
|---|---|---|
| **Inhalational anesthetics** Isoflurane Sevoflurane Desflurane | Produce general anesthesia. Distributed as a liquid. Each agent has a specific vaporizer | Patients are more sensitive. Usually takes longer to get gas in and out of elderly patients. |
| **Hypnotics** Thiopental/Pentothal | Use in a large bolus to induce anesthesia. Almost no current use as a sedative. Occasionally used to maintain coma in ICU. | Induction dose reduced by 15% |
| Propofol | Currently the primary induction agent when used in large bolus doses. Produces controlled levels of sedation when used in lower doses. Frequently used as a continuous infusion in OR and ICU. | Induction dose reduced by 20% (slower induction requires lower doses) (20-year-old: 2.0–3.0 mg/kg IV; 80-year-old: 1.7 mg/kg IV). Emergence: slightly faster. |
| Midazolam | Intravenous sedative. Can be used in small boluses or continuous infusion. | Sedation/induction dose reduced by 50% Elderly can become disinhibited rather than sedated. Recovery: delayed (hours). |
| Etomidate | Alternative induction agent used in patients who are less hemodynamically stable. | Induction dose reduced by 20%. Central clearance; volume of distribution. Affects adrenal function. |
| Ketamine | Can be used for induction of anesthesia (high dose) or sedation (low dose) in combination with midazolam. | Used with hemodynamically unstable patients as it typically does not cause a drop in blood pressure. Use with caution: hallucinations, seizures, mental disturbance, release of catecholamines: avoid in combination with levodopa (tachycardia, arterial hypertension). |
| Dexmedetomidine | Sedation of intubated patients; becoming popular as an adjunct to general anesthesia and an OR sedative. | Bolus doses frequently cause hypotension and bradycardia in the elderly, begin infusion without bolus. |
| **Opioids** Fentanyl, alfentanil, sufentanil | Synthetic opioids, produce analgesia, only minor sedation. | Induction dose reduced by 50%. Maintenance doses reduced by 30–50%. Emergence: may be delayed. |

*(continued)*

**Table 24.1** *(continued)*

| Remifentanil | Ultra-short-acting potent analgesic. Must be given by continuous infusion. | Induction dose reduced by 50%. Maintenance dose reduced by 70%. Emergence: may be delayed. |
|---|---|---|
| Morphine | Intermediate acting. Analgesia with sedation. | Induction dose reduced by 50%. Maintenance doses reduced by 30–50%. |
| Meperidine (Demerol) | Bad reputation as an analgesic for elderly. Used effectively to reduce shivering following general anesthesia (12.5 mg). | Currently not recommended for elderly except for shivering. |
| **Reversal agents** | | |
| Neostigmine, pyridostigmine | Antagonize cholineseterase, increasing the clearance of muscle relaxants. | Doses not substantially changed. |
| Edrophonium | Antagonize cholineseterase, increasing the clearance of muscle relaxants. | No changes. |
| **Local anesthetics** | Sensitivity of the nervous tissue (?) | Epidural (and spinal) dose requirements. Duration of spinal and epidural anesthesia seems clinically independent of age, toxicity (percentage free drug). |

Morphine remains a useful narcotic for general anesthesia. Occasionally, morphine administration is followed by profound histamine release and hypotension. Morphine may provide somewhat more of a sedative sensation that fentanyl and has been used successfully to sedate intubated and ventilated patients.

Meperidine (Demerol) was an extremely popular narcotic analgesic that is used in sedation regimens. It has not been used in large doses because of the presence of a metabolite that may cause seizures. In addition, meperidine in the elderly has been linked to the development of delirium (Marcantonio et al., 1994) (see the text that follows). Meperidine would probably have disappeared altogether from the anesthesia workplace, but it has retained a role in low doses (12.5 mg) to treat shivering after anesthesia. This is the only one of the narcotics that is effective in this role and its mechanism is not clear.

## Muscle Relaxants

There are two general classes of muscle relaxants. Both are more appropriately referred to as blockers of neuromuscular transmission because they don't directly relax muscle, rather they take away the neural input that generates contraction. Succinylcholine is a *depolarizing* muscle relaxant. This drug causes the neuromuscular junction to release transmitter-causing fasciculation (uncoordinated writhing contractions) followed by profound lack of muscle tone. Succinylcholine remains the fastest acting agent and remains popular in trauma and other emergency care scenarios. It has been associated with profound release of potassium and cardiac arrest when it is used for subsequent (but not initial) care of traumatic patients. Patients frequently complain of sore muscles after succinylcholine administration.

The *nondepolarizing* muscle relaxants block neuromuscular transmission but do not stimulate the receptor, so there are no fasciculations. The original drug in this class was curare, which is no longer in clinical use. Muscle relaxants currently in use are listed in Table 24.2. In general, the shorter acting agents have become very popular as they are relatively easy to control and have almost no hemodynamic side effects. For most operations requiring endotracheal intubation, the anesthesia team will administer a sedative hypnotic (typically propofol), ascertain that it is possible to adequately ventilate the patient while he or she is asleep and then administer an intubating dose (see typical induction protocol) of a nondepolarizing agent understanding that they will have to wait about 2 to 3 minutes until the patient is adequately relaxed to easily intubate.

The patient can be monitored by stimulating a nerve and muscle group and evaluating the twitches. The most common method is to use a small battery-powered nerve stimulator on the ulnar nerve and to evaluate contraction of the abductor pollicis muscles (thumb). If you stimulate a normal nerve four times, you will see four strong contractions of the thumb (train of four). With nondepolarizing muscle relaxants, the number and strength will fade. When they start to return, additional drug can be administered if necessary. This same device can easily be used to evaluate a patient in the ICU who has been treated with muscle relaxants.

At the end of surgery, full muscle strength is needed to successfully extubate the patient. This is assessed by clinical criteria (the ability of the patient to maintain his or her head elevated, tidal volume, respiratory rate, etc.) and with the neuromuscular blockade monitor (i.e., full return of four twitches). Muscle relaxant can be allowed to wear off based on pharmacokinetics. There are also antagonists that can assist in reversing the action of neuromuscular blockade. These drugs are cholinesterase inhibitors that inhibit the breakdown of acetylcholine. The neuromuscular blockers compete with acetylcholine for the neuromuscular junction. If acetycholine is not broken down, its concentration increases, and it is able to more effectively compete for binding sites. These drugs, neostigmine and edrophonium, tend to cause bradycardia, so they are coadministered with glycopyrolate and atropine, respectively to prevent severe slowing of the heart rate. It is not routinely required to administer reversal agents to all patients who are given neuromuscular blockers.

A patient who is extubated with muscle relaxant activity still present may have a very difficult time breathing. She or he might not even be able to tell you that she or he is having a hard time breathing if there is insufficient air movement to generate speech. Frequently patients manifest uncoordinated general movements that have been compared to a fish out of water. These patients need to have their ventilation assisted while additional antagonist is administered. Occasionally, these patients need to be reintubated.

## Dexmedetomidine (Precedex in Europe)

In recent years, a sedative analgesic drug that is an alpha 2 agonist has provided an interesting interface between ICU sedation and the OR. Dexmedetomidine was initially approved only for the sedation of intubated patients in the ICU (Carollo, Nossaman, & Ramadhyani, 2008). As such, patients would be started on dexmedetomidine infusions prior to the end of surgery, primarily cardiac surgery, and brought to the ICU intubated. The patient would then be extubated at which point the dexmedetomidine is discontinued. As an alpha 2 agent, dexmedetomidine produces a type of sedation that is

## 24.2   Some Properties of Muscle Relaxants

| Drug | Intubation Dose (mg/kg) | Time Until Ready to Intubate After Intubating Dose (min) | Duration of Intubating Dose (min) | Maintenance Dosing by Infusion (mg/kg/min) |
|---|---|---|---|---|
| Rocuronium | 0.6–1.0 | 1.5 | 35–75 | 9–12 |
| Mivacurium | 0.2–0.25 | 2.5–3.0 | 15–20 | 4–15 |
| Atracurium | 0.5–0.6 | 2.5–3.0 | 30–45 | 5–12 |
| Cisatracurium | 0.15–0.2 | 2.0–3.0 | 40–75 | 1–2 |
| Vecuronium | 0.–0.2 | 2.0–3.0 | 45–90 | 1–2 |
| Pancuronium | 0.08–0.12 | 2.0–3.0 | 60–120 | N/A |
| Pipecuronium | 0.08–0.1 | 2.0–3.0 | 80–120 | N/A |
| Doxacurium | 0.05–0.07 | 4.0–5.0 | 90–150 | N/A |

distinct from benzodiazepines or other sedative hypnotics in that the patient appears more like a person taking a nap. Patients awaken with less drowsiness. Dexmedetomidine has been shown to decrease the incidence of ICU delirium (see below, and chapter 26 this text) and is currently under study to prevent postoperative delirium. Dexmedetomidine is also becoming popular for certain surgical procedures, such as deep brain stimulator implantation.

### Hemodynamic Stability During Anesthesia

Maintaining an appropriate blood pressure and heart rate is a core goal of anesthesia and one of the more challenging aspects of anesthetic care for older patients. Blood pressure commonly decreases in all patients following the induction of general anesthesia. The decrease in blood pressure occurs primarily because of a decrease in sympathetic tone, which in turn is associated with a lower heart rate, decrease systemic vascular resistance, and consequent peripheral pooling of blood, which will lower cardiac preload and hence cardiac output. There is also some direct myocardial depression. All of these effects are exaggerated in older adults, particularly hypertensive elderly patients. When the blood pressure is very low, the anesthetic level can only be decreased so far before the patient either moves or has recall of intraoperative events. Movement is frequently prevented with muscle relaxants, but, just like in the ICU, it is vital to provide amnesia when the patient is paralyzed. It is possible to use vasopressor infusions during general anesthesia. Supporting the blood pressure allows the use of general anesthetic agents. Very unstable patients, however, will not tolerate volatile anesthetics. In those cases, either a benzodiazepine, typically midazolam, or scopolamine will be administered to minimize recall (Silverstein & McLeskey, 1996).

Intravenous fluids are administered in larger quantities and more consistently than any other drug in the operating room. There are large varieties of intravenous fluids available. Most anesthesia teams use a multiple electrolyte solution (Na+, Cl-, Mg++, K+) with some base precursor (lactate, gluconate, or acetate). Some solutions, such as Ringer's lactate, contain calcium. Solutions containing primarily salts are called crystalloids (normal saline, Ringer's lactate, Plasmalyte, etc.). When administered, these fluids distribute widely throughout the body. The other major class of fluids contains large molecules that attract or maintain fluid in the intravascular space and are therefore called colloids (hetastarch, gelatin, albumin). The argument over whether to give crystalloids or colloids has been raging in the anesthesia and surgical literature for almost 50 years. Local practices still vary significantly. In the last few years, a number of investigators have suggested that too much fluid is administered to patients during and after surgical procedures, particularly for the older adult (Holte & Kehlet, 2006). Both excess and insufficient fluids are more noticeable in geriatric patients; however, there is no consensus on a means of determining an appropriate amount of fluid. Recent evidence suggests that excess fluid is commonly administered in the operating room and the first 72 hours of intensive care stay. Excess salt and water can be associated with morbidity and mortality in the intensive care unit and specifically with pulmonary edema, postoperative ileus, and delayed wound healing. The restricted fluid regimens tend toward a total of 2 liters of fluid per day, as opposed to 3 or more in most standard regimens. The most recent tendency among anesthesia personnel appears to favor less fluid (Brandstrup et al., 2003; Holte & Kehlet, 2006; Shields, 2008).

The most commonly used drug to elevate blood pressure for a short period of time is ephedrine. Ephedrine stimulates both alpha and beta receptors and effectively raises pressure, but, because it acts by stimulating the release of catecholamines from the nerve ending, the effect wears off. Ephedrine cannot be used as an infusion. Phenylephrine, a pure alpha agonist, can be conveniently given as either a bolus or a low-dose infusion and effectively maintains blood pressure. Phenylephrine appears to be more popular among anesthesia personnel than norepinephrine, the drug that is most similar. All pressors have potential adverse effects, of course, but serious problems from their use are infrequent.

The elderly have less capacity to defend their core body temperature than younger patients (Sessler, 2008). The elderly are particularly prone to thermal disturbance during anesthesia, with hypothermia being the most common problem. Anesthetic drugs impair the ability to maintain normal body temperature. These same systems appear diminished in aging. In the absence of some effort to warm the patient, the elderly will lose 2 to 4 °C, over a 1 to 2 hour surgical case. Hypothermia causes shivering and decreases drug metabolism, slowing emergence from anesthesia. Outcomes research suggests that hypothermia is associated with an increased incidence of myocardial infarction, increased infections, increased blood loss, and longer hospitalization (Sessler, 1993). Therefore maintaining a normal body temperature, usually with forced air warming blankets, is considered a standard of care.

Atelectasis occurs in almost all patients undergoing general anesthesia and older adults are particularly vulnerable. Blood flow through the lungs is controlled to perfuse those alveoli that are ventilated, but the effectiveness of hypoxic pulmonary vasoconstriction is reduced by volatile anesthetics. In addition, mechanical ventilation disturbs the normal pattern of diaphragmatic breathing in the supine patient, altering normal ventilation/perfusion matching. Ciliary action, which is responsible for the removal of particulate mater from the respiratory tract, is diminished into the postoperative period by both volatile anesthetics and the placement of an endotracheal tube. Very frail patients are at increased risk for ventilatory failure postoperatively. Finally, silent regurgitation and aspiration are more common in older patients (Smetana, Lawrence, & Cornell, 2006). Aspiration is much more likely to occur postoperatively than in the operating room. Aspiration will present with some evidence of dysfunction (e.g., hypoxia) within a few hours of the aspiration.

Most pulmonary problems occur after surgery. End tidal and arterial $CO_2$ are frequently increased in the immediate postoperative period, particularly if narcotics were administered. This finding is usually benign and an indication of good analgesia. Supplemental oxygen should be administered and the patient watched carefully. Supplemental oxygen should be considered for a longer period of time after surgery in older patients. Pneumonia is the most common and important complication in the elderly and the ability to prevent it is limited. Deep breathing and vigorous coughing by the patient are thought to help prevent pneumonia, but postoperative pain and pain medication may make these maneuvers difficult. Improved pain control may be one mechanism by which epidural analgesia improves perioperative outcome (see section on Postoperative Analgesia) (Lawrence, Cornell, & Smetana, 2006). The role of silent aspiration in the development of postoperative pneumonia is unclear and warrants closer examination.

# Regional Anesthesia

Regional anesthesia techniques include topical anesthesia (surface), infiltration, plexus block, epidural (extradural) block, and spinal anesthesia. Many procedures in the elderly, such as cataract surgery, can be done with local anesthetic drops and no additional sedation. Neuraxial blocks, including spinal and epidural anesthesia, are considered complete anesthetics; no other supplemental treatment is necessary. Most patients request sedation and anesthesia practitioners usually provide some additional sedation. Spinal anesthesia differs from epidural anesthesia in the location of anesthetic administration, the amount of anesthetic used, and on the resulting clinical manifestations of treatment. With spinal anesthesia, the local anesthetic is injected into the cerebrospinal fluid, inside the dura and arachnoid space, where it quickly diffuses into the spinal nerves. Small doses of local anesthetic effectively block all nerve fibers, including motor, touch, and sympathetic nerves. The results are anesthesia, paralysis, and sympathetic blockade.

Epidural anesthetic is usually administered through a catheter placed just outside the dura mater. In the epidural space, spinal nerves are covered with a thick connective tissue, so large quantities of anesthetic are needed and the onset is much slower. By using different concentrations of the injected local anesthetic, nerve types can be differentially blocked. This is important for postoperative analgesia, where partial blockade of pain fibers is desired, but sensation and motor activity need to be preserved.

Regional anesthetic techniques can be combined with general anesthesia. In combined general/regional anesthesia, the patient is first given a high thoracic epidural anesthetic following which general anesthesia is induced. Because the epidural provides complete analgesia, very little general anesthetic is required and the patient wakes up pain free. The epidural catheter is then used to manage postoperative pain. It is also common to place an epidural catheter exclusively for postoperative pain control, which is not used as part of the anesthesia and only activated at the end of surgery.

## Regional Versus General Anesthesia

Regional and general anesthesia are such different approaches that it is hard to believe that the outcomes for these procedures would be the same. Some anesthesia team members are extremely partial to one technique or another. Markers of stress such as cortisol, catecholamines and cytokines become elevated during and after surgery with a general anesthetic, whereas spinal and epidural anesthesia markedly attenuate these changes during surgery, and much of the attenuation will continue after surgery if epidural analgesia is continued postoperatively (Bonnet, 1993). Multiple studies comparing regional versus general anesthesia have attempted to show a benefit to one over the other (usually the authors believe regional is superior). Several of the studies demonstrated lower mortality and morbidity with respect to cardiac and pulmonary complications. Other studies have demonstrated additional benefits of regional anesthesia, including reduced blood loss during hip-replacement surgery, a decreased incidence of deep vein thrombosis and pulmonary emboli, and a reduction in early graft thrombosis in peripheral vascular surgery. Not all studies demonstrate consistent benefits, however (Silverstein, 2008). On balance, the current evidence of the benefit of postoperative epidural analgesia is weak, as is the evidence of the superiority of neuraxial anesthesia over general anesthesia as the primary anesthetic technique. Nevertheless, better pain relief is usually achieved by regional techniques, and it is still possible that some medical benefits exist with this approach.

## Postoperative Delirium and Postoperative Cognitive Dysfunction

Although ICU delirium and long-term cognitive change following ICU care are an important and related issue (see: www.icudelirium.org), it is valuable for the ICU nurse to be aware of the distinctions among emergence delirium, postoperative delirium, and postoperative cognitive dysfunction (POCD) (Silverstein, Timberger, Reich, & Uysal, 2007). In a variety of patients, perhaps primarily in children, emergence is associated with extreme disinhibition and inability to follow direction. Patients may wake up extremely agitated, trying to get off the OR table, and pulling out intravenous lines. This phenomenon is called emergence delirium or emergence excitation. It is not common in the elderly and is rarely found to have any long-term consequences. Such patients usually respond well to additional sedation and a slower emergence from anesthesia (Silverstein et al.).

After an interval of lucidity, elderly patients have a tendency to develop delirium 24 to 72 hours following surgery. Delirium is a disturbance in consciousness that is not accounted for by dementia and that develops in a short time and fluctuates during the day. The hyperactive form of delirium is easily noted by even casual observers; however, the hypoactive form, in which the patient is disoriented but quiet, is frequently ignored or misdiagnosed as depression or dementia. Postoperative delirium is associated with poor outcomes and additional medical costs. Interventions by geriatricians, including the management of multiple medications and attention to geriatric issues, have decreased the incidence of delirium in hip-fracture patients, but this activity has not spread to the ICU (Marcantonio et al., 2001).

Postoperative cognitive dysfunction (see chapter 26, this volume), unlike delirium, is not a clinical diagnosis but rather a research finding. Although much discussed, patients must undergo preoperative neurocognitive testing to determine if deterioration is present. Most patients do not have such tests in the absence of a research study. Nonetheless, in elderly patients, depending on when the patient is tested, some level of measureable impairment is found. In the largest studies of elective major surgery under general anesthesia, approximately 10% of patients have measureable decline 3 months following surgery (Monk et al., 2008). Whether postoperative delirium leads to cognitive decline and is a means to prevent cognitive change awaits future research.

## Summary

Perioperative care of older adult patients is a new area of focus for anesthesiologists and surgeons. We hope that within the next decade we will be making decisions based on high-quality evidence. Until that time, a fair amount of information has permitted surgeons and anesthesiologists to operate on progressively older patients with good success. As such, these patients will be coming to the ICU and some will be coming from the ICU to the operating room. ICU nurses will improve their ability to care for the elderly surgical patient by understanding the interests and concerns of the anesthesia team and serving as professional communicator among the many professionals caring for ICU patients today.

## References

Bonnet, F. (1993). Endocrine-metabolic response to abdominal aortic surgery: A randomized trial of general anesthesia versus general plus epidural anesthesia. Invited commentary. *World Journal of Surgery, 17*, 606–607.

Brandstrup, B., Tonnesen, H., Beier-Holgersen, R., Hjortso, E., Ording, H., Lindorff-Larsen, K., et al. (2003). Effects of intravenous fluid restriction on postoperative complications: Comparison of two perioperative fluid regimens: A randomized assessor-blinded multicenter trial. *Annals of Surgery, 238*(5), 641–648.

Carollo, D. S., Nossaman, B. D., & Ramadhyani, U. (2008). Dexmedetomidine: A review of clinical applications. *Current Opinion in Anaesthesiology, 21*(4), 457–461.

Hilton, D., Iman, N., Burke, G. J., Moore, A., O'Mara, G., Signorini, D., et al. (2001). Absence of abdominal pain in older persons with endoscopic ulcers: A prospective study. *American Journal Gastroenterology, 96*(2), 380–384.

Holte, K., & Kehlet, H. (2006). Fluid therapy and surgical outcomes in elective surgery: A need for reassessment in fast-track surgery. *Journal of the American College of Surgeons, 202*(6), 971–989.

Kaarlola, A., Tallgren, M., & Pettila, V. (2006). Long-term survival, quality of life, and quality-adjusted life-years among critically ill elderly patients. *Critical Care Medicine, 34*(8), 2120–2126.

Kleinpell, R. M., & Ferrans, C. E. (2002). Quality of life of elderly patients after treatment in the ICU. *Research in Nursing & Health, 25*(3), 212–221.

Lawrence, V. A., Cornell, J. E., & Smetana, G. W. (2006). Strategies to reduce postoperative pulmonary complications after noncardiothoracic surgery: Systematic review for the American College of Physicians. *Annals of Internal Medicine, 144*(8), 596–608.

Lawrence, V. A., Hazuda, H. P., Cornell, J. E., Pederson, T., Bradshaw, P. T., Mulrow, C. D., et al. (2004). Functional independence after major abdominal surgery in the elderly. *Journal of the American College of Surgeons, 199*(5), 762–772.

Lawton, M. P., & Brody, E. M. (1969). Assessment of older people: Self-maintaining and instrumental activities of daily living. *The Gerontologist, 9*, 179–186.

Lindeman, R. D. (1993). Renal physiology and pathophysiology of aging. *Contributions to Nephrology, 105*, 1–12.

Marcantonio, E. R., Flacker, J. M., Wright, R .J., & Resnick, N .M. (2001). Reducing delirium after hip fracture: A randomized trial. *Journal of the American Geriatrics Society, 49*(5), 516–522.

Marcantonio, E. R., Juarez, G., Goldman, L., Mangione, C. M., Ludwig, L. E., Lind, L., et al. (1994). The relationship of postoperative delirium with psychoactive medications [see comments]. *Journal of the American Medical Association, 272,* 1518–1522.

Monk, T. G., Weldon, B. C., Garvan, C. W., Dede, D. E., van der Aa, M.T., Heilman, K. M., et al. (2008). Predictors of cognitive dysfunction after major noncardiac surgery. *Anesthesiology, 108*(1), 18–30.

Muravchick, S. (1997). *Geroanesthesia. Principles for management of the elderly patient.* St. Louis: Mosby.

Parker, L. J., Vukov, L. F., & Wollan, P. C. (1997). Emergency department evaluation of geriatric patients with acute cholecystitis. *Academic Emergency Medicine, 4*(1), 51–55.

Reuben, D. B., Herr, K. A., Pacala, J. T., Pollock, B. G., Potter, J. F., & Semla, T .P. (2006). *Geriatrics at your fingertips.* New York: American Geriatrics Society.

Sessler, D. I. (1993). Perianesthetic thermoregulation and heat balance in humans. *FASEB Journal, 7,* 638–644.

Sessler, D. I. (2008). Perioperative thermoregulation. In J. H. Silverstein, G. A. Rooke, J. G. Reves, & C. H. McLeskey (Eds.), *Geriatric anesthesiology* (pp. 107–122) New York: Springer Publishing Company.

Shields, C. J. (2008). Towards a new standard of perioperative fluid management. *Therapeutics and Clinical Risk Management, 4*(2), 569–571.

Silverstein, J. H. 2008. The practice of geriatric anesthesia. In J. H. Silverstein, G. A. Rooke, J. G. Reves, & C. H. McLeskey (Eds.), *Geriatric anesthesiology* (pp. 3–14). New York: Springer Publishing Company.

Silverstein, J. H., & McLeskey, C. H. (1996). Geriatric trauma. *Current Opinion in Anaestesiology 9,* 192–197.

Silverstein, J. H., Timberger, M., Reich, D. L., & Uysal, S. (2007). Central nervous system dysfunction after noncardiac surgery and anesthesia in the elderly. *Anesthesiology, 106*(3), 622–628.

Smetana, G .W., Lawrence, V. A., & Cornell, J. E. (2006). Preoperative pulmonary risk stratification for noncardiothoracic surgery: Systematic review for the American College of Physicians. *Annals of Internal Medicine, 144*(8), 581–595.

# Acute Respiratory Failure and Mechanical Ventilation in the Elderly

# 25

Jill Kamen

## Case Study

Mr. R. is a 74-year-old former smoker who presented to the emergency department with acute shortness of breath and a fever. He has a long history of smoking, chronic obstructive pulmonary disease (COPD), hypertension, hypercholesterolemia, and congestive heart failure. The medications he takes at home are a bronchodilator, Hydrochlorthiazide, Simvastatin and Altase. Mr. R. stopped smoking 6 years ago and uses supplemental oxygen at home. He lives alone with his two dogs, which he walks several times per day. His son lives nearby with a wife and two young children, ages 14 and 9. Mr. R.'s daughter lives 4 hours away.

Mr. R. was placed on 4 L of oxygen via a nasal cannula. He was awake, alert, oriented but anxious. His vital signs were blood pressure (BP) 144/90, sinus tachycardia 108, arterial oxygen saturation (SaO)$_2$ of 90%, respiratory rate (RR) of 32, and temperature of 102.4°F. His breath sounds revealed distant breath sounds in his right lower lobe and rhonchi. He says that he had been coughing up sputum for several weeks, having fevers, and feeling fatigued. Blood work, including an arterial blood gas, was obtained as well as a sputum sample. A chest X-ray was ordered.

While awaiting the results of the lab tests Mr. R.'s $SaO_2$ decreased to 88%. Despite his son's efforts to reassure him, Mr. R. became agitated. When asked about a health care directive, his son said that his father did not want one and that he wanted to return to his dogs and watch his grandson's baseball games. Noninvasive positive pressure ventilation was initiated via face mask on assist control with pressure support. Mr. R. kept removing the face mask and a nasal mask was attempted. The respiratory therapist and nurse monitored Mr. R. for a decrease in dyspnea, tachypnea, and a return to his baseline mental status. After 20 minutes a blood gas was obtained indicating a worsening of acidemia and hypercarbia from the baseline results obtained on arrival to the emergency department.

Mr. R. was sedated, intubated, and transferred to the ICU. Mr. R.'s blood gases stabilized using the assist-control mode, pressure support, and positive end expiratory pressure (PEEP). Right lower lobe pneumonia was noted on the chest X-ray and antibiotics were started. A nasogastric tube was inserted and placed on intermittent suction. The medical, nursing staff, and respiratory therapists monitored Mr. R. closely for his fever to resolve and his chest X-ray to improve. On the fifth day of ICU care, the physicians decided to observe Mr. R. for several more days before deciding on a tracheotomy.

On day 7, Mr. R. was alert, afebrile, and his X-ray showed marked improvement. His tube feedings and sedation were discontinued and his ventilator settings were weaned to about half of what they had been. A spontaneous breathing trial was performed for 60 minutes on continuous positive airway pressure (CPAP). The nurse stayed with Mr. R. during the trial providing reassurance and closely monitoring him for ominous signs of hemodynamic instability, increased dyspnea, tachypnea, and discomfort. Mr. R. tolerated the trial and was extubated.

Mr. R. was transferred out of the ICU and placed on a progressive care unit for monitoring. Plans were made to eventually discharge Mr. R. home with his son. He was looking forward to being reunited with his dogs, which were being cared for at his son's house. Mr. R.'s long-term plans included securing a health care directive and attending his grandson's baseball game the following summer.

---

Elderly patients comprise 48% of all critical care admissions, with respiratory failure as the primary reason for critical care admissions (El Solh & Ramadan, 2006). As the prevalence of serious respiratory disease (chronic obstructive pulmonary disease [COPD], pneumonia) increases with age, older adults are increasingly likely to develop respiratory failure requiring mechanical ventilation (Sevransky & Haponik, 2003). Improved medical therapies in the treatments of myocardial infarction, congestive heart failure, renal failure, neurological disorders, and cancer have led to increased patient survival in an aging population with compromised pulmonary reserve resulting from the usual aging processes (Sevransky & Haponik). The decision to provide mechanical ventilation to an elderly patient is multidimensional and patient and family decisions and outcomes must be weighed carefully. A team approach that

| 25.1 | Normative Physiological Alterations of the Respiratory System With Aging | |
|---|---|---|
| **Structural** | | |
| Chest wall | Decreased compliance | |
| | Barrel chest | |
| | Decreased diaphragm strength | |
| | Increased energy needed for work of breathing | |
| Lung parenchyma | Decreased elasticity | |
| | Distal airway collapse sooner in expiration | |
| | Fewer gas exchange surfaces | |
| **Lung function** | | |
| Spirometry | Increased residual volume (RV) | |
| | Increased functional residual capacity (FRC) | |
| | Decreased vital capacity (VC) | |
| | Decreased forced expiratory volume in 1 sec./forced vital capacity ($FEV_1$/FVC) | |
| | Decreased maximal expiratory flow | |
| Blunted responses to breathing regulation | Decreased perception of hypoxia | |
| | Decreased perception of hypercarbia | |
| | Decreased tidal volume at rest | |
| | Decreased respiratory rate at rest | |
| Alterations in defense | Reduced cough effectiveness | |
| | Decrease in mucociliary clearance | |
| | Altered mucous gland activity | |
| | Decreased immune function | |

*Note.* From Jindal (2006) and Sue (2000).

includes geriatric specialists is essential to coordinate the skills of multiple health care professionals.

## Pathophysiology

Usual aging affects the structure, function, response to breathing regulation, and lung defenses. Structural changes include those affecting the parenchyma and chest wall and are functionally significant. Changes in lung function include alterations in lung volumes and capacities as reflected in pulmonary function studies. Changes occur in the ability to regulate breathing and to defend against invading organisms. A summary of changes may be found in Table 25.1. The anatomical and physiological changes of the respiratory system that occur with usual aging greatly affect the occurrence and course of disease process in the elderly. More than any other body system, it is difficult to distinguish among usual age-related changes in the respiratory system, make accurate predications of a rate of decline, and define age-appropriate norms (Zeleznik, 2003). Although changes in the respiratory system associated with usual aging may become evident in situations in which physiologic demand reaches the limits of supply, there is no evidence that they impact day-to-day function of the older adult (Zeleznik).

## Chest Wall and Lung Parenchyma

The most important physiological changes associated with aging are a decrease in elastic recoil of the lung, a decrease in compliance of the chest wall, a decrease in respiratory muscle strength and endurance, early alveolar collapse on exhalation, and fewer gas exchange surfaces (Janssens, Pache, & Nicod, 1999; Resnick, 2005). Chest wall compliance decreases progressively with age because of structural changes of the rib cage, including calcification of the joints of the ribs with the sternum and spinal column and osteoporosis of vertebrae leading to age-related kyphosis (El Solh & Ramadan, 2006; Janssens et al.). The increased rigidity leads to an increased chest anteroposterior diameter and a barrel chest appearance. An increased anteroposterior diameter flattens the curve of the diaphragm requiring increased amounts of energy for the same amount of respiratory work. Diaphragmatic strength is reduced by approximately 10 to 20% in healthy older adults with a mean age of 73 (Polkey et al., 1997). These changes are compounded by a loss of type II A muscle fibers (Resnick) and degenerative changes in the nutritional status (Berend, 2005). The result is a decrease in muscle strength and endurance and an increased work of breathing (El Solh & Ramadan; Resnick; Sevransky & Haponik, 2003). Moreover, those who are inactive, such as those receiving mechanical ventilation, lose more muscle mass than those who are active and of a similar age (Hébuterne, Bermon, & Schneider, 2001). The increased amount of energy needed for respiratory work predisposes the elderly to difficulties in ventilator weaning and respiratory ailments (El Solh & Ramadan).

In addition to changes in the chest wall, changes occur in the lung parenchyma. Changes that occur with aging in the lung parenchyma relate to changes in the elastic fiber network with a resultant loss of elastic recoil (Berend, 2005; Janssens et al., 1999). This results in an increase in the diameter of alveolar ducts, whereas the alveolar sacs become wider and shallower (Berend; El Solh & Ramadan, 2006; Janssens et al.; Resnick, 2005). The flattening of the alveoli is associated with a loss of as much as 20% of the alveolar surface area (Berend; Janssens et al.; Resnick). The dilatation of the alveolar ducts and enlargement of the airspaces produce similar changes in lung compliance to that of emphysema, but is more homogeneous and differs histologically from emphysema (Janssens et al.). All of these changes result in a tendency for distal airway collapse sooner in expiration and fewer gas exchange surfaces.

## Laboratory Tests

Pulmonary function tests (PFTs) measure lung volumes and airflow and change with usual aging. Structural changes in both the lung parenchyma as well as the chest wall lead to predictable alterations in PFTs (see Table 25.1). The stiffer, less compliant chest wall combined with the more distensible lungs result in an increased residual volume of 50% caused by air trapping between the ages of 20 to 70 (Janssens et al., 1999). The residual volume (RV) is the amount of air remaining in the lungs after forced expiration. The functional residual capacity (FRC) is the volume of air remaining in the lungs at the end of a normal exhalation. Both the RV and the FRC increase in the elderly (El Solh & Ramadan, 2006; Janssens et al.; Jindal, 2006; Resnick, 2005). The forced vital capacity (FVC) is the amount of air that can be quickly and forcefully exhaled after maximum inspiration and the forced expiratory volume (FEV)$_1$ is the FVC in 1 second. The $FEV_1$ decreases by 10 to 30 mL per year beginning at age 30 (Burrows, Knudsen,

<table>
<tr><td colspan="5">

**25.2** Arterial Blood Gas Reference Values* for Healthy Elderly Persons

</td></tr>
</table>

| | Men | | Women | |
|---|---|---|---|---|
| | Mean (*SD*) | Lower Limit | Mean (*SD*) | Lower Limit |
| PaO$_2$ mmHg | 77.0 (9.1) | 62 | 73.5 (8.4) | 59.6 |
| SaO$_2$% | 95.3 (1.4) | 93 | 94.8 (1.7) | |
| PaCO$_2$ mmHg | 39.0 (3.0) | 39.8 (3.6) | | |

*Clinical application of these values may need to be validated for each laboratory.

*Note.* Adapted with permission from Hardie et al. (2004).

Camilli, Lyle, & Lebowitz, 1987) and is accelerated in smokers. The FEV$_1$/FVC ratio decreases by approximately 0.2% each year (Janssens et al.). Changes in the FVC and the peak expiratory flow rate, the maximum airflow rate during forced expiration, are related to changes in body weight and strength as opposed to changes in the lung parenchyma (Resnick). There is a decrease in vital capacity (VC), the maximum volume of air exhaled after a maximum inspiration (El Solh & Ramadan; Jindal; Resnick) by about 75% of best values. Changes in PFTs reflect changes in lung tissue, body weight, and strength.

Accurate reference values for arterial blood gases in the elderly have been the subject of much discussion over the past decade (Janssens et al., 1999; Zeleznik, 2003). Aging was classically thought to be accompanied by a decline in PaO$_2$ (Resnick, 2005; Sorbini, Grassi, Slinas, & Muiesan, 1968; Sue, 2000), however, recent studies (Cerveri et al., 1995; Guenard & Marthan, 1996; Hardie, Vollmer, & Buist, 2004) have found no significant correlation between PaO$_2$ and age. The American Thoracic Society advocates that reference values be based on subjects who are representative of the general healthy population (American Thoracic Society, 1991). The deviations in reference values from past findings are thought to relate to the extrapolations of values from the inclusion of young subjects and those with pulmonary disease and comorbidities, the variability of the blood gas analyzers, and the position of the subject during blood gas sampling (Hardie et al.). Hardie et al. measured arterial blood gases and spirometry values in 146 healthy elderly subjects ranging from 70 years of age to more than 90 years and found that PaO$_2$ and the SaO$_2$ are age independent, but gender specific (values for women are lower than for men) with no significant changes with age in the PaCO$_2$ (see Table 25.2). Caution must be used in interpreting these results as clinical application of these values may need to be validated for each laboratory and ideally each laboratory should establish its own reference values (Hardie et al.). The presence of hypercarbia and respiratory acidosis should always be considered pathological (El Solh & Ramadan, 2006; Zeleznik).

## Breathing Regulation

Breathing regulation alters in the elderly (Janssens et al., 1999; Jindal, 2006; Sue, 2000). Normal elderly persons have a minute ventilation identical to that of younger persons at rest, but use lower tidal volumes and higher respiratory rates (Janssens et al.). Ventilatory responses to hypoxemia and hypercarbia decrease with aging (Jindal; Sevransky & Haponik, 2003) and make older persons vulnerable to effects of sedation. Aging is also associated with a decline in the ability to perceive bronchoconstriction (Janssens et al.). Blunting of the hypoxia and hypercapnia responses as well as a lower ability to perceive bronchoconstriction decreases the elders' protective mechanisms (Janssens et al.)

## Defense Against Invading Organisms

The respiratory system in the older adult is particularly prone to infection. The changes are caused by decreased mechanical function as well as immunological changes. Reduced cough effectiveness along with a decrease in mucociliary clearance and altered mucous gland activity predispose elderly patients to pneumonia (Jindal, 2006; Sue, 2000). Malnutrition further predisposes the elderly to infections as a result of impaired cellular and humoral immunity. Decreased respiratory muscle strength is a consequence of protein–calorie, trace element, and vitamin deficiency (Sue). Diminished nutritional intake may stem from a disinterest in eating, social problems, financial limitations, chronic illness, and gastrointestinal problems (Sue). A lack of antioxidant vitamins and trace elements has been associated with lung injury. Patients who are malnourished are more likely to have respiratory failure and patients with chronic lung diseases who have respiratory failure are more likely to be malnourished (Sue). Furthermore, because of a decreased dietary intake of antioxidants, the elderly may have a suboptimal immune function and so have less protection against infection (Sue).

## Respiratory Failure

The elderly are predisposed to ventilatory failure because of decreased elastic recoil of the lungs, loss of supporting airway structure, stiffening of the rib cage, and decreased muscle mass (McNally, 2000). Acute respiratory failure (ARF) refers to the inablity to eliminate $CO_2$ (hypercapneic) or bring in $O_2$ (hypoxic) (McNally). Common causes of hypercapnic respiratory failure in the elderly are chronic obstructive pulmonary disease, asthma, sedation, as well as central nervous system (stroke) and neuromuscular disorders (Arbour, 2007; Delerme & Ray, 2008; Sevransky & Haponik, 2003; Sue, 2000). Common causes of hypoxemic respiratory failure include pneumonia, cardiogenic pulmonary edema, and acute respiratory distress syndrome (ARDS) (Arbour; Delerme & Ray; Sevransky & Haponik; Sue). Conditions associated with ARDS include noncardiogenic pulmonary edema, aspiration of gastric contents, sepsis, hypotension, shock, and inhalation of toxic gas (Arbour). Acute respiratory failure has traditionally been defined as a partial pressure of oxygen in arterial blood ($PaO_2$) < 60 mmHg and/or a partial pressure of carbon dioxide in arterial blood ($PaCO_2$) > 45 mmHg (Delerme & Ray; Urden, Stacy, & Lough, 2006). These values serve as a general guide and must be placed within the context of the patient's history and clinical findings. The most common cause of ventilatory failure in the elderly is most likely an increased work of breathing (WOB) associated with COPD (McNally). Other causes include decreased respiratory muscle strength, a lack of a central drive to breathe (e.g., drug toxicity), and an increased $CO_2$ production as a result of fever or agitation. In addition to blood gas analysis, clinical criteria indicative of ARF include a gradual worsening of symptoms such as polypnea > 30 per minute, contraction of the accessory (inspiratory) muscles, abdominal respiration, orthopnea, cyanosis, and asterixis (Delerme & Ray; McNally, 2000). The incidence of endotracheal intubation following hypoxic ARF may be as high as 40%, therefore, patients should be managed in an area where intensive care unit (ICU) staff and equipment are immediately available (Confalonieri et al., 1999).

# Mechanical Ventilation

Positive pressure ventilation (PPV) is the mainstay treatment for respiratory failure. Positive pressure provides sufficient minute ventilation to those whose ventilatory requirements exceed their sustained ventilator capacities because of increased work of breathing, respiratory muscle fatigue, and inefficient gas exchange. Positive pressure ventilation may be provided through cuffed orotracheal or nasotracheal intubation or noninvasively through nasal or face mask.

The goal of mechanical ventilation is to correct gas exchange and rest the respiratory muscles while concomitant pharmacologic intervention is administered to correct the underlying condition that resulted in the respiratory failure (Abou-Shala & Meduri, 1996). During the past decade, a great deal of research has focused on the effectiveness of noninvasive means of delivering positive pressure ventilation. Traditionally, an endotracheal tube is inserted into the trachea to deliver the ventilator breath to the lungs, however, noninvasive ventilation delivered through a face or nasal mask is a safe and effective means of ventilatory support for many patients with acute respiratory failure, especially related to COPD and should be considered prior to endotracheal intubation (Abou-Shala & Meduri; Evans et al., 2001; Girault et al., 2003; Peter, Moran, & Phillips-Hughes, 2002). Although it is often difficult to determine which patients with acute respiratory failure will require prolonged mechanical ventilation (PMV), endotracheal intubation remains the undisputed treatment of choice for long-term support (Abou-Shala & Meduri). To determine the delivery method of mechanical ventilation, the overall clinical status of the patient is considered, including the deterioration of mental status, signs of respiratory muscle fatigue, and/or deterioration of blood gases (Abou-Shala & Meduri).

## Noninvasive Positive Pressure Ventilation

The decision to begin noninvasive positive pressure ventilation (NPPV) for patients in acute respiratory failure depends on the presence of dyspnea, tachypnea, use of accessory muscles, paradoxical abdominal motion, and arterial blood gases (Abou-Shala & Meduri, 1996). The response and duration of treatment for those receiving NPPV cannot be predicted by the severity of the underlying lung disease or by arterial blood gas values obtained prior to the initiation of treatment (Abou-Shala & Meduri, 1996) . As opposed to traditional endotracheal intubation, the noninvasive nature of NPPV allows for easy, rapid application in the clinical setting.

NPPV has been used in patients with acute exacerbations of COPD, chronic respiratory failure secondary to COPD, postextubation or postoperative ARF, asthma, noncardiogenic and cardiogenic pulmonary edema, community-acquired pneumonia,

## 25.3 Contraindications for Noninvasive Mechanical Ventilation

Absent respirations

High oxygen requirements (advanced ARDS)

Facial trauma

Hemodynamic or electrocardiographic instability, including unstable angina or acute MI

Inability to maintain a patent airway

Inability to properly fit the mask resulting in air leakage

Poor patient cooperation

Morbid obesity (>200% of ideal body weight)

Patients unable to remove the mask in the event of vomiting (including those restrained)

*Note.* From Abou-Shala and Meduri (1996), Fenstermacher and Hong (2004), Rady (2005), and Urden et al. (2006).

opportunistic pneumonia in AIDS patients, obesity hypoventilation syndrome, and obstructive sleep apnea (Abou-Shala & Meduri, 1996; Fenstermacher & Hong, 2004), however, the efficacy of NPPV in patients with hypercapnic COPD has demonstrated the best results so far. NPPV successfully avoids intubation in patients with varied etiologies of ARF between 50 to 65% of the time (Benhamou, Girault, Faure, Portier, & Muir, 1992; Girault et al., 2003; Honrubia et al., 2005; Richard et al., 1999). NPPV may be used for patients in acute respiratory failure who refuse endotracheal intubation but still desire some palliative ventilatory support, such as those patients with COPD. It is estimated that as many as 20% of all hospitalized patients may be candidates for NPPV (Plant, Owen, & Elliot, 2000a). NPPV decreases the work of breathing without the need for endotracheal intubation and therefore avoids complications associated with intubation such as barotraumas, injury to the upper airways between the endotracheal tube or cuff and the mucosa, nosocomial infections, ventilator-associated pneumonia, the need for continuous sedation, and prolonged immobility (Fenstermacher & Hong). NPPV allows greater patient comfort, is better tolerated, permits talking, and requires less sedation (Fenstermacher & Hong).

NPPV is not appropriate for patients with absent respirations, excessive secretions, high oxygen requirements (advanced ARDS), facial trauma, hemodynamic or electrocardiographic instability (see Table 25.3) (Fenstermacher & Hong, 2004; Rady, 2005). Other contraindications may include the inability to properly fit the mask resulting in air leakage, poor patient cooperation, morbid obesity (more than 200% of ideal body weight), unstable angina, and a patient's inability to remove the mask in the event of vomiting (Abou-Shala & Meduri). Patient cooperation for NPPV is essential to voluntarily synchronize respiratory efforts with the ventilator. Anxiety is common in patients experiencing dyspnea but generally subsides soon after instituting NPPV (Abou-Shala & Meduri, 1996). Patients experiencing extreme anxiety and an inability to cooperate should be sedated and endotracheally intubated.

# Ventilator Modes and Settings

The type of ventilator and choice of mode is based on local expertise and familiarity, and is tailored to the etiology and severity of illness and location of care (Evans et al., 2001). NPPV is commonly delivered using continuous positive airway pressure (CPAP), volume-cycled and pressure-limited modes (see Table 25.4). Ventilatory settings are adjusted to provide the lowest inspiratory pressure or volume needed to produce improved patient comfort as evidenced by the respiratory rate and respiratory muscle unloading, and gas exchange (Evans et al.). CPAP is delivered by a flow generator with a high pressure gas source or using a portable compressor. CPAP prevents the patient's airway pressure from falling to zero and thereby restores the functional residual capacity (FRC). CPAP may be used in the treatment of hypoxemic ARF if the patient has spontaneous respirations.

Pressure-limited modes may be used with NPPV using pressure-controlled ventilation (PCV). Pressure-support ventilation (PSV) may be used when there is poor inspiratory effort. Biphasic positive airway pressure (BiPAP), available on modern ventilators, is effective in the treatment of asthma (Soroksky, Stav, & Shpirer, 2003) and superior to CPAP in the treatment of COPD (Panacek & Kirk, 2002; Wood, 1998). PSV can ensure reliable NPPV provided that lung compliance remains constant. PSV enhances patient comfort and minimizes the side effects incurred with volume-cycled modes. Patients must be closely monitored for hypercapnia as well as air leaks.

NPPV can be delivered using volume modes whereby a ventilator delivers a set tidal volume for each breath with varying inflation pressures. The assist/control mode assists the spontaneously breathing patient by delivering a full preset tidal volume either imposed on or in the presence of inspiratory efforts (Evans et al., 2001). Volume-cycled support can be safely used in patients with changing respiratory impedance, but because peak mask pressure is not limited, there is an overall complication rate of about 10% (Abou-Shala & Meduri, 1996). Complications associated with volume-cycled NPPV include more susceptibility to leaks, pressure sores, and about a 7 to 10% chance of skin necrosis (Abou-Shala & Meduri). Early use of a clear dressing is indicated to prevent skin necrosis that heals spontaneously within 2 to 7 days after discontinuing the mask. Gastric distension, aspiration, conjunctivitis, and pneumothorax occur in <1 to 2% of those receiving NPPV (Abou-Shala & Meduri).

Whereas barotrauma is damage to alveoli caused by high pressure, volutrauma is damage to alveoli caused by high volumes. The elderly may be at greater risk for barotrauma, pulmonary $O_2$ toxicity, and hemodynamic compromise from positive pressure ventilation and positive end-expiratory pressure (PEEP) than younger patients with ARDS of similar severity (Sue, 2000). Therefore, ventilator settings are selected to provide the lowest inspiratory pressures or volumes needed to improve the respiratory rate, respiratory muscle unloading (patient comfort), and gas exchange (Evans et al., 2001). Appropriate ventilator settings are needed to avoid excessive muscle loading and patient–ventilator asynchrony. Common ventilator settings are listed in Table 25.5.

# Patient–Ventilator Interfaces

In acute respiratory failure, NPPV is delivered through use of an oronasal (full-face) mask or a nasal mask (see Table 25.6). NPPV administered through a properly fitted

| 25.4 Common Ventilator Modes | | | |
|---|---|---|---|
| **Mode** | **Description** | **Clinical Application** | **Set by Clinician** |
| Controlled mandatory ventilation (CMV) or control ventilation (CV) | Breaths are delivered at a set rate per minute and a set $V_t$ | Rarely used; patient cannot take spontaneous breaths; used only when patient has no drive to breathe (anesthetized, paralyzed) | Rate, $V_t$, inspiratory time and PEEP |
| Assist control (AC) or assisted mandatory ventilation (AMV) | Machine breaths and spontaneous patient breaths are delivered at the preset $V_t$ | Used in patients when first intubated or emerging from anesthesia, also with neuromuscular disorders, pulmonary edema, and ARF | Rate, inspiratory time, PEEP, sensitivity; patient can be hyperventilated if the rate or $V_t$ are set too high or hypoventilated if the rate or $V_t$ are set too low. The sensitivity must be set so it is not too difficult for the patient to initiate a breath or the patient may tire or develop asynchrony with the ventilator |
| Intermittent mandatory ventilation (IMV) and synchronized intermittent mandatory ventilation (SIMV) | Patient can take spontaneous breaths in between preset machine breaths. Spontaneous patient breaths are at patient's own rate and $V_t$. If synchronized, the ventilator synchronizes patient's spontaneous breaths with the preset ventilator breaths. | Used as a weaning mode. Patient takes on more work of breathing, preventing muscle atrophy, however, patient must be monitored for fatigue associated with spontaneous breathing efforts. May be used with PSV to ease work of breathing. | Rate, $V_t$, inspiratory time, sensitivity, PEEP preset rate must be adequate if patient's spontaneous rate is low to provide adequate ventilation. |

*(continued)*

face or nasal mask can be as effective as mechanical ventilation delivered through an endotracheal tube in patients with acute respiratory failure (Abou-Shala & Meduri, 1996) and uses lower pressures than those needed to overcome the resistance of an endotracheal tube (Abou-Shala & Meduri). Face masks should fit firmly, but not tightly (Evans et al.). Claustrophobia can occur with face masks. In a randomized control (Evans et al., 2001) study of 70 patients, Kwok found oronasal masks to be better tolerated than nasal masks, mainly because of greater air leakage through the mouth associated with nasal masks (Kwok, McCormack, Cece, Houtchens, & Hill, 2003). Both masks performed similarly in relieving respiratory symptoms, improving vital signs, and gas exchange. Face masks may be more effective for severe hypoxic ARF. Nasal

**Table 25.4 (continued)**

| Mode | Description | Clinical Application | Set by Clinician |
|---|---|---|---|
| Pressure support ventilation (PSV) | Provides a preset positive pressure on inspiration to a spontaneously breathing patient. | May be used as a primary mode; patient must be monitored for hypercapnia; may be used with continuous ventilation and with SIMV during weaning to lessen the work of breathing. | Inspiratory pressure level, PEEP, and sensitivity; patient's spontaneous breathing determines rate, length of inspiration and $V_t$ flow rate must be set greater than patient's inspiratory flow rate. |
| Pressure-controlled ventilation (PCV) | Machine breaths are delivered at a set pressure. | Used to control plateau pressure where compliance is decreased and the risk of barotrauma is high (ARDS). Used for oxygenation problems despite a high $FIO_2$ and PEEP. | $V_t$ varies with compliance and must be monitored; inspiratory pressure level, sensitivity; must monitor for hypercapnia. |
| Pressure controlled inverse ratio ventilation (PC-IRV) | Inspiratory-to-expiratory time is greater than 1:1. | Normal I:E ratio is 1:2; a prolonged positive pressure is applied increasing the inspiratory time. Progressively expands collapsed alveoli. Patient requires sedation with or without paralysis. Indicated for ARDS for those with refractory hypoxemia despite high levels of PEEP. | I:E ratio may be increased from 1:1 to 4:1. Must monitor for auto-PEEP. |
| Continuous positive airway pressure (CPAP) | Positive pressure is continuous during inspiration and expiration. | Restores functional residual capacity. | Airway pressure |

*(continued)*

plugs and pillows are reserved for nonacute use. A variety of interfaces should be readily available for immediate use.

## Use of NPPV for Specific Patient Populations

NPPV can improve arterial blood gases, respiratory rate, dyspnea, and use of accessory muscles in ARF (Antonelli et al., 1998, 2000). Inspiratory muscle fatigue is thought to be the cause of ARF in patients with severe COPD (Abou-Shala & Meduri, 1996). NPPV is an effective adjunct to usual medical care in the management of respiratory

**Table 25.4 *(continued)***

| Mode | Description | Clinical Application | Set by Clinician |
|---|---|---|---|
| Bilevel positive airway pressure (BiPAP) | Different positive pressures for inspiration and expiration are delivered; provides a higher inspiratory positive airway pressure (IPAP) and lower expiratory positive airway pressure (EPAP). | Prevents alveolar collapse; offsets buildup of intrinsic PEEP. | Inspiratory and expiratory airway pressure. |

$V_t$—Tidal volume; PEEP—positive-end-expiratory pressure

*Note.* From Bucher and Seckel (2007) and Charlebois, Earven, Fisher, Lewis, and Merrel (2005).

## 25.5 Common Ventilator Settings to Be Individualized

| Parameter | Description | Typical Setting |
|---|---|---|
| Oxygen ($FIO_2$) | Fraction of inspired oxygen delivered to the patient | 21–100% |
| Respiratory rate (RR) | Machine breaths/min | 12–20/min, or 4 breaths per minute less than patient's breath rate |
| Tidal volume (TV) | Volume of gas delivered with each machine breath | 6–10 ml/kg to minimize lung injury; 10-12 ml/kg if needed |
| PEEP | Positive pressure at end-expiration of machine breaths to prevent atelectasis | 3–5 cm $H_2O$ |
| Pressure support (PS) | Positive pressure on inspiration | 5–10 cm $H_2O$ |
| Inspiratory flow rate and time | Speed with which TV is delivered | 40–80 L/min 0.8–1.2 secs |
| Sensitivity | Determines amount of effort to draw a machine breath | Pressure trigger 0.5–1.5 cm $H_2O$ below baseline pressure Flow trigger: 1–3 L/min below baseline flow |
| High pressure limit | Max pressure to deliver TV | 10–20 cm $H_2O$ above peak inspiratory pressure |

*Note.* From Charlebois et al. (2005), Fenstermacher and Hong (2004), Urden et al. (2006).

| 25.6 | Comparison of Noninvasive Positive Airway Pressure Patient–Ventilator Interfaces | | |
|---|---|---|---|
| **Device** | **Advantages** | **Disadvantages** | |
| Oronasal mask | For acute respiratory failure<br>Better tolerated than nasal | Less air leakage than nasal masks<pa Permits mouth breathing; better for patients with dyspnea<br>Requires less patient cooperation | Less comfortable<br>Claustrophobic reactions<br>Interferes with oral intake, speech, expectoration<br>Pressure necrosis of nasal bridge |
| Nasal mask | Mostly used for chronic respiratory failure, more recently for acute respiratory failure<br>Requires patent nasal passages<br>Requires mouth closure to minimize air leaks<br>Interferes with oral intake, speech, expectoration | Not as well tolerated as oronasal mask due to more air leakage through mouth resulting in less reliable air pressures to lungs<br>Pressure necrosis of nasal bridge | |
| Nasal plugs or pillows | Reduce dead space<br>Reduce $pCO_2$ as effectively as face masks<br>May be used for "rest" periods to relieve pressure on nasal bridge | | |

*Note.* From Fenstermacher and Hong (2004); Kwok et al. (2003).

failure secondary to acute exacerbations of COPD and should be considered early to avoid endotracheal intubation, reduce mortality, and hospital length of stay (Keenan, Sinuff, Cook, & Hill, 2003; Lightowler, Wedzicha, Elliott, & Ram, 2003; Peter et al., 2002; Ram, Picot, Lightowler, & Wedzicha, 2004). A recent study of elderly COPD patients with associated severe hypercapnic neurological dysfunction revealed a mortality rate of 33% for those receiving invasive mechanical ventilation (age 70.1 ± 8.9) as compared with 16.7% for those receiving NPPV (age 71.2 ± 5.3) (Claudett et al., 2008). A meta-analysis of 15 randomized controlled trials using 793 patients revealed a reduced mortality, reduced need for mechanical ventilation, and shorter hospital length of stay among patients with COPD in acute respiratory failure receiving NPPV (Peter et al., 2002). NPPV is less successful in cases of ARDS and cardiogenic pulmonary edema. Further research is needed to evaluate the effectiveness in the treatment of asthma.

## Use at the End-of-Life

NPPV is indicated for those with ARF who are poor candidates for endotracheal intubation such as those with advanced directives. Several studies have achieved a 35 to 43% survival-to-discharge rate among patients with do-not-intubate status receiving NPPV (Levy et al., 2004; Schettino, Altobelli, & Kacmarek, 2005) and one study revealed a 30% 1-year survival among patients with COPD in ARF with a do-not-intubate status (Chu et al., 2004). Early discussions of the use of NPPV among patients and their physicians as an option for life support that can easily be discontinued are recommended (Schettino et al.). Because sedation is usually not required with NPPV, the patient may remain capable of receiving continued informed consent (Schettino et al.). In a study of 131 do-not-intubate-status patients, all of the patients accepted the option of NPPV (Schettino et al.) to provide symptomatic relief of dyspnea (Abou-Shala & Meduri, 1996; Schettino et al.). NPPV may be used for urgently needed ventilatory support while the patient, family, and physician work through this difficult decision-making period.

## Collaborative Care

Ongoing monitoring of patients receiving NPPV is determined by the patient's condition and site of care, however, most patients receiving NPPV should be managed in an ICU or within an environment capable of providing high-level monitoring (Evans et al., 2001). A potential benefit of NPPV is the ability to apply the treatment early, outside of the ICU setting, to prevent complications until the patient is transferred to the ICU (Plant, Owen, & Elliott, 2000b). Patients must be closely monitored for patient and ventilator-related complications, including gas leaks from around the mask. The respiratory rate, use of accessory muscles, patient comfort, and oxygenation status are continually monitored. Other assessments include checks for cyanosis, tachycardia, blood pressure, and level of consciousness (Evans et al.). The first hour of NPPV is labor intensive and a dedicated respiratory therapist familiar with NPPV is important for success (Abou-Shala & Meduri, 1996). Patient reassurance is provided as well as instructions on how to breathe *with* the ventilator. Continuous oximetry with appropriately set alarm parameters should be provided. Blood gases are monitored and an arterial catheter is recommended for severe hypercapnia (Abou-Shala & Meduri). Unlike correction of hypercapnia for intubated patients that is expected to occur within the first hour, correction of hypercapnia may require several hours (Abou-Shala & Meduri). The patient's subjective response to dyspnea and comfort is assessed and ongoing emotional support provided. The level of consciousness is monitored for changes reflective of the overall status of treatment. It is recommended that the head of the bed be elevated at > 45 degrees to improve the effectiveness of the treatment and to minimize aspiration (Abou-Shala & Meduri). The patient is closely monitored for gastric distention and a nasogastric tube is placed for decompression if necessary. The patient's ability to manage expectorated secretions is assessed. Treatment is discontinued if the patient does not improve or if the patient becomes unstable. Patients with acute hypoxemia, persistent acidosis or nonrespiratory organ system involvement, or whose condition deteriorates require a higher level of monitoring, including placement of a central venous and/or arterial catheter. Factors essential to the successful outcomes of NPPV are skilled staff, the capacity for adequate monitoring, experience in teaching patients about NPPV, knowledge of equipment, and awareness of potential complications (Abou-Shala & Meduri).

## Intubation

The elderly must be assessed for complications from endotracheal intubation. Complications from endotracheal intubation contribute to ventilator dependence (MacIntyre et al., 2005). Complications associated with intubation include injury to the upper airways between the point of contact and the mucosa (Abou-Shala & Meduri, 1996; Fenstermacher & Hong, 2004; Liesching, Kwok, & Hill, 2003). Nosocomial infections include ventilator-associated pneumonia and sinusitis (Abou-Shala & Meduri; Fenstermacher & Hong; Liesching et al.). Sinusitis with or without tenderness and purulent nasal drainage should be suspected in mechanically ventilated patients with an unexplained fever or bacteremia (Abou-Shala & Meduri). Despite the use of low-pressure artificial airways with high-volume tracheostomy tube cuffs, as many as 10% of patients receiving PMV may develop tracheal injury and 5% may develop distal tracheal obstruction (Rumbak, Walsh, Anderson, Rolfe, & Solomon, 1999). Swallowing dysfunction, often to the result of silent aspiration, may contribute to weaning difficulties (Elpern, Scott, Petro, & Ries, 1994; Rumbak et al., 1997; Schonhofer, Barchfeld, Haidl, & Kohler, 1999; Tolep, Getch, & Criner, 1996). Discomfort and pain during the intubation procedure itself or from the ongoing endotracheal tube placement are a major source of distress in intubated patients as is the inability to verbally communicate with relatives and the medical and nursing staff (Abou-Shala & Meduri; Fenstermacher & Hong).

## Weaning

Discontinuing ventilatory support begins with a thorough assessment of the recovery status from acute respiratory failure and any causes that may contribute to ventilator dependence. Frequent assessments of those ready to wean and appropriate reductions in ventilatory support are essential (MacIntyre et al., 2001; Scheinhorn, Chao, Stearn-Hassenpflug, & Wallace, 2001) because unnecessary delays in the weaning process lead to increased complications such as pneumonia, airway trauma, discomfort, as well as increased costs (MacIntyre et al.). Criteria for weaning must be individualized and include adequate oxygenation, hemodynamic stability, capacity to initiate inspiration, and patient comfort. In a study of 40 trauma and surgical intensive care unit (SICU) patients aged 60 and above, those successfully weaned from ventilators were weaned earlier and had lower daily and cumulative fluid balances as well as decreased central venous pressures during the time leading up to their extubations (Epstein & Peerless, 2006). A rapid shallow breathing index is the respiratory rate divided by the tidal volume ($f/V_T$), and has been shown to be an accurate predictor of weaning success in the elderly. A study of 59 patients (more than 70 years of age) showed a threshold value of $f/V_T < 130$ as an appropriate predictor for weaning success and that serial measurements increase the accuracy of prediction (Krieger, Isber, Breitenbucher, Throop, & Ershowsky, 1997).

Methods for discontinuing support include gradual reductions in intermittent mandatory ventilation and/or pressure support, spontaneous breathing trials, and NPPV. Although the optimal method of weaning the elderly is not known (Sevransky & Haponik, 2003), discontinuation and weaning protocols that are designed for nonphysician health care professionals such as respiratory therapists and nurses can reduce the time a patient receives mechanical ventilation. In a study of 252 predominantly elderly patients (mean age of 71) in a long-term acute-care facility, a therapist-implemented weaning protocol reduced the weaning time from 29 days to 17 days. The literature supports that it is the use of a standardized approach as opposed to a specific discontinuation protocol that improves outcomes and that institutions must customize their protocols to local practice and patient populations (MacIntyre et al., 2001).

Suggested approaches for weaning the elderly that have been used in long-term acute-care facilities include weaning combinations of pressure support (PS), synchronized intermittent mechanical ventilation/intermittent mechanical ventilation (SIMV/IMV), and assisted control ventilation (ACV) before beginning daily spontaneous breathing trials (Scheinhorn et al., 2001; Schonhofer, Euteneuer, Nava, Suchi, & Kohler, 2002; Sevransky & Haponik, 2003). All patients, regardless of approach, are closely observed for respiratory compromise, including the respiratory pattern, $SaO_2$ via pulse oximetry, heart rate and blood pressure, and patient comfort (MacIntyre et al., 2001). Spontaneous breathing trials consist of increasing time periods whereby the patient is completely taken off ventilatory support for increasing lengths of time. Patients are then most typically placed on CPAP or pressure support. Discontinuing ventilatory support for those tolerating a spontaneous breathing trial (SBT) of 30 to 120 minutes should be considered; this approach has a success rate of 77% (MacIntyre et al., 2001).

Elderly patients failing a SBT should have all possible causes corrected and returned to a stable level of support to avoid muscle overload, optimize comfort (including sedation), and avoid complications. Patients are reassessed for a subsequent trial every 24 hours as daily SBTs shorten the discontinuation period as opposed to strategies that do not include daily SBTs (MacIntyre et al., 2001). The assessment for subsequent SBTs should include adequacy of pain control, the appropriateness of sedation, fluid status, bronchodilator needs, control of myocardial ischemia, as well as other disease processes (MacIntyre et al.). Esteban et al. (1995) found that in patients (median ages of 65 and 63 for patient groups) who initially failed one SBT, subsequent SBTs with stable support between trials permitted faster ventilatory discontinuation than gradual reductions in pressure support or intermittent mandatory ventilation. Recently, NPPV has been used as a weaning modality from mechanical ventilation (Abou-Shala & Meduri, 1996; Nava et al., 1998; Udwadia, Santis, Steven, & Simonds, 1992). One study (Girault et al., 2003) demonstrated a success rate of 68% for elderly (mean age 70 + 11) patients with respiratory failure caused by COPD. Like other modes of weaning, patients being weaned from NPPV must be closely monitored for signs of distress. Criteria for discontinuing NPPV weaning are listed in Table 25.7. More widespread use of NPPV as a weaning modality is being examined.

## Prolonged Mechanical Ventilation

Mechanical ventilation is the major critical care treatment modality that extends beyond ICUs, establishing a continuum of care in step-down units and long-term care hospitals (Scheinhorn, Votto, Epstein, & Petrak, 2007). In 2004, The National Association for Medical Direction of Respiratory Care (NAMDRC) defined PMV as > 21 consecutive days of mechanical ventilation for > 6 hours per day (MacIntyre, Epstein, Carson, Scheinhorn, & Muldoon, 2005). In a study of 181 patients examining patients

## 25.7   Criteria to Discontinue Noninvasive Ventilation

Inability to tolerate the mask

Inability to improve gas exchange or dyspnea

Need for endotracheal intubation to manage secretions or protect the airway

Electrocardiographic instability such as dysrhythmias and signs of cardiac ischemia

Failure to improve mental status within 30 minutes of initiating NPPV in those lethargic from $CO_2$ retention or agitated from hypoxemia

*Note.* From Abou-Shala and Meduri (1996).

aged 70 and older, receiving mechanical ventilation (for > 3 days), the overall in-hospital mortality rate was 57% and no one older than 85 years of age survived (Meinders, van der Hoeven, & Meinders, 1996).

The etiology of ventilator dependence is often multifactorial and valid approaches to predict weaning outcomes are needed (MacIntyre et al., 2005). Excessive breathing load capacity and diminished respiratory muscle capacity have been found among patients requiring PMV. During spontaneous breathing, indexes of excessive loading and/or impaired capacity include a lower maximal inspiratory pressure and high respiratory frequency/tidal volume ratios ($f/V_T$) (MacIntyre et al.)

Coexistent nonpulmonary diseases are associated with poor outcomes. In 2004, Scheinhorn studied more than 1,400 patients in a multicenter study of 23 long-term acute-care (LTAC) facilities. The average patient was 72 years of age and the mean admission APACHE (acute physiology and chronic health evaluation) III score was 36. Forty-three percent of the patients had COPD; however, 54% also had coronary artery disease or congestive heart failure. Other comorbidities associated with poor outcomes in those requiring prolonged mechanical ventilation included hemodialysis, cardiac ischemia or left ventricular dysfunction, hypoalbuminemia, an abnormal mental status or emotional status, and sleep deprivation (MacIntyre et al., 2005). Over a period of 8 years, APACHE III scores increased in long-term acute-care (LTAC) facilities indicating a higher patient acuity in LTAC facilities (Scheinhorn, Chao, Stearn-Hassenpflug, Heltsley, & LaBree, 1997). Moreover, as many as 23 to 48% of patients with nonpulmonary comorbidities outside of short-term acute-care (STAC) facilities are readmitted to STAC ICUs (Chan, Mehta, & Vasishtha, 1999; MacIntyre et al., 2004; Nasraway, Button, Rand, Hudson-Jinks, & Gustafson, 2000). Identification of reversible factors is crucial to successful outcomes.

The most common complication of mechanical ventilation is nosocomial infection. In a multicenter study (Scheinhorn et al., 2004) of patients requiring PMV, 32% of patients had urinary tract infections, 28% had lower respiratory tract infections, 18% had clostridium difficile, and 12% had an infection related to a central line. The length of hospital stay and weaning times were substantially longer for patients with infections.

Elderly patients requiring prolonged mechanical ventilation have special needs and consumption patterns (MacIntyre et al., 2005). Whereas the care in an acute ICU setting entails the addition of life-support measures to sustain life, PMV care focuses on the reduction of support already in place. Specialized care facilities, management strategies, and reimbursement methods are rapidly emerging.

## Outcomes

Most outcomes have been studied in long-term acute-care settings. In the multicenter study of elderly patients mentioned previously (median age of 71.8), 54.1% were weaned at discharge, 20.9% remained ventilator dependent, and 25% died (Scheinhorn et al., 2007). Long-term survival of 1 year following PMV is 23 to 76% (Carson, Bach, Brzozowski, & Leff, 1999; Scheinhorn et al., 1997; Stoller, Meng, Mascha, & Rice, 2003). The large range is attributable to varied patient populations and definitions of PMV. Accurate models and other predictors of survival and quality of life are needed to help physicians and other health care members provide patients and families with realistic expectations for outcomes. Models and predictors could greatly facilitate resource and end-of-life planning as well as assist hospitals, postacute facilities and payers plan appropriately (MacIntyre et al., 2005). Current approaches to estimates of acute ICU survival have not greatly influenced decisions whether or not to provide aggressive care (SUPPORT Investigators, 1995). Some studies have shown age to be a poor predictor of survival (Dematte-D'Amico, et al., 2003; Ely, Evans, & Haponik, 1999), whereas in 2004, Chelluri and colleagues (2004) showed that age and comorbidities are the primary risk factors after 14 days of mechanical ventilation. Along with survival, comorbidities, prolonged critical illness, suffering, and permanent functional impairment must be considered in determining outcomes of aggressive respiratory support.

## Transitioning From Short-Term Acute Care

Patients with underlying cardiorespiratory diseases and/or slowly resolving cardiorespiratory illnesses transition from being acutely ill to chronically critically ill. Alternatives to short-term acute-care (STAC) venues must be considered early or when the need for a tracheostomy is first considered (MacIntyre et al., 2005). The focus of care shifts from a life-support focus to a more comprehensive patient-focused rehabilitative process of care (see Table 25.8) (Criner, 2002; O'Bryan, Von Rueden, & Malila, 2002) that may provide increased ventilator weaning safety (Jefferies Equity Research, 2003). Nurses must be competent in the management of ventilators, suctioning, and tracheostomy care, as well as indwelling lines, feeding tubes, and bladder catheters. A multispecialty approach includes physicians, case managers, nutritionists, respiratory therapists, pharmacists, physical, occupational and speech therapists, as well as psychological and social services.

Although there is no clear evidence when weaning from PMV is futile, several authorities agree that patients who have been on ventilatory support for 3 months will most likely not be successfully weaned (MacIntyre et al., 2001, 2005). PMV has been shown to be associated with frustration, dyspnea, discomfort, anxiety, sleep disturbances, depression, and inability to communicate (Nasraway et al., 2000).

## 25.8   Potential Benefits of a Long-Term-Care Venue

Relative quiet environment

Day/night cycles with outdoor view

Roomy environment with personal objects encouraged

Supportive visitation encouraged

Increased independence and mobility

Comprehensive reconditioning program

Reliance on patient interaction as opposed to technology

Focus on staff nurturing

Comprehensive counseling program

Palliative care

Home-geared discharge planning

*Note.* From MacIntyre et al. (2005).

Options include continued ventilatory support with additional or limited care or withdrawal of support. Decisions to discontinue weaning include treatment progress, repeated failures to wean, and a realization that the patient's functional capacity and quality of life are unacceptable even if weaned (MacIntyre et al.). Consensus among the care team, patient, and family should be obtained and consultation by palliative care, social, and pastoral services may be useful. Palliative care can play a significant role in STAC ICUs as well as PMV venues in the relief of pain, dyspnea, anxiety, and other symptoms commonly associated with chronic critical illness (Nelson, Nierman, & Meier, 2001). The development of predictive models for ventilator weaning success, hospital discharge, survival, functional status, quality of life, and costs are urgently needed. Strategic research will ultimately benefit older adult patients by contributing to their comfort and appropriate management of acute and chronic respiratory failure.

## Summary

With older adults comprising nearly half of all critical care admissions and respiratory failure as the primary cause, comprehensive gerontologic care is essential. Although endotracheal intubation remains the gold standard for long-term ventilatory support, noninvasive positive pressure ventilation should be considered for short-term use to relieve dyspnea, improve arterial blood gases, and as an adjunct to palliative care. The older adult in respiratory failure must be carefully monitored, treated, and evaluated. A thoughtful approach involving the patient, family, and geriatric health care specialists that addresses survival, prolonged critical illness, suffering, and permanent function is crucial to bringing about acceptable outcomes.

# References

Abou-Shala, N., & Meduri, G. U. (1996). Noninvasive mechanical ventilation in patients with acute respiratory failure. *Critical Care Medicine, 24,* 705–715.

American Thoracic Society. (1991). Lung function testing: Selection of reference values and interpretative strategies. *American Review of Respiratory Disease, 144,* 1202–1218.

Antonelli, M., Conti, G., Bufi, M., Costa, M. G., Lappa, A., & Rocca, M., et al. (2000). Noninvasive ventilation for treatment of acute respiratory failure in patients undergoing solid organ transplantation: A randomized trial. *Journal of the American Medical Association, 283,* 235–41.

Antonelli, M., Conti, G., Rocco, M., Bufi, M., de Biasi, R. A., & Vivino, G., et al. (1998). A comparison of noninvasive positive-pressure ventilation and conventional mechanical ventilation in patients with acute respiratory failure. *New England Journal of Medicine, 339,* 429–35.

Arbour, R. B. (2007). Respiratory failure and acute respiratory syndrome. In S. L. Lewis, M. M. Heitkemper, S. R. Dirksen, P. G. O'Brien, & L. Bucher (Eds.), *Medical-surgical nursing: Assessment and management of clinical problems* (7th ed., pp. 1799–1820) St. Louis: MO: Mosby Elsevier.

Beers, M. H. (Ed.). (2000). Pulmonary disorders: Respiratory failure. In *The Merck Manual of Geriatrics.* (3rd ed.). Retrieved December 27, 2008, from http://www.merck.com/mkgr/mmg/sec10/ch79/ch79a.jsp

Benhamou, D., Girault, C., Faure, C., Portier, F., & Muir, J. F. (1992). Nasal mask ventilation in acute respiratory failure: Experience in elderly patients. *Chest, 102,* 912–917.

Berend, N. (2005). Normal ageing of the lung: Implications for diagnosis and monitoring of asthma in older people. *Medical Journal of Australia, 183*(1 Suppl.), S28–S29.

Bucher, L., & Seckel, M. (2007). Critical care: Nursing management. In F. M. Lewis, M. M. Heitkemper, S. R. Dirksen, P. G. O'Brien, & L. Bucher (Eds.), *Medical-surgical nursing: Assessment and management of clinical problems* (7th ed., pp. 1733–1771). St. Louis: MO: Mosby Elsevier.

Burrows, B., Knudsen, R. J., Camilli, A. E., Lyle, S. K., & Lebowitz, M. D. (1987). The horse racing effect and predicting decline in forced expiratory volume in one second from screening spirometry. *American Review of Respiratory Disease, 135,* 788–796.

Carson, S. S., Bach, P. B., Brzozowski, L., & Leff, A. (1999). Outcomes after long-term acute care: An analysis of 133 mechanically ventilated patients. *American Journal of Respiratory Critical Care Medicine, 159,* 1568–1573.

Cerveri, I., Zoia, M. C., Fanfulla, F., Spagnolatti, L., Berrayah, L., & Grassi, M., et al. (1995). Reference values of arterial oxygen tension in the middle-aged and elderly. *American Journal of Respiratory Critical Care Medicine, 152,* 934–941.

Chan, M., Mehta, R., & Vasishtha, N. (1999). Ventilator care in a nursing home [abstract]. *American Journal of Respiratory Critical Care Medicine, 159,* A374.

Charlebois, D. L., Earven, S. S., Fisher, C. A., Lewis, R., & Merrel, P. K. (2005). Patient management: Respiratory system. In P. G. Morton, D. K. Fontaine, C. M. Hudak, & B .M. Gallo (Eds.), *Critical care nursing: A holistic approach* (8th ed., pp. 517–565). Philadelphia: Lippincott Williams & Wilkins.

Chelluri, L., Im, K. A., Belle, S. H., Schutz, R., Rotondi, A., & Donahoe, M., et al. (2004). Long-term mortality and quality of life after prolonged mechanical ventilation. *Critical Care Medicine, 32,* 61–69.

Chu, C. M., Chan, V. L., Wong, I. W., Leung, W. S., Lin, A. W., & Cheung, K. F. (2004). Noninvasive ventilation in patients with acute hypercapnic exacerbation of chronic obstructive pulmonary disease who refused endotracheal intubation. *32,* 372-377.

Claudett, K. H., Claudett, M. H., Wong, M. A., Andrade, M. G., Cruz, C. X., & Esquinas, A., et al. (2008). Noninvasive mechanical ventilation in patients with chronic obstructive pulmonary disease and severe hypercapnic neurological deterioration in the emergency room. *European Journal of Emergency Medicine, 15,* 127–133.

Confalonieri, M., Potena, A., Carbone, G., Porta, R. D., Tolley, E. A., & Meduri, G. U. (1999). Acute respiratory failure in patients with severe community-acquired pneumonia: A prospective randomized evaluation of noninvasive ventilation. *American Journal of Respiratory Critical Care Medicine, 160,* 1585–1591.

Criner, G. J. (2002). Care of the patient requiring invasive mechanical ventilation. *Respiratory Care Clinics of North America, 8,* 575–592.

Delerme, S., & Ray, P. (2008). Acute respiratory failure in the elderly: Diagnosis and prognosis. *Age and Ageing, 37,* 251–257.

Dematte-D'Amico, J. E., Donnelly, H. K., Mutlu, G. M., Feinglass, J., Javanovic, B. D., & Ndukwu, I. M. (2003). Risk assessment for inpatient survival in the long-term acute care setting after prolonged critical illness. *Chest, 124,* 1039–1045.

El Solh, A., & Ramadan, F. (2006). Overview of respiratory failure in older adults. *Journal of Intensive Care Medicine, 21*(6), 345–347.

Elpern, E. H., Scott, M. G., Petro, L., & Ries, M. H. (1994). Pulmonary aspiration in mechanically ventilated patients with tracheostomies. *Chest, 105,* 563–566.

Ely, E. W., Evans, G. W., & Haponik, E. F. (1999). Mechanical ventilation in a cohort of elderly patients admitted to an intensive care unit. *Annals of Internal Medicine, 131,* 96–104.

Epstein, C. D., & Peerless, J. R. (2006). Weaning readiness and fluid balance in older critically ill surgical patients. *American Journal of Critical Care, 15,* 54–77.

Esteban, A., Frutos, F., Tobin, M. J., Inmaculada, A., Solsona, J. F., & Vallverdu, I., et al. (1995). A comparison of four methods of weaning patients from mechanical ventilation: The Spanish lung failure collaborative group. *New England Journal of Medicine, 332,* 345–350.

Evans, T. W., Albert, R. K., Angus, D. C., Bion, J. F., Chich, J. D., & Epstein, S. K., et al. (2001). International consensus conferences in intensive care medicine: Noninvasive positive pressure ventilation in acute respiratory failure. *American Journal of Respiratory Critical Care Medicine, 163*(283), 291.

Fenstermacher, D., & Hong, D. (2004). Mechanical ventilation: What have we learned? *Critical Care Nursing Quarterly, 27,* 258–294.

Girault, C., Briel, A., Hellot, M. F., Tamion, F., Woinet, D., & Leroy, J., et al. (2003). Noninvasive mechanical ventilation in clinical practice: A 2-year experience in a medical intensive care unit. *Critical Care Medicine, 31,* 552–559.

Guenard, H., & Marthan, R. (1996). Pulmonary gas exchange in elderly subjects. *European Respiratory Journal, 9,* 2573–2577.

Hardie, J. A., Vollmer, W. M., & Buist, S. (2004). Reference values for arterial blood gases in the elderly. *Chest, 125,* 2053–2060.

Hébuterne, X., Bermon, S., & Schneider, S. M. (2001). Ageing and muscle: The effects of malnutrition, re-nutrition, and physical exercise. *Current Opinion in Nutrition and Metabolic Care, 4,* 295–300.

Honrubia, T., Lopez, F. J., Franco, N., Mas, M., Guevara, M., & Daguerre, M., et al. (2005). Noninvasive vs conventional mechanical ventilation in acute respiratory failure: A multicenter randomized controlled trial. *Chest, 128,* 3916–3924.

Janssens, J. P., Pache, J. C., & Nicod, L. P. (1999). Physiological changes in respiratory function associated with ageing. *European Respiratory Journal, 13,* 197–205.

Jefferies Equity Research. (2003). *Long term acute care hospitals: An opportunity in change.* Long Island, NY: Jefferies and Company.

Jindal, S. K. (2006). *Pulmonary disease in elderly.* Retrieved January 4, 2008, from http://ezproxy.library.nyu.edu:24934/show/127/Pulmonary_Disease_in_Elderly/Pulmonary_Disease_in_Elderly

Keenan, S. P., Sinuff, T., Cook, D. J., & Hill, N. S. (2003). Which patients with acute exacerbation of chronic obstructive pulmonary disease benefit from noninvasive positive-pressure ventilation? A systematic review of the literature. *Annals of Internal Medicine, 138,* 861–870.

Krieger, B. P., Isber, J., Breitenbucher, A., Throop, G., & Ershowsky, P. (1997). Serial measurements of the rapid-shallow-breathing index as a predictor of weaning outcome in elderly medical patients. *Chest, 112,* 1029–1034.

Kwok, H., McCormack, J., Cece, R., Houtchens, J., & Hill, N. S. (2003). Controlled trial of oronasal versus nasal mask ventilation in the treatment of acute respiratory failure. *Critical Care Medicine, 31,* 468–473.

Levy, M., Tanios, M. Z., Nelson, D., Short, K., Senechia, A., & Vespia, J., et al. (2004). Outcomes of patients with do-not-intubate orders treated with noninvasive ventilation. *Critical Care Medicine, 32,* 2002–2007.

Liesching, T., Kwok, H., & Hill, N. S. (2003). Acute applications of noninvasive positive pressure ventilation. *Chest, 124,* 699–713.

Lightowler, J. V., Wedzicha, J. A., Elliott, M. W., & Ram, F. S. (2003). Non-invasive positive pressure ventilation to treat respiratory failure resulting from exacerbations of chronic obstructive pulmonary disease: Cochrane systematic review and meta-analysis. *British Medical Journal, 326,* 1–5.

MacIntyre, N. R., Cook, D. J., Ely, E. W., Epstein, S. K., Fink, J. B., & Heffner, J. E., et al. (2001). Evidence-based guidelines for weaning and discontinuing ventilatory support: A collective task force facilitated by the American college of chest physicians, the American association for respiratory care, and the American college of critical care medicine. *Chest, 120* (Suppl.), 375S–395S.

MacIntyre, N. R., Epstein, S. K., Carson, S., Scheinhorn, K. C., & Muldoon, S. (2005). Management of patients requiring prolonged mechanical ventilation: Report of a NAMDRC consensus conference. *Chest, 128*, 3937–3954.

McNally, D. (2000). Respiratory failure. In M. H. Beers (Ed.), *The Merck manual of geriatrics* (3rd ed.). Retrieved December 27, 2008, from http://www.merck.com/mkgr/mmg/sec10/ch79/ch79a.jsp

Meinders, A. J., van der Hoeven, J. G., & Meinders, A. E. (1996). The outcome of prolonged mechanical ventilation in elderly patients: Are the efforts worthwhile? *Age and Ageing, 25*, 153–159.

Nasraway, S. A., Button, G. J., Rand, W. M., Hudson-Jinks, T., & Gustafson, M. (2000). Survivors of catastrophic illness: Outcome after direct transfer from intensive care to extended care facilities. *Critical Care Medicine, 28*, 19–25.

Nava, S., Ambrosino, N., Clini, E., Prato, M., Orlando, G., & Vitacca, M., et al. (1998). Noninvasive mechanical ventilation in the weaning of patients with respiratory failure due to chronic obstructive pulmonary disease. *Annals of Internal Medicine, 128*, 721–728.

Nelson, J., Nierman, D., & Meier, D. (2001). The symptom burden of chronic critical illness [abstract]. *American Journal of Respiratory Critical Care Medicine, 163*, A62.

O'Bryan, L., Von Rueden, K., & Malila, F. (2002). Evaluating ventilator weaning best practice: A long-term acute care hospital systemwide quality initiative. *AACN Clinical Issues, 13*, 567–576.

Panacek, E. A., & Kirk, D. J. (2002). Role of noninvasive ventilation in the management of acutely decompensated heart failure. *Review of Cardiovascular Medicine, 3*, S35–S40.

Peter, J. V., Moran, J. L., & Phillips-Hughes, J. (2002). Noninvasive ventilation in acute respiratory failure—A meta-analysis update. *Critical Care Medicine, 30*, 555–562.

Plant, P. K., Owen, J., & Elliot, M. W. (2000a). One-year prevalence study of acidosis in patients admitted to hospital with an exacerbation of COPD-implications for noninvasive ventilation. *Thorax, 55*, 550–554.

Plant, P. K., Owen, J. L., & Elliott, M. W. (2000b). Non-invasive ventilation (NIIV) in acute exacerbations of COPD-the Yorkshire non-invasive ventilation trial. *Lancet, 355*, 1931–1935.

Polkey, M. I., Harris, M. L., Hughes, P. D., Rafferty, G. F., Moxham, J., & Green, M. (1997). The contractile properties of the elderly human diaphragm. *American Journal of Respiratory Critical Care Medicine, 155*, 1560–1564.

Rady, M. Y. (2005). Bench-to-bedside review: Resuscitation in the emergency department. *Critical Care, 9*, 170–176.

Ram, F. S. F., Picot, J., Lightowler, J., Wedzicha, J. A. (2004). Non-invasive positive pressure ventilation for treatment of respiratory failure due to exacerbations of chronic obstructive pulmonary disease. *Cochrane Database of Systematic Reviews,* Issue 3. Art. No.: CD004104. DOI: 10.1002/14651858.CD004104.pub3

Resnick, B. (2005). The critically ill older patient. In P. G. Morton, D. K. Fontaine, C .M. Hudak, & B. M. Gallo (Eds.), *Critical care nursing: A holistic approach* (8th ed., pp. 150–174). Philadelphia: Lippincott Williams & Wilkins.

Richard, J. C., Carlucci, A., Wysocki, M., Chastre, J., Beliot, C., & Lepage, E., et al. (1999). French multicenter survey: Noninvasive versus conventional mechanical ventilation {abstract}. *American Journal of Respiratory Critical Care Medicine, 159*, A367.

Rumbak, M. J., Graves, E. E., Scott, M. P., Sporn, G. K., Walsh, F. W., & Anderson, W. M., et al. (1997). Tracheostomy tube occlusion protocol predicts significant tracheal obstruction to air flow in patients requiring prolonged mechanical ventilation. *Critical Care Medicine, 25*, 413–417.

Rumbak, M. J., Walsh, F. W., Anderson, W. M., Rolfe, M. W., & Solomon, D. A. (1999). Significant tracheal obstruction causing failure to wean in patients requiring prolonged mechanical ventilation. *Chest, 115*, 1092–1095.

Scheinhorn, D. J., Chao, D. C., Stearn-Hassenpflug, M., Doig, G. S., Epstein, S. K., & Knight, E. B., et al. (2004). Infectious complications in weaning from prolonged mechanical ventilation at long-term hospitals: Preliminary report from a multicenter study [abstract]. *American Journal of Respiratory Critical Care Medicine, 169*, A44.

Scheinhorn, D. J., Chao, D. C., Stearn-Hassenpflug, M., Heltsley, D. J., & LaBree, L. D. (1997). Post-ICU mechanical ventilation: Treatment of 1,123 patients at a regional weaning center. *Chest, 111*, 1654–1659.

Scheinhorn, D. J., Chao, D. C., Stearn-Hassenpflug, M., & Wallace, W. A. (2001). Outcomes in post-ICU mechanical ventilation: A therapist-implemented weaning protocol. *Chest, 119*, 236–242.

Scheinhorn, D. J., Votto, J. J., Epstein, S. K., & Petrak, R. A. (2007). Post-ICU mechanical ventilation at 23 long-term care hospitals. *Chest, 131*, 85–93.

Schettino, G., Altobelli, N., & Kacmarek, R. M. (2005). Noninvasive positive pressure ventilation reverses acute respiratory failure in select "do-not-intubate" patients. *Critical Care Medicine, 33,* 1976–1982.

Schonhofer, B., Barchfeld, T., Haidl, P., & Kohler, C. (1999). Scintigraphy for evaluating early aspiration after oral feeding in patients receiving prolonged ventilation via tracheostomy. *Intensive Care Medicine, 25,* 311–314.

Schonhofer, B., Euteneuer, S., Nava, S., Suchi, S., & Kohler, D., et al. (2002). Survival of mechanically ventilated patients admitted to a specialized weaning center. *Intensive Care Medicine, 28,* 908–916.

Sevransky, J. E., & Haponik, E. F. (2003). Respiratory failure in elderly patients. *Clinics in Geriatric Medicine, 19,* 205–224.

Sorbini, C. A., Grassi, V., Solinas, E., & Muiesan, G. (1968). Arterial oxygen tension in relation to age in health subjects. *Respiration, 25,* 3–13.

Soroksky, A., Stav, D., & Shpirer, I. (2003). A pilot, prospective randomized placebo-controlled trial of bilevel positive airway pressure in acute asthmatic attack. *Chest, 123,* 1018–1025.

Stoller, J. K., Meng, X., Mascha, E., & Rice, R. (2003). Long-term outcomes for patients discharged from a long-term hospital-based weaning unit. *Chest, 124,* 1892–1899.

Sue, D. Y. (2000). Acute respiratory failure. In T. T. Yoshikawa & D. C. Norman (Eds.), *Acute emergencies and critical care of the geriatric patient* (pp. 243–268). New York: Marcel Dekker.

SUPPORT Investigators. (1995). A controlled trial to improve care for seriously ill hospitalized patients: The study to understand prognoses and preferences for outcomes and risks of treatments (SUPPORT). *Journal of the American Medical Association, 274,* 1591–1598.

Tolep, K., Getch, C. L., & Criner, G. J. (1996). Swallowing dysfunction in patients receiving prolonged mechanical ventilation. *Chest, 109,* 167–172.

Udwadia, Z. F., Santis, G. D., Steven, M. H., & Simonds, A. K. (1992). Nasal ventilation to facilitate weaning in patients with chronic respiratory insufficiency. *Thorax, 47,* 715–718.

Urden, L. D., Stacy, K. M., & Lough, M. E. (2006). Pulmonary disorders. *Critical care nursing: Diagnosis and management* (5th ed., pp. 617–656). St. Louis: Mosby Elsevier.

Wood, K. (1998). The use of noninvasive positive pressure ventilation in the emergency department. *Chest, 113,* 1339–1346.

Zeleznik, J. (2003). Normative aging of the respiratory system. *Clinics in Geriatric Medicine, 19,* 1–18.

# Delirium in Critical Illness

# 26

Marquis D. Foreman
Marieke Schuurmans
Koen Milisen

## Introduction

Delirium is a common syndrome in critically ill older patients; estimates of its occurrence range as high as 87% depending on patient characteristics, local sedation practices, severity of illness, the confounding influence of medication-associated coma, and the methods used for case finding (Ouimet, Kavanagh, Gottfried, & Skrobik, 2007; Pandharipande, Jackson, & Ely, 2005). More important, delirium is consistently linked to poorer outcomes of care at higher costs, with persistent impairment in cognitive abilities (Jackson et al., 2003). Yet, delirium is frequently underrecognized or misattributed to the effects of aging or the presence of dementia, thereby missing opportunities of prevention through identifying modifiable risk factors (Foreman & Milisen, 2004). Because of its common occurrence and poor outcomes at higher costs, in this chapter we discuss the nature of delirium, the factors that place an individual at risk of developing delirium in critical illness, methods of assessment for identifying delirium, and currently accepted strategies for preventing and managing delirium in older critically ill patients.

The nature of delirium is complex and contributes to the challenge of its recognition. By nature, delirium is a fluctuating disturbance in consciousness and disorganized

## 26.1   Criteria for Delirium, According to the Diagnostic and Statistical Manual of Mental Disorders (DSM-IV)

■ Disturbance of consciousness (i.e., reduced clarity of awareness of the environment) with reduced ability to focus, sustain, or shift attention.

■ Change in cognition (such as memory deficit, disorientation, or language disturbance) or the development of a perceptual disturbance that is not better accounted for by a preexisting, established, or evolving dementia.

■ The disturbance develops over a short period of time (usually hours to days) and tends to fluctuate over the course of the day.

■ There is evidence from the history, physical examination, or laboratory findings that the disturbance is caused by the direct physiological consequences of a general condition, by an intoxication substance, by medication use or by more than one etiology.

*Note.* Adapted from the American Psychiatric Association (2000).

thinking that develops rapidly with evidence of an underlying pathophysiologic or medical condition (American Psychiatric Association [APA], 2000) (see Table 26.1).

These criteria are manifested as the cardinal symptoms of memory loss, attention deficit, disorientation, language disturbance, or the development of a perceptual disturbance, for exmple, misinterpretations or hallucinations (APA, 2000) (see Table 26.2). The hallmark characteristics helping to differentiate delirium from other forms of cognitive impairment are that delirium develops over a short period of time and that the cardinal symptoms fluctuate in severity over the course of the day. As a result, at different times during the day the patient may appear to be functioning normally, whereas at others may seem extremely disoriented and exhibiting grossly incoherent and rambling conversations. Moreover, the individual's behavior may appear unusual for the individual or inappropriate to the situation (see Table 26.2)

Little is known about subsyndromal delirium in patients who are critically ill. Subsyndromal delirium is a condition in which patients exhibit one or more symptoms, for example, disorientation, inattention, or perceptual disorder, but fail to manifest all symptoms of delirium (Levkoff, Yang, & Liptzin, 2004; Meagher, 2009). Subsyndromal delirium is important as it may be prodromal to an overt episode of delirium, or it may indicate the incomplete resolution of delirium with the persistence of some symptoms, for example, persistent memory loss (Jackson et al., 2003). Clinically, risk factors for subsyndromal delirium are the same as those associated with an overt episode of delirium, as is a poorer prognosis and worse outcomes; for example, disability outcomes that are intermediate between normal and delirious patients (Cole, McCusker, Dendukuri, & Han, 2003; Kiely, Jones, Bergmann, & Marcantonio, 2007; Levkoff et al.; Morandi, Jackson, & Ely, 2009, Ouimet, Riker, et al., 2007). Thus, it seems prudent to routinely monitor for subsyndromal delirium in this patient population as it may increase the potential to prevent adverse outcomes or improve outcomes (Cole et al., 2003; Morandi et al., 2009, Ouimet, Riker, et al.).

Recognition of delirium is even more complex as a result of its highly variable presentation. Three subtypes of delirium have been identified (Meagher & Trzepacz, 2000; Morandi et al., 2009; Peterson et al., 2006): hypoalert–hypoactive; hyperalert–hyperactive, and mixed. The hypoalert–hypoactive subtype of delirium is most prevalent in older persons, occurring in about 40 to 60% of delirious patients (Pandharipande

## 26.2 A Comparison of the Clinical Features of Delirium, Dementia, and Depression

| Clinical Feature | Delirium | Dementia | Depression |
|---|---|---|---|
| Onset | Sudden/abrupt; depends on cause; often at twilight | Insidious/slow and often unrecognized; depends on cause | Variable, often coincides with major life changes; often abrupt but can be gradual |
| Course | Short; diurnal fluctuations in symptoms; worse at night, in darkness, with fatigue and on awakening | Long; no diurnal effects, symptoms progressive yet relatively stable over time, may see deficits with increased stress | Diurnal effects, typically worse in the morning; situational fluctuations in symptoms but less than with delirium |
| Progression | Abrupt | Slow and uneven | Variable; rapid or slow but generally even |
| Duration | Typically hours to a few days; however, some symptoms persist for up to 6 months | Months to years | Generally at least 6 weeks, can be several months to years |
| Consciousness | Altered | Clear until last stages | Clear |
| Alertness | Fluctuates from stuporus to hypervigilant | Generally normal, until last stages | Generally normal |
| Attention | Inattentive; easily distractible and may have difficulty shifting from one focus to another | Generally normal | Minimal impairment but is distractible |
| Orientation | Generally impaired; should not be disoriented to person | Normal in beginning stage | Generally unimpaired; selective disorientation |
| Memory | Recent and immediate impaired; unable to recall events of hospitalization and current illness; forgetful, unable to recall instructions | Recent and remote impaired without inattention | Selective or "patchy" impairment; "islands" of intact memory, evaluation often difficult due to low motivation |
| Thinking | Disorganized; rambling, irrelevant and incoherent conversation; unclear or illogical flow of ideas | Difficulty with abstraction, thoughts impoverished; judgment impaired; words difficult to find | Intact but with themes of hopelessness, helplessness, or self-deprecation |

*(continued)*

**Table 26.2** *(continued)*

| Clinical Feature | Delirium | Dementia | Depression |
|---|---|---|---|
| Perception | Perceptual disturbances such as illusions and visual and auditory hallucinations; misperceptions of common people and objects | Misperceptions usually absent in beginning stage; Frequently paranoid | Intact, delusions and hallucinations absent except in severe cases. |
| Psychomotor behavior | Irregular and unpredictable variability; hypoactive, hyperactive, or mixed | Normal, but may have apraxia | Variable; psychomotor retardation or agitation but not to the extreme seen with delirium |
| Associated features | Variable affective changes; symptoms of autonomic hypo-hyper arousal | Affect tends to be superficial, inappropriate, and labile; attempts to conceal deficits in intellect; personality changes; aphasia, agnosia may be present; lacks insight | Affect depressed; dysphoric mood, exaggerated and detailed complaints; preoccupied with personal thoughts; insight present; verbal elaboration; somatic complaints; poor hygiene and neglect of self |
| Assessment | Distracted from task; fails to remember instructions, frequent errors without notice | Failings highlighted by family, frequent 'near miss' answers, struggles with test, great effort to find an appropriate reply, frequent requests for feedback on performance | Failings highlighted by individual; frequent "don't know" answers; little effort; frequently gives up; indifferent toward test; does not care or attempt to find answer |

*Note.* Adapted from Braes, Milisen, and Foreman (2008).

et al., 2007, Peterson et al.), and is characterized by profound lethargy, inattention, decreased responsiveness, and little body movement. These individuals are quiet and cooperative with care; strong physical or verbal stimuli (e.g., vigorous shaking or shouting) are needed to arouse the patient, and despite these stimuli arousal is incomplete and transient at best. As a consequence, this subtype frequently goes unrecognized or is attributed to sedation or depression (Inouye, Foreman, Mion, Katz, & Cooney, 2001; Peterson et al.), and as a result patients manifesting the hypoalert–hypoactive subtype have the worst prognosis and outcomes (Morandi et al., Peterson et al.) Patients who tend to manifest the hypoalert–hypoactive subtype of delirium tend to be older and to have some form of dementia (Inouye et al.). Conversely, the hyperalert–hyperactive subtype is rare; occurring in about 2% of delirious patients (Peterson et al.), and is characterized by hypervigilance, extreme restlessness, and combative behavior. Such behavior is problematic to providers and thus is readily detected, recognized, and treated. As a consequence, patients manifesting the hyperalert–hyperactive subtype of delirium tend to have a better prognosis and better outcomes (Morandi et al., Peterson et al.) The occurrence of the third subtype varies between 6 and 55% of patients with delirium, depending on patient characteristics (e.g., surgical and trauma intensive care unit [ICU] patients versus patients admitted to the medical intensive care unit [MICU]) (Pandharipande et al.; Peterson et al.). The mixed subtype is characterized by behavior that fluctuates between the two extremes of hypoalert–hypoactive and hyperalert–hyperactive subtypes. It is this variability in the presentation of delirium that contributes to the difficulties in detecting and recognizing this condition. The clinical value of subtypes is speculative at the moment. Several authorities speculate that how delirium presents is indicative of the underlying etiology(ies). It is thought that how patients manifest delirium might facilitate the identification of the underlying cause of the delirium and thereby expedite its treatment. To date, however, the evidence linking the behavioral manifestation of delirium with causes remains unsubstantiated.

Given the acuity of older patients in ICUs worldwide, it is not surprising that the incidence [newly developed after admission to the ICU] of delirium is high in this patient population. The incidence of delirium in critically ill older patients has been reported to range from a low of 21.7% (Lin et al., 2008) to a high of 81.7% (Ely, Inouye, et al., 2001). The incidence tends to be lower in patient populations that are younger and healthier, for example, in older patients admitted for elective surgery incidence is reported to be about 21.7 to 24% (Koebrugge, Koek, van Wensen, Dautzenberg, & Bosscha, 2009; Lin et al.), whereas higher rates of incidence are associated with older age and greater physiologic instability, for example, 81.7% in patients who are sedated and mechanically ventilated (Ely, Inouye, et al.).

Delirium in this patient population tends to occur by the third day of intensive care with a mean duration of 3 to 4 days (Ely, Inouye, et al., 2001). Some researchers have reported worse outcomes with longer duration. There have been attempts to link the severity of delirium with outcomes; however, severity of delirium tends to be measured by the behavioral manifestations of delirium, which are not linked to the underlying physiologic instability, and, as a result, quantifying the severity of delirium currently has no clinical value (Foreman & Milisen, 2004).

Of great concern is the fact that delirium is frequently underrecognized or misattributed to the effects of aging or the presence of dementia or depression. Patients who manifest the hypoalert–hypoactive subtype of delirium are older, have vision impairment, and have a 20-fold risk of not having their delirium recognized by nurses (Inouye et al., 2001). Similarly, Han and colleagues (2009) found that 76% of older people in an emergency department who presented with delirium were not recognized as delirious by the health care staff. More alarming is the fact that 36% of these delirious patients were discharged from the emergency department to home, despite the fact that many consider delirium to be akin to acute myocardial infarction (Holmes, 2009; Lipowski, 1990). So it should not be surprising that such patients have poorer prognosis and experience worse outcomes.

It is essential that all health care providers working with older patients who are critically ill, that is, those in emergency departments and intensive care units, be equipped to detect delirium in these patients, as delirium has been repeatedly demonstrated to independently contribute to poorer outcomes for patients, health care providers, and for society (Holmes, 2009). Morandi et al. (2009) reported that delirious patients were more likely to self-extubate and remove other therapeutic devices, to require prolonged stays both in the ICU as well as post-ICU hospitalization, be discharged more frequently to continued care environments, and to experience greater morbidity and mortality not only while in the ICU but in the post-ICU period as well. Medically ventilated patients who experience delirium in the ICU have a threefold increased risk of death in 6 months, even after controlling for preexisting comorbidities, severity of illness, coma, and the use of sedative and analgesic medicines. Each additional day of delirium contributes a 20% increased risk of remaining in hospital and a 10% increased risk of death (Ely et al., 2004).

Although delirium is often defined as a transient organic mental syndrome this does not guarantee that survivors return to their premorbid cognitive state. In some cases patients' cognitive dysfunction may persist over time. Apart from these factors, many ICU patients recall experiences of vivid dreams, hallucinations, or delusions that can be persecutory in nature and sometimes very frightening. These postdischarge remembrances possibly stem from the times when the patient was experiencing delirium (Jackson et al., 2003).

As a result of the symptoms of delirium, patients put a serious burden on nursing care and demand one-on-one nursing care to guarantee patient safety (Breitbart, Gibson, & Tremblay, 2002; Milisen, Cremers, et al., 2004). For family members the delirious episode is very stressful (Brajtman, 2003; Breitbart et al.). On top of the threat of death or disability from the critical illness, families must cope with behavior they do not understand, that is embarrassing, frightening, and adds significantly to the suffering of patients (Brajtman; Breitbart et al.).

The consequences of delirium also are severe in terms of economic costs. Delirium is associated with higher ICU ($22,346 vs. $13,332) and hospital costs ($41,836 vs. $27,106) (Milbrandt et al., 2004), costs that are incrementally greater as the severity and duration of delirium increases (Milbrandt et al.) Milbrandt and colleagues attributed these costs to the protracted stay in both the ICU and hospital and not to an increased intensity of resource use. However, this just reflects the short-term economic consequences of delirium. Leslie et al. (2005) calculated costs beyond hospitalization to be an additional $60,000 to $64,000 per patient per year. Given the incidence of delirium in this patient population, the additional health care costs of delirium are estimated to exceed $38 billion annually (Leslie et al.). Posthospital costs are in part the result of the fact that these individuals are frail with a very limited functional ability and as a result require a higher level of care, many times requiring institutionalization or protracted home care (Bellelli, Bianchetti, & Trabucchi, 2008).

## Monitoring Delirium

In summary, delirium is extremely common with critical illness in older patients; however, it is associated with profound consequences for patients, their families, health care providers and institutions, and society. Thus, the routine monitoring or this health emergency must be an integral component of the standard of care.

Routine monitoring for delirium enables the identification of individuals at risk of developing delirium; the prompt and early diagnosis and treatment of the underlying cause can prevent negative outcomes (Young & Inouye, 2007). These screening methods are also useful for monitoring progress and response to treatment over time (Michaud et al., 2007).

However, the assessment of delirium of a critically ill patient is not an easy task. Monitoring and assessment are more complex with critically ill older patients, as these patients are frequently nonverbal (e.g., intubated), and experiencing a reduced and fluctuating level of consciousness.

The first step in the assessment of delirium is the determination of the individual's level of consciousness or sedation (Jacobi et al., 2002; Pun et al., 2005). Although there are several scales developed for the determination of sedation and agitation in critically ill patients, for example, the Ramsay Scale (RS; Ramsay, Savege, Simpson, & Goodwin, 1974), Motor Activity Assessment Scale (MAAS; Devlin et al., 1999), and the Sedation–Agitation Scale (SAS; Riker, Fraser, Simmons, & Wilkins, 2001), only the Richmond Agitation–Sedation Scale (RASS; Ely et al., 2003; Ely, Margolin, et al., 2001; Sessler et al., 2002) is able to detect changes in sedation over consecutive days of intensive care (Ely et al.). As a consequence, the RASS is ideal for identifying and monitoring alterations in an individual's level of consciousness as a basis for delirium assessment (Sessler et al.) and response to treatment (Jacobi et al.). Training videos for the RASS can be found at www.ICUdelirium.org.

In selecting an instrument to monitor or assess for delirium, it is recommended that a standardized tool that has been validated in a critically ill population be used. The tool also should: (a) have acceptable validity and reliability in critically ill patients, especially those patients with communication impairments, for example, those who are endotracheally intubated for the administration of mechanical ventilation; (b) be quick and easy to use for patients and providers; (c) offer results that are easy to interpret; (d) generate results that are clinically meaningful; and (e) not require extensive training for use by any health care provider (Braes, Milisen, & Foreman, 2008; Devlin, Fong, Fraser, & Riker, 2007; Pandaripande et al., 2005). Given these characteristics there are three commonly used instruments for detecting delirium in critically ill patients: (a) the Confusion Assessment Method-ICU (CAM-ICU; Ely, Gautam, et al., 2001; Ely, Inouye, et al., 2001), (b) the Intensive Care Delirium Screening Checklist (ICDSC; (Bergeron, Dubois, Dumont, Dial, & Skrobik, 2001), and (3) the NEECHAM Confusion Scale (Neelon, Champagne, Carlson, & Funk, 1996). Each instrument is discussed in the text that follows.

## CAM-ICU

The Confusion Assessment Method (CAM; Inouye et al., 1990) was originally developed for detection of delirium in general hospitalized patients, but recently was modified for use with physically restrained and/or nonverbal [mechanically ventilated], critically ill patients (Ely, Gautam, et al., 2001; Ely, Inouye, et al., 2001). As with the original CAM, the CAM-ICU measures the four cardinal features of delirium: (a) acute onset of mental status change or fluctuating course, (b) inattention, (c) disorganized thinking, and (d) altered level of consciousness. Delirium is present when features 1, 2, and 3 or 4 are present. Simple nonverbal tasks such as picture recognition, the vigilance A test (Foreman & Vermeersch, 2004), yes/no logic questions, and simple commands are used to rate the presence of the four cardinal features of delirium. The CAM-ICU is usually accompanied with use of the RASS (Ely et al., 2003; Sessler et al., 2002), as recommended by the Society of Critical Care Medicine (Jacobi et al., 2002) to capture information about a patient's level of consciousness.

Overall, the CAM-ICU is quick and easy to use with critically ill patients, and makes few diagnostic errors (Devlin et al., 2007; Pun & Ely, 2007); however, the CAM-ICU is not as sensitive as the CAM in picking up mild or subtle symptoms of delirium (McNicoll, Pisani, Ely, Gifford, & Inouye, 2005). As a result, if the patient is capable of verbally responding, the original CAM should be used instead. Training videos for the CAM-ICU can be found at www.ICUdelirium.org.

## ICDSC

The ICDSC was developed based on the *Diagnostic and Statistical Manual of Mental Disorders (DSM-IV)* criteria (APA, 1994) as an easy-to-use bedside screening tool for patients who do not verbally communicate. It consists of eight items that are rated as present or absent; one point is assigned when an item is rated as present. A score of four or higher out of eight is considered evidence of delirium. It is recommended that ratings of the ICDSC should ideally be based on observations of the patient over a 24-hour period. The ICDSC is reputed to be easily incorporated into the daily routine nursing care in a busy unit of critically ill patients who have communication impairments. The ICDSC is able to detect almost all delirious patients (sensitivity of 99%), but generates a considerable portion of false-positive patients (specificity of 64%) (Bergeron et al., 2001). Additional benefits of the ICDSC include high agreement rates with the CAM-ICU (kappa = 0.80; Plaschke et al., 2008); each of the eight items comprising the ICDSC is highly discriminating for the diagnosis of delirium (Marquis, Ouimet, Riker, Cossette, & Skrobik, 2007); and the ICDSC is sufficiently sensitive to detect subsyndromal delirium (Ouimet, Riker, et al., 2007).

## NEECHAM Confusion Scale

The NEECHAM Confusion Scale (Neelon et al., 1996) was originally developed for assessment of delirium in general hospitalized patients, but recently has been adapted for use with critically ill patients (Csokasy, 1999; Devlin et al., 2007; Immers, Schuurmans, & van de Bijl, 2005). The NEECHAM Scale was developed to be scored using information from routine clinical observations of patient behavior while providing routine nursing care in a busy inpatient unit (Neelon et al.); it can be rapidly scored taking less than 4 minutes on average to complete (Immers et al.), provide clinically meaningful scores, and guide intervention (Neelon et al.). The Scale consists of nine items covering three different categories: (a) ability to process information, (b) behavior, and (c) physiological functioning. The total score ranges between 0 and 30; scores between 19 and zero indicate delirium. The NEECHAM has high agreement rates with the CAM-ICU (Van Rompaey et al., 2007), detects almost all delirious ICU patients (sensitivity of 97%), and generates an acceptable portion of false-positive patients (specificity of 83%).

## Proxy Ratings

In instances in which patients are admitted to the critical care unit and are unable to be evaluated because they are currently experiencing an altered level of consciousness, either because of sedation, analgesia, or preexisting cognitive impairment, use of the measures just described to identify and monitor delirium becomes problematic. In such instances, it is recommended to obtain proxy assessments of a patient's usual cognitive state to enable the health care team to be able to monitor progress and response to treatment (Pisani, Redlich, McNicholl, Ely, & Inouye, 2003). When it is impossible to directly assess an individual's cognitive abilities, the Modified Blessed Dementia rating Scale (MBDRS; Blessed, Tomlinson, & Roth, 1968) or the Informant Questionnaire on Cognitive Decline in the Elderly (IQCODE; Jorm, 1994) can be used to query proxy respondents. If the proxy has at least 5 years knowledge of the patient, then the MBDRS is preferred; otherwise the IQCODE is recommended. In either event, administration of either instrument takes about 3 to 5 minutes (Pisani et al).

## Neuropathogenesis

Historically, numerous physiological and/or structural abnormalities were thought to cause delirium (Lipowski, 1990). However, since the early 1990s there has been increasing effort to identify a "final common pathway" (Trzepacz, 1999). The currently accepted hypothesis for the neuropathogenesis of delirium is widespread brain dysfunction, especially in the subcortical, occipital, and brainstem areas, resulting from global hypoperfusion (Gunther, Morandi, & Ely, 2008; Trzepacz). This global hypoperfusion creates imbalances in the synthesis, release, and degradation of selected neurotransmitters, notably the underactivity of the cholinergic system, with a relative increase in the dopamine system (Gunther et al.; Trzepacz). Support for this hypothesis is from metabolic, pharmacologic, and structural evidence (Gunther et al; Trzepacz); however, the exact neurophysiological mechanisms underlying the pathogenesis of delirium are not yet identified (Gunther et al; Trzepacz). As a result, interventions to prevent and treat delirium are inexact and have limited efficacy.

## Prevention of Delirium

Because the actual neurophysiological mechanisms underlying the pathogenesis of delirium are not fully identified and understood, the primary focus for the prevention of delirium is modification of a person's risk for delirium by eliminating or minimizing the risk factor (Milisen, Lemiengre, Braes, & Foreman, 2005). In general, older patients admitted to an ICU should be considered at extremely high risk for delirium because of the presence of multiple risk factors for developing delirium—the greater the number of risk factors, the greater the risk for delirium (Inouye, Viscoli, Horwitz, Hurst, & Tinetti, 1993); it is not rare that a critically ill older adult would have 10 or more risk factors for delirium (Pandharipande et al., 2005). As a consequence, knowledge of the most important risk factors on admission to the ICU will help caregivers target those at highest risk for delirium (Pandharipande et al.; Pisani, Murphy, Van Ness, Araujo, & Inouye, 2007). To date, there's only one study highlighting the most important admission risk factors to identify older ICU patients at greatest risk (Pisani et al.). The risk factors identified at admission include dementia, receipt of benzodiazepines immediately before ICU admission (i.e., in the ED or other parts of the hospital), elevated creatinine level (> 2 mg/dL), and low arterial pH (< 7.35). Furthermore,

| 26.3 Predisposing and Precipitating Risk Factors for Delirium in Critically Ill Patients | |
| --- | --- |
| **Predisposing Risk Factors (Baseline Vulnerability)** | **Precipitating Risk Factors** |
| ■ Advanced age<br>■ History of alcoholism<br>■ History of smoking<br><br>Comorbidities<br>■ Pre-existing cognitive impairment<br>■ Pre-existing functional impairment<br>■ History of hypertension<br>■ Affective disorders, esp. depression | Effects of critical illness<br>■ Greater severity of illness<br>■ Anemia<br>■ Sepsis<br>■ Hypoxia<br>■ Dehydration<br>■ Renal dysfunction<br>■ Acidemia<br><br>Effects of the treatment for the critical illness or iatrogenesis<br>■ Unrelieved pain<br>■ Too high dose of analgesics<br>■ Immobilizing devices/Use of physical restraints<br>■ Anticholinergic medications<br>■ Long-acting benzodiazepines<br><br>Effects of the care environment<br>■ Visual/hearing impairment<br>■ Busy, noisy, brightly lit unit<br>■ Frequent nighttime interruptions<br>■ Sleep deprivation |

*Note.* Compiled from Dubois et al. (2001); Han et al. (2009); Pandharipande et al. (2005, 2006); Peterson et al. (2006); Pisani et al. (2007); Ouimet, Riker, et al. (2007).

distinction should be made between predisposing (nonmodifiable/baseline host vulnerability) and precipitating (modifiable/iatrogenic) factors (see Table 26.3).

As suggested by a multifactorial model for delirium (Inouye & Charpentier, 1996), which represents the complex interrelationship between a vulnerable patient with numerous predisposing factors and noxious insults or precipitating factors, a highly vulnerable patient (e.g., advanced age, dementia) may develop delirium with even relatively benign precipitating factors, such as a single dose of psychoactive medication (e.g., sedative and analgesic medications such as lorazepam, fentanyl, morphine, and propofol) or a noisy environment that disrupts sleep. There have been few studies of risk factors for delirium in critically ill patients. In this highly vulnerable patient population, predisposing factors for delirium include: advanced age and greater comorbidities, such as preexisting functional, cognitive, and sensory impairments. Predisposing factors tend not to be modifiable and therefore not amenable to intervention. Precipitating risk factors, or those than can be modified, fall into three categories: (a) effects of the critical illness, for example, hypoxia, sepsis, dehydration, and severity of illness; (b) effects of the treatment for the critical illness or iatrogenesis, for example, sedatives, analgesics, and medications with anticholinergic effects (see Table 26.4); and (c) effects of the care environment, for example, disrupted sleep (Dubois, Bergeron, Dumont, Dial, & Skrobik, 2001; Han et al., 2009; Pandharipande et al., 2005, 2006;

## 26.4  Deliriogenic Medications Commonly Used in ICUs*

**Analgesics**
- Codeine
- Meperdine
- Fentanyl
- Morphine
- Penthidine

**Antiarrhythmic agents**
- Disopyramide
- Quinidine
- Tocainide

**Anticholinergic agents**
- Atropine
- Benztropine
- Homatropine
- Hyoscine
- Orphenadrine
- Scopolamine

**Anticonvulsants**
- Carbamazepine
- Phenytoin
- Phenobarbital
- Valproic acid

**Antidepressants**
- Amitriptyline
- Doxepin
- Fluoxetine
- Paroxetin
- Paroxetine

**Antiemetics**
- Diphenhydramine
- Hydroxyzine
- Meclazine
- Metoclopramide
- Prochlorperazine
- Promethazine

**Antihistamines**
- Brompheniramine
- Chlorphenamine
- Diphenhydramine
- Phenylpropanolamine
- Promethazine
- Pseudoephedrine

**Antihypertensive agents**
- Atenolol
- Clonidine
- Diltiazem
- Metoprolol
- Methyldopa
- Nifedipine
- Prazosin
- Propranolol
- Timolol
- Verapamil

**Antipsychotics**
- Chlorpromazine
- Fluphenazine
- Haloperidol
- Thioridazine
- Trifluperazine

**Corticosteroids**
- Dexamethasone
- Hydrocortisone
- Methylprednisone
- Prednisone

**$H_2$ receptor antagonists**
- Cimetidine
- Famotidine
- Nizatidine
- Ranitidine

**Sedative-hypnotic agents**
- Benzodiazepines, especially longer acting ones
- Chlordiazepoxide
- Chloral hydrate
- Thiopental

*Please note that this list is not exhaustive.

Compiled from Borthwick et al. (2006), Fick et al. (2003), and the Registered Nurse Association of Ontario (2003).

Peterson et al., 2006; Pisani et al., 2007; Ouimet, Kavanaagh, et al., 2007), see Table 26.3 for a more comprehensive list of risk factors. Knowing a patient's risk profile at the time of admission to a critical care unit assists care providers in targeting those patients at highest risk for delirium (Pisani et al.; Pandharipande et al.).

Strategies for risk modification include:

- **Hydration protocol**: Calculation and delivery of daily hydration needs tailored to patient status (Inouye et al., 1999; Marcantonio, Flacker, Wright, & Resnick 2001; Michaud et al., 2007; Young, Leentjens, George, Olofsson, & Gustafson, et al., 2008).

- **Nonpharmacologic sleep protocol**: Unit-wide noise-reduction strategies; rescheduling procedures to maximize sleep times; diurnal variation in lighting and activity; sleep-promoting activities, for example, relaxation tapes, music, or back massage (Inouye et al.; Marcantonio et al.; Michaud et al.; Mistraletti et al., 2008; Young et al.).
- **Early mobilization**: Progressive increase in activity as tolerated by patient from passive range-of-motion exercises three times a day with minimal use of immobilizing equipment, to ambulation in the hallways as tolerated (Bailey et al., 2007; Inouye et al.; Marcantonio et al.; Michaud et al.; Morris et al., 2008; Needham, 2008; Pitkala, Laurila, Strandberg, & Tilvis, 2006; Timmerman, 2007; Young et al.) (also see chapter 9, this volume).
- **Cognitive-stimulation protocol**: Stimulation such as discussion of daily events, structured reminiscence, and communication to provide orientation provide stimulation (Borthwick, Bourne, Craig, Egan, & Oxley, 2006; Inouye et al.; Lundstrom et al., 2005; Marcantonio et al.; Michaud et al.; Pitkala et al.; Young et al.).
- **Sensory impairment protocol emphasizing hearing and visual impairment**: Use amplification devices as necessary, and hearing and visual aids as appropriate (Inouye et al., Marcantonio et al., Milisen et al., 2001; Young et al.).
- **Dose reduction or elimination of unnecessary medications**: see Table 26.4 (Borthwick et al.; Inouye et al.; Marcantonio et al.; Pitkala et al., Young et al.)
- **Appropriate and adequate treatment of pain** (Marcantonio et al.; Milisen et al.; Morrison et al., 2003; Young et al.).

Unfortunately risk modification has only shown to be efficacious with patients at moderate risk for delirium, that is, those with one or two risk factors, and has not shown sustained benefits 6 months after the episode of hospitalization (Bogardus et al., 2003; Inouye et al., 1999).

In addition to risk modification, pharmacological strategies have been examined. These pharmacological strategies have consisted primarily of the prompt cessation of deliriogenic drugs (Borthwick et al., 2006; Inouye et al., 1999). For example Inouye et al. accomplished this by advocating a nonpharmacologic approach to sleep promotion resulting in a reduced reliance on sedative-hypnotic drugs that as a class of drugs are well known to be deliriogenic (Borthwick et al., Fick et al., 2003; Registered Nurses Association of Ontario, 2003). Generally, benzodiazepines are to be avoided as they have been implicated in increasing an individual's risk for delirium (Gadreau, Gagnon, Roy, Harel, & Tremblay, 2005); moreover, the risk for delirium increases with the duration of effect of the drug (Tropea, Holmes, Gorelik, & Brand, 2009). However, benzodiazepines have been effective in treating delirium resulting from alcohol withdrawal (Longergan, Britton, Luxenberg, & Wyller, 2007; Longergan, Luxenberg, Areosa Sastre, & Wyller, 2009). Other drugs known to be deliriogenic and, therefore to be avoided, are listed in Table 26.4.

There has been limited success with prophylactic low-dose haloperidol in reducing the severity and duration in the episodes of delirium (Siddiqi, Holt, Britton, & Holmes, 2009); low-dose haloperidol has been more efficacious in managing the symptoms of delirium once it has developed (see discussion that follows). Overall, the evidence on the efficacy of pharmacological interventions to prevent delirium is sparse (Siddiqi et al.).

# Treatment of Delirium

Treatment guidelines for delirium in critically ill older adults consists of two components: (a) nonpharmacological approaches, and (b) pharmacological approaches.

## Nonpharmacological Approaches

The principle behind the nonpharmacological approaches to the treatment of delirium in critically ill older adults is to (a) identify and treat or eliminate the underlying etiology(ies), and (b) provide supportive care (APA, 1999; Meagher, O'Hanlon, O'Mahoney, & Casey, 1996; Michaud et al., 2007; Milisen et al., 2005).

Strategies for identifying and treating or eliminating the underlying etiologies begin with a comprehensive history and physical examination, followed by appropriate blood chemistry and imaging studies (Michaud et al., 2007). One caveat with the elderly is that the underlying pathophysiologic abnormality might be so small as to seem clinically irrelevant, but clearly is the cause of the delirium.

- **Hydration protocol:** Calculation and delivery of daily hydration needs tailored to patient status (Inouye et al., 1999; Marcantonio et al., 2001; Michaud et al., 2007; Young et al., 2008);
- **Elimination of unnecessary medications** (Borthwick et al., 2006; Inouye et al.; Marcantonio et al.; Pitkala et al., 2006, Young et al);
- **Treatment of infection** (Michaud et al.).

The provision of supportive care includes:

- **Environmental modification:** Unit-wide noise reduction strategies; rescheduling procedures to maximize sleep times; diurnal variation in lighting and activity; sleep-promoting activities, for example, relaxation tapes, music, or back massage (Inouye et al.; Marcantonio et al.; Meagher et al., 1996; Michaud et al.; Mistraletti et al., 2008; Young et al.);
- **Early mobilization:** Progressive increase in activity as tolerated by patient from passive range-of-motion exercises three times a day with minimal use of immobilizing equipment, to ambulation in the hallways as tolerated (Bailey et al., 2007; Inouye et al.; Marcantonio et al.; Michaud et al.; Morris et al., 2008; Needham, 2008; Pitkala et al., 2006; Timmerman, 2007; Young et al.) (also see chapter 9, this text);
- **Cognitive-stimulation protocol:** Activities such as discussion of daily events, structured reminiscence, and communication to provide orientation help patients avoid delirium (Borthwick et al., 2006; Inouye et al.; Lundstrom et al., 2005; Marcantonio et al.; Michaud et al.; Pitkala et al.; Young et al.);
- **Sensory-impairment protocol emphasizing hearing and visual impairment:** Provide amplification devices as necessary, and hearing and visual aids as appropriate (Inouye et al., Marcantonio et al., Milisen et al., 2001; Young et al.); and
- **Appropriate and adequate treatment of pain** (Marcantonio et al.; Milisen et al.; Morrison et al., 2003; Young et al.).

## Pharmacological Approaches

The second component of an effective treatment protocol for delirium in critically ill older adults is the selection of appropriate pharmacological treatment for behavioral symptoms, as necessary (APA, 1999; Michaud et al., 2007), also see chapter 21, this text. Haloperidol has been a recommended component of the treatment of delirium for many years (APA, 1999; Lonergan et al., 2007), even though the evidence supporting this recommendation is inconclusive (Marcantonio et al., 2001; Young, 2008). Although optimal doses of haloperidol have not been determined, initial doses in the range of 1 to 2 mg every 2 to 4 hours as needed have been used with success (APA, 1999), however, lower doses are recommended with older patients, but higher doses may be required with patients who are agitated (doses of haloperidol should not exceed 20 mg in a 24-hour period). The rationale for recommending haloperidol is based in part on the observation of the fact that after administration of haloperidol, patients with agitation tend to become more docile. In addition, haloperidol is known to affect dopamine receptors, one of the hypothesized neuropathogenetic mechanisms. However, high-dose haloperidol is associated with a greater incidence of side effects, primarily extrapyramidal in nature, and in 2007, Johnson and Johnson, the manufacturer of haloperidol, notified the FDA that they recently learned that the IV administration of haloperidol (an off-label usage but the one used to treat delirium) is associated with a greater risk of sudden death, QT prolongation, and Torsades de Pointes (TdP), which should be monitored regularly (USFDA, 2007). Lorazepam may be added for delirious patients with extreme agitation, as the combination adds to the sedation more rapidly and also may decrease extrapyramidal effects of haloperidol (Breitbart & Alici, 2008).

Newer atypical antipsychotics (risperidone, olanzapine, and quetiapine) are gaining interest in the treatment of delirium and may be preferred as they are associated with fewer adverse side effects as compared to conventional antipsychotics (e.g., haloperidol). However, most of the studies examining the efficacy of the atypical antipsychotics, that is, risperidone, olanzapine, quetiapine, and, more recently, ziprasidone, have not been rigorous enough or used sufficient samples (Michaud et al., 2007), and clozapine should be avoided because of the risk of agranulocytosis (Breitbart & Alici, 2008). Support for atypical antipsychotics arises chiefly from their broad potential for therapeutic efficacy with minimal sedation and extrapyramidal side effects (Leso & Schwartz, 2002), and haloperidol is associated with a higher rate of mortality (Schneeweiss, Setoguchi, Brookhart, Dormuth, & Wang, 2007). Moreover, these newer atypical antipsychotics target dopamine $D_2$ and $D_3$ receptors and serotonin 5HT2A, 2C, and 1D receptors, and alpha1 adrenergic receptors—those currently hypothesized as underlying the pathogenesis of delirium.

Although part of the hypothesized neuropathophysiological mechanism includes acetylcholine and cholinesterase inhibitors, for example, donepezil, they have not been shown to be effective in the treatment of delirium (Overshott, Karim, & Burns, 2009). Overall, there is no consensus about a standard pharmacologic approach to the treatment of delirium (Straker, Shapiro, Muskin, 2006). Moreover, most of these studies were undertaken with acutely ill rather than critically ill older patients.

Another pharmacologic strategy for the treatment of delirium is derived from a study by Milisen et al. (2001). Although not specific to treating the symptoms of delirium, Milisen et al. demonstrated that a scheduled pain protocol (as part of a multi-component intervention program) in postoperative patients was effective in lessening the duration and severity of delirium. The scheduled pain protocol consisted of a short-acting, weak opioid analgesic in combination with a nonopioid analgesic that was administered intravenously for the first 24 hours and then orally for the next 4 days.

## Case Study With Discussion

Mrs. O. is a 79-year-old retired nurse who lives at home with her husband who is physically frail. Mrs. O. was diagnosed with probable Alzheimer's disease approximately 3 years ago. In addition, she has type II diabetes that is generally well controlled on Actoplus (pioglitazone hydrochloride and metformin hydrochloride). She and her husband are able to remain living in their own home because of help from their children, neighbors, friends, and a monthly visit from a home health nurse. Mrs. O. is quite mobile but recently has begun to wander at times. Her husband reports that she has been more confused over the past few days and has fallen twice since yesterday. There is evidence of minor physical injury, which Mrs. O. insists is "nothing." Her husband also is concerned that she has not been taking her Actoplus as prescribed; although she has been eating okay, he is concerned that she has not been drinking enough. Because of these concerns, he calls the home health nurse to come and evaluate the situation, as he is concerned that his wife may need urgent attention. [Mr. O.'s concerns are real and the call to the home health nurse is appropriate].

When the nurse arrives, she assesses Mrs. O., including her cognitive functioning. The results of her assessment indicate that Mrs. O.'s cognitive functioning has deteriorated significantly since the nurse's visit 2 weeks ago. Mrs. O. is more disoriented to time and place, more easily distracted, her conversation is disorganized, and she has greater difficulty following commands and remembering simple objects. In talking with the husband, the nurse learns that these changes occurred in the past 2 days. The nurse suspects delirium as evidenced by the sudden and dramatic decline in Mrs. O.'s cognitive abilities. The nurse thinks that Mrs. O. may be severely dehydrated because her diabetes is no longer controlled, and is concerned about impending hyperosmolar, nonketotic coma. The nurse seeks an emergency admission to the local hospital for further diagnostic work to determine the cause for her suspected delirium; is she hyperglycemic and dehydrated? [The nurse's suspected diagnosis is certainly a health emergency warranting further diagnostic workup to confirm a diagnosis of delirium and the identification of the underlying causes.]

Mrs. O. is admitted to the ICU with a diagnosis of mental status changes, and impending hyperosmolar, nonketotic coma. On admission to the hospital, the nurse describes Mrs. O. as "cooperative, lying quietly in bed, but being slow to respond." Being short staffed that day and given Mrs. O.'s history of dementia, the nurse decides that these changes are merely a worsening of her dementia and nothing new. The nurse moves on to other patients and more "critical" patient care concerns. A couple of hours later, the nurse goes back to check on Mrs. O. only to find her obtunded, unresponsive to physical stimuli, hypotensive, and tachycardic. The nurse calls a code, but Mrs. O. fails to respond and dies. [What went wrong here? It is likely that the assessment performed by the home health nurse was not transmitted to the nurse in the hospital. Thus, vital information was missing, and the nurse in the hospital was working at a disadvantage.] In addition, it is not uncommon for health care providers to assume because an older person is "confused," that this confusion is either a result of age or an exacerbation of underlying dementia or both (Fick & Foreman, 2000). However, this is an erroneous assumption, and in this case dangerous as the undetected worsening of Mrs. O.'s cognitive impairment resulted in lack of treatment of the underlying hyperglycemia and severe dehydration leading to her eventual death. The cascade of mortal events could have been prevented with detection of the impairment, diagnosis of delirium, and prompt treatment of the underlying cause (adapted from Braes et al., 2008).

## Summary and Conclusions

Delirium is a syndrome that is common with critical illness in older patients that is consistently linked with poor outcomes and greater costs of care. Thus, it is imperative to promptly identify those patients at risk for delirium, and to maintain vigilance by routinely monitoring for delirium using instruments validated for use with critically ill patients. Pharmacologic and nonpharmacologic strategies for preventing or treating delirium in this highly vulnerable patient population must be initiated on admission to the critical care environment.

## Selected Web Resources for Delirium

American Psychiatric Association. (2006). *Practice guidelines for the treatment of patients with delirium.*
　　Retrieved October 13, 2008, from
　　http://www.guideline.gov/summary/summary.aspx?doc_id=2180
British Geriatrics Society. (2001). *Guidelines for the prevention, diagnosis, and management of delirium in older people in hospital.*
　　Retrieved October 13, 2008, from http://www.bgs.org.uk/Publications/Clinical%20Guidelines/clinical_1-2_fulldelirium.htm
European Delirium Association. (2009).
　　http://www.europeandeliriumassociation.com
Hartford Institute for Geriatric Nursing. This Web site provides access to several clinical resources useful for delirium: there is the *Try This* series featuring among others the use of the Mini-Mental State Examination (MMSE), the Confusion Assessment Method (CAM), and the Confusion Assessment Method for the ICU (CAM-ICU) Retrieved October 13, 2008, from
　　http://www.hartfordign.org/
Hospital Elder Life Program (HELP) at Yale University. This Web site provides information about recognizing, preventing, and managing delirium in hospitalized older people. Available at
　　http://www.elderlife.med.yale.edu/public/public_main.php?pageid=01.00.00

National Guideline Clearinghouse, of the U.S. Dept. of Health and Human Services, Agency for Healthcare Research and Quality (AHRQ). *Assessing cognitive function* (2007). Retrieved October 13, 2008, from

http://www.guideline.gov/summary.aspx?doc_id=12266&nbr=006350&string= delirium

*Delirium: Prevention, early recognition, and treatment.* (2007). Retrieved October 13, 2008, from     http://www.guideline.gov/summary.aspx?doc_id=12261&nbr=006345& string=delirium

Registered Nurses' Association of Ontario. A section of this Web site is dedicated to nursing best practice guidelines of which the following are two examples: *Screening for delirium, dementia, and depression in older adults.* (2003). Retrieved October 13, 2008, from

http://www.rnao.org/Page.asp?PageID=924&ContentID=818

*Caregiver strategies for older adults with delirium, dementia and depression.* Retrieved October 13, 2008, from

http://www.rnao.org/Page.asp?PageID=924&ContentID=797

Vanderbilt ICU Delirium and Cognitive Impairment Study Group. (2008). This Web site provides access to a wealth of information about delirium in the ICU, including several videos that feature the use of the CAM-ICU and the RASS among others. Available at http://www.icudelirium.org/delirium

# References

American Psychiatric Association. (1994) *Diagnostic and statistical manual of mental disorders,* (4th ed., pp. 124–133). Washington, DC: American Psychiatric Press.

American Psychiatric Association. (1999). *Practice guideline for the treatment of patients with delirium.* Washington, DC: American Psychatric Press.

American Psychiatric Association. (2000) *Diagnostic and statistical manual of mental disorders* (4th ed., text rev., pp. 135–147). Washington, DC: American Psychiatric Press.

Bailey, P., Thomsen, G. E., Spuhler, V. J., Blair, R., Jewkes, J., Bezdjian, L., et al. (2007). Early activity is feasible and safe in respiratory failure patients. *Critical Care Medicine, 35,* 139–145.

Bellelli, G., Buanchetti, A., & Trabucchi, M. (2008). Delirium and costs of informal home care. *Archives of Internal Medicine, 163,* 1717.

Bergeron, N., Dubois, M. J., Dumont, M., Dial, S. P., & Skrobik, Y. (2001). Intensive Care Delirium Screening Checklist: evaluation of a new screening tool. *Intensive Care Medicine, 27*(5), 859–864.

Blessed, G., Tomlinson, B. E., & Roth, M. (1968). The association between quantitative measures of dementia and senile changes in the cerebral grey matter of elderly subjects. *British Journal of Psychiatry, 114,* 797–811.

Bogardus, S. T., Desai, M. M., Williams, C. S., Leo-Summers, L., Acampora, D., & Inouye, S.K. (2003). The effects of a targeted multicomponent delirium intervention on post-discharge outcomes for hospitalized older adults. *American Journal of Medicine, 114,* 383–390.

Borthwick, M., Bourne, R., Craig, M., Egan, A., & Oxley, J. (2006, June). *Detection, prevention, and treatment of delirium in critically ill patients.* United Kingdom Clinical Pharmacy Association. Available at http://www.ics.ac.uk/icmprof/downloads/UKCPA%20Delirium%20Resourc e%20 June%202006%20v1%202.pdf

Braes, T., Milisen, K., & Foreman, M. D. (2008). Assessing cognitive function. In. E. Capezuti, D. Zwicker, M. Mezey, & T. Fulmer (Eds.), *Evidence-based geriatric nursing protocols for best practice* (3rd ed., pp. 41–56). New York: Springer Publishing Company.

Brajtman, S. (2003). The impact on the family of terminal restlessness and its management. *Palliative Medicine, 17,* 454–460.

Breitbart, W., & Alici, Y. (2008). Agitation and delirium at the end of life: "We couldn't manage him." *Journal of the American Medical Association, 300*(24), 2898–2910.

Breitbart, W., Gibson, C., & Trembley, A. (2002). The delirium experience: Delirium recall and delirium-related distress in hospitalized patients with cancer, their spouses/caregivers, and their nurses. *Psychosomatics, 43*, 183–194.

Cole, M., McCusker, J., Dendukuri, N., & Han, L. (2003). The prognostic significance of subsyndromal delirium in elderly medical inpatients. *Journal of the American Geriatrics Society, 51*(6), 754–760.

Csokasy, J. (1999). Assessment of acute confusion: The use of the NEECHAM Confusion Scale. *Applied Nursing Research, 12*, 51–55.

Devlin, J. W., Boleski, G., Mlynarek, M., Nerenz, D. R., Peterson, E., Jankowski, M., et al. (1999). Motor Activity Assessment Scale: A valid and reliable sedation scale for use with mechanically ventilated patients in an adult intensive care unit. *Critical Care Medicine, 27*(7), 1271–1275.

Devlin, J. W., Fong, J. J., Fraser, G. L., & Riker, R. R. (2007). Delirium assessment in the critically ill. *Intensive Care Medicine. 33*, 929–940.

Dubois, M. J., Bergeron, N., Dumont, M., Dial, S., & Skrobik, Y. (2001). Delirium in an Intensive care unit: A study of risk factors. *Intensive Care Medicine, 27*(8), 1297–1304.

Ely, E. W., Gautam, S., Margolin, R., Francis, J., May, L., Speroff, T., et al. (2001). The impact of delirium in the intensive care unit on hospital length of stay. *Intensive Care Medicine, 27*, 1892–1900.

Ely, E. W., Inouye, S. K., Bernard, G. R., Gordon, S., Francis, J., May, L., et al. T (2001). Delirium in mechanically ventilated patients: Validity and reliability of the confusion assessment method for the intensive care unit (CAM-ICU). *Journal of the American Medical Association, 286*(21), 2703–2710.

Ely, E. W., Margolin, R., Francis, J., May, L., Truman, B., Dittus, R., et al. (2001). Evaluation of delirium in critically ill patients: validation of the Confusion Assessment Method for the Intensive Care Unit (CAM-ICU). *Critical Care Medicine, 29*(7), 1370–1379.

Ely, E. W., Shintani, A., Truman, B., Speroff, T., Gordon, S. M., Harrell, F. E., Jr., et al. (2004). Delirium as a predictor of mortality in mechanically ventilated patients in the intensive care unit. *Journal of the American Medical Association, 291*(14), 1753–1762.

Ely, E. W., Truman, B., Shintani, A., Thomason, J. W. W., Wheeler, A.P., Gordon, S., et al. (2003). Monitoring sedation status over time in ICU patients. Reliability and validity of the Richmond Agitation-Sedation Scale (RASS). *Journal of the American Medical Association, 289*(22), 2983–2991.

Fick, D. M., Cooper, J .W., Wade, W. E., Waller, J. L., Maclean, R., & Beers, M. H. (2003). Updating the Beers criteria for potentially inappropriate medication use in older adults. *Archives of Internal Medicine, 163*, 2716–2724.

Fick, D. M., & Foreman, M.D. (2000). Consequences of not recognizing delirium superimposed on dementia in hospitalized elderly individuals. *Journal of Gerontological Nursing, 26*, 30–40.

Foreman, M. D., & Milisen, K. (2004). Improving recognition of delirium in the elderly. *Primary Psychiatry, 11*, 46–50.

Foreman, M. D., & Vermeersch, P. E. H. (2004). Measuring cognitive status. In M. Frank-Stromborg & S. J. Olsen (Eds.), *Instruments for clinical health care research* (3rd ed., pp. 100–127). Sudbury, MA: Jones and Bartlett.

Gadreau, J.-D., Gagnon, P., Roy, M.-A., Harel, F., & Tremblay, A. (2005). Association between psychoactive medications and delirium in hospitalized patients: A critical review. *Psychosomatics, 46*, 302–316.

Gemert van, L. A., & Schuurmans, M. J. (2007). The NEECHAM Confusion Scale and the Delirium Observation Screening Scale: Capacity to discriminate and ease of use in clinical practice. *BMC Nursing, 6*:3 (doi:10.1186/1472-6955-6-3).

Gunther, M. L., Morandi, A., & Ely, E. W. (2008). Pathophysiology of delirium in the intensive care unit. *Critical Care Clinics, 24*, 45–65.

Han, J. H., Zimmerman, E. E., Cutler, N., Schnelle, J., Morandi, A., Dittus, R. S., et al. (2009). Delirium in older emergency department patients: Recognition, risk factors, and psychomotor subtypes. *Academic Emergency Medicine, 16*, 1–8.

Holmes, J. (2009). Delirium: A clarion call. *International Review of Psychiatry, 21*(1), 4–7.

Immers, H. E., Schuurmans, M. J., & van de Bijl, J. J. (2005). Recognition of delirium in ICU patients: A diagnostic study of the NEECHAM confusion scale in ICU patients. *BMC Nursing, 4*, 7.

Inouye, S. K., Bogardus, S. T., Jr., Charpentier, P. A., Leo-Summers, L., Acampora, D., Holford, T. R., et al. (1999). A multicomponent intervention to prevent delirium in hospitalized older patients. *New England Journal of Medicine, 340*, 669–676.

Inouye, S. K., & Charpentier, P. A. (1996). Precipitating factors for delirium in hospitalized elderly persons. Predictive model and interrelationship with baseline vulnerability. *Journal of the American Medical Association, 275*(11), 852–857.

Inouye, S. K., Foreman, M. D., Mion, L. C., Katz, K. H., & Cooney, L. M., Jr. (2001). Nurses' recognition of delirium and its symptoms: Comparison of nurse and researcher ratings. *Archives of Internal Medicine, 161*(20), 2467–2473.

Inouye, S. K., Van Dych, C. H., Alessi, C. A., Balkin, S., Siegal, A. P., & Horwitz, R. I. (1990). Clarifying confusion: The Confusion Assessment Method; A new method for detection of delirium. *Annals of Internal Medicine, 113*, 941–948.

Inouye, S. K., Viscoli, C. M., Horwitz, R. I., Hurst, L. D., & Tinetti, M. E. (1993). A predictive model for delirium in hospitalized elderly medical patients based on admission haracteristics. *Annals of Internal Medicine, 119*(6), 474–481.

Jackson, J. C., Hart, R. P., Gordon, S. M., Shintani, A., Truman, B., May, L., et al. (2003). Six-month neuropsychological outcome of medical intensive care unit patients. *Critical Care Medicine, 31*, 1226–1234.

Jacobi, J., Fraser, G. L., Coursin, D. B., Riker, R. R., Fontaine, D., Wittbrodt, E. T., et al. (2002). Clinical practice guidelines for the sustained use of sedatives and analgesics in the critically ill adult. *Critical Care Medicine, 30*(1), 119–141.

Jorm, A. (1994). A short form of the Informant Questionnaire on Cognitive Decline in the Elderly (IQCODE): Development and cross-validation. *Psychological Medicine, 24*, 145–153.

Kiely, D. K., Jones, R. N., Bergmann, M. A., & Marcantonio, E. R. (2007). Association between psychomotor activity delirium subtypes and mortality among newly admitted post-acute facility patients. *Journal of Gerontology, A: Biological Science and Medical Science, 62*(2), 174–179.

Koebrugge, B., Koek, H. L., van Wensen, R. J. A., Dautzenberg, P. L. J., & Bosscha, K. (2009). Delirium after abdominal surgery at a surgical ward with a high standard of delirium care: Incidence, risk factors, and outcomes. *Digestive Surgery, 26*, 63–68.

Leslie, D. L., Zhang, Y., Bogardus, S. T., Holford, T. R., Leo-Summers, L. S., & Inouye, S. K. (2005). Consequences of preventing delirium in hospitalized older adults on nursing home costs. *Journal of the American Geriatrics Society, 53*, 405–409.

Leso, L., & Schwartz, T. L. (2002). Ziprasidone treatment of delirium. *Psychosomatics, 43*, 61–62.

Levkoff, S. E., Yang, F. M., & Liptzin, B. (2004). Delirium: The importance of subsyndromal states. *Primary Psychiatry, 11*, 40–44.

Levkoff, S. E., Evans, D. A., Liptzin, B., Cleary, P. D., Lipsitz, L. A., Wetle, T. T., Reilly, C. R., et al. (1992). Delirium. The occurrence and persistence of symptoms among elderly hospitalized patients. *Archives of Internal Medicine, 152*(2), 334–340.

Lin, S. M., Hueang, C. D., Liu, C. Y., Wang, C. H., Huamg, P. Y., Fang, Y. F., et al. (2008). Risk factors for the development of early-onset delirium and the subsequent clinical outcome in mechanically ventilated patients. *Journal of Critical Care, 23*, 372–379.

Lipowski, Z. J. (1990). *Delirium: Acute confusional states.* New York: Oxford University Press.

Longergan, E., Britton, A. M., Luxenberg, J., & Wyller, T. (2007). Antipsychotics for delirium. *Cochrane Collaboration, 2*, 1–24.

Longergan, E., Luxenberg, J., Areosa Sastre, A., & Wyller, T. B. (2009). Benzodiazepines for delirium. *Cochrane Collaboration, 1*, 1–11.

Lundstrom, M., Edlund, A., Karlsson, S., Brannstrom, B., Bucht, G., & Gustafson, Y. (2005). A multifactorial intervention program reduces the duration of delirium, length of hospitalization, and mortality in delirious patients. *Journal of the American Geriatrics Society, 53*, 622–628.

Marcantonio, E. R., Flacker, J. M., Wright, J., & Resnick, N. M. (2001). Reducing delirium after hip-fracture: A randomized trial. *Journal of the American Geriatrics Society, 49*, 516–522.

Marquis, F., Ouimet, S., Riker, R., Cossette, M., & Skrobik, Y. (2007). Individual delirium symptoms: Do they matter? *Critical Care Medicine, 35*(11), 2533–2537.

McNicoll, L., Pisani, M. A., Ely, E. W., Gifford, D., & Inouye, S. K. (2005). Detection of delirium in the intensive care unit: Comparison of confusion assessment method rating. *Journal of the American Geriatrics Society, 53*, 495–500.

McNicoll, L., Pisani, M. A., Zhang, Y., Ely, E. W., Siegel, M. D., & Inouye, S. K. (2003). Delirium in the intensive care unit: occurrence and clinical course in older patients. *Journal of the American Geriatrics Society, 51*(5), 591–598.

Meagher, D. (2009). Motor subtypes of delirium: Past, present, and future. *International Review of Psychiatry, 21*, 59–73.

Meagher, D. J., & Trzepacz, P. T. (2000). Motoric subtypes of delirium. *Seminars in Clinical Neuropsychiatry, 5*(2), 75–85.

Meagher, D. J., O'Hanlon, D., O'Mahony, E., & Casey, P. R. (1996). The use of environmental strategies and psychotropic medication in the management of delirium. *British Journal of Psychiatry, 168*, 512–515.

Michaud, L., Bula, C., Berney, A., Camus, V., Voellinger, R., Stiefel, F., et al. (2007). Delirium: Guidelines for general hospitals. *Journal of Psychosomatic Research, 62*, 371–383.

Milbrandt, E. B., Deppen, S., Harrison, P. L., Shintani, A. K., Speroff, T., Stiles, R. A., et al. (2004). Costs associated with delirium in mechanically ventilated patients. *Critical Care Medicine, 32*(4), 955–962.

Milisen, K., Cremers, S., Foreman, M. D., Vandevelde, E., Haspeslagh, M., De Geest, S., et al. (2004). The Strain of Care for Delirium Index: A new instrument to assess nurses' strain in caring for patients with delirium. *International Journal of Nursing Studies, 41*, 775–783.

Milisen, K., Foreman, M. D., Abraham, I. L., De Geest, S., Godderis, J., Vandermeulen, E., et al. (2001). A nurse-led interdisciplinary intervention program for delirium in elderly hip-fracture patients. *Journal of the American Geriatrics Society, 49*, 523–532.

Milisen, K., Lemiengre, J., Braes, T., & Foreman, M.D. (2005). Multicomponent intervention strategies for managing delirium in hospitalized older people: A systematic review. *Journal of Advanced Nursing, 52*(1), 79–90.

Mistraletti, G., Carloni, E., Cigada, M., Zambrelli, E., Taverna, M., Sabbatici, G., et al. (2008). Sleep and delirium in the intensive care unit. *Minerva Anaesthesiology, 74*, 329–333.

Morandi, A., Jackson, J. C., & Ely, E. W. (2009). Delirium in the intensive care unit. *International Review of Psychiatry, 21*, 43–58.

Morris, P. E., Goad, A., Thompson, C., Taylor, K., Harry, B., Passmore, L., et al. (2008). Early intensive care unit mobility therapy in the treatment of acute respiratory failure. *Critical Care Medicine, 36*, 2238–2243.

Morrison, R. S., Magaziner, J., Gilbert, M., Koval, K. J., McLaughlin, M. A., Orosz, G., et al. (2003). Relationship between pain and opioid analgesics on the development of delirium following hip fracture. *Journal of Gerontology: Medical Sciences, 58A*, 76–81.

Needham, D. M. (2008). Mobilizing patients in the intensive care unit. Improving neuromuscular weakness and physical function. *Journal of the American Medical Association, 300*(14), 1685–1690.

Neelon, V. J., Champagne, M. T., Carlson, J. R., & Funk, S. G. (1996). The NEECHAM Confusion Scale: Construction, validation and clinical testing. *Nursing Research, 45*, 324–330.

Ouimet, S., Kavanagh, B. P., Gottfried, S. B., & Skrobik, Y. (2007). Incidence, risk factors and consequences of ICU delirium. *Intensive Care Medicine. 33*(1), 66–73.

Ouimet, S, Riker, R., Bergeron, N., Cossette, M., Kavanagh, B., & Skrobik, Y. (2007). Subsyndromal delirium in the ICU: Evidence for a disease spectrum. *Intensive Care Medicine, 33*(6), 1007–1013.

Overshott, R., Karim, S., & Burns, A. (2009). Cholinesterase inhibitors for delirium. *Cochrane Collaboration, 1*, 1–12.

Pandharipande, P., Cotton, B. A., Shintani, A., Thompson, J., Costabile, S., Pun, B. T., et al. (2007). Motoric subtypes of delirium in mechanically ventilated surgical and trauma intensive care unit patients. *Intensive Care Medicine. 33*(10), 1726–1731.

Pandharipande, P., Jackson, J., & Ely, E.W. (2005). Delirium: Acute cognitive dysfunction in the critically ill. *Current Opinions in Critical Care, 11*(4), 360–368.

Pandharipande, P., Shintani, A., Peterson, J., Pun, B.T., Wilkinson, G.R., Dittus, R.S., et al. (2006). Lorazepam is an independent risk factor for transitioning to delirium in intensive care unit patients. *Anesthesiology, 104*, 21–26.

Peterson, J. F., Pun, B. T., Dittus, R. S., Thomason, J. W., Jackson, J. C., Shintani, A .K., et al. (2006). Delirium and its motoric subtypes: A study of 614 critically ill patients. *Journal of the American Geriatric Society, 54*(3), 479–484.

Pisani, M. A., Murphy, T. E., Araujo, K. L. B., Slattum, P., Van Ness, P. H., & Inouye, S. K. (2009). Benzodiazepine and opioid use and the duration of intensive care unit delirium in an older population. *Critical Care Medicine, 37*, 177–183.

Pisani, M. A., Murphy, T. E., Van Ness, P. H., Araujo, K. L., & Inouye, S. K. (2007). Characteristics associated with delirium in older patients in a medical intensive care unit. *Archives of Internal Medicine, 167*(15), 1629–1634.

Pisani, M. A., Redlich, C., McNicoll, L., Ely, E. W., & Inouye, S. K., (2003). Underrecognition of preexisting cognitive impairment by physicians in older ICU patients. *Chest, 124*, 2267–2274.

Pitkala, K. H., Laurila, J. V., Strandberg, T. E., & Tilvis, R. S. (2006). Multicomponent geriatric intervention for elderly inpatients with delirium: A randomized, controlled trial. *Journal of Gerontology: Medical Sciences, 61A*, 176–181.

Plaschke, K., von Haken, R., Scholz, M., Engelhardt, R., Brobeil, A., Martin, E., et al. (2008). Comparison of the confusion assessment method for the intensive care unit (CAM-ICU) with the intensive care delirium screening checklist (ICDSC) for delirium in critical care patients gives high agreement rate(s). *Intensive Care Medicine, 34*, 431–436.

Pun, B. T., & Ely, E. W. (2007). The importance of diagnosing and managing ICU delirium. *Chest, 132,* 624–636.

Pun, B. T., Gordon, S. M., Peterson, J. F., Shintani, A. K., Jackson, J. C., Foss, J., et al. (2005). Large-scale implementation of sedation and delirium monitoring in the intensive acre unit: A report from two medical centers. *Critical Care Medicine, 33*(6), 1199–1205.

Ramsay, M. A., Savege, T. M., Simpson, B. R. & Goodwin, R. (1974). Controlled sedation with alphazalone-alphadolone. *British Medical Journal, 2,* 656–659.

Registered Nurses Association of Ontario. (2003). *Screening for delirium, dementia, and depression in older adults.* Available at http://www.rnao.org/Page.asp?PageID=924&ContentID=818

Riker, R .R., Fraser, G. L., Simmons, L. E., & Wilkins, W. L. (2001). Validating the Sedation-Agitation Scale with the Bispectral Index and Visual Analogue Scale in adult ICU patients after cardiac surgery. *Intensive Care Medicine, 27*(5), 853–858.

Schneeweiss, S., Setoguchi, S., Brookhart, A., Dormuth, C., & Wang, P. S. (2007). Risk of death associated with the use of conventional versus atypical antipsychotics drugs among elderly patients. *Canadian Medical Association Journal, 176,* 627–632.

Sessler, C. N., Gosnell, M. S., Grap, M. J., Brophy, G. M., O'Neal, P. V., Keane, K. A., et al. (2002). The Richmond Agitation-Sedation Scale. Validity and reliability in adult intensive care unit patients. *American Journal of Respiratory and Critical Care Medicine, 166,* 1338–1344.

Siddiqi, N., Holt, R., Britton, A. M., & Holmes, J. (2009). Interventions for preventing delirium in hospitalized patients. *Cochrane Collaboration. 1,* 1–46

Straker, D. A., Shapiro, P. A., & Muskin, P. R. (2006). Aripiprazole in the treatment of delirium. *Psychsomatics, 47,* 385–391.

Timmerman, R. A. (2007). A mobility protocol for critically ill adults. *Dimensions of Critical Care Nursing, 26*(5), 175–179.

Tropea, J., Holmes, A. C. N., Gorelik, A., & Brand, C. A. (2009). Use of antipsychotic medications for the management of delirium: An audit of current practice in the acute care setting. *International Psychogeriatrics, 21,* 172–179.

Trzepacz, P. T. (1999). Update on the neuropathogenesis of delirium. *Dementia and Geriatric Cognitive Disorders, 10,* 330–334.

U.S. Food and Drug Administration. (2007). *FDA Alert: Information for healthcare professionals: Haloperidol.* Medwatch; available at http://www.drugs.com/news/fda-medwatch-haloperidol-marketed-haldol-haldol-decanoate-haldol-lactate-new-warnings-revised-6861.html

Van Rompaey, B., Schuurmans, M. J., Shortridge-Baggett, L. M., Truijen, S., Elseviers, M., & Bossaert, L. (2007). A comparison of the CAM-ICU and the NEECHAM Confusion Scale in intensive care delirium assessment: An observational study in non-intubated patients. *Critical Care, 12*:R16 (doi:10.1186/cc6790).

Young, J., & Inouye, S. K. (2007). Delirium in older people. *British Medical Journal, 334* (7598), 842–846.

Young, J., Leentjens, A. F., George, J., Olofsson, B., & Gustafson, Y. (2008). Systematic approaches to the prevention and management of patients with delirium. *Journal of Psychosomatic Research, 65,* 267–272.

# Index